T0176555

The Veterinary Dental Patient

The Veterinary Dental Patient

A Multidisciplinary Approach

Edited by

Jerzy Gawor
DiplAVDC, Dipl EVDC, FAVD, DVM PhD
Krakow
Poland

Brook Niemiec
DiplAVDC, Dipl EVDC, FAVD
San Diego, CA
USA

WILEY Blackwell

This edition first published 2021
© 2021 John Wiley & Sons Ltd

All rights reserved. No part of this publication may be reproduced, stored in a retrieval system, or transmitted, in any form or by any means, electronic, mechanical, photocopying, recording or otherwise, except as permitted by law. Advice on how to obtain permission to reuse material from this title is available at http://www.wiley.com/go/permissions.

The right of Jerzy Gawor and Brook Niemiec to be identified as the authors of the editorial material in this work has been asserted in accordance with law.

Registered Offices
John Wiley & Sons, Inc., 111 River Street, Hoboken, NJ 07030, USA
John Wiley & Sons Ltd, The Atrium, Southern Gate, Chichester, West Sussex, PO19 8SQ, UK

Editorial Office
9600 Garsington Road, Oxford, OX4 2DQ, UK

For details of our global editorial offices, customer services, and more information about Wiley products visit us at www.wiley.com.

Wiley also publishes its books in a variety of electronic formats and by print-on-demand. Some content that appears in standard print versions of this book may not be available in other formats.

Limit of Liability/Disclaimer of Warranty
The contents of this work are intended to further general scientific research, understanding, and discussion only and are not intended and should not be relied upon as recommending or promoting scientific method, diagnosis, or treatment by physicians for any particular patient. In view of ongoing research, equipment modifications, changes in governmental regulations, and the constant flow of information relating to the use of medicines, equipment, and devices, the reader is urged to review and evaluate the information provided in the package insert or instructions for each medicine, equipment, or device for, among other things, any changes in the instructions or indication of usage and for added warnings and precautions. While the publisher and authors have used their best efforts in preparing this work, they make no representations or warranties with respect to the accuracy or completeness of the contents of this work and specifically disclaim all warranties, including without limitation any implied warranties of merchantability or fitness for a particular purpose. No warranty may be created or extended by sales representatives, written sales materials or promotional statements for this work. The fact that an organization, website, or product is referred to in this work as a citation and/or potential source of further information does not mean that the publisher and authors endorse the information or services the organization, website, or product may provide or recommendations it may make. This work is sold with the understanding that the publisher is not engaged in rendering professional services. The advice and strategies contained herein may not be suitable for your situation. You should consult with a specialist where appropriate. Further, readers should be aware that websites listed in this work may have changed or disappeared between when this work was written and when it is read. Neither the publisher nor authors shall be liable for any loss of profit or any other commercial damages, including but not limited to special, incidental, consequential, or other damages.

Library of Congress Cataloging-in-Publication Data

Names: Gawor, Jerzy, author. | Niemiec, Brook A., author.
Title: The veterinary dental patient : a multidisciplinary approach / Jerzy Gawor, Brook Niemiec.
Description: Hoboken, NJ : Wiley-Blackwell, 2021. | Includes bibliographical references and index.
Identifiers: LCCN 2020021098 (print) | LCCN 2020021099 (ebook) | ISBN 9781118974735 (hardback) | ISBN 9781118974698 (adobe pdf) | ISBN 9781118974681 (epub)
Subjects: MESH: Dentistry–veterinary | Veterinary Medicine | Practice Management, Veterinary
Classification: LCC SF867 (print) | LCC SF867 (ebook) | NLM SF 867 | DDC 636.089/763–dc23
LC record available at https://lccn.loc.gov/2020021098
LC ebook record available at https://lccn.loc.gov/2020021099

Cover Design: Wiley
Cover Image: Courtesy of Jerzy Gawor

Set in 9.5/12.5pt STIXTwoText by SPi Global, Pondicherry, India

Printed in Singapore
M098318_170621

Contents

List of Contributors *vii*
Preface *ix*
Acknowledgments *xi*
About the Companion Website *xiii*

Part I General Considerations: How to Start Dentistry *1*

1 Establishing a Dental Presence within a General Veterinary Practice *3*
Jerzy Gawor

2 Marketing and Communication in Veterinary Dentistry *27*
Rachel Perry

3 Teaching Veterinary Dentistry *37*
Zlatko Pavlica, Jerzy Gawor, and Lisa Mestrinho

4 Distribution of Tasks Around the Dental Patient in General Practice: Receptionists, Technicians, and Other Veterinary Team Members *45*
Mary Berg

5 Prophylactic Program for Oral Health *59*
Brook Niemiec

6 Nutrition, Oral Health, and Feeding Dental Patients *75*
Michał Jank

7 Antimicrobials in Veterinary Dentistry *87*
J. Scott Weese

8 Dental Patient Welfare *109*
Kymberley C. McLeod

Part II The Dental Patient *119*

9 Local, Regional, and Systemic Complications of Dental Diseases *121*
Jerzy Gawor and Brook Niemiec

10 Hereditary Oral Disorders in Purebred Dogs and Cats *133*
Jerzy Gawor

11 Pain Management in the Dental Patient *139*
Paulo Steagall and Peter Pascoe

12 Anesthesia of the Dental Patient *169*
Victoria M. Lukasik

13 The Dental Patient and Its General Conditions: Cardiac Disease, Diabetes Mellitus, Pregnancy, History of Seizures, and Brachycephalic Syndrome *189*
Eva Eberspächer-Schweda

14 Ophthalmic Considerations in the Veterinary Dental Patient *201*
Jamie J. Schorling

15 Oral Health in the Context of Other Planned Surgeries *211*
Daniel Koch

16 Systemic Diseases Influencing Oral Health and Conditions *219*
Jerzy Gawor

17 Common Situations of Malpractice and Mistakes, and How Best to Avoid Them *233*
Jerzy Gawor and Brook Niemiec

18   **Dentistry Through Life: Pediatric and Geriatric Dentistry**   *245*
     Jerzy Gawor and Brook Niemiec

Part III   Dentistry in Daily Practice: What Every Veterinarian Should Know   *259*

19   **Management of the Dental Patient**   *261*
     Jerzy Gawor and Brook Niemiec

20   **Professional Dental Cleaning**   *269*
     Brook Niemiec

21   **Oral and Maxillofacial Surgery: What's the Difference?**   *291*
     Jerzy Gawor

22   **Extraction Techniques and Equipment**   *305*
     Brook Niemiec

23   **Oral Emergencies**   *319*
     Jerzy Gawor

24   **Feline Dentistry**   *339*
     Jerzy Gawor and Brook Niemiec

Part IV   When to Call the Specialist   *363*

25   **A Brief Introduction to Specific Oral and Dental Problems that Require Specialist Care**   *365*
     Jerzy Gawor

26   **How to Cooperate with a Specialist**   *373*
     Brook Niemiec

Useful Algorithms for the Management of Oral Problems   *377*
Jerzy Gawor

Appendix A: Drugs and Doses   *387*
Margo Karriker

Appendix B: Instruments Handling and Sharpening   *393*
Jerzy Gawor

Appendix C: Abbreviations and Dental Charts   *399*
Jerzy Gawor

Appendix D: List of Hereditary Problems and Breed Predispositions in Dogs and Cats   *409*
Jerzy Gawor

Appendix E: Tolerance of Malocclusion and Dental Abnormalities in Dogs   *419*
Jerzy Gawor

Appendix F: Assisted Feeding in Dental Patients (website)   *423*
Michał Jank and Jerzy Gawor

Index   *429*

List of Contributors

Mary Berg
Beyond the Crown Veterinary Education, Lawrence, KS, USA

Eva Eberspächer-Schweda
Anaesthesiology and Perioperative Intensive Care, Department for Companion Animals and Horses, University of Veterinary Medicine Vienna, Vienna, Austria

Jerzy Gawor
Veterinary Clinic Arka, Kraków, Poland

Michał Jank
Division of Pharmacology and Toxicology, Department of Preclinical Sciences, Institute of Veterinary Medicine, Warsaw University of Life Sciences (WULS-SGGW), Warsaw, Poland

Margo Karriker
University of California Veterinary Medical Center, San Diego, CA, USA

Daniel Koch
Daniel Koch Small Animal Surgery Referrals, Diessenhofen, Switzerland

Victoria M. Lukasik
Southwest Veterinary Anesthesiology, Tucson, AZ, USA
University of Arizona College of Veterinary Medicine, Oro Valley, AZ, USA

Lisa Mestrinho
Assistant professor, Faculty of Veterinary Medicine, University of Lisbon, Portugal

Kymberley C. McLeod
Conundrum Consulting, Toronto, ON, Canada

Brook Niemiec
Veterinary Dental Specialties and Oral Surgery, San Diego, CA, USA

Peter Pascoe
Professor emeritus, Department of Surgical and Radiological Sciences, School of Veterinary Medicine, University of California, Davis, CA, USA

Zlatko Pavlica
University of Ljubljana, Ljubljana, Slovenia

Rachel Perry
Perry Referrals, Brighton, UK and Royal Veterinary College, London, UK

Jamie J. Schorling
American College of Veterinary Ophthalmologists, San Diego, CA, USA

Paulo Steagall
Department of Clinical Sciences, Faculty of Veterinary Medicine, Université of Montréal, Saint-Hyacinthe, QC, Canada

J. Scott Weese
Ontario Veterinary College, University of Guelph, Guelph, ON, Canada

Preface

Being doctors, we do not treat diseases: we treat patients. Our patients' quality of life, functionality, and welfare are the most important goals of treatment.

Controlling periodontal disease is a complex action that requires the joint efforts of several people, including the first-contact vet, the dentist, and the nurse.

Oral injuries and tooth fractures always require general anesthesia, in order to save the patient stress and provide the opportunity for appropriate assessment and treatment. It is again a team effort to carry the patient through all procedures safely.

Oral problems can affect almost *all* veterinary patients. Over 10% will become emergency patients and require immediate action.

Dentistry is a very important and interesting subject, but regardless of the technique, instrumentation, skills, and materials, it is *all* about the patient.

Many oral pathologies are camouflaged or go undiagnosed due to patient behaviors (animals do not express their discomfort), limitations in good access to the oral cavity, and prejudices among veterinarians and pet owners. Therefore, it is very important to educate veterinarians and urge them to pay attention not only to obvious signalments but also to signs of coming problems.

Almost every veterinary practice will claim, "We Do Dentistry" or "We Descale Teeth", but the overall quality of service is poor. Students lack dental education, and as graduates and young veterinarians they go on to neglect dentistry. More is needed than just a book, but we can at least point out herein what we expect from universities.

Pet owners accept the presence of human dentistry as a separate medical discipline, but for some reason they treat veterinary dentistry as a cosmetic addendum to veterinary services.

There is one thing worse than neglecting dental problems: performing poor dentistry. Thus the aim of this book is thus to present the standards of good dentistry in the most common applications. We hope to remind you that every patient is a dental patient, and to offer advice on how to properly manage them. You should maintain an appropriate attitude toward dental and oral problems in dogs and cats. We offer an interdisciplinary approach to the dental patient, providing perspectives from such disciplines as oncology, cardiology, anesthesiology, and radiology.

In order for our profession to continue to improve in protecting and improving the oral and general health of our patients, I believe two things are required. First, clinicians in general practice need to ensure that they have adequate training and are suitably equipped with dental diagnostic tools, from periodontal probes to X-ray machines. Second, and perhaps more importantly, the curriculum in our veterinary undergraduate programs needs to include practical training in dental and oral diagnostics.

My professional experiences are different from those of most specialists. Over 60% of the dental patients I see come from education, promotion, and prophylaxis. The remainder come through referral. My perspective is thus non-academic; I deal with patients at all different levels every day. I hope I may be of help to those in developing countries as well as to graduates and professionals in the developed world.

Jerzy Gawor

Acknowledgments

The two things in life which give me the greatest pleasure are my family and my profession. Without the support and encouragement of the former, I would never have been able to achieve so much or have the motivation to go still further in the latter. Furthermore, the daily interaction I have with my clients and patients has given me tremendous job satisfaction and allowed me to become the man I am.

I owe my patients a debt of gratitude which surpasses that due to my professional discipline of veterinary dentistry. I always strive to be a better veterinarian and dentist by putting my patients' welfare first, and to this day, difficult cases teach me humility and challenge my skills. Throughout my career, I have become increasingly aware of the need for the entire practice team to focus on the requirements of the dental patient.

Teaching is an important part of being a specialist, and writing this book as an educational tool has presented a unique set of challenges to myself and my associates. Special thanks go to Emilia Klim, my mentee who contributed to the selection and production of pictures; my friend Brook, who is always ready to share projects, challenges, and commitments; my wife Grażyna and our kids Jerzy, Antoni, and Mela; and my parents and brothers.

Finally, to all my veterinary dental patients of all species, small and large, old and young: my heartfelt thanks.

Jerzy Gawor

About the Companion Website

This book is accompanied by a companion website:

www.wiley.com/go/gawor/veterinary-dental-patient

The website includes:

- Further content on 'Assisted feeding in dental patients'

Scan this QR code to visit the companion website.

Part I

General Considerations

How to Start Dentistry

1

Establishing a Dental Presence within a General Veterinary Practice
Jerzy Gawor

Veterinary Clinic Arka, Kraków, Poland

1.1 Introduction

This chapter will cover the creation of a dental presence within a general practice. In addition, it will discuss how to create a business plan and how to design a consulting room and dental operatory. It will describe all the necessary equipment, instrumentation, and materials. Finally, it will cover the practical use of instruments.

1.2 General Considerations: How to Begin Offering Dentistry

There are many reasons why creating a dental presence within a general practice is a natural, necessary, and reasonable move in the development of a small-animal veterinary business. Some are listed in this chapter, and they should provide more than enough motivation for the practice manager or owner to provide dental services. However, this book focuses on the dental patient, and the proposed solutions will thus emphasize the benefits to the patient, not the business. The author believes that it is very important to combine a focus on the patient with the commercial side of dentistry.

Studies have shown that most of our patients require immediate dental care. By the age of just two years, 80% of dogs and 70% of cats have some level of periodontal disease (Lund et al. 1999); more recent studies have reported the incidence at closer to 90% of all patients: (Fernandes et al. 2012; Stella et al. 2018). Some 10% of dogs presented to veterinary clinics have pulp exposure, while the prevalence of teeth resorption in cats is estimated at 28–62% (Reiter and Mendoza 2002). The oral cavity is the fourth most common place to find oral cancer. There are proven links between periodontal disease and pathologic findings in the liver, kidney, and myocardium (DeBowes 1998). Thus,

with this obvious systemic impact of dental problems, we must not neglect dentistry in our general preventative care program for dogs and cats under our care.

Three major areas cover approximately 75% of dental procedures offered in small-animal dentistry: **diagnostics**, **prophylactic procedures**, and **extractions**. These also make up a significant part of the day-to-day work of specialty clinics.

Having a dental presence within a general practice means having the ability and equipment to properly perform these three groups of procedures. Each area present challenging cases, and therefore it is necessary to have a good relationship with the relevant specialists. Currently, the internet provides a very fast and easy means of communication, in addition to professional portals offering specialty consultations based on submitted radiographs, videos, photographs, and other resources.

The vast majority of small-animal patients require what is known by the general public as "dental" or "prophy." The Veterinary Internet Network (VIN) refers to this instead as "comprehensive oral health assessment and treatment" (COHAT), which much better describes the essence of prophylactic procedure. According to American Veterinary Dental College (AVDC) nomenclature, the current preferred term is "professional dental cleaning". This procedure will be detailed in Chapter 20.

It is possible to perform professional dental cleanings within a general practice with a dedicated and well-equipped dental room along with a skilled veterinarian and personnel. Considering the number of dental cases which may or should be performed daily in our practices, a dental X-ray, high-speed dental unit, sonic or ultrasonic scaler, and polisher are at the top of the list of profitable equipment to obtain for a surgery, and the fastest to pay for themselves.

A clinic's investment plan and equipment selection should be the result of a thorough deliberation on what kind and

The Veterinary Dental Patient: A Multidisciplinary Approach, First Edition. Edited by Jerzy Gawor and Brook Niemiec.
© 2021 John Wiley & Sons Ltd. Published 2021 by John Wiley & Sons Ltd.
Companion website: www.wiley.com/go/gawor/veterinary-dental-patient

range of dentistry it wants to offer. Most procedures belong to one of the three aforementioned groups, but the fundamental one is diagnostics. Without appropriate diagnostics, the number and degree of mistakes and the likelihood of malpractice become unacceptably large. Therefore, sufficient investment in diagnostic tools is very important. With improvement in skills and equipment, additional procedures can be performed; however, the majority of cases will still be part of the main three core ones.

The most critical diagnostic element of veterinary dentistry is **radiography**. One can obtain sufficiently good radiographs with conventional full-body X-Ray when exposing intraoral films or plates. For many indications in dental and maxillofacial conditions, such a device is likewise useful. For intraoral exposures, dental radiology is more convenient and appropriate. Ideally, practices should have both modalities: dental and conventional full-body X-ray machines. The next thing to consider in diagnostic radiography is the selection of a system that will both provide the radiation (generator) and create the image. Analog dental films, which require a darkroom and chemicals, are slowly leaving the market, and being replaced by digital systems. There are numerous products available, and it is not easy to decide between them based exclusively on manufacturer information and advertising.

A **professional dental cleaning** includes a thorough examination in both the conscious and the sedated patient, radiography (preferably intraoral), a dental exam including periodontal probing and dental charting, supragingival and subgingival deposit removal with the use of mechanical scalers and hand instruments, polishing, and gingival sulcus lavage. An important part of prophylaxis is the establishment of homecare, composed of both active and passive methods: toothbrushing, diet, supplements, dental chews, and toys. To properly perform dentistry in a clinic, it is necessary to carry out all these tasks at a standardized level.

The provision of dental services in private practice should include all necessary parts of the business plan. For most such plans, it is useful to follow the "SMART" acronym:

Specific: Specify what exactly is needed. Dentistry is a large subject, and for novices it can be quite confusing. Election of a range of dental procedures to implement at the outset is necessary to the design of a good plan. In addition to equipment investments, the education required to utilize them should also be considered.

Measurable: Plan expenses on an appropriate level. Consummate with the local market, select prices that will provide a relatively quick recoup of expenses without driving away clients. At the same time, the quality of purchased equipment must be high. Skimping on quality, warranty, or durability often works out to be more expensive in the long run.

Achievable: There are no limits to possible expenses, so it is important at the outset to establish the minimum amount of money that it will be necessary to invest according to local prices and stock.

Realistic: Buy what is necessary according to the skills available at the practice, its specific features, human resources, and the practice's general business plan.

Time-bound: Be realistic. Plan timing and deadlines, then make them real. Use **promotion**. If possible, plan future development and evaluate its results.

1.3 Education

The educational opportunities listed in this section may not be available in every country, but e-learning is becoming ever easier to access, and its quality is steadily increasing. Teaching dentistry is the subject of Chapter 3, so here we will only emphasize the critical need for education prior to establishing a dental presence and the importance of continuous further development.

Dental Program During Veterinary School: See Chapter 3

Self-Education: This can include books, articles, journals, training, and cooperation with a referral vet. Despite there being just one journal dedicated to veterinary dentistry – the *Journal of Veterinary Dentistry* (https://journals.sagepub.com/home/jov)– dental articles can be found frequently in Journal of American Veterinary Medical Association (JAVMA), Journal of Small Animal Practitioner (JSAP), European Journal of Companion Animal Practitioners (EJCAP), Journal of Feline Medicine and Surgery (JFMS), Frontiers in Veterinary Science and its section: Veterinary Dentistryand Oromaxillofacial Surgery and other publications. Textbooks are available both from traditional publishers and from smaller, independent ones, or in e-formats like those offered by the International Veterinary Information Service (IVIS). Finally, the Dental Guidelines of the World Small Animal Veterinary Association (WSAVA) offer a comprehensive overview of the veterinary dentistry field.

Associations: The European Veterinary Dental Society (https://www.evds.org), Foundation for Veterinary Dentistry (https://veterinarydentistry.org), and British Veterinary Dental Association (https://www.bvda.co.uk) offer many educational opportunities via their websites, publications, and conferences.

Continuing Education: Courses organized and tutored by specialists are often available. The really good ones combine a practical component with theoretical prerequisites. Additionally, dentistry streams are offered by the WSAVA and Federation of European Companion Animals Veterinary Associations (FECAVA), and during national congresses, seminars, and conferences dedicated to dentistry.

Continuing Professional Development (CPD) Courses: These are offered by pre-congress wetlabs, the European School for Advanced Veterinary Studies (ESAVS) or Accesia Academy, and training centers (e.g. the San Diego Veterinary Dental Training Center).

Certifications and Specializations: These are offered by the European Veterinary Dental College (EVDC), American Veterinary Dental College (AVDC), and Australian and New Zealand College of Veterinary Scientists (ANZCVS).

Nursing: Lack of nurse education may be a major limitation in dental service development. However, there are an increasing number of CPD events dedicated to nurses, and Accreditation Committee for Veterinary Nurse Education (ACOVENE)-accredited nursing schools provide dentistry-oriented profiles.

1.4 Promotion

Although important, promotion may not be seen as such by the public or the veterinary community. It is performed differently in Europe, where many countries have specific regulations on advertising veterinary services, than in the North America. Marketing will be the subject of Chapter 2; our purpose here is only to highlight the importance of certain policy related to promotional efforts.

Should we promote the various services we offer? Should the major goal of marketing be focused on making customer say "Yes," or should it present the benefits of oral health and of releasing the patient from pain and infection? Both aspects are important, and a balance is required.

The follow techniques are worth considering.

a) Participate in educational events like National Pet Dental Health Month and the Pet Smile Campaign.
b) Make use of oral care products and merchandising provided by pet food companies: models, posters, leaflets, brochures, and so on. It is not easy to select high-quality dental hygienic products based exclusively on manufacturer information, so turn to institutions like the Veterinary Oral Health Council (VOHC) http://www.vohc.org for information. Products with the VOHC seal are more reliable that those with just a marketing logo. Additionally, there are a growing number of evidence-based medicine studies evaluating the effectiveness and mechanism of oral hygiene products (See more in Chapter 5).
c) Provide information on your website and in your waiting room and reception on standards, safety, and the importance of oral health

d) Make dental care part of your prophylacitc/preventative/wellness program, together with vaccination, deworming, senior care, and so on.

1.5 Equipment Considerations

1.5.1 Waiting Room

Depending on the types of patient you typically see, the waiting area should be arranged in such a way as to handle animals of all different sizes and types at the same time. Regarding dentistry, communication should start with examples of the problems that create pain and infection. Pictures demonstrating procedures and patients should not be too scary or dramatic, however, as children and some other customers may find them upsetting. A TV screen displaying information about the quality of oral hygiene, anesthesia, and surgery provided by the practice is very useful, especially for those clients who have to wait some time for consultation or for discharge of their pet (Figure 1.1). However, too many advertisements may have the effect of alienating customers, so be careful not to overdo it.

1.5.2 Consulting Room

This is where the examination is performed in the conscious patient, which is a very important part of the dental consultation. In clinics that respect the International Society of Feline Medicine (ISFM) recommendations and standards, it is necessary to have separate rooms for cats where dogs are not allowed to enter (Figure 1.2). This really makes a huge difference in examination comfort, particularly in sensitive cats with a fragile mentality. A list of cat-friendly clinics is available online.

The dental consulting room does not have to be large, but the ability to examine the patient in good light is required. For the presentation of radiographs, it is convenient to reduce daylight by closing window blinds.

Space should be available in which to watch the patient's behavior. The examination table should have access to daylight or to a diagnostic lamp that provides near-natural light. Plaque-disclosing solution, a toothbrush, and examples of hygienic solutions are very helpful for establishing oral hygiene strategies. Instrumentation should be available to demonstrate additional diagnostic modalities. However, very few patients allow for conscious examination with a periodontal probe or mirror. Having dental models or educational posters and presentations available will be of excellent benefit when explaining what treatments will be performed to the pet owner (Figure 1.3).

It is confusing when the veterinarian must leave the room repeatedly to fetch equipment, so it is wise to store all of the equipment in one place. It is also important to keep

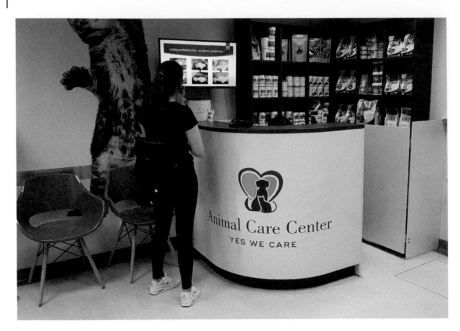

Figure 1.1   Waiting room TV screen with informational dental presentation.

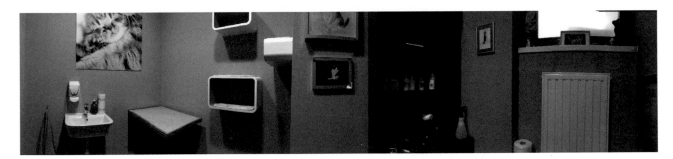

Figure 1.2   Feline cabinet, following the standards of a cat-friendly clinic.

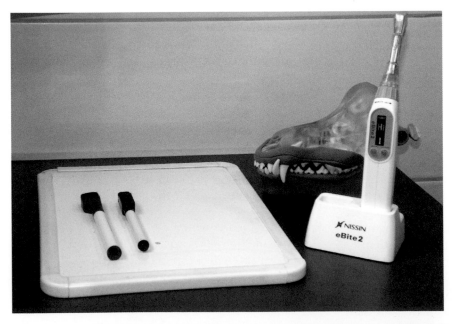

Figure 1.3   Dental models and instruments as well as a small whiteboard can be helpful in explaining dental problems to owners.

the equipment and models clean and sterile (e.g. for tooth-brushes or probes).

Even novices should be able to describe the outline of a problem in an understandable way (e.g. brief pathogenesis, diagnostics and the goal of treatment). Education of the pet owner is very helpful when done in an inoffensive way and adapted to the individual. White boards and a set of colors markers will improve the explanation (Figure 1.4). Posters presenting occlusal problems, the importance of radiography, and the most commonly diagnosed problems are available (Figure 1.5). So too are iPad applications containing easy-to-follow and customer-friendly movies on the most common dental problems (Figure 1.6).

Good-quality flat-screen computer monitors are important for the presentation of radiographs and other illustrations during discussion with the client, especially for those who prefer visual communication. Others may prefer logic and quiet verbal communication. Additionally to make important notes withdrawn from the clinical interview a paper and a pen is needed.

As a safety consideration, animals' teeth are a part of their defensive apparatus. A patient may bite as a result of aggression, fear, stress, or frustration, and in most of the cases we cannot blame them for doing so. Before an oral examination in a conscious animal, it is reasonable to ask the owner about its attitude toward strangers. There is a device available that protects the fingers, but in the author's experience it is better to stop an examination rather than force it until the patient begins to fight (Figure 1.7). Depending on local regulations, the veterinarian may be responsible for any injuries that happen to the pet owner within the consulting room, including being bitten by their own pet. Therefore, anesthesia should be performed in any circumstances where the owner cannot assure assistance or where such assistance may create a hazardous situation.

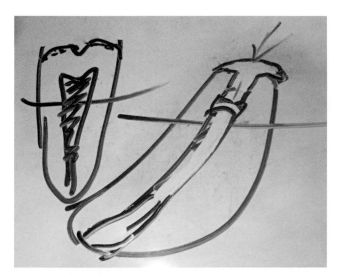

Figure 1.4 White board drawings explaining a crown height-reduction procedure.

Finally, here is a list of useful equipment to install in the consulting room:

1) Dental models of a dog and a cat
2) Educational posters
3) Diagnostic flashlight
4) High-quality screen or tablet
5) Paper and pen
6) Whiteboard and markers (or tablet)

1.6 Dental Operatory

The first step in organizing a dental presence at a practice might be to install a dental corner/table in the preparation room. However, it is much better to have a separate dental operatory (Figure 1.8). During dental procedures, significant contamination will be produced, including of an infectious aerosol. This is a specific situation in dentistry and thus it is important to separate the dental department from the rest of the surgical operatory. At the same time, all procedures will be performed under general anesthesia, so it is mandatory to provide the infrastructure for safe anesthesia (Figure 1.9).

Water plays a very important role in dental procedures, not only as a coolant, but also as a cleaning and flushing (lavage) medium. A source of demineralized water is necessary for the dental unit when using air-driven handpieces, as the minerals in water can cause damage to them. Demineralized water provided by three-way syringe or mechanical scalers can be supplied via containers attached to these devices. The water used for postoperative washing of the patient may be tap water, and it is convenient to have separate preparation and postoperative care tables with hot and cool water, a shower, and a bath (Figure 1.10a). Water used during dental procedures causes rapid loss of body temperature of the anesthetized patient, so the dental room must be equipped with all devices necessary for body temperature maintenance.

Central distribution of compressed air or nitrogen and of oxygen, as well as a central vacuum cleaner with convenient distribution of ports, will improve comfort and reduce noise and dirt (Figure 1.10b).

The small operating field must be well illuminated, using a light source as close as possible to natural.

Dental X-ray is necessary for almost every dental procedure, so the X-ray equipment must be close to the operating table and preferably wall-mounted. Dental X-ray generators do not require frequent changes of patient recumbency or position. Having a computer with radiography software in the operatory provides an easy way to evaluate digital scans immediately after exposure. Handheld devices may

The Importance of
Dental Radiographs

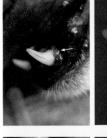

Figure 1: Normal dental radiograph, feline mandible.
- Mandibular symphysis (a).
- Canine roots (b).

Roots of the canine teeth comprise the majority of the mandible.

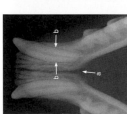

Figure 2: Normal dental radiograph, canine mandible.
- Bone fills furcation (a) and extends to CEJ (b)
- The periodontal ligament (c) is even in width around the root.
- The root canals are all visible and of comparable size (d)

Similar teeth should have similar radiographic anatomy.

Figure 3: Advanced periodontal disease of the mandible.
- Severe periodontal disease of the right lower quadrant is evident on physical examination (upper).
- Radiograph reveals thin bone in the area of the first molar (lower).

Dental radiographs can help prevent iatrogenic damage (such as jaw fractures) during extractions.

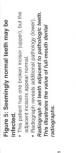

Figure 4: Small enamel fractures are very common.
- Apparently healthy tooth with a small cusp fracture (upper).
- This tooth is endodontically infected, as noted by the dark areas around the root tip (lower).
- This infection would be missed without dental radiographs

Dental radiographs are required for all fractured teeth to rule out hidden pathology.

Figure 5: Seemingly normal teeth may be infected.
- This patient has one broken incisor (upper), but the adjacent incisors appear normal.
- Radiograph reveals additional pathology (lower).

Radiograph all teeth adjacent to pathologic teeth. This illustrates the value of full-mouth dental radiographs.

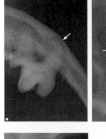

Figure 6: Feline tooth resorption (TR) is very common.
- Minimal clinical evidence of pathology (upper)
- Painful pathology missed without radiographs (lower)

Full mouth radiographs are recommended for all feline patients.

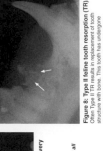
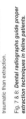

Figure 7: Type I feline tooth resorption (TR).
- Complete extraction of all roots is required for Type I TR.
- These teeth have significant coronal resorption (a), but normal root structure (b).

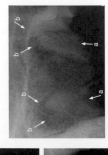

Figure 8: Type II feline tooth resorption (TR).
Often Type II TR results in replacement of tooth structure with bone. This tooth has undergone significant replacement resorption and may be treated with crown amputation, which is less traumatic than extraction.

Fig. 7 & 8: *Dental radiographs guide proper extraction techniques in feline patients.*

Figure 9: Worn teeth are common.
- Both canine teeth are worn (upper).
- The left lower canine tooth is non-vital (dead) as evidenced by the wider root canal (a) compared to the other side (b). The tooth is also likely infected, as evidenced by periapical lucency (c).

All worn teeth should be radiographed.

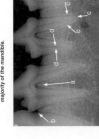

Figure 10: Oral neoplasia is common in veterinary patients.
- Large masses may be benign and small masses may be malignant.
- A small, benign appearing growth (upper).
- The radiograph reveals the tumor to be very large and aggressive (lower).

All oral masses should be radiographed and biopsied. Dental radiographs were instrumental in formulating the correct treatment plan to save this patient's life.

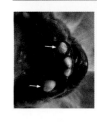

Figure 11: Dental radiographs are essential for primary (baby) tooth extraction.
- Clinically normal teeth may have undergone resorption, making extraction very difficult.
- Significant resorption just under the gum line (upper), which may cause the root to fracture, requiring surgical extraction.
- A completely resorbed root facilitates simple extraction (lower).

Dental radiographs can save the pet from an unnecessary surgery or a painful retained root.

Figure 12: Anatomic variation can result in very difficult extractions.
- This radiograph of a mandibular left first molar reveals severe root curvature and thin apical bone (upper) around the apex of the mesial (front) root.
- This maxillary right third premolar has an extra middle root (lower).

Radiographs are recommended for all teeth prior to extraction.

Figure 13: Retained roots may be painful and/ or infected.
- Retained and infected roots (a) following an extraction attempt.
- Dark areas around the roots (b) indicate likely infection, which requires complete extraction of the roots.

Post-operative radiographs are used to confirm complete extraction.

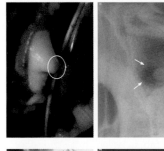

VDR

VETDENTALRAD.COM

YOUR DENTAL TELERADIOLOGY PARTNER.

© 2008 VetDentalRad.com. All Rights Reserved.

Educational posters avaliable at www.vetdentalrad.com.

Figure 1.5   Educational posters avaliable at www.vetdentalrad.com.

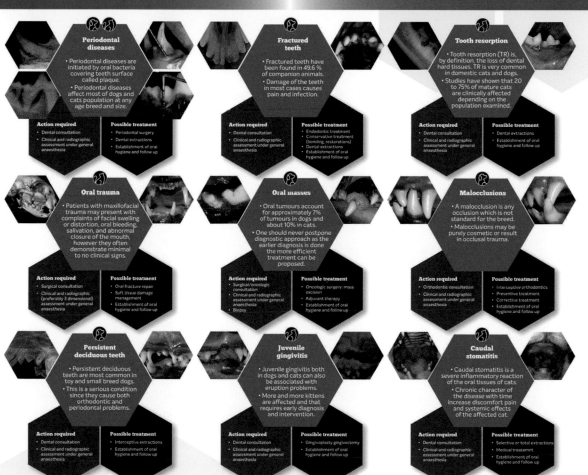

TOP 10 ORAL PATHOLOGIES IN CATS AND DOGS

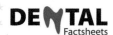
DENTAL Factsheets

Key points

1. **Dental, oral, and maxillofacial diseases** are the most common clinical problems in small animal veterinary practices.

2. A complete oral exam should be performed during every patient exam. **Every patient every time.**

3. Oral disease is a tremendously **underdiagnosed and undertreated** disease process world-wide.

Most common canine oral pathologies

1. Periodontal diseases
2. Persistent deciduous teeth
3. Fractured teeth
4. Malocclusions
5. Oral masses

Most common feline oral pathologies

1. Periodontal diseases
2. Juvenile gingivitis
3. Tooth resorption
4. Caudal stomatitis
5. Oral trauma

Periodontal diseases
- Periodontal diseases are initiated by oral bacteria covering teeth surface called plaque.
- Periodontal diseases affect most of dogs and cats population at any age breed and size.

Action required
- Dental consultation
- Clinical and radiographic assessment under general anaesthesia

Possible treatment
- Periodontal surgery
- Dental extractions
- Establishment of oral hygiene and follow up

Fractured teeth
- Fractured teeth have been found in 49.6 % of companion animals.
- Damage of the teeth in most cases causes pain and infection.

Action required
- Dental consultation
- Clinical and radiographic assessment under general anaesthesia

Possible treatment
- Endodontic treatment
- Conservative treatment (bonding, restorations)
- Dental extractions
- Establishment of oral hygiene and follow up

Tooth resorption
- Tooth resorption (TR) is, by definition, the loss of dental hard tissues. TR is very common in domestic cats and dogs.
- Studies have shown that 20 to 75% of mature cats are clinically affected depending on the population examined.

Action required
- Dental consultation
- Clinical and radiographic assessment under general anaesthesia

Possible treatment
- Dental extractions
- Establishment of oral hygiene and follow up

Oral trauma
- Patients with maxillofacial trauma may present with complaints of facial swelling or distortion, oral bleeding, salivation, and abnormal closure of the mouth, however they often demonstrate minimal to no clinical signs.

Action required
- Surgical consultation
- Clinical and radiographic (preferably 3 dimensional) assessment under general anaesthesia

Possible treatment
- Oral fracture repair
- Soft tissue damage management
- Establishment of oral hygiene and follow up

Oral masses
- Oral tumours account for approximately 7% of tumours in dogs and about 10% in cats.
- One should never postpone diagnostic approach as the earlier diagnosis is done the more efficient treatment can be proposed.

Action required
- Surgical/oncologic consultation
- Clinical and radiographic assessment under general anaesthesia
- Biopsy

Possible treatment
- Oncologic surgery: mass excision
- Adjuvant therapy
- Establishment of oral hygiene and follow up

Malocclusions
- A malocclusion is any occlusion which is not standard for the breed.
- Malocclusions may be purely cosmetic or result in occlusal trauma.

Action required
- Orthodontic consultation
- Clinical and radiographic assessment under general anaesthesia

Possible treatment
- Interceptive orthodontics
- Preventive treatment
- Corrective treatment
- Establishment of oral hygiene and follow up

Persistent deciduous teeth
- Persistent deciduous teeth are most common in toy and small breed dogs.
- This is a serious condition since they cause both orthodontic and periodontal problems.

Action required
- Dental consultation
- Clinical and radiographic assessment under general anaesthesia

Possible treatment
- Interceptive extractions
- Establishment of oral hygiene and follow up

Juvenile gingivitis
- Juvenile gingivitis both in dogs and cats can also be associated with eruption problems.
- More and more kittens are affected and that requires early diagnosis and intervention.

Action required
- Dental consultation
- Clinical and radiographic assessment under general anaesthesia

Possible treatment
- Gingivoplasty gingivectomy
- Establishment of oral hygiene and follow up

Caudal stomatitis
- Caudal stomatitis is a severe inflammatory reaction of the oral tissues of cats.
- Chronic character of the disease with time increase discomfort pain and systemic effects of the affected cat.

Action required
- Dental consultation
- Clinical and radiographic assessment under general anaesthesia

Possible treatment
- Selective or total extractions
- Medical treatemnt
- Establishment of oral hygiene and follow up

Jerzy Gawor,
MRCVS, DVM PhD,
Dipl. AVDC, Dipl. EVDC

Brook A. Niemiec,
DVM, Dipl. AVDC,
Dipl. EVDC

= statistically most common in this species

Lund EM, Armstrong PJ, Kirk CA, Kolar LM, Klausner JS. Health status and population characteristics of dogs and cats examined at private veterinary practices in the United States. J Am Vet Med Assoc. 1999 May 1;214(5):1336–41. PMID: 10319174.
Marshall MD, Wallis CV, Milella L, Colyer A, Tweedie AD, Harris S. A longitudinal assessment of periodontal disease in 52 Miniature Schnauzers. BMC Vet Res. 2014 Sep 1;10:166. doi: 10.1186/1746-6148-10-166. PMID: 25179569; PMCID: PMC4236762.
Niemiec BA. Oral pathology. Top Companion Anim Med. 2008 May;23(2):59–71. doi: 10.1053/j.tcam.2008.02.002. PMID: 18482706.
Niemiec BA: Small Animal Dental, Oral & Maxillofacial Disease. Manson Publishing Ltd., London; 2011.
Peralta S, Verstraete FJ, Kass PH. Radiographic evaluation of the types of tooth resorption in dogs. Am J Vet Res. 2010 Jul;71(7):784–93. doi: 10.2460/ajvr.71.7.784. PMID: 20594081.
Roux, P, Howard, J. (2010) The evaluation of dentition and occlusion in dogs. European Journal of Companion Animal Practice. 20(3):241–51.
Soukup JW, Hetzel S, Paul A. Classification and Epidemiology of Traumatic Dentoalveolar Injuries in Dogs and Cats: 959 Injuries in 660 Patient Visits (2004–2012). J Vet Dent. 2015 Spring;32(1):6–14. doi: 10.1177/0898756415030200101. PMID: 26197685.
Wiggs RB, Lobprise HB: Periodontology. In Veterinary Dentistry. Principals and Practice. Philadelphia, PA, Lippincott – Raven. 1997: pp 186–231

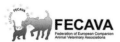
FECAVA
Federation of European Companion Animal Veterinary Associations

Figure 1.5 (Continued)

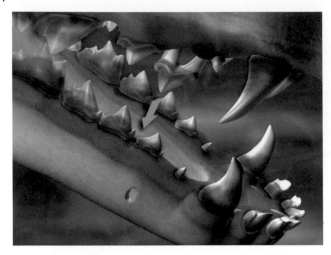

Figure 1.6 Educational video shown on a tablet in a waiting room. *Source:* Courtesy of Vetoquinol.

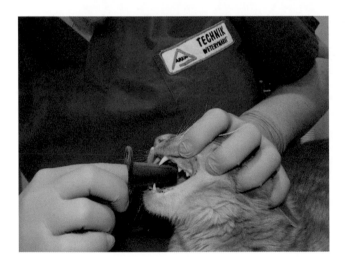

Figure 1.7 Finger protection during feline oral cavity assessment.

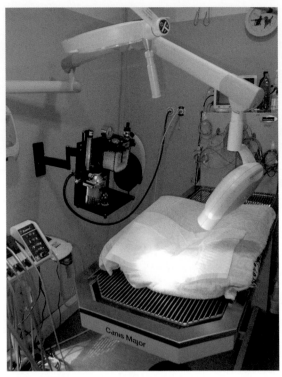

Figure 1.8 Dental operatory.

be kept clean and the walls can be disinfected. It should also have an air circulation with slightly negative pressure in order to enable the evacuation of toxic remnants of anesthetic gas and infectious aerosols, and to protect the rest of the clinic against contamination. Hazardous material containers should be easy accessible, correctly labeled, and highly visible (Figure 1.13).

1.7 Ergonomy, Organization, and Functionality

Ergonomic solutions for operator and assistant include numerous items, beginning with the organization of the room, which should have easy access to equipment, materials, and instrumentation. This solution must be planned from the onset and discussed with the designer prior to construction.

An operating table with adjustable height and comfortable access to the patient's head is important. Such a table should enable the utilization of copious amount of water, with the possibility for its drainage and evacuation of liquids. Chairs that provide proper and relaxed positioning during long procedures should be provided. A central vacuum and gas delivery with oxygen source and central suction will be very convenient. Again, this should be planned for prior to construction, as redesigning is more expensive.

be very practical for a limited number of exposures or when the dentist must operate in a variety of places or in exotic locations without electricity supply, but this solution may be a safety concern in some countries (Figure 1.11).

Anesthesia equipment, including a cardiorespiratory monitor, should be placed so that it is visible to both the assistant or anesthesiologist and the surgeon or veterinarian. A portable anesthetic machine will be convenient if the clinic has several places where anesthesia is needed. The mounted version saves space, but it should be attached to a movable platform in order that it can be utilized in different sizes of patient (Figure 1.12). Anesthesia equipment is described in detail in Chapter 12.

Hygienic requirements are presented in Chapter 7, but in general the dental room should have good access so it can

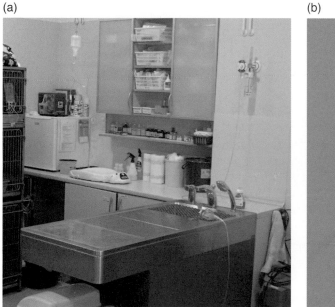

Figure 1.9 Protection of the patient during sedation.

(a)   (b)

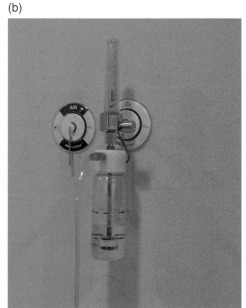

Figure 1.10 Central distribution of (a) water in preparation and postoperative care tables with hot and cool water, a shower, and a bath and (b) air or oxygen.

The more adjustable and flexible the positions of the anesthesia machine, table, and dental unit, the easier their use and the greater their adaptability to different operators (e.g., left- or right-handed, tall or short) and patient sizes (Figure 1.14).

Currently, high-speed internet and computer database networks are common features of every veterinary practice.

They allow the utilization of electronic dental charting systems such as electronic Veterinary Dental Scoring (eVDS), as well as the sending of digital radiographs from the X-ray or operator room to the consulting room.

Size, height, air conditioning, light, intensity of water access, and the presence of windows and doors may be specified by legal regulations, which will vary from country

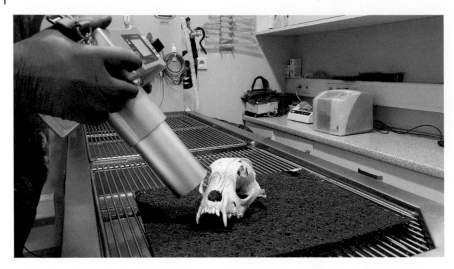

Figure 1.11   Handheld X-ray generator.

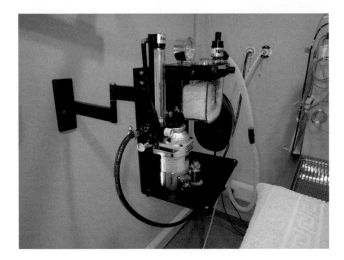

Figure 1.12   Wall-mounted anesthesia machine.

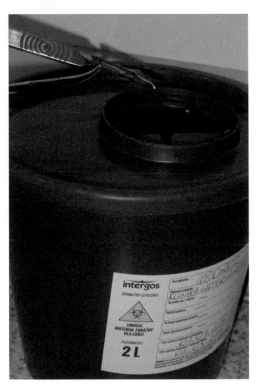

Figure 1.13   Hazardous materials have to be stored in dedicated containers and described.

to country, with no recognized international standards. In general, it is easier to control the microclimate in a larger room, so it may be easier to organize a larger room than a smaller one. This author has experienced many different rooms in his career, some organized in a perfect and functional way, some in a very nonpractical or even unacceptable way. Some of the best solutions are presented in this section.

The organization of all materials, instruments, and surgical kits, as well as all cleaning, sterilizing, and sharpening procedures, should ideally be under the control of the nurses or technicians. This will insure that clean, sharp, and autoclaved instruments are delivered on time, necessary materials appear almost immediately, and spare burs, probes, brushes, and photostimulable phosphor (PSP) radiographic plates are available in seconds, not minutes.

One important consideration in communication with the pet owner pertains to their presence in the dental room: is this desirable, optional, or not allowed? Some specialists prefer presenting the patient under anesthesia and demonstrating any conditions directly in their mouth, as well as reviewing the radiographs in person (Figure 1.15). Alternatively (and this is this author's preference), all details may be discussed and presented in consulting room.

(a)

(b)

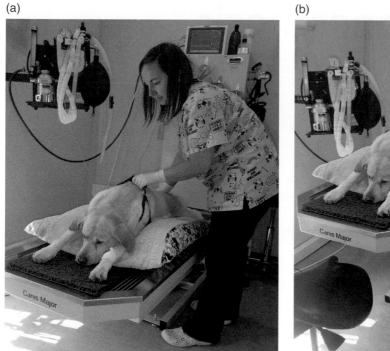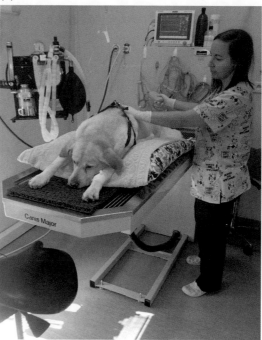

Figure 1.14   An adjustable table is helpful when working on with larger patients. (a) Placement is easier when the position is low. (b) The height can then be adjusted to "operating" level.

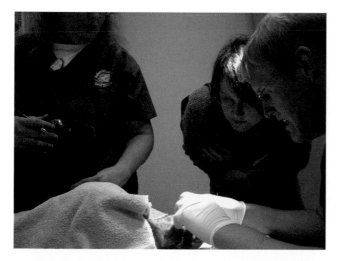

Figure 1.15   Veterinary dentist demonstrating the pathology to the pet owner.

Pictures and radiographs can be displayed on a computer screen, and the dental chart and medical records should also be available (Figure 1.16). This is an easy process when the IT infrastructure is well organized and efficient. For those owners who want to see how the operating area is organized, a PowerPoint presentation can be prepared and

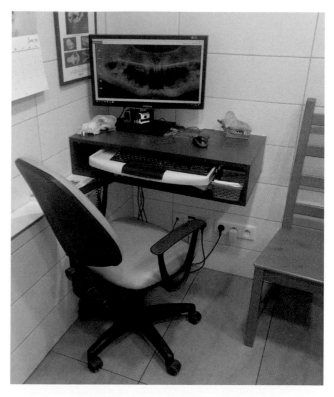

Figure 1.16   Discussion in the consulting room is easier when a high-quality screen and medical database are available.

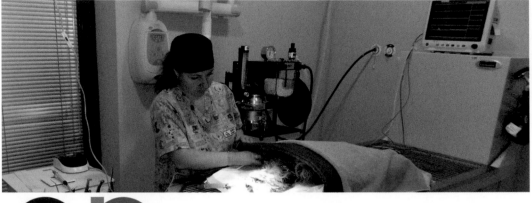

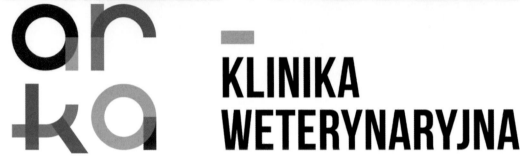

Figure 1.17   Presentation displayed in the waiting room explaining the safety of anesthesia.

displayed in the consulting or waiting room. Safe anesthesia requirements, prophylactic procedures, and standards of hygiene and practice might also be displayed (Figure 1.17).

1.8   How to Choose the Proper Equipment

There are two options when investing in modern techniques: purchase the machines and then learn how to use them or learn how to use them first and then purchase them. In this author's experience, the better option is to first get the skills, and then select the most suitable technology or specific brand for their use. Ideally, the supplier will offer the required education and future service, which continues with cooperation in regard to regular upgrades of equipment. Therefore, the best thing before making a final decision is to participate in courses where one can try several different machines and manufacturers before committing to a purchase. The intention of organizers is often to provide the widest review of available instrumentation and equipment. Following two or three days of use, it is easier to understand if some particular equipment is worth the investment.

Here are some helpful hints in deciding about equipment:

1) Better equipment is more expensive, but much more reliable, effective, and long-lasting.
2) Better equipment usually provides a wider range of possibilities and enables a higher quality of clinical results.
3) Technical support from the supplier is invaluable. Professional representatives should advise and select the optimal equipment and its configuration to match the facility, skills, and expectations of the practitioner. During use, the practice should have continuous backup when problems occur, with prompt response, service, and substitution. From the author's experience, the best advice is always received from those representatives who are responsible for the service of the equipment they have sold.
4) Approximately 95% of dental procedures require a professional dental cleaning. Be sure that your equipment fully covers everything necessary to perform this critical procedure.
5) Participation in a practical workshop providing a selection of different units and types of equipment is very

Table 1.1 Suggested business plan for the equipment of the dental part of a practice.

Requirements service level	Radiology	Dental equipment	Instruments and materials	Knowledge	Case log
Hygienic and diagnostic	X-ray machine, dental oral films	Scaler and polisher	Diagnostic kit Basic surgical kit	Basic educational dental modules offered by the European Veterinary Dental Society (EVDS), American Veterinary Dental Society (AVDS), or dental specialists Books and other educational resources	Participation in oral health campaigns Two or three patients a week
Daily dentistry	X-ray machine, dental oral films, or a digital system	Air-driven dental unit with scaler and polisher	Extended surgical periodontal diagnostic kits, as well as materials corresponding to offered dental services	Selection of ESAVS or EVDS/AVDS courses Books and other educational resources	Common contact with dental patients and dental problems 20% of the week dedicated to dentistry
Enthusiast of dentistry	Dental X-ray, phosphoric plates, or sensors in all dental sizes	National specialization requirements	National specialization requirements	Complete ESAVS courses National specialization requirements Books and other educational resources	40% of the week dedicated to dentistry
Dental specialist	Dental X-ray, phosphoric plates, or sensors in all dental sizes	EVDC or AVDC list of requirements	EVDC or AVDC list of requirements	EVDC or AVDC diplomat Books and other educational resources	Daily contact with dental patients More than 50% of the workload dedicated to dentistry

beneficial. Apart from the previously mentioned advantages, some teachers offer their students distance follow-up in terms of advice in consultations and other suggestions.

Table 1.1 provides advice on how to make a business plan for the equipment of a dental room. The data and information listed are only estimates, and the service level presented in the first column is a subjective proposal of the author and does not carry any guarantees.

Radiography is a critical part of a dental, oral, and maxillofacial assessment. Different systems of digital radiography may deliver different speeds and accuracies of diagnosis. The quality of the equipment present at the clinic should be linked to the number of dental procedures carried out: the more are performed, the more radiographs are exposed, and so the greater the income from radiography. Simultaneous with the development of skills, the range of services that can be offered increases and a better quality of radiographs is produced.

In dental radiography, two digital systems are available: indirect and direct. Both have their advantages and limitations, and in the author's experience, at advanced levels of practice, the best solution is to have both available. Indirect radiography utilizes phosphor plates in different sizes (from 0 through 1, 2, 4, or 5) (Figure 1.18); for rabbits and rodents, one can also customize the plates to expose intraoral projections. The quality of radiographs obtained is very good, but the process of scanning takes from 20 to 40 seconds. Direct radiography uses only sizes 1 and 2, but it produces a picture in a much shorter amount of time: most systems can create an image within 1.5 seconds. An additional benefit is the possibility of adjusting the radiographic technique with the tubehead, and of performing a series of radiographs with the sensor in the same position. The former is very helpful in periodontology, the latter in endodontics.

Ideally, the screen presenting exposed radiographs should be located in a position which allows review at any moment of the procedure without additional effort.

Depending on how the facility is designed, it may be possible to integrate the digital radiographic system with the clinic database. This makes it possible to send files to the consulting room and to show them to the owner while discussing the treatment plan and estimates, or to send them by email on request.

Currently, 3D imaging plays an increasingly important role in dental and maxillofacial diagnostics. There is evidence that 3D imaging provides more and better information in terms of accurate diagnosis of oral trauma, oncology, developmental defects, and temporomandibular joint disorders (Bar-Am et al. 2008; Ghirelli 2013; Nemec et al. 2015)

(a)
(b)

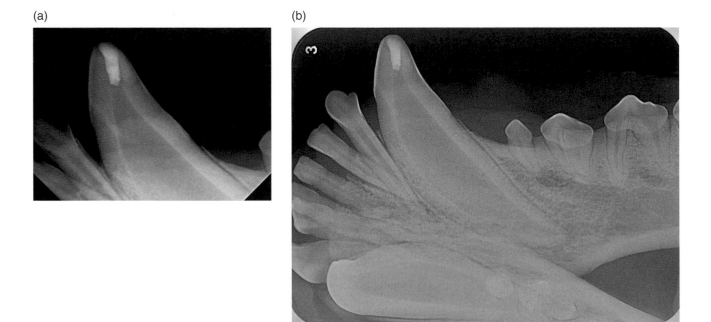

Figure 1.18 An object (e.g., a treated tooth) can be radiographically assessed in a smaller (direct radiography) or larger format (indirect radiography). The larger format generally provides a wider perspective and makes reading easier and diagnosis more accurate. (a) is the standard #2 size of digital sensor and (b) is size 4 of the phosphoric plate.

(Figure 1.19). Nevertheless, investment needs to be justified according to the competence and experience of the team and their caseload.

1.9 Power Dental Equipment

Combined mechanical scalers and polishers are still available on the market, but they limit dental procedures to prophylaxis with no possibility for surgical extraction, which is limiting and will prove insufficient over time (Figure 1.20). Simple devices may be used in emergency situations, when the major equipment is out of order. Therefore, it is worth considering investment in a dental unit equipped with low- and high-speed handpieces and a three-way syringe. Such a configuration is quite common and easily available on the market. Some manufacturers offer scalers separately, while others provide the scaling handpieces as part of a dental unit. Many units have their own compressors, some with wall-mounted versions that requires attachment into a central compressed-air system or vacuum (Figure 1.21).

Progress in technology and continuous cooperation between manufacturers and specialists are producing better and better solutions for veterinary dentistry. Selection of the optimal supplier is an individual decision. Before that decision is made, a trial is strongly recommended.

1.10 Dental Instrumentation

Specific instruments are necessary to perform oral surgery and dentistry. One cannot compromise patient care by using instruments inappropriately or using nonmedical instruments. The decision about which types or brands should be purchased is based on individual preferences. However, the author can recommend some based on experience and personal needs. Most instruments can be organized in groups (kits) dedicated to specific procedures or specific species or sizes of animal. A very important part of the correct use of any instrument is having a proper grasp. Also important is maintaining the correct shape of working surface or tip, which is associated with sharpening and conservation. Ensuring that instruments are always clean, ready, and sharp is a must, not only in the dental world, but in all of medicine.

This section presents the absolute basic instruments that every general practice offering any form of dentistry should be equipped with.

1.10.1 Diagnostic Kit

An explorer and periodontal probe are very often combined, having one side of the instrument being an explorer and the other being a probe. For dogs, a combination of a UNC 17 periodontal probe with a shepherd hook explorer is this author's preference (Figure 1.22). In cats, a finer explorer ODU or Orban explorer combined with a Michigan probe with Williams markings will better adapt to the feline gingival sulcus and smaller oral cavity. Additionally, evaluation of areas suspected of tooth resorption is more convenient with this explorer (Figure 1.23).

Mouth props are preferred to gags as they do not apply additional force to the temporomandibular joint area, and in cats they diminish the risk of complications of excessive jaws opening (Stiles et al. 2012) (Figure 1.24).

For conscious patient examination, finger protectors are very useful where there is danger of the patient hurting the assessor (see Figure 1.7).

Mirrors can be used to visualize the palatal and lingual surfaces of teeth, the caudal part of the oral cavity, the pharynx, and the choanae. The most caudal areas can be illuminated by light reflection from the mirror (Figure 1.25).

Revealing small lesions or details during oral examination is easier with the use of magnification combined with lightening (Figure 1.26). For beginners, 2.5 dental loupes are a good choice. With time, 3.5× magnification may be preferred. It is important to understand that using magnification will not immediately improve the quality of a procedure. It takes experience and training, but magnification will become an invaluable support for the operator, help to avoid errors, and expose small details during operations.

The next step in magnifying the operating area is the use of an operating microscope, which further improves the assessment of surgical tissues.

During oral assessment, it is important to record all observations on a dental chart appropriate to the species and age of the patient. Regardless of whether two- or four-handed dentistry (i.e., with or without an assistant) is performed, filling in the chart is obligatory (Figure 1.27).

High-quality photography can further augment the diagnostic process. It can be used for presentation to the owner, for communication with a referring veterinarian, for comparison at distant follow-up, and for illustration of publications or presentations. This is a matter of personal preference, but the camera should preserve natural colors and provide sufficient magnification and focal distance. The latter can be difficult in compact cameras, which require very small distances for macro mode, where lenses and external optics may get foggy from the humid oral environment.

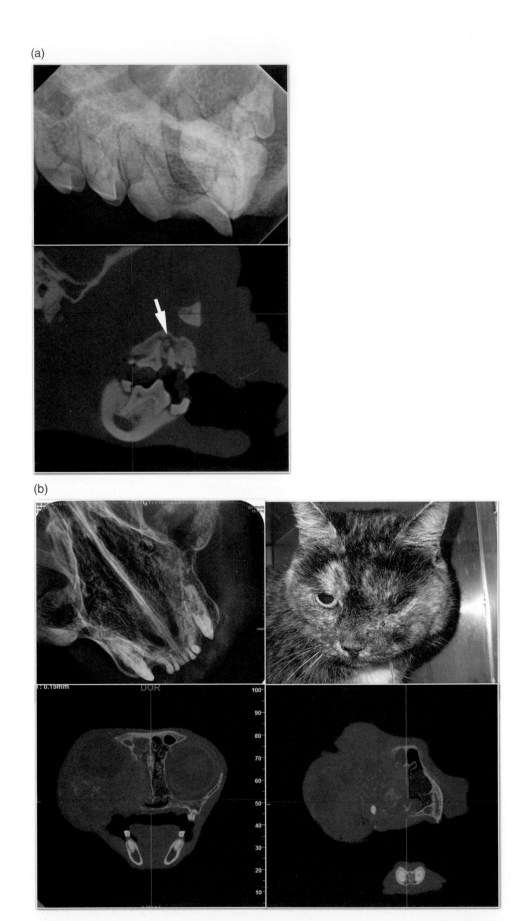

Figure 1.19 Advantages of 3D versus 2D imaging. (a) The sequestrum revealed next to the infected root of the 208 (arrow) would not be identified in a standard radiograph. (b) The extent of neoplastic growth is better assessed in 3D than in intraoral radiograph.

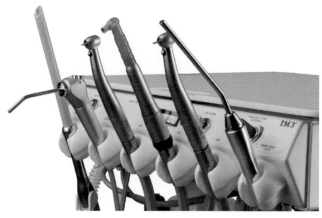

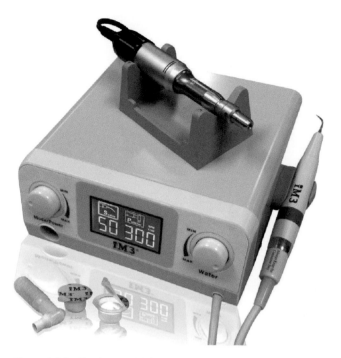

Figure 1.21 Dental unit main board, including (from left) suction, three-way syringe, high-speed handpiece, low-speed handpiece, second high-speed handpiece, and illuminating wand.

Figure 1.20 Device combining a scaler and a polisher.

(a)

(b)

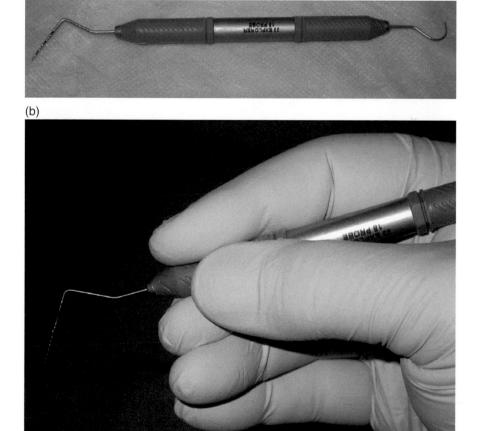

Figure 1.22 (a) Combination of a UNC probe and explorer in a single instrument. (b) and its pen grasp.

(a)

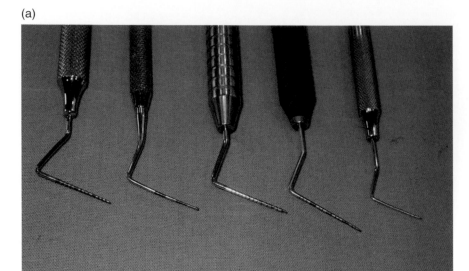

(b)

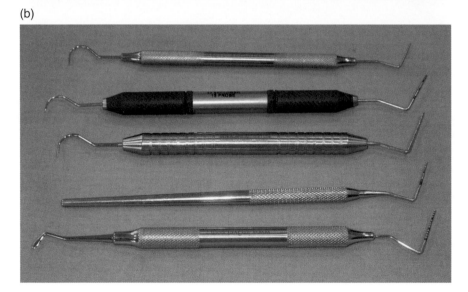

Figure 1.23 Series of combined probes and explorers. (a) Probes. From left: UNC 15, Michigan, Niemiec, UNC 17, Williams. (b) Whole instruments.

1.10.2 Surgical Kit

In most cases, oral surgery will mean extraction. More information on this topic is provided in Chapter 22. The oral surgery kit has been developed and presented in textbooks by several specialists (Niemiec, Verstraete, Reiter), and oral surgeons have their own preferences in terms of type, size, and brand. Nevertheless, all agree that the following should always be included: blade holder, tissue forceps, periosteal elevator, tissue scissors, suture scissors, and needle holder (Figure 1.28). The part of the needle holder that grasps the suture should be delicate or it can weaken the material, causing it to break after a few sutures.

Oral needle holders must not be used for materials larger than 4/0 or they will immediately lose good attachment to sutures and needle.

Tissue scissors with serrated cutting edges provide a better margin of the cut mucosa and gums, but they should never be used for sutures. Suture scissors should preferably be blunt-ended in order not to harm the tissue while cutting the sutures.

The surgical kit may have medium/large canine and cats/small dogs variations and be packed together with diagnostic instruments. For surgery in the caudal area of the mouth or oropharynx, instruments must be long enough for comfortable operation.

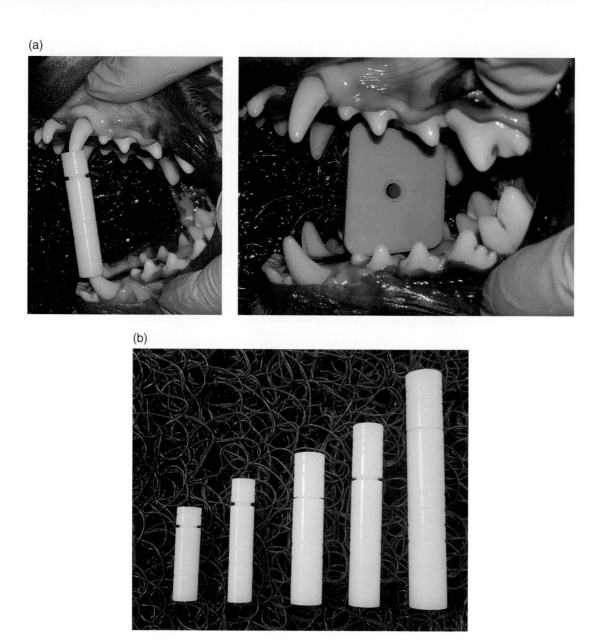

Figure 1.24   (a) Mouth props extending a dog's jaws. (b) Selection of props in different sizes for dogs and cats.

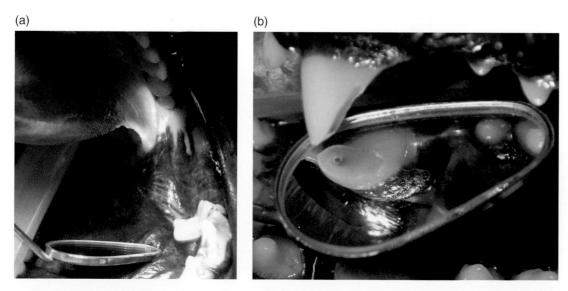

Figure 1.25   Mirror (a) reflecting light into the caudal part of the oral cavity and (b) showing the other side of a tooth.

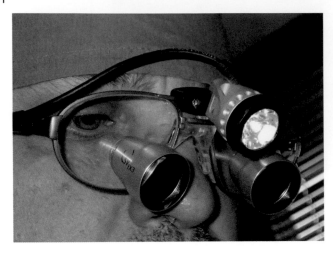

Figure 1.26 Magnification helps greatly with dental procedures.

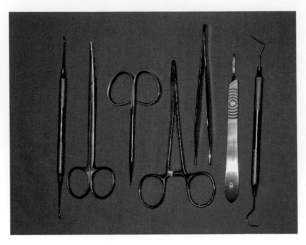

Figure 1.28 The oral surgical general kit includes, from left: periosteal elevator, suture scissors, tissue scissors, needle holder tissue forceps, blade holder, and periodontal probe.

(a)

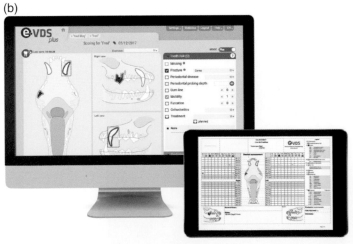

(b)

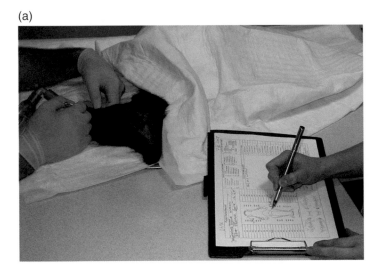

Figure 1.27 Charting: filling in (a) a paper dental chart and (b) an electronic veterinary dental scoring system.

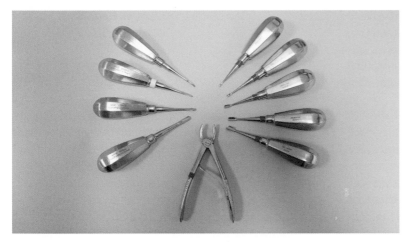

Figure 1.29 Extraction kit: luxators (left) and elevators (right), as well as extraction forceps. *Source:* Emilia Klim.

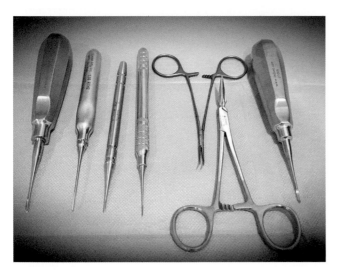

Figure 1.30 Rescue kit - From left: four superslim luxators and elevators, mosquito titanium forceps, root tip forceps, and root tip elevator.

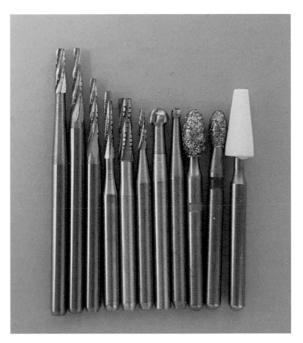

Figure 1.31 Selection of burs for extraction. *Source:* Emilia Klim.

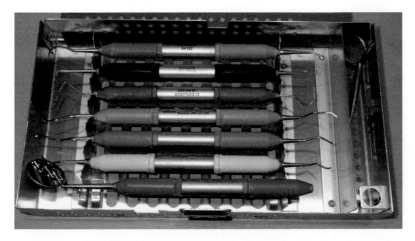

Figure 1.32 Periodontal kit. From bottom: mirror, three curettes, periodontal probe, and two scalers.

A necessary addition to this kit is an extraction package that contains an assortment of luxators and elevators, as well as extraction forceps (Figure 1.29), and possibly a separate set of instruments dedicated to solving complications, such as root-tip forceps and root-tip elevators (Figure 1.30).

There is also an option for a combination luxator and elevator, called an extractor. In this author's hands, it does not fulfill expectations, but it may be worth trying, particularly under the supervision of someone familiar with its use.

An additional element of an extraction kit is a selection of burs, typically used during surgical extractions. The most common varieties of burs are round, pear-shaped, and fissure, in both standard and surgical lengths (Figure 1.31).

1.10.3 Periodontal Kit

A manual scaler (either Jacquette or sickle) is a good addition for removing supragingival deposits. For subgingival deposits (plaque and calculus) and granulation tissue debridement, curettes are utilized. There are two major types of curettes: universal and area-specific. Universal curettes have a blade with two cutting edges and can be adapted to all regions in the mouth and dentition (Figure 1.32); however, there are smaller and larger versions enabling the working to reach every small area of interest. Area-specific curettes are designed differently, with only one cutting edge and 70° angulation of the face (Figure 1.33). The most popular set is the Gracey series.

In all kinds and variations of surgical instruments, the key to successful use is good working conditions and correct application, which includes: handling, adequate surface use, and proper movement of working tip and the hand.

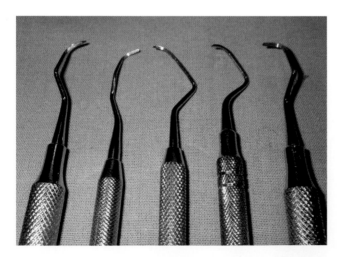

Figure 1.33 Area-specific curettes.

1.10.4 Instrument Care and Sharpening

See Appendix B.

1.10.5 Materials Required

Generally, absorbable monofilament suture materials are recommended for oral surgery, size 5/0 for cats and 4/0 for dogs. These materials result in less irritation of local soft tissues and fewer cases of infection. Polyglecapron 25 is the most popular material, and due to its relatively long time of absorption, it is a good option even in wounds where slow healing may be anticipated.

Suture needles for oral surgery must be the swaged-on type. Needle curvature is either 3/8 or 1/2, with the latter more indicated in the caudal part of the oral cavity. A reverse-cutting needle is best for suturing gingiva and mucosa, but for delicate mucosa, a taper point may be optimal. In the author's experience, colored sutures are easier to handle than transparent ones; the most commonly available color is blue.

Polishing paste is routinely used for final cleaning and smoothing of the rough crown surface after descaling. Flour of pumice is a very popular product for this. It is often stored in large containers, but disposable mini containers are also available. In most cases, fine-grit paste is preferred. Some polishing pastes contain fluoride and some are colored so as to be more easily identifiable following the final flush of the mouth.

Chlorhexidine (CHX) solution is used to flush the mouth before descaling and to provide antimicrobial action if potential infection is significant (Figure 1.34). Premade concentrated CHX bottles can be added to water tanks in dental units. It is important to follow manufacturer instructions and apply the solution only if it is accepted by your particular model and type of handpiece.

Plaque-disclosing solutions are helpful in identifying plaque coverage on tooth crowns. They can be presented to pet owners when discussing oral hygiene methods or applied as a quality control after scaling of teeth to reveal remnants of dental deposits (Figure 1.35).

Pharyngeal packs can be made of gauze or sponge and are inserted into the pharynx around the endotracheal tubes or esophageal probe to protect the respiratory tract against aspiration of water and other contamination that occurs during professional dental cleaning. They must not be too tight as this can compromise lymphatic or blood-vessel circulation and cause edema. To avoid leaving them in after the procedure, it is helpful to have a thread left hanging outside the mouth that can be used to pull them out (Figure 1.36).

Personal protective equipment is described in detail in Chapter 7.

Oral hygienic products are described in Chapter 5.

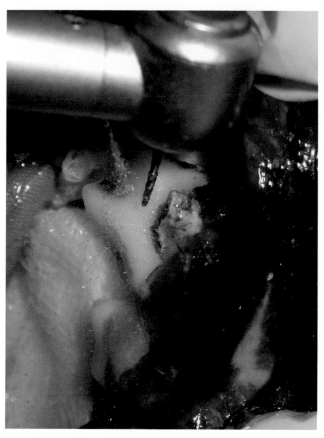

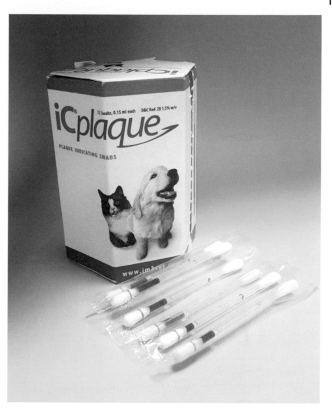

Figure 1.35 Plaque-disclosing solution. *Source:* Emilia Klim.

Figure 1.34 Use of CHX solution during extraction of a badly infected mouth.

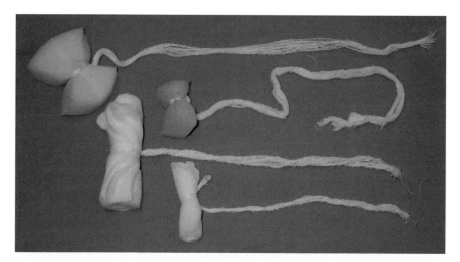

Figure 1.36 Disposable custom-made pharyngeal packs made of gauze or sponge.

References and Further Reading

Bar-Am, Y., Pollard, R.E., Kass, P.H. et al. (2008). Diagnostic yield of conventional radiographs and CT in dogs and cats with MFT (maxillofacial trauma). *Vet. Surg.* 37 (3): 294–299.

Bellows J. Small Animal Dental Equipment, Materials and Techniques Blackwell, 2004

DeBowes L. Mosier D., Lofan E et al. Association of periodontal disease and histologic lesions in multiple organs from 45 dogs *J.Vet.Dent* 1996; 13 (2)

DeBowes LJ. The effects of dental disease on systemic disease. Vet Clin North Am Small Anim Pract. 1998 Sep;28(5):1057-62. doi: 10.1016/s0195-5616(98)50102-7. PMID: 9779540.

Fernandes, N.A., Batista Borges, A.P., Carlo Reis, E.C. et al. (2012). Prevalence of periodontal disease in dogs and owners' level of awareness – a prospective clinical trial. *Revista Ceres* 59: 446–451.

Ghirelli, O. (2013). Comparison of standard radiography and CT in 21 dogs with maxillary masses. *JVD* 30 (2): 72–76.

Harvey CE, Emily PP. Small Animal Dentistry. St. Louis: Mosby -Year Book, 1993.

Holmstrom SE, Frost P, Eisner ER. Veterinary Dental Techniques for the Small Animal Practitioner, 3rd ed. Philadelphia: WB Saunders, 2004.

Lund, E.M., Armstrong, P.J., Kirk, C.A. et al. (1999). Health status and population characteristics of dogs and cats examined at private veterinary practices in the United States. *J. Am. Vet. Med. Assoc.* 214: 1336–1341.

Mulligan TW, Aller MS, Williams CA. Atlas of Canine and Feline Dental Radiography, Trenton. Veterinary Learning Systems, 1998.

Nemec, A., Daniaux, L., Johnson, E. et al. (2015). Craniomaxillofacial abnormalities in dogs with congenital palatal defects: computed tomographic findings. *Vet. Surg.* 44: 417–422.

Niemiec B, Gawor J, Nemec A, Clarke D, McLeod K, Tutt C, Gioso M, Steagall PV, Chandler M, Morgenegg G, Jouppi R. World Small Animal Veterinary Association Global Dental Guidelines. J Small Anim Pract. 2020 Jul;61(7):E36-E161. doi: 10.1111/jsap.13132. PMID: 32715504.

Reiter AM and Gracis M. BSAVA Manual of Canine and Feline Dentistry and Oral Surgery BSAVA 2018.

Reiter AM, Mendoza KA. Feline odontoclastic resorptive lesions an unsolved enigma in veterinary dentistry. Vet Clin North Am Small Anim Pract. 2002 Jul;32(4):791-837, v. doi: 10.1016/s0195-5616(02)00027-x. PMID: 12148312.

Stella, J.L., Bauer, A.E., and Croney, C.C. (2018). A cross-sectional study to estimate prevalence of periodontal disease in a population of dogs (*Canis familiaris*) in commercial breeding facilities in Indiana and Illinois. *PloS One* 13: e0191395.

Stiles, J., Weil, A.B., Packer, R.A. et al. (2012). Post-anesthetic cortical blindness in cats: twenty cases. *Vet. J.* 193 (2): 367–373.

Tutt C. Small Animal Dentistry a manual of techniques Blackwell Publishing 2006.

Verstraete FJM, Lommer MJ Oral and Maxillofacial Surgery in Dogs and Cats Saunders 2012.

Wiggs RB, Lobprise HB. Dodd JR; Wiggs's Veterinary Dentistry: Principles and Practice, Philadelphia: Wiley & Sons 2019.

2

Marketing and Communication in Veterinary Dentistry

Rachel Perry[1,2]

[1] *Perry Referrals, Brighton, UK*
[2] *Royal Veterinary College, London, UK*

2.1 Introduction

For many years, the education of veterinary dentistry at the university level has been limited, especially when compared to the frequency with which oral and dental problems are encountered in practice (Perry 2014). Veterinarians can therefore leave university and start practicing veterinary dentistry with limited skills and knowledge (Clark et al. 2002; Greenfield et al. 2004). Techniques may then be learned from older colleagues, who themselves received little or no training in the subject. Without a formal, structured continuing professional development (CPD) program that includes small-animal dentistry, the subject can be overlooked. Many veterinarians feel ill-equipped to diagnose oral and dental problems and make meaningful treatment recommendations to their clients (Perry 2014). They may understandably be afraid of performing dental procedures if they have limited understanding of the skills and equipment involved. Furthermore, when one's understanding of a subject is limited, it can be difficult to make accurate self-assessments of one's skill and knowledge levels (Kruger and Dunning 1999).

It is therefore not surprising that veterinarians struggle to adequately market their veterinary dentistry services (if they do so at all) or to make compelling recommendations for treatments at appropriate stages of the oral/dental disease process. This may result in:

1) A welfare issue as pets either do not receive the dental treatment they require, or receive suboptimal treatment (WSAVA 2018).
2) Demotivated professionals considering the "dental" as a chore, or as something that new graduates or students perform (Perry 2014).

3) Clients who perceive poor value for money when they present their pets for treatment ("We cleaned the teeth, and pulled the rotten ones").
4) Financial underperformance of the clinic due to missed opportunities for dental treatment, lack of chargeable diagnostic and therapeutic items (such as dental radiographs, regional anesthesia, and multiparameter anesthetic monitoring), or undercharging (as "it's just a dental").
5) Clients electing for "dental" proposals from nonveterinary/lay sources or investing in worthless or damaging products and procedures such as anesthesia-free dentistry or dentistry performed by groomers.

The reasons these things may occur include (see Figure 2.1):

- Unconscious incompetence (veterinarian is unaware they do not possess the necessary skills/knowledge) (Kruger and Dunning 1999)
- Lack of correct equipment and tools to carry out diagnostic tests and perform treatments (e.g., periodontal probe, dental radiography, dental unit, Luxator/elevators, periosteal elevators)
- Lack of enthusiasm for booking dental procedures due to dislike/fear
- Lack of time allotted to dental procedures (leading to stress)
- Lack of confidence (leading to the inability to make meaningful recommendations, or to inappropriate undercharging for services)
- Lack of conviction (disbelief) that a treatment is truly required (may be detected by the client in the veterinarian's unconscious body language)
- Lack of confidence around the ability to provide safe general anesthesia (leading veterinarians not to make recommendations for dental treatment)

The Veterinary Dental Patient: A Multidisciplinary Approach, First Edition. Edited by Jerzy Gawor and Brook Niemiec.
© 2021 John Wiley & Sons Ltd. Published 2021 by John Wiley & Sons Ltd.
Companion website: www.wiley.com/go/gawor/veterinary-dental-patient

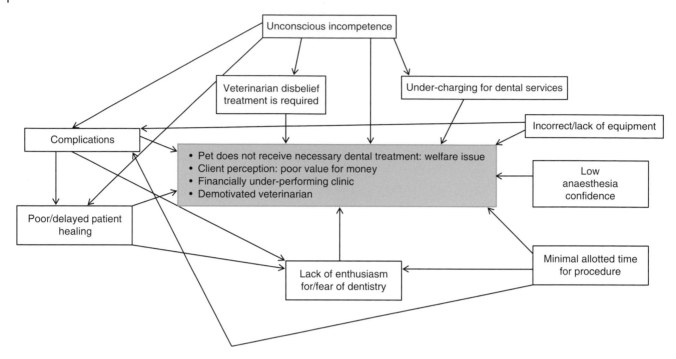

Figure 2.1 Scheme illustrating problems associated with selling veterinary dental services.

- Ignorance (leading to prejudices and misconceptions in both the public and veterinary communities, such as: animals do not feel pain; it is impossible to anesthetize an older patient; tartar is a natural phenomenon; bad breath is normal in dogs and cats)

Rather than making a convincing argument for dental assessment and treatment, the veterinarian may inadvertently send a very confusing message to their clients. A statement such as "Rusty's teeth are pretty dirty. He could do with a dental within the next 6 months" does not motivate the client to take immediate action. Rather, it invalidates the need for intervention: "dirty" is not a medical term, and implies a cosmetic solution, while the timescale (six months) suggests the pet does not have a *real* problem and there is no need to take any action.

This unfortunately leads to our profession being *reactive* when it comes to oral and dental care in pets, rather than *proactive* (like our human dental counterparts). This may be compounded by the fact that oral and dental problems are hidden from the owner's view, halitosis is normalized, and pets invariably continue to eat despite oral pain and infection. It is therefore not uncommon for patients to be finally booked in for treatment at the end stages of the disease process: a fractured maxillary fourth premolar causing facial swelling despite having been painful for a number of months/years; halitosis becoming unbearable for the owner; advanced periodontitis leading to pathologic jaw fracture.

2.2 Compliance

In order to provide a proactive approach to oral and dental care in pets, we must take action before the disease process starts. To achieve this, our clients must be compliant with our recommendations. **Compliance** essentially describes the act of agreeing to and obeying a certain proposal. Medically, it can be thought of as the extent to which a patient's behaviors coincide with medical advice (e.g. taking medication, making lifestyle or dietary changes) (Evangelista 1999). Veterinary compliance describes the percentage of pets receiving a treatment, screening, or procedure in line with current accepted veterinary healthcare advice (AAHA 2003, 2009). **Adherence** describes the extent to which clients administer prescribed medications at the correct dose for the correct time, completing the course and refilling any long-term prescription (AAHA 2009). In veterinary dentistry, we would like to see both compliance and adherence at various times: booking a pet in for assessment and treatment under general anesthesia after we have made a recommendation; giving medications for treatment; performing preventative home care; possibly making dietary changes; and attending re-call appointments/treatments.

The traditional concept of compliance, however, may be described as being **paternalistic**: the health professional gives the patient/client instructions that they must follow, and can label the patient/client as noncompliant when there may be many reasons why they are not complying. The side-effects of a particular drug might be too unbearable for the patient, so they do not complete the course of drug. By definition, they are noncompliant. An elderly patient with arthritis might not be able to remove the lid of a tablet container in order to take their medication. Therefore, again, they are noncompliant.

Relationship-centered care is a new concept in healthcare, which emphasizes the bond between client and veterinarian and between client and pet, and involves a negotiation of outcomes, allowing the client to voice concerns while ultimately recognizing the position that the pet plays within the client's family (Shaw 2006) (Figure 2.2). This shared approach to decision-making may be termed **concordance**.

In an American Animal Hospital Association (AAHA) study into compliance in 2003, practice teams felt that simply giving information about a service was enough for clients to accept their advice and follow through. Estimations of compliance levels were higher than actual values (54% vs. 35%). If the client was noncompliant, it was the client's failure, and was probably due to the anticipated cost. Clients' perspectives were very different, however. Cost was not seen as a barrier to compliance, but rather the *failure to make a recommendation* or the *failure to explain the importance of the recommended treatment*. In addition, had a follow-up call or reminder occurred, clients claimed they would have been far more likely to follow the advice.

In 2006, a task force consisting of health industry providers, healthcare professionals, and associations gathered to assess companion animal practice growth amidst industry struggles. The research focused on the effect of the bond between client and pet and client and veterinarian in terms of the care that the pet received (Lue et al. 2008). It was shown that the greater the bond between client and pet, the higher the level of care expected, regardless of cost. In addition, clients with strong bonds with their pets visited the veterinarian more often and were more likely to seek preventive healthcare.

Owners were likely to display stronger bonds to dogs than to cats, resulting in more frequent clinic visits for dogs (Figure 2.3). Cat owners, however, were likely to be better educated and more researched about their pet's disease. In multi-pet households, dogs were more likely to be taken to the veterinarian than cats. It is important to acknowledge and not judge these client–pet bonds. The veterinarian should enquire about other pets in the household and make recommendations for examination of any cats.

The bond between client and veterinarian is positively affected by good communication, interaction with the pet, and ability to educate. Clients who feel their veterinarian communicates well are more likely to follow their recommendations. This includes thorough explanations and recommendations, which increase the client perception that the veterinarian is recommending *something that their pet needs*. Cost was not cited as a barrier to following a recommendation in the AAHA study. The things that contributed to poor compliance instead included confusion, misunderstanding, and uncertainty. Clients may not have felt that there was a need for treatment, or were not made aware of the value of performing a procedure.

Figure 2.2   Client–pet and client–veterinarian bonds.

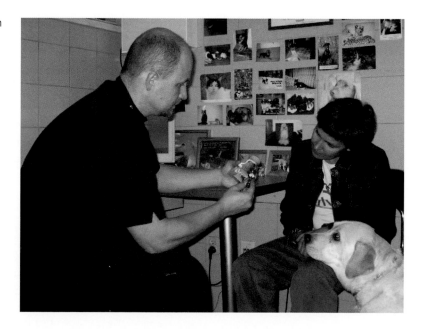

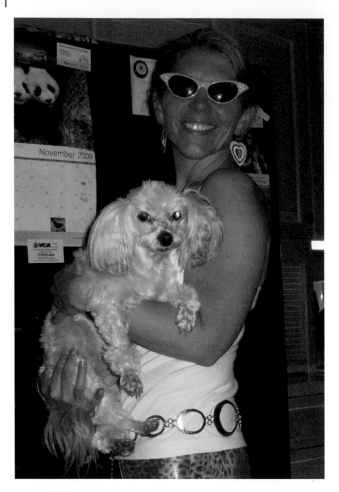

Figure 2.3 Example of a human–dog bond, with humanization efforts.

The effect of veterinarian–client–pet interactions on adherence to a dentistry recommendation has also been studied (Kanji et al. 2012). This research assessed whether relationship-centered care and client satisfaction were positively associated with client adherence. Overall, the odds of a client adhering to a clear rather than an ambiguous recommendation were seven times greater. Adhering clients were shown to be significantly more satisfied following an interaction. The emotional tones used by the veterinarian also had an impact. Sympathetic and empathic tones were more likely to result in adherence than hurried, angry, nervous, or dominant tones.

2.3 To Sell Is Human

In Daniel H. Pink's *To Sell Is Human* (2012), he argues that we are all intrinsically designed to be sellers. That is, we are hardwired to motivate or persuade someone to take action. He describes how one in nine people in the United States

work in sales. The other eight, however, work in a *non-sales selling*. As a medical profession, we are involved in non-sales selling every day, whether of vaccines, a worming protocol, a diet food, a pre-anesthetic blood test, dental treatment under anesthesia, or tooth extraction. We need to persuade people to take action based on our recommendations.

Rather than selling the client something that they or their pet does not need, we can instead use evidence-based veterinary medicine to guide us toward such recommendations (Schmidt 2007).

2.4 Making Persuasive Recommendations

Persuasion is the act of inducing someone to do something via reasoning: motivating them to take action. This could be going on a dinner date, attending a conference, or buying (and reading) a new veterinary dentistry textbook. Persuasion relies on a sense of **trust**, a display of **empathy**, and a **logical** argument (Borg 2010).

2.4.1 Trust

Trust in the medical profession has been widely studied (Hall et al. 2002). It may be displayed as trust in the profession or trust in a particular clinician. The latter involves confidence in their competence and belief in their honesty. Displaying professional qualifications and thank-you cards in waiting and consulting areas can help to strengthen a client's feelings of trust (Figures 2.4 and 2.5). However, the decision on whether or not to trust someone is based very much on *gut feelings*. It is an unconscious decision.

2.4.2 Empathy

Empathy is the ability to understand a client's emotions and feelings, and to reflect them back to them in a supportive way. It is an essential communication skill for the clinician to learn and utilize. The good news is that the skills required to come across as trustworthy and empathic can be learned and improved by practice.

2.4.3 Logic

Logic encompasses the actual words we use and the explanations we give of diseases and treatments, which are *consciously* assimilated by the client. In the Internet age, clients can be incredibly well educated about their pet's clinical signs and disease. If a client is seeking information from Google (where unprofessional opinions abound), try

Figure 2.4   Diplomas in the waiting room.

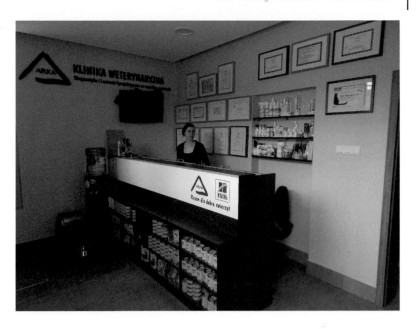

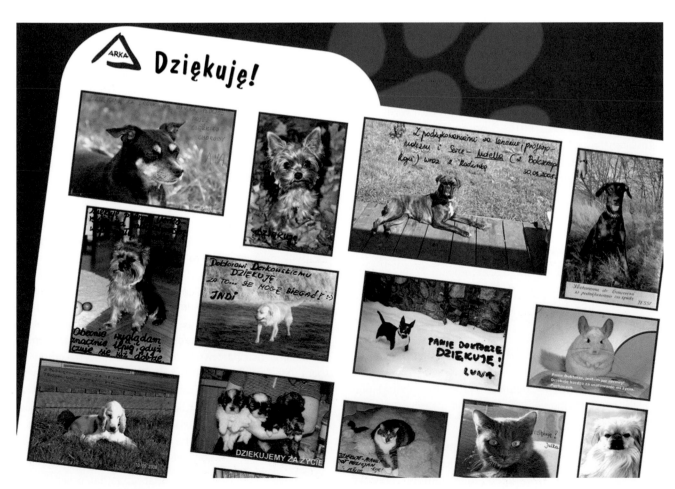

Figure 2.5   Array of thank-you pictures.

instead to direct them to Google Scholar for more objective, scientific information.

We must strive to educate the client. Indeed, this has been shown to increase levels of satisfaction and compliance (Lue et al. 2008). During the consultation process, use whiteboards, a pen and paper, or digital tools (tablets) to explain disease processes, and show the show client dental radiographs, slideshows, or pictures. Provide a scrapbook in the waiting area and collect client testimonials. Have a "dental pet of the month" on a display board. Produce professional leaflets explaining dental diseases for clients to take away and read. Ensure your website is up to date and contains useful information and videos ("How to Brush my Dog's/Cat's Teeth"). Ensure that your own skills and knowledge meet current recommended standards (Holmstrom et al. 2013). This is best achieved through a combination of theory and practical CPD courses. The whole team must voice the same message (see Chapter 4).

Logic allows a client to validate their gut-feelings gained from the unconscious messages of trust and empathy.

2.5 Communication Skills

Communication should be thought of as a *clinical* skill essential to clinical competence – one that can be learned and improved (Beck et al. 2002; Shaw et al. 2004; Shaw 2006; Kanji et al. 2012). Communication skills are significantly associated with outcomes of patient care, including patient health, patient and physician satisfaction, and malpractice risk (Shaw 2006). There are three principal types:

- **Content Skills:** The content of questions and information given.
- **Process Skills:** Verbal (words chosen) and nonverbal communication, including vocal indicators (speech tone and pace, rhythm, inflections, sounds used to convey understanding [uh-huh, ahh, mm], volume, laughing, yawning, etc.), facial expressions, eye contact, posture, touch (beware of intense cultural differences), gestures (pointing), body movement (foot or finger tapping), smell, and appearance.
- **Perceptual Skills:** Cognitive (problem solving) and relationship (personal awareness and awareness of others) skills.

Shaw (2006) identified four core communication skills that highly effective practitioners should possess: nonverbal communication, open-ended questioning, reflective listening, and displays of empathy.

2.5.1 Nonverbal Communication

Nonverbal and verbal communication should complement one another. If their messages are contradictory, the receiver (client) will instinctively trust the nonverbal signs as the true message (Mehrabian 1981). For instance, a veterinarian might say that a pet needs dental treatment because of signs of advanced periodontal disease, but if they are shifting in their seat and not maintaining eye contact with the client, this will not be a credible recommendation.

Miscommunication is much more likely to occur when nonverbal communication is lacking (e.g., emails and telephone calls).

> Increase sensitivity to clients' nonverbal cues. Reflecting them back to the client in a supportive way can help display empathy (e.g., "I can see that you are concerned about the safety of a general anesthetic for Monty, so may I explain how we reduce the risks?"). Empathy is a positive predictor of consultation outcomes, including client satisfaction and compliance (Beck et al. 2002).

Increase awareness of your own nonverbal cues, which can include eye contact, gaze, body posture, orientation toward client, gesturing, and nodding.

Sincere smiling and appropriate eye contact can enhance your communication and display of empathy. Smiling reduces stress, increases positivity, and is infectious – when clients smile back, they feel more positive themselves. Eye contact can indicate attention and sincerity, but inappropriate gazing may come across as being aggressive and can negatively impact the physician–patient interaction (Beck et al. 2002) (Figure 2.6).

2.5.2 Open-Ended Questioning

Open-ended questions allow the client to elaborate and impart as much relevant information as possible. They start with words such as "What. . .?", "How. . .?", and "Tell me. . ." (e.g., "How has Misty been since I last saw you?). Closed questions, on the other hand, demand a one-word answer ("Is Fluffy vomiting?"). Both styles are useful during the consultation process, but starting with an open question allows the client to voice all of their perceived problems and concerns, allowing them to feel fully heard. If the clinician can listen effectively (and not interrupt), they can reflect this back to the client, again showing empathy. Closed questions can be used later in the process to gain further details and clarification.

2.5.3 Reflective Listening

Effective listening is an essential skill that practitioners must learn. A good listener seeks to *understand* before

(a)

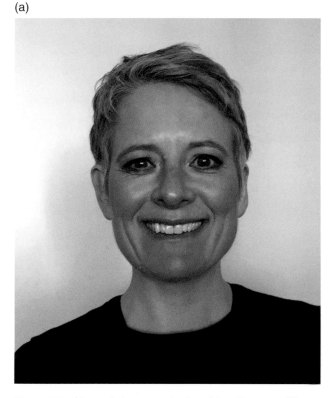

(b)

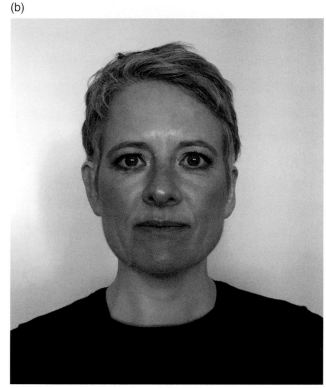

Figure 2.6   Nonverbal communication: (a) smile versus (b) non-smile.

being *understood*. It is important that you and the client agree that what you understand is a true representation of what the client was saying. Listening is very different from hearing. It can be challenging because our brains move much faster than we talk, thinking ahead and formulating diagnostic and treatment plans. Beckman and Frankel found in 1984 that in 69% of medical consultations, the patient was interrupted within 18 seconds of speaking to a doctor. When this happens, the patient loses their flow of thought, may repeat things that they have already said, and may go on to omit essential information.

Reflective listening returns back to the client both the words and the emotions that they themselves have conveyed. It shows that they have been heard *and* understood, and allows them to correct, clarify, or add additional details. It can be achieved via paraphrasing and summarizing:

a) **Paraphrasing** is restating the content and emotion of the client's message in your own words: "It must have been very distressing for you to see Milo paw at his face so aggressively."

b) **Summarizing** presents to the client what you have understood so far: "So, Coco seems to be going off dry food, but is still keen on wet food. Her breath smells, but she seems well in herself. Is there anything else?"

2.5.4   Displays of Empathy

Empathy is different from sympathy, which entails concern from outside the client's position. The practitioner must be able to identify what the client is feeling, or what emotions they are displaying (sadness, worry, anger, shock, denial). An empathic statement could sound like: "I can see that you are worried about the prospect of Willy having his teeth extracted" (Figure 2.7). You may want to explore exactly what the client is concerned about – perhaps they are worried their pet may not be able to eat properly. This message can be strengthened when combined with nonverbal signals, including facial expression, tone of voice, and even touch. This display of empathy is integral to building rapport with the client and enabling true relationship-centered care because the client feels completely understood and has their concerns validated. In addition, it can help to build a trusting relationship. Trust is also integral to relationship-centered care, and is a vital tool in being persuasive. It appears, however, that veterinarians may miss vital opportunities to display empathy (Shaw et al. 2004). The clinician should therefore try to identify these opportunities and practice displaying empathy.

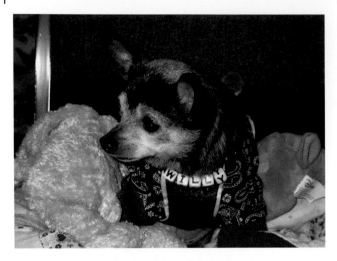

Figure 2.7 A centralized position of the patient is necessary to display empathy and accept the unusual bond between owner and animal.

Table 2.1 Verbal behaviors significantly associated with positive or negative outcomes during consultation.

Positive Outcome	Negative Outcome
Empathy	Formal behavior
Reassurance	High level of biomedical questioning
Support	Interruptions
Encouragement of questions	Irritation
Friendliness	One-way flow of information *to* patient
Courtesy	
Positive reinforcement of patient actions	
Psychosocial talk	
Increased encounter length	
Listening	
Orientation during physical examination	
Summarization	

Source: Adapted from Beck et al. (2002).

In 2002, a systematic review of the existing primary-care research was conducted in order to study the impact of the verbal and nonverbal behaviors of physicians on patient outcomes, including intention to comply, actual compliance, trust, quality of life, health status, and satisfaction (Beck et al. 2002). The findings are summarized in Tables 2.1 and 2.2.

Table 2.2 Nonverbal behaviors significantly associated with positive or negative outcomes during consultation.

Positive Outcome	Negative Outcome
Forward lean	Backward lean
Head nodding	Indirect body orientation
Direct body orientation	Crossed arms
Uncrsossed arms	Frequent touch
Uncrossed legs	
Less mutual gaze	

Source: Adpated from Beck et al. (2002).

2.6 Marketing Dental Services

Clients have a choice about which veterinary practice to attend with their beloved pet and will often perform Internet searches when looking for a new one. This choice is not necessarily based solely on cost (Lue et al. 2008). Clients will often seek out practitioners with a special interest or particular qualifications in dentistry. It is therefore worthwhile advertising the full extent of your dental services: does your practice offer dental radiography, dental charting, surgical extractions, local anesthetic nerve blocks, or multiparameter anesthetic monitoring? The local clinic offering "budget dentistry" may well forego these vital items, but the client may not realize this unless you advertise it on your website or in a newsletter.

Consider having a waiting-room display of the dental services you offer or the "dental pet of the month," including a client testimonial of how treatment has improved their pet's well-being. Client testimonials can be very motivating for others to read. If they can see their peers have had the same concerns as them but were ultimately pleased with the treatment outcome under your care, it can help to strengthen your message.

We are used to receiving dental check-up reminders from our own dentists every 6–12 months, and this can easily become part of your practice reminder system. It is vital that clients understand that periodontal disease is managed and not cured by one professional cleaning. Regular check-ups are vital, and veterinary nurses/technicians can play an important role in the ongoing preventative health-care regimen. The efficacy of home care efforts can be monitored, advice can be given regarding adjunctive methods such as dental diets or chews, and clients' motivation for toothbrushing can be enhanced or renewed. This can also lead to increased overall practice-bonding. Once individual treatment plans are agreed upon, reminders about dental checks and professional prophylaxis treatments can be sent.

2.7 Conclusion

Veterinary dental services are offered by nearly all small-animal practices. When performed to current gold standards (WSAVA 2018), they provide a unique opportunity for improving small-animal health and welfare, alleviating pain, increasing client bonding to the practice, enhancing practice profitability, and augmenting practitioners' own professional satisfaction. Communication skills are an integral part of this service, and can be learned and practiced just like any other clinical skill. You should challenge yourself to actively display empathy in every consultation.

It can be a useful exercise to film a series of consultations with clients (obviously, with their explicit permission) and constructively appraise your own consulting communication skills. How did you come across (bored/angry/rushed/approachable)? Did you display empathy? Did you interrupt the client? By developing our communication skills, we can ensure that pets receive the correct dental treatment. After all, it does not matter how good our surgical extraction skills are if we are not given permission to anesthetize the patient. Implementing evidence-based veterinary medicine and current global guidelines ensures we can act in our patients' best interests at all times.

References

AAHA (2003). *The Pathway to High-Quality Care.* Lakewood, CO: AAHA Press.

AAHA (2009). *Compliance: Taking Quality Care to the Next Level.* Lakewood, CO: AAHA Press.

Beck, R.S., Daughtridge, R., and Sloane, P.D. (2002). Physician–patient communication in the primary care office: a systematic review. *J. Am. Board Fam. Pract.* 15: 25–38.

Beckman, H. and Frankel, R. (1984). The effect of physician behavior on the collection of data. *Ann. Intern. Med.* 101 (5): 692–696.

Borg, J. (2010). *Persuasion: The Art of Influencing People.* Harlow: Pearson Education.

Clark, W.T., Kane, L., Arnold, P.K., and Robertson, I.D. (2002). Clinical skills and knowledge used by veterinary graduates during their first year in small animal practice. *Aust. Vet. J.* 80: 37–40.

Evangelista, L.S. (1999). Compliance – a concept analysis. *Nurs. Forum* 34 (1): 5–11.

Greenfield, C.L., Johnson, A.L., and Schaeffer, D.J. (2004). Frequency of use of various procedures, skills, and areas of knowledge among veterinarians in private small animal exclusive or predominant practice and proficiency expected of new veterinary school graduates. *J. Am. Vet. Med. Assoc.* 224 (11): 1780–1787.

Hall, M.A., Camacho, F., Dugan, E., and Balkrishnan, R. (2002). Trust in the medical profession: conceptual and measurement issues. *Health Serv. Res.* 37 (5): 1419–1439.

Holmstrom, S.E., Bellows, J., Juriga, S. et al. (2013). AAHA dental care guidelines for dogs and cats. *J. Am. Anim. Hosp. Assoc.* 49: 75–82.

Kanji, N., Coe, J.B., Adams, C.L., and Shaw, J.R. (2012). Effect of veterinarian–client–patient interactions on client adherence to dentistry and surgery recommendations in companion animal practice. *JAVMA* 240 (4): 427–436.

Kruger, J. and Dunning, D. (1999). Unskilled and unaware of it: how difficulties in recognizing one's own incompetence lead to inflated self-assessments. *J. Pers. Soc. Psychol.* 77 (6): 1121–1134.

Lue, T., Pantenburg, D.P., and Crawford, P.M. (2008). Impact of the owner–pet and client–veterinarian bond on the care that pets receive. *JAVMA* 232 (4): 531–540.

Mehrabian, A. (1981). *Silent Messages: Implicit Communication of Emotion and Attitude.* Belmont, CA: Wadsworth.

Perry, R. (2014). Final year veterinary students' attitudes towards small animal dentistry: a questionnaire-based survey. *J. Small Anim. Pract.* 55 (9): 457–464.

Pink, D.H. (2012). *To Sell Is Human.* New York: Riverhead.

Schmidt, P.L. (2007). Evidence-based veterinary medicine: evolution, revolution or repackaging of veterinary practice? *Vet. Clin. Small Anim.* 37: 407–417.

Shaw, J.R. (2006). Four core communication skills of highly effective practitioners. *Vet. Clin. Small Anim.* 36: 385–396.

Shaw, J.R., Adams, C.L., Bonnett, B.N. et al. (2004). Use of the roter interaction analysis system to analyze veterinarian–client–patient communication in companion animal practice. *JAVMA* 225 (2): 222–229.

WSAVA (2018) Global Dental Guidelines. Available from https://wsava.org/global-guidelines/global-dental-guidelines/ (accessed July 5, 2020).

3

Teaching Veterinary Dentistry

Zlatko Pavlica[1], Jerzy Gawor[2], and Lisa Mestrinho[3]

[1] *University of Ljubljana, Ljubljana, Slovenia*
[2] *Veterinary Clinic Arka, Kraków, Poland*
[3] *Faculty of Veterinary Medicine, University of Lisbon, Portugal*

3.1 Introduction

This chapter was written for several reasons. First, to highlight the importance of education to the proper development of veterinary dentistry. Second, to present the current situation, which is plagued by a lack of systemic solutions, leading to low competence among veterinary graduates in the field of dentistry. And third, to discuss the requirement to provide efficient veterinary dental education.

Dentistry is part of the clinical sciences: a vast field of veterinary science based on practical learning and training.

In clinical disciplines, students should acquire skills based on the model of Miller's pyramid of clinical competence (Miller 1990), from the *knows*, to the *knows how*, to the *shows how*, to the *does*. At the base of this pyramid is fact gathering, progressing to an upper level of interpretation and application, followed by demonstration of learning, and finally performance integrated into practice (Figure 3.1).

There are several aspects and fields of veterinary dental education in which Miller's principles are applied. Teaching at university or college (addressed to future veterinarians or nurses) is key to achieving graduate competence. Continuous professional development (CPD) helps in the development and extension of skills. Finally, public education improves awareness of the importance of oral health among pet owners.

3.2 Veterinary Dentistry in Europe's University Curricula

Several current documents list the minimum requirements for veterinary education among establishments of higher education (Directive 78/1027) and regulate professional qualification (Directive 2005/36), but without defining or describing veterinary specialization as they would for human doctors. At all European universities, veterinarians must qualify after a five- or six-year curriculum, comprising a bachelor degree (three years) plus a master's degree (two years), as set out in the Bologna Process (2005).

The first Global Conference in Paris (2009) identified the need to define minimum competences that newly graduated veterinarians must have in order to provide veterinary services. The recommendations on veterinary day-one competencies were first produced by the World Organization of Animal Health (OIE 2012). Although such recommendations do not have a legal power, nowadays, with the work of the European Association of Establishments of Veterinary Education (EAEVE), through the certification of European universities, they have improved the institutional education throughout Europe.

The Joint European Veterinary Dental Society (EVDS)/European Veterinary Dental College (EVDC) Statement on Clinical Competencies in Small Companion Animal Dentistry and Oral Surgery states the following:

> Veterinarians must possess scientific knowledge and be able to demonstrate practical skills in order to perform basic diagnostic and treatment procedures in veterinary dentistry and oral surgery, independently, at the time of graduation. At a minimum, veterinary graduates must be competent in providing entry-level dental and oral health care for small companion animals. The veterinary university/school/college must provide training for students to meet day-1 and for veterinarians to meet year-1 and year-3 competencies in small companion animal dentistry and oral surgery. Academic institutions

The Veterinary Dental Patient: A Multidisciplinary Approach, First Edition. Edited by Jerzy Gawor and Brook Niemiec.
© 2021 John Wiley & Sons Ltd. Published 2021 by John Wiley & Sons Ltd.
Companion website: www.wiley.com/go/gawor/veterinary-dental-patient

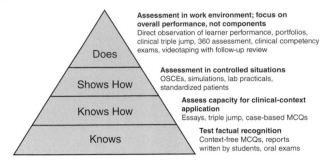

Figure 3.1 Framework for clinical assessment. *Source:* Based on Miller (1990).

that provide evidence for offering appropriate learning and continuing education opportunities in that regard may – upon thorough review of these opportunities – be awarded an endorsement by EVDS/EVDC. (EVDS and EVDC 2014)

Day-one skills include the following veterinary dental procedures (www.evds.org):

- Obtain a history for a dentistry and oral surgery patient
- Perform an oral examination in a conscious and anesthetized patient
- Distinguish between normal and abnormal oral and maxillofacial anatomy
- Utilize nomenclature accepted in dentistry and oral surgery
- Use the modified Triadan system for numbering teeth
- Identify and name normal anatomical structures on a dental radiograph
- Interpret and fill out an oral examination assessment form
- Demonstrate the use of a dental explorer, periodontal probe, and dental mirror
- Perform a professional dental cleaning with scaling and polishing
- Explain and demonstrate home oral care/hygiene measures
- Recognize and relieve pain in dentistry and oral surgery patients
- Understand the rational use of antibiotics in dentistry and oral surgery
- Know when and how to refer a dentistry and oral surgery patient to a specialist

It is remarkable that there are no surgical skills on this list, despite extraction being a very frequent surgical oral procedure. These skills are intentionally included in year-1 and year-3 competencies for the veterinarian as a part of their CPD.

3.3 How Is Veterinary Dentistry Taught in Universities? What Is Missing?

Since oral health must be incorporated into primary care, dentistry should be an obligatory subject (as opposed to an elective) for all small-animal-oriented students. However, there seems to be a disconnection between the required classes in the standard veterinary curriculum and the skills required in everyday practice.

Regardless of the OIE recommendations concerning the competencies needed for graduating veterinarians – in addition to publications from the scientific community – veterinary dentistry is still severely undertaught in veterinary school. The situation regarding the teaching of veterinary dentistry was the subject of a survey among students of veterinary faculties at 28 universities across 24 European countries (Austria, Belgium, Croatia, Czech Republic, Denmark, Estonia, Finland, France, Germany, Greece, Hungary, Italy, Latvia, Netherlands, Norway, Poland, Portugal, Romania, Serbia, Slovenia, Spain, Switzerland, the United Kingdom, Ukraine) in 2010 (Gawor 2011). The first question was, "Is veterinary dentistry taught in your school?" Replies showed that small-animal and equine dentistry were taught at 68% of schools, just small-animal at 18%, and no dentistry at 14%. Meanwhile, 63% of faculties that provided veterinary dentistry had it as compulsory and 33% as optional, with 4% indicating it was both. The majority of schools offered dentistry at the fourth and fifth year of education, with 70% providing a combination of theoretical and practical classes compared with 26% providing only theory. In 59% of establishments, dentistry was a part of the surgical department, in 23% it was provided independently, and in the rest it was a part of small-animal clinics. In 24% of surveyed schools, the dental program was provided by the diplomate of the veterinary dental college, in 38% by a veterinarian practicing only or mostly dentistry, in 10% by a human dentist, and in the remaining 28% by random veterinarians.

There are few veterinary faculties worldwide that include dentistry in the regular curriculum. Only a few locations in Europe provide a veterinary dental program, in terms of number of hours and lecturer competence: Aristotle University of Thessaloniki, Veterinarmedizinische, Fakultet der Universitat Leipzig, Univerza v Ljubljani Veterinarska fakulteta, the Faculty of Life Science at the University of Copenhagen, and the Faculty of Veterinary Medicine at the University of Helsinki. A handful more offer veterinary dentistry as an elective/optional course, usually with limited enrolment (Perry 2014). The situation of veterinary dentistry in North america is very similar to that in Europe. Currency, only about 20% of Veterinary Universities have a

Board Certified veterinary dentist on staff. Some have "Board Qualified" or "enthusiast" level faculty, however for the most part dentistry is taught (to the extent that it is) by general practitioners in the community practice section. A few have veterinary dentists who are associated with the University, but this is becoming more rare. Finally, there are still some that have human dentists teach veterinary dentistry. Didactic learning is often part of the internal medicine or surgery department offerings in most schools. Therefore, like Europe, unless the student is in one of the few universities with a dentist on staff the education is poor. Even those universities who have a dentist on staff, dentistry continues to be an elective. Luckily, this is about to change. As of November 2020, instruction in veterinary dentistry is REQUIRED by the AVMA. We look forward to improved dental care as a result of this excellent (but overdue) directive (AVMA Council on Education 2020).

3.4 Veterinary Dental Education Today

At universities, dentistry appears to be fragmented across the five to six years of a degree, from anatomy, physiology, and pathology to the clinic. It can be either species- or discipline-oriented. It is traditionally included in the medical or surgical disciplines and can be divided academically into small animal, equine, and exotic/zoo animal. Regardless of how the complex of academic activities within the subject are divided, there are three major areas: education, clinical services, and research.

The focus should be on practical skills. The hands-on wetlab part of dental education is of paramount importance. In addition to the basic theoretical knowledge, practical tutored time with feedback should be provided. Some universities offer dentistry services in small-practice teaching hospitals or clinics, but unfortunately this is usually the only time that students come in contact with a clinical dental case.

Other means of teaching dentistry should be considered as complementary or additional. From lectures and interactive sessions to books and e-learning tools, it is important to remember that the acquisition of practical skills requires an intermediate step. A "do-it-yourself" manual can lead to confusion or complications, including iatrogenic damage.

In, general teaching methods include the following:

- **E-learning:** Webinars, movies, quizzes, journal clubs, and virtual handbooks (Figure 3.2).
- **Face-to-Face:** One-on-one or in small groups. Maximum ratio is eight to ten students per tutor, but lowering the ratio will improve interaction and experience (Figure 3.3).
- **Interactive Sessions:** No audience limit, but it is important to involve the entire audience. The use of scoring or polling applications is encouraged for the collection of feedback (Figure 3.4).
- **Indirect Contact:** Via books, journals, and posters.

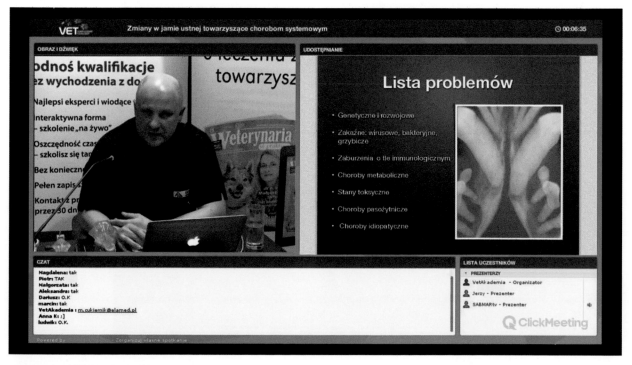

Figure 3.2 Webinar in dentistry.

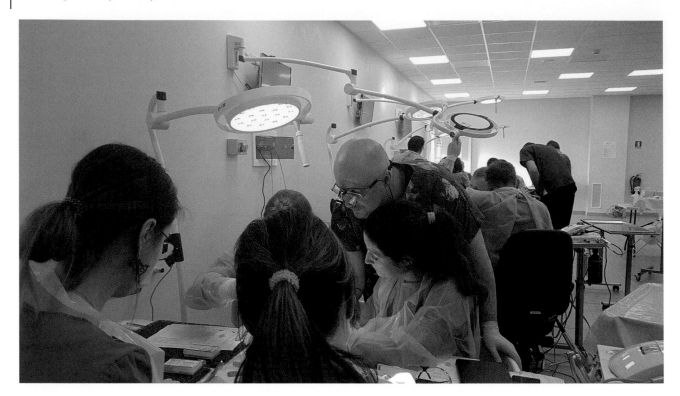

Figure 3.3   Face-to-face learning.

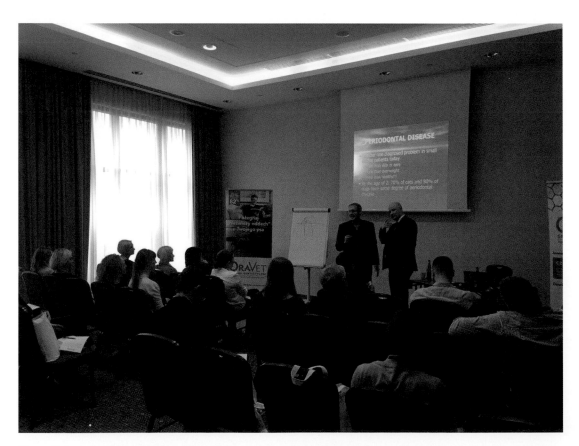

Figure 3.4   Interactive session.

The e-learning concept uses technology such as electronic instruments and web platforms, organized as webinars, videos, quizzes, journal club discussions, virtual books, and presentations. These techniques are cheap to develop, allow for flexible timing, have no need of travel, and can be recorded and stored in a searchable database. Over time, with further development of electronic communication instruments, e-learning will improve and become more common. The major limitation is that only theoretical education can be performed in this manner and supplementation with a practical workshop is necessary. Another issue might be language barriers. E-learning is great solution for the theoretical part of dentistry and an effective prerequisite for practical (hands-on) workshops and wetlabs under specialist supervision. The journal club formula is getting more and more popular and may become the most important way of learning and teaching, provided *all* participants have a serious attitude. Educational films are very helpful in allowing students to understand concepts such as active home care, the correct handling of instruments, and basic procedures. They can be addressed to students, veterinarians, or even the general public. If it is necessary to present a structured problem such as the safety of anesthesia, a PowerPoint presentation appears to be the best way of communication.

The teaching of dentistry cannot be performed *ex cathedra* without discussion and based purely on theoretical lectures and knowledge, however. Hands-on labs are a necessary part of dental education. In regard to the relationship between teachers and students, the best model is that of mentor/mentee, as it provides the most efficient means of sharing experiences and provides the student with individual attention. This relationship is typical for specialty courses but is not available in many cases and can be quite expensive to implement. At universities, a student's performance in dentistry can be supervised by tenured (or tenure-track) faculty, residents, non-tenure-track faculty, or a private practitioner who is employed part-time – ideally, a specialist. For practical workshops, a very important consideration is the student–instructor ratio. In most cases, one tutor per eight participants is the maximum that still allows for good supervision and quality control.

The teaching of dentistry is thus done through both theoretical and practical methods. Theory is presented in lectures, interactive sessions, and seminars, which can be very attractive and efficient when properly structured and supported by a quality lecturer, especially with good audiovisual components. Even difficult or complicated information can be explained in an understandable way. In order to allow the participation of every attendee, it is necessary to have a smaller group. This will also enable the tutor to know whether each student has understood the most important messages.

Textbooks, chapters, and articles should follow the evidence-based medicine (EBM) concept. The practice of EBM is a process of lifelong, self-directed, problem-based learning with an emphasis on delivering reliable knowledge that helps the recipient reach the correct decision. It is not a "cookbook" of recipes, simple solutions, and straightforward hints. Application of EBM means relating individual clinical signs and experiences with the best scientific evidence obtained through clinical research (Sackett et al. 2000).

3.5 Examples of Teaching

One of the few European universities with a veterinary dentist on staff is the University of Ljubljana, Slovenia. The veterinary dentistry curriculum for DVM students offers three components in their final year:

1) **Theoretical Part:** Lectures are supported with audiovisual equipment (PowerPoint presentations and videotapes). The course presents special topics on oral and dental diseases of dogs and cats, as well as horses, rodents, and lagomorphs. Comparative dentistry (herbivores, carnivores, omnivores) is also included. The theoretical part includes the following aspects of dentistry: anatomical and histological characteristics of the oral cavity with an emphasis on teeth and periodontal tissues; the proper performance of dental procedures and treatment outcome(s); and physiology and pathophysiology of the oral cavity, periodontal tissues, and teeth with an emphasis on the relationship between the oral cavity and the patient.

2) **Three Practical Cadaver-Based Sessions For Small Groups:** This introductory laboratory course covers the principles of oral examination, oral radiography, routine periodontal treatment, and dental extraction techniques. In addition, diagnostic and treatment procedures for the most common oral problems are discussed. Groups should be no more than three or four students per tutor. Program outline:

- **Session 1:** Oral examination, dental charting and periodontal assessment, routine periodontal treatment performed on canine and feline specimens; proper use of periodontal manual instruments and power equipment
- **Session 2:** Principles of oral radiology and radiography; intraoral and extraoral film/sensor positioning

in the dog and cat; film processing; dental radiograph interpretation: film orientation, normal radiologic anatomy, and common pathologic findings.

- **Session 3:** Local nerve blocks, aseptic techniques, simple and surgical extraction techniques performed on canine specimens; appropriate use and handling of extraction instruments.

3) **Two-Week Elective Clinical Rotation:** After having completed the clinical rotation in dentistry and oral surgery, the student should fulfill all requirements described in the Joint EVDS/EVDC Statement on Clinical Competencies in Small Companion Animal Dentistry and Oral Surgery (EVDS and EVDC 2014).

3.6 Student Chapters

In order to increase students' interest in and knowledge of veterinary dentistry, the EVDS and EVDC have jointly created a program for Student Chapters of the European Veterinary Dental Society (SCEVDS) at veterinary schools. Similar initiative is present in the USA veterinary faculties. The aim is to help students who wish to increase their knowledge of veterinary dentistry. Through this scheme, students can attend lectures and wetlabs held by EVDC diplomates or veterinarians who have a special interest in veterinary dentistry, and they are given access to a step-by-step compendium written by veterinary dentists. The program also encourages exchanges and cooperation between universities in Europe. As long as most veterinary schools offer scant education in dentistry to their students, the EVDS/EVDC think it is important to give our future colleagues an opportunity to gain knowledge of veterinary dentistry. This will benefit us all, as it increases the status and the quality of our specialty. Further information is available at www.evds.info.

3.7 Postgraduate Education and Specialization

Since universities do not provide postgraduate continuing education, and in the absence of an EU directive defining veterinary specialization (as is done in the human medical field), professionals continue to develop their skills and clinical specialization regardless of the absence of official EU bylaws. Some European countries, like Germany, have their own national specialization recognition system, but the requirements are not equivalent across countries, according to what is stated in the veterinary EU Directive 2005/36. Specialization can also be interpreted academi-

cally as PhD training, but such a degree is of low interest for the veterinary practitioner.

Small-animal practitioners can find an enormous number of continuing-education courses in response to their need to acquire advanced veterinary professional skills. The level and quality of these courses are extremely variable and cannot be compared with the professional specialization process.

To show the need for postgraduate professional requirements at the general practitioner level, a small group of specialists created a document describing the fundamentals of small-animal dentistry, the World Small Animal Veterinary Association Global Dental Guidelines (WSAVA) (Niemiec et al. 2017) (Figure 3.5).

Intensive courses of three to five days' duration cover different aspects of oral and dental therapy. They are organized in a systemic way and taught by board-certified dental specialists. All available educational methods are used, with a focus on practical solutions. There are two programs for small-animal dentistry in Europe and Asia offering comprehensive education, aimed at general practitioners and nurses who want to develop their dental skills. Courses are dedicated to selected subjects and the participants can select those that are most interesting to them after obtaining basic knowledge of oral diagnostic, prophylaxis, and surgery.

3.8 Veterinary Dental Specialists

A diplomate of the American Veterinary Dental College (AVDC) or EVDC is a veterinarian who has been certified as having demonstrated specialist knowledge and expertise in veterinary dentistry. In order to qualify, they must complete all training requirements and successfully pass an examination; only then can they be considered veterinary dentists (specialists in veterinary dentistry) and practice veterinary dentistry at a specialist level.

Specialization in the veterinary medical profession can be species- or discipline-oriented. At this level, the European and American Boards of Veterinary Specialization (EBVS and ABVS) provide a common umbrella to assure a homogenous postgraduate education to veterinarians who want to become specialists. Like the AVDC in North America, the EVDC is a transversely recognized institution.

3.9 Veterinary Dental Education in the Future

To respond properly to the needs of all patients suffering from oral diseases, meet market expectations, and follow ongoing trends in veterinary business, a new veterinary dental education system must be implemented. The key

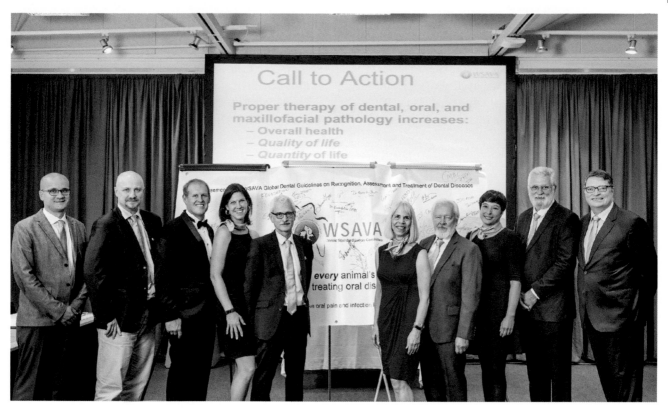

Figure 3.5 WSAVA Dental guidelines team From left: Paulo Stegall DACVAA (Canada), Jerzy Gawor DAVDC, DEVDC, FAVD (Poland), Brook A. Niemiec DAVDC, DEVDC, FAVD (USA), Kymberley Stewart (Canada) Gottfried Morgenegg (Switzerland), Marge Chandler DACVN, DACVIM, DECVIM-CA (UK), Rod Jouppi (Canada), Ana Nemec DAVDC, DEVDC (Slovenia), Cedric Tutt, DEVDC (South Africa), David Clarke DAVDC (Australia).

points of the WSAVA chapter dedicated to education are worth citation here (Niemiec et al. 2017):

- Veterinary dentistry is a largely neglected field in the veterinary medicine curriculum in most of the universities.
- Teaching veterinary dentistry at an undergraduate level should include lectures and hands-on workshops on basic examination techniques, most common oral/dental diseases and treatments.

- Teaching hospitals should establish a veterinary dentistry department, striving at providing dentistry services at a specialist level to create the necessary teaching environment.
- Postgraduate training in veterinary dentistry should include residency training, ideally in the future combined with PhD training.
- Effective teaching of veterinary dentistry in the veterinary school is the key to progression in this field of veterinary medicine.

References

AVMA Council on Education (2020) JAVMA 257 (9): 881

Bologna Process (2005). A Framework for Qualifications of the European Higher Education Area. In: Bergen Conference of European Ministers Responsible for Higher Education. May 19–20, 2005. Bergen, Norway. Available from http://ecahe.eu/w/images/7/76/A_Framework_for_Qualifications_for_the_European_Higher_Education_Area.pdf (accessed July 5, 2020).

EVDS and EVDC (2014). Competencies in Dentistry and Oral Surgery for Small Companion Animals. Available from https://www.evds.org/images/pdf/Competencies.pdf (accessed July 5, 2020).

Gawor, J. (2011). Dentistry in European Veterinary Faculties. Proceedings of European Congress of Veterinary Dentistry Chalkidiki.

Miller, G.E. (1990). The assessment of clinical skills/competence/performance. *Acad. Med.* 65 (9): 63–67.

Niemiec B.A., Gawor J., Nemec A., et al. (2017). Kymberley Stewart World Small Animal Veterinary Association Global Dental Guidelines. Available from

https://wsava.org/wp-content/uploads/2020/01/
Dental-Guidleines-for-endorsement_0.pdf (accessed
July 5, 2020).

OIE (2012) OIE recommendations on the competencies of
graduating veterinarians ("day 1 graduates") to assure
high-quality of national veterinary services. Paris: World
Organization for Animal Health.

Perry, R. (2014). Final year veterinary students' attitudes
toward small animal dentistry: a questionnaire-based
survey. *J. Small Anim. Pract.* 55 (9): 457–464.

Sackett, D.L., Richardson, W.S., Rosenberg, W. et al. (2000).
Evidence-Based Medicine: How to Practice and Teach, 2e.
Edinburgh: Churchill-Livingstone.

4

Distribution of Tasks Around the Dental Patient in General Practice

Receptionists, Technicians, and Other Veterinary Team Members

Mary Berg

Beyond the Crown Veterinary Education, Lawrence, KS, USA

4.1 Introduction

Companion animals have become an important part of our lives, and many people consider their pet a part of their family. This bond is important to the veterinarian and their team as it has made clients more interested in dental care for their pets. It is essential that communication remains open between all parties and that the entire veterinary team project the same message to the client. All members of the veterinary team must be excited and motivated. The veterinarian and their team must educate the client about the need for dentistry and demonstrate the importance of good oral hygiene to the overall health of their pet. Clients need to hear the same message seven times to ensure they retain and understand the meaning. In this author's experience, 25% of your clients will accept whatever you say immediately; 60% will take a little time to accept your recommendations; and the remaining 15% will never accept your suggestions. As veterinary professionals, we need to concentrate on the 60% to ensure they understand the need for dental care.

4.2 Receptionists

The receptionist is the first and last person the client sees in the practice (Figure 4.1). They must be friendly and confident, and must provide the client with accurate information. They demonstrate their interest in the client and pet through body language and words. A receptionist who projects a positive attitude regarding dentistry and home care is essential for success. The acceptance of dentistry within a practice can be greatly affected if the receptionist isn't fully on board.

This interaction may begin with a telephone conversation. All practices have phone shoppers who are seeking the best deal on dental care. It is very important that the receptionist be trained on the how to handle such calls (Bellows 1999). When asked how much the practice charges for a dental procedure, the answer must be, "It depends upon the degree of oral disease present." The receptionist should avoid quoting prices over the phone. It is best to explain that it is difficult to determine the true extent of oral disease until each tooth has been examined under general anesthesia and radiographs have been evaluated, after which a treatment plan can be formulated and accurate fees calculated. A script that can be used for phone shoppers would be something like: "We are unable to give you an accurate estimate for a dental treatment over the phone as the cost depends upon the degree of treatment necessary to give your pet the very best care possible. It is essential that we exam your pet to give you a more accurate idea of the cost."

It is very important to remember that an oral examination and dental cleaning is rarely a routine procedure. The receptionist should be able to discuss the basic safety of anesthesia and address any concerns the pet owner may have about the procedure. It is advisable for the receptionist to understand the complications and limitations of nonanesthetic dental (NAD) procedures. They should emphasize that NADs do not allow for cleaning below the gumline, where disease can lead to destruction of the supporting tissues and bone, posing a risk of injury to both the pet and the individual performing the procedure. Complete oral exams and dental radiographs are not possible without general anesthesia (See more in Chapter 8 Section 8.12).

In many veterinary practices, the receptionist is responsible for scheduling appointments and procedures.

The Veterinary Dental Patient: A Multidisciplinary Approach, First Edition. Edited by Jerzy Gawor and Brook Niemiec.
© 2021 John Wiley & Sons Ltd. Published 2021 by John Wiley & Sons Ltd.
Companion website: www.wiley.com/go/gawor/veterinary-dental-patient

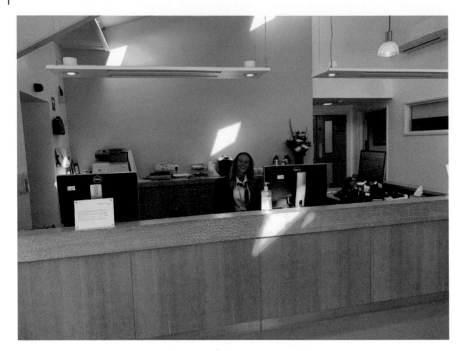

Figure 4.1 The first impression when a client enters the clinic: North Downs Specialist Referrals reception desk. *Source:* Rachel Perry.

Give them guidance on how to efficiently work with your schedule. If a patient has had a conscious oral examination, the anticipated level of disease should be recorded. This level will help the receptionist know the correct amount of time to allot for a future procedure.

The receptionist should be encouraged to watch a procedure from start to finish, in order that they understand the importance of proper dental care. Each step should be explained as you go. An option might be to perform the procedure on the receptionist's own pet and let them see the effect on its overall health. This will allow them to speak from personal experience as to the benefits of a comprehensive dental procedure.

The receptionist is the bridge between the client and the rest of the veterinary team. They will often be the person who schedules a procedure, and likely the person who meets and receives the patient on the day. They should collect contact information from the client, provide them with an informed consent form and get their signature, reassure the client that their pet will be well cared for, and inform the client that the veterinarian will contact them once the oral exam and radiographs are complete with an updated treatment plan. If the client is not readily available by phone during the day, the receptionist should schedule a time for them to contact the practice for an update, and communicate this information to the dental team for proper scheduling.

The receptionists should maintain a clean and pleasing waiting room; however, the current trend is to move the patient and client to an examination room as soon as possible. While the client waits, the receptionist should offer them reading material or videos covering the value of good oral home care options, the safety of anesthesia, periodontal and other common oral diseases, and – if appropriate – dental care for exotic pets.

The receptionist can be also responsible for putting together estimates and collecting dental fees. This can be a positive experience for the client, and they may thank the team for an exceptional experience – or it can be a negative experience, if the client feels they have been overcharged or not kept informed of the cost of treatment. A positive outcome can be ensured by discussing financial concerns early on and revisiting the status of the case frequently. Ideally, the veterinarian or nurse will discuss the findings and review the dental radiographs and (hopefully) photographs with the client before billing them out. A positive, well-informed, and educated receptionist can reassure the client over costs and explain any additional items should the client question them at discharge.

The receptionist is also responsible for ensuring that all referral paperwork is complete and gets sent to the specialist in a timely manner. It is helpful to teach them how to send digital dental X-rays and dental charts.

Many practices are moving to online scheduling for appointments and procedures. The receptionist must be versed in the use of such systems, as well as any text messaging systems: calling or texting clients to remind them of their next appointment is also their responsibility.

4.3 Kennel Assistants

Many veterinary practices offer boarding services for their patients. It is important that kennel assistants be trained to examine patients' teeth when the client brings them in for boarding (Figure 4.2). They should show the client any calculus or red, swollen gums and ask if they would like their pet to have a more advanced oral examination and possible dental cleaning and treatment while they are boarding. They should also examine for damaged teeth upon intake, as this can avoid a complaint of teeth breaking during boarding, which is not an uncommon occurrence (Figure 4.3). The kennel staff should be empowered to discuss the importance of good oral home care with the client and offer to brush the pet's teeth or perform other home care while boarding. They can be taught to recognize basic pathology and bring it to the attention of the veterinarian. They can also inform the client if the type of treats or chews they have brought for their pet might cause dental injuries, and recommend safe, effective alternatives. These simple things can help emphasize the importance of oral care to the client.

4.4 Veterinary Care Assistants

The veterinary care assistant plays a huge role in dentistry within the practice. Their work can be divided into three areas: preoperative, intraoperative, and postoperative.

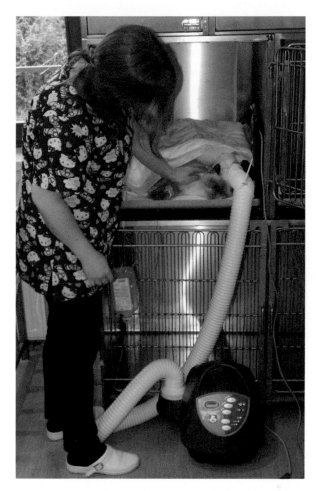

Figure 4.2   The kennel assistant, a first-line dental team member.

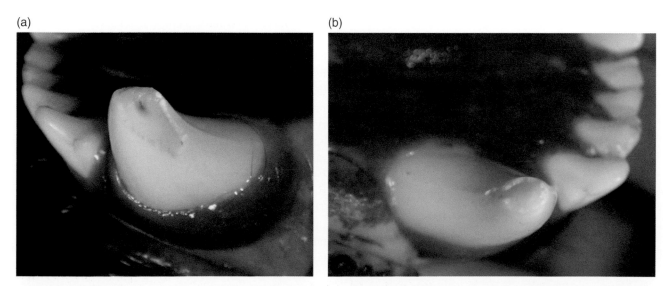

(a)   (b)

Figure 4.3   (a) This patient came to boarding with a fractured 304. (b) An uncomplicated crown fracture in 404 was identified on evaluation.

Preoperatively, the veterinary care assistant should be trained to ensure that the dental suite is cleaned, fully stocked, organized, and set up and ready for each patient. They should inform the veterinary nurse or practice manager when an instrument needs sharpening or replacement. In addition, they should pay attention to when ultrasonic tips or burs require replacement, as well as any supplies that need to be ordered. Finally, they should organize and pack the dental kits to optimize use for the veterinarian (Figure 4.4).

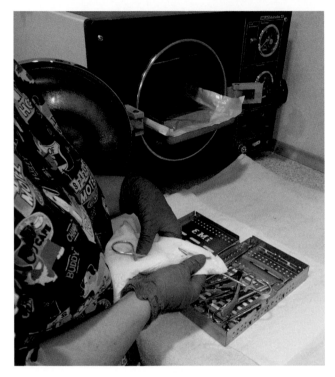

Figure 4.4   Veterinary care assistant packing a dental kit.

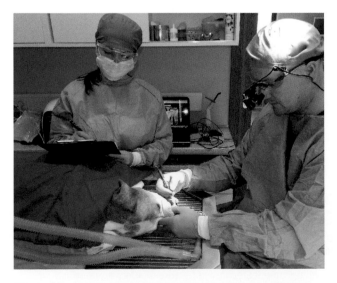

Figure 4.5   Four-handed dentistry: examination and charting.

Intraoperatively, the veterinary care assistant serves as the technician/nurse's assistant in dental procedures by recording findings on the dental chart, helping with patient positioning, and assisting with pre- and postoperative dental photos and X-rays. Four-handed dentistry, in which two people work together to record findings on the dental chart and operate the dental software during X-ray can decrease the procedure time and ensure a thorough dental examination and cleaning (Niemiec 2010) (Figure 4.5). The assistant should also transcribe findings into the practice management software, upload photos and X-rays, and help with the preparation of the discharge paperwork.

Postoperatively, the veterinary care assistant should ensure that the patient is cleaned and ready for discharge prior to release. The patient should be dry, their hair should be brushed, and any remnants of blood should be removed prior to their being presented to their owner. Taking a few extra minutes to perform these tasks can ensure the client feels that this was a pleasant and important procedure. The veterinary care assistant should also perform maintenance on the dental equipment, including cleaning and autoclaving the instruments, assessing the sharpness of the instruments, cleaning and preforming routine maintenance on the dental unit by releasing the pressure of the compressor, lubricating the handpieces, and preparing the operatory for the next patient (Figure 4.6).

4.5   Credentialed Veterinary Technicians/Nurses

Credentialed veterinary technicians/nurses are essential member of the dental team, as pet advocates and client educators. They are often eager to be empowered, and dentistry is one of the areas of the veterinary practice where technicians/nurses can be fully utilized. It is important to remember that a credentialed technician/nurse can do everything but diagnose, perform surgery, prescribe drugs, and give a prognosis. Empowering a veterinary technician/nurse to become the dental go-to at a practice allows for both professional growth and pride in their chosen profession, as well as increasing the practice's dental revenue. The dental technician/nurse will be the source for all things dental and have responsibility for the training of the entire staff so that everyone understands the importance of good oral health.

Every practice should have a veterinary technician/nurse whose main emphasis and training are in dentistry (Bellows 1999). The veterinarian is the only person who

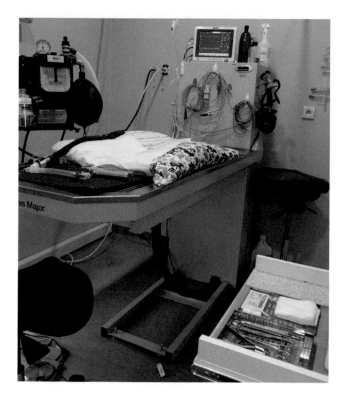

Figure 4.6 Preparation of the operatory.

can make a diagnosis of disease, but a credentialed veterinary technician/nurse with training in dentistry can assist them by gathering an accurate history and recognizing abnormalities and pathology and bringing them to their attention.

This technician's responsibilities include:

- patient history gathering
- patient intake
- performing oral examination
- dental prophylaxis and cleaning procedures
- charting
- taking dental radiographs
- assisting in oral surgeries and other dental procedures
- recording information in the patient's medical record
- delivering postoperative instructions
- ensuring the dental operatory is stocked and the equipment is well maintained.

They should also be allowed to thoroughly discuss home care, client education, and follow-up visits with pet owners.

4.5.1 History Gathering

The veterinary technician/nurse can help the veterinarian gather the information needed to determine a treatment plan. The veterinarian will use a combination of education and observation, comparing abnormal findings with normals (Niemiec 2010). The veterinary technician/nurse has responsibility for gathering the relevant dental information and obtaining an accurate overall health history. This allows the veterinarian to enter the exam room with an understanding of the oral condition and overall health of the patient and to work with the technician and client to prepare the best treatment options for them.

Some clients are educated and recognize that there is a problem with their pet's oral cavity, but the majority seem to be unaware when there may be a dental concern (Bellows 1999; Niemiec 2010; Perrone 2012). When a client suspects their pet has a problem, it is necessary to interview them to gather the needed information as well as to perform an oral exam of the pet. Veterinary professionals have to rely on information regarding the symptoms of the pet as it is provided by the owner (Perrone 2012). The most common symptom noticed by owners is malodor, but many owners (and veterinary professionals) think that halitosis is normal in pets. Occasionally, they may notice excessive salivation, inappetence, swelling, difficulty swallowing, or indications of oral pain or discomfort (Niemiec 2010; Perrone 2012). All these signs, along with the complete history including past oral examinations and treatments, diet, chewing habits, and home care, are pieces of a puzzle that must be put together (Perrone 2012).

Most commonly, owners are unaware that there is any problem with their pet's mouth. Dental issues may instead be discovered during the oral portion of an examination. The client may have noticed a change but not thought it important. This is the perfect time for the veterinary technician/nurse to educate them on oral disease and its importance to an animal's overall health, as well as the typical lack of clinical signs.

The past history of the patient is valuable information that can assist the veterinarian in determining the treatment plan (Bellows 1999). Having a complete history of past oral examinations, extractions, and treatments helps the veterinarian understand the patient's present oral condition and predict the outcome of any procedure. Age is not the most significant factor determining the stage of periodontal disease: frequency of dental cleaning is more important. For example, a seven-year-old Yorkshire terrier that has not had any previous oral examinations or treatments is likely to have severe oral disease, while a similar patient that has had annual dental cleanings may only have a mild form (Figure 4.7).

The veterinary technician should ask many questions when interviewing the client about their pet's oral health.

(a)

(b)

(c)

(d)

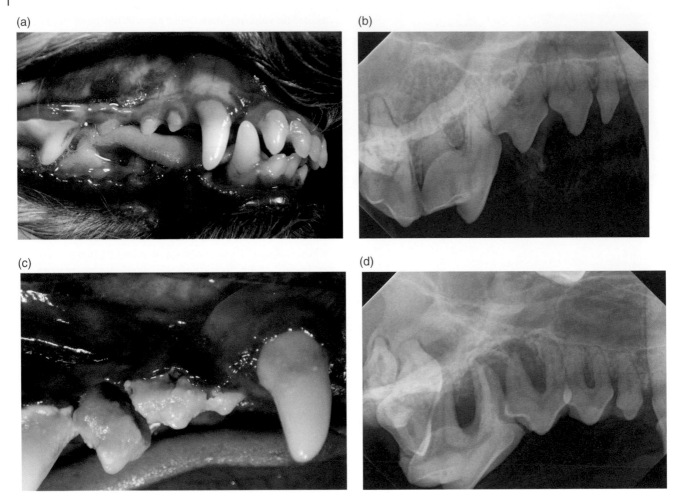

Figure 4.7 (a, b) Seven-year-old Yorkshire terrier that has received annual comprehensive oral health assessment and treatment (COHAT) all its life. (c, d) Seven-year-old Yorkshire terrier presenting for the first time.

Open-ended questions are best. If a client is not aware of any problems with their pet's oral cavity, they should be asked the following:

- "Tell me about any previous dental work?" The client should be allowed time to volunteer information. If they respond with, "Yes, they had two teeth extracted at my previous veterinarian," more direct questions can be asked regarding the cause of the extractions, when the procedure was performed, and so on.
- "What are your pet's chewing habits?" Some pets are very orally fixated, while others may not be chewers. Toys such as tennis balls, ice, cow hooves, pig ears, and hard nylon bones can cause serious trauma in the mouth (Bellows 1999). Clients may not realize the harm that could be caused by what they think is a great toy. This is an opportunity to educate them.

If the client is aware of a dental problem, ask them when they first noticed it. Again, many owners think that bad breath is normal and are not aware that periodontal disease is likely responsible for the malodor (Lobprise and Wiggs 2000).

The following questions should be asked in situations where the owner is concerned about a problem:

- "What are your pet's eating habits?"
- "Does the patient seem to salivate excessively?"
- "Does the patient appear to have problems drinking or swallowing?"
- "Has there been a change in the patient's habits or behavior? Do they rub their face on the carpet or paw at their face?" Face rubbing, apart from being a common signalment of allergy, can also be a sign of oral pain or inflammation.

4.5.2 Oral Examination: The Conscious Patient

A general health exam must be performed by the veterinarian. The entire animal should be examined, nose to tail. A thorough exam should include the eyes, ears, skin, heart, lung, and abdomen. If anesthesia is planned, it is highly recommended to perform blood and urine analysis.

In a well-managed practice (i.e. one that effectively utilizes lay staff), the veterinary technician/nurse can perform the initial oral examinations on both the conscious and the anesthetized patient and report their findings to the veterinarian (Figure 4.8). The conscious exam is limited to olfactory, visual, and tactile examination.

Is the head symmetrical? Do both sides appear to be uniform or does one look different to the other? (Niemiec 2010) Is there swelling in any area of the mouth/head? If swelling appears below the eye, look for a fractured maxillary fourth premolar. Do the jaws appear symmetrical? If one side of the jaw is swollen or asymmetrical, rule out mandibular or tooth fractures, or oral masses.

Feel the head. Palpate the bones of the head, including the zygomatic arch and mandibles. Feel for the presence of abnormalities. Evaluate the lymph nodes, including the sublingual and submandibular nodes. Inflammation in the oral cavity can contribute to swelling of these nodes. The temporomandibular joint should also be palpated for indications of pain or discomfort.

A detailed oral exam should be performed prior to anesthesia, if possible. Check for occlusion, tooth fractures, gingival recession, and inflammation, as well as missing,

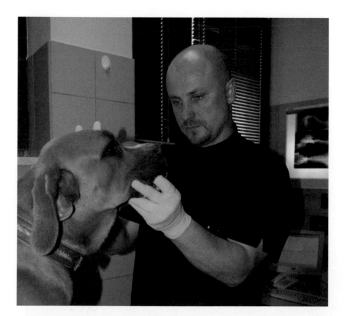

Figure 4.8 Concious animal assessment.

supernumerary, or loose teeth. Count the teeth. This task can be difficult as not every patient is willing to allow a complete examination, especially if they are head shy or young. Each tooth should be evaluated for fractures, mobility, and the amount of plaque and calculus present.

While it is most important to evaluate the gingiva under general anesthesia when the gingival index and pocket depth can be evaluated, it is important too to observe the gingiva to determine a preliminary degree of periodontal inflammation. Healthy gingiva is pink with defined margins, while inflammation is indicated by red, swollen gums. Gingival recession or enlargement is a key element of periodontal disease and should be noted.

A complete examination can only be completed under general anesthesia, but examination of the conscious patient can yield vital information that can help create the initial treatment plan and client estimate (Figure 4.9).

4.5.3 Treatment Plan

Even the best veterinarian may not practice their dental skills if the owner does not give permission. The client needs to understand the pathology and the reason for therapy. The technician plays a vital role in providing this education.

The treatment plan should be itemized and must be as accurate as possible. The technician should go through it with the client, explaining the reason for and value of each item. For example, preanesthetic blood work can sometimes locate systemic problems that have a bearing on the anesthesia protocol, as well as determining the patient's anesthetic risk. Dental radiographs are necessary to determine whether there is pathology that is not visible to the naked eye.

Explaining the treatment plan line by line helps the client understand the need for and importance of the treatment. Clients can see and understand pathology more easily in pictures, models, and videos than directly in the oral cavity of their pet. The treatment plan should also address the patient's anesthetic risk level and explain the precautions necessary for a positive outcome.

It is good practice to provide a treatment plan or estimate to the client prior to every procedure. This prevents distress over unexpected expenses and helps the client understand that the procedure is important to their pet's health. Providing an estimate in advance can also help the client make arrangements for payments.

An exact treatment plan cannot be determined on a conscious patient, but a close estimation can be created from the oral exam. The veterinary technician/nurse should explain that the treatment plan is only an estimate and that a more accurate one can be prepared once the animal is

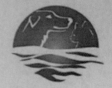

Veterinary Dental Specialties & Oral Surgery
5775 Chesapeake Court
San Diego, California, 92123
P 858-279-2108
F 858-573-8607
Email staff@scvds.com

DESCRIPTION	QTY	TOTAL
Dental Prophy [SupItem]	1 → 1	$0.00 → $0.00
Exam - No Charge	1 → 1	$0.00 → $0.00
Diazepam/Midazolam Inj.	1 → 1	$55.68 → $55.68
Dexmedetomidine Inj.	0 → 1	$0.00 → $57.00
Opioid Analgesic Premedication	0 → 1	$0.00 → $57.00
IV Catheter	1 → 1	$65.00 → $65.00
IV Fluids/Liter	1 → 1	$42.01 → $42.01
Anesthesia Induction	1 → 1	$125.00 → $125.00
Propofol Inj./mL	6 → 12	$21.00 → $42.00
Gas Anesthesia Maintenance/15 min.	6 → 8	$302.28 → $403.04
Surgical Monitoring - ECG/Pulse Ox/BP/Ca	1 → 1	$100.00 → $100.00
Dental Prophylaxis, Exam & Charting	1 → 1	$120.16 → $120.16
Oravet Professional Application	1 → 1	$64.17 → $64.17
Nail Trim Courtesy	1 → 1	$0.00 → $0.00
Dental Radiograph [First]	1 → 1	$43.34 → $43.34
Dental Radiograph [Each Add'l]	8 → 12	$200.00 → $300.00
Meloxicam Inj.	0 → 1	$0.00 → $54.58
Cerenia Inj./mL	1 → 1	$42.76 → $42.76
Waived Consultation Fee	1 → 1	-$50.00 → -$50.00

Total

$1131.40→$1521.74

This estimate is not a firm quote and as such is subject to change due to unforeseen circumstances. Due to the complex nature of most cases we see, the final charges may vary from this estimate. We will make every effort to inform you should your pet's changing condition require substantial procedures or diagnostic work not outlined in the above estimate. As part of our ongoing commitment to your pet's health, we encourage you to call if you have any questions. Please call the hospital at 858-279-2108.

I have read, understand and accept the estimate and terms above.

Signed (☐OWNER or ☐AGENT) 10-01-2019
Witness 10-01-2019

Figure 4.9 Client estimate, prepared based on a filled-in dental chart.

under anesthesia and a complete oral exam and dental radiographs have been performed.

Creating an estimate that is higher than anticipated can have a twofold benefit. First, it provides for an allowance if the periodontal disease turns out to be more advanced than is thought from the initial exam. Second, the client may be pleasantly surprised to receive a lower bill than expected. If the client would like a more precise estimate prior to the procedure, a "worst-case scenario" can be prepared, but this should be properly explained to them.

The veterinary technician/nurse should develop an understanding of the client's commitment and ability to perform home care, which will help develop the treatment plan (Bellows 1999). The veterinarian may thus plan to refer the patient to a dental specialist for periodontal surgery in order to save their teeth, or else to extract the teeth in the patient's best interest.

4.5.4 Oral Examination: The Anesthetized Patient

Prior to the anesthetic procedure, the veterinary technician/nurse should ensure that the operatory is prepared and check all parts of the anesthetic machine and monitoring devices. As stated earlier, a thorough oral examination can only be completed under general anesthesia (Figure 4.10). The veterinarian and veterinary technician/nurse should work together to determine the best anesthetic protocol for the patient. The technician/nurse will prepare and administer the drugs for sedation and induction and perform preoxygenation prior to inducing and intubating the patient. They will then induce anesthesia with the assistance of the veterinary assistant or another veterinary technician/nurse. (In some countries, nurses are not allowed to induce anesthesia, so the veterinarian

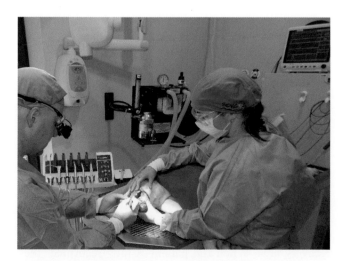

Figure 4.10 Anaesthetised animal assessment.

will have to do it themselves.) The technician/nurse must ensure the patient is correctly connected to monitors and that heating devices have been properly placed and the patient is at a surgical stage of anesthesia prior to beginning the oral examination.

One of the most common reasons clients are resistant to dental procedures is the fear of anesthesia. It is important to explain that each patient will be fully evaluated and the best protocol will be used for their particular needs. It is also reassuring for the client to know that a dedicated anesthetist will be on hand during the entire procedure. The anesthetist will closely monitor the patient, ensure they are kept warm to prevent hypothermia, and keep detailed records of the anesthesia event.

A veterinary technician/nurse who has received a decent amount of dental training should perform a thorough examination on each tooth in the oral cavity while the veterinary assistant records the findings on a dental chart. Each tooth should be evaluated for gingivitis, periodontal pockets, gingival recession, mobility, and furcation involvement (on multirooted teeth). Any extra or missing teeth should be noted, along with abnormalities. This chart will be presented to the veterinarian along with the dental X-rays to allow them to assess potential problem areas and develop a more detailed treatment plan.

The veterinary technician/nurse will also take the dental X-rays. It is highly recommended that full mouth X-rays be taken for every pet every year. The veterinary technician/nurse must be provided with training in order to successfully take diagnostic X-rays in a timely manner and must be able to assess whether the position and technique of radiography are correct. In more advance practices, the veterinary technician/nurse should assist with other imaging modalities such as CT scan, CBCT, MRI, and contrast studies.

4.5.5 Professional Dental Cleaning

Professional dental cleaning should be completed by the veterinary technician/nurse. They must have knowledge of how to properly and safely use each instrument involved in the procedure and must continually evaluate and train the rest of the staff on the proper techniques in the dental operatory.

The full step-by-step cleaning procedure will be addressed in Chapter 20. For now, it is important just to remember the gold standards of cleaning and polishing. In this section, therefore, we present a few helpful tips on how to perform efficient and effective dental cleaning.

Gross calculus can be removed by using a calculus removal forceps. Ultrasonic or sonic scalers are useful for

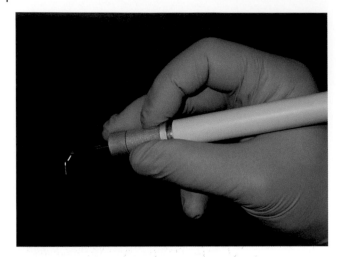

Figure 4.11   Modified pen grasp of a scaling handpiece.

removing the remainder of the supragingival calculus deposits. The instrument should be grasped lightly in a modified pen grasp, with the handpiece balanced on the index or middle finger (Figure 4.11). The instrument, not the hand, must be allowed to do the work – the hand is merely a guide. The handpiece should be used with a light touch and with minimal pressure, keeping the tip moving on the tooth. Stopping in any one area can cause damage.

The side of the wide tip (beaver tail) should be used for cleaning and held parallel to the long axis of the tooth. Never hold the tip at a 90° angle to the tooth surface as this can damage the tooth and provides less of a cleaning surface, making it less effective. Ultrasonic scalers can create a tremendous amount of heat. It is important to ensure that they have adequate water for cooling to prevent overheating of the tooth and potential pulp damage.

The most important part of the dental cleaning procedure is ensuring that the tooth is cleaned below the gumline. A curette or specific subgingival ultrasonic scaler tip should be used to remove subgingival plaque and calculus. Several companies make scaler tips that are specifically designed for this procedure. Removal of this subgingival plaque is vital to the success of the treatment. If it is not removed, bacteria will continue the inflammatory process, leading to the destruction of the periodontium and further bone loss and eventual tooth loss (Westfelt et al. 1998).

Hand scaling of the root to remove subgingival calculus deposits should be performed if a periodontal ultrasonic tip is not available. A curette is used for this procedure. This instrument has a sharp side (the face) and a rounded side, where the sharp side is held toward the tooth surface and the round side toward the gingival tissue. It should adapt to the curvature of the tooth surface; if it does not, the opposite end should be used. The curette is inserted into the pocket with the sharp side facing the root surface. It is moved over the calculus and positioned so that the cutting

surface is under the calculus. A rocking pull stroke is used to remove the calculus from the root surface. This procedure is repeated until all calculus is removed.

An explorer should be used to check the tooth surface for remaining calculus. The crown can be inspected for missed plaque by the application of a disclosing solution or for missed calculus by air drying, which will make the calculus appear chalky white. Disclosing solutions should be applied then gently rinsed with water to show any remaining plaque or calculus. This technique must be used with care as it may cause staining of the hair around the patient's mouth.

Polishing with a prophy cup and paste applied with an electrical or air-powered polisher is an important step. This will remove any missed plaque and smooth out the microscopic scratches on the tooth surface (Bellows 2004). When etching occurs, it gives the plaque bacteria more surface area to attach to the tooth. The prophy cup on a low-speed handpiece moves at approximately 3000 rpm. Using a higher rpm or staying on a tooth longer than approximately 10 seconds can lead to overheating of the tooth and pulp damage (Holmstrom et al. 1998). Disposable prophy cups are available and inexpensive. The advantage is they don't need to be cleaned after each use.

An inexpensive prophy paste can be made by mixing flour pumice with water or glycerin. There are many commercially available prophy pastes on the market that are more convenient to use, however. These range in grit and hardness from fine to extra course. Fine or flour grit pumice is recommended to ensure the enamel is as smooth as possible.

Irrigation of the mouth following calculus removal and polishing is vital. All pieces of calculus and prophy paste must be removed from the mouth to avoid aspiration upon recovery. This can be done with a spray bottle filled with water or chlorhexidine gluconate. The gingival sulcus should be irrigated to remove debris. Saline or diluted chlorhexidine gluconate (0.12%) can be used. The advantage of chlorhexidine is its substantivity (its ability to adhere to oral tissues and release its agents over an extended period).

The veterinary technician/nurse should be trained and prepared to assist the veterinarian in any additional dental procedures that may need to be performed. This includes the retraction of tissue, handing of instruments, and blotting of blood to keep the work area clear. An experienced veterinary technician/nurse should anticipate the next steps in the procedure and be prepared to assist when needed. They should also properly record the procedure and findings in the patient's medical record.

Postoperatively, the veterinary technician/nurse should postoxygenate and ensure that the back of the mouth is clean, then extubate the patient and provide a comfortable recovery area. When the patient is fully recovered, they should supervise the move from the recovery area to the hospital ward. They should work with the veterinarian to determine appropriate dietary recommendations and postoperative pain management.

4.5.6 Home Care Instructions

The client who understands the importance of and is willing to perform oral home care to ensure that their pet's mouth heals and remains healthy will be happier in the long run. The veterinary technician/nurse should work with them to develop a strong relationship between them and the clinic. Explaining to the client why home care is important and demonstrating how to administer such care is critical to gaining compliance. Home care instructions must include postoperative medications, dietary restrictions or recommendations, an explanation of the procedure, and after care needs, as well as long-term dental home care recommendations.

Follow-up visits can often be a technician appointment. It is strongly recommended that all dental patients have a postoperative follow-up within one to two weeks to allow the technician to evaluate healing, but also to reinforce the need for dental home care. Home care techniques can be evaluated and discussed with the client during these visits.

Some practices use a color-coding system for continuing follow-up examinations: a red code means the patient needs to have a follow-up every three months, orange means every six months, and green means every year. Patients can be up- or downgraded from one code to another depending upon the results (Figure 4.12).

Handouts should be individualized to the patient, and are another way of showing the client the importance of dental health. They should include a simplified dental chart for making notations (e.g., on depth, furcation exposure, or missing/extracted teeth), the prescribed treatment

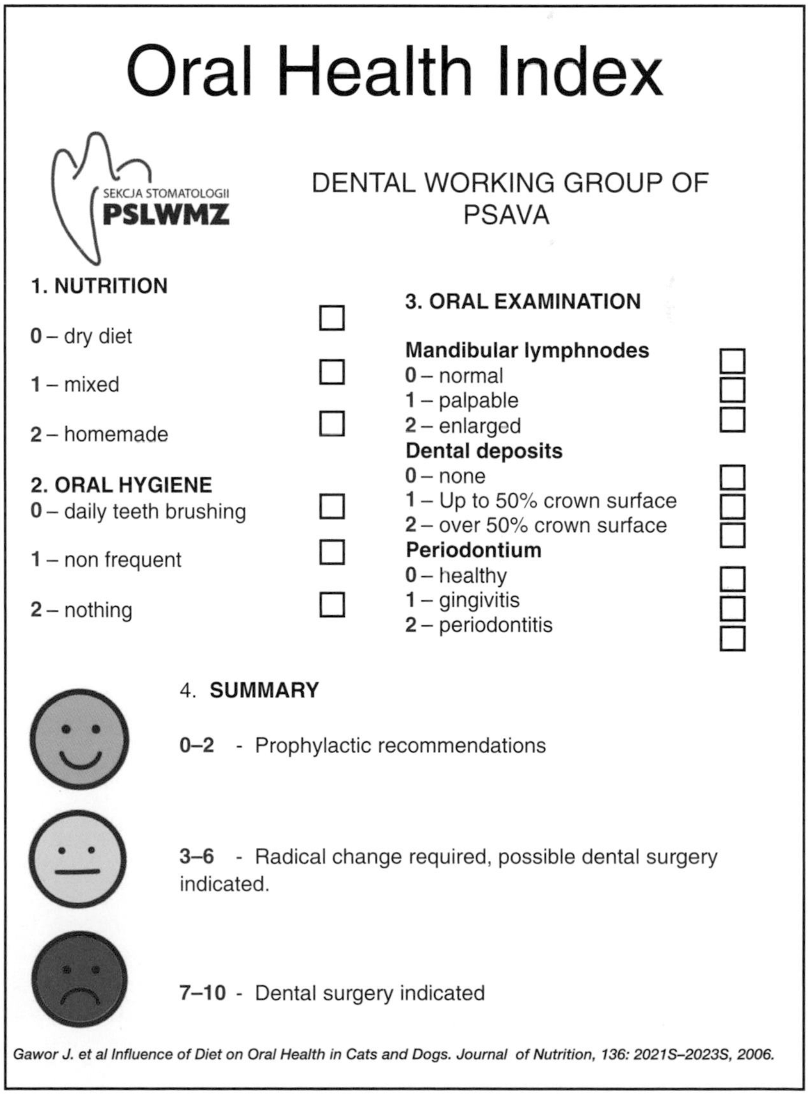

Figure 4.12 Color coding of patients for follow-up visits.

Oral Health Index

SEKCJA STOMATOLOGII
PSLWMZ

DENTAL WORKING GROUP OF PSAVA

1. NUTRITION

0 – dry diet ☐

1 – mixed ☐

2 – homemade ☐

2. ORAL HYGIENE
0 – daily teeth brushing ☐

1 – non frequent ☐

2 – nothing ☐

3. ORAL EXAMINATION

Mandibular lymphnodes
0 – normal ☐
1 – palpable ☐
2 – enlarged ☐
Dental deposits
0 – none ☐
1 – Up to 50% crown surface ☐
2 – over 50% crown surface ☐
Periodontium
0 – healthy ☐
1 – gingivitis ☐
2 – periodontitis ☐

4. **SUMMARY**

0–2 - Prophylactic recommendations

3–6 - Radical change required, possible dental surgery indicated.

7–10 - Dental surgery indicated

Gawor J. et al Influence of Diet on Oral Health in Cats and Dogs. Journal of Nutrition, 136: 2021S–2023S, 2006.

plan, a discharge form, and a copy of the dental X-rays. Handouts on common dental problems, home care options, and treatments can be created by the veterinary technician/nurse. These should be sent home with the client after discussing the procedure or problem with them in the exam room.

The veterinary technician/nurse, along with the rest of the veterinary team, should see themselves as public educators. This not only helps more pets receive better dental care but can show that a practice has embraced dentistry and its importance to patient well-being. There are now many options for getting the word out about the importance of oral health. Social media posts can contain trivia questions, important information, and even interesting cases (with client permission). Consider your audience when posting cases, however, and leave out the bloody gore, even though this can be a useful tool for raising owner awareness of dental conditions.

Be creative. There are many opportunities to educate the public about the importance of oral health for pets. Here are a few ideas:

- Hold an open house and tours of the dental suite for clients, visitors, and youth groups
- Provide informational brochures in waiting rooms (Figure 4.11)
- Offer a video on your website explaining the client/patient experience on the day of a dental procedure at your practice
- Create a smile book with before and after photos and a pictorial step-by-step of a dental cleaning procedure (Figure 4.12)
- Write an article for a local newspaper
- Visit an elementary school with a dog that loves to have its teeth brushed
- Offer a program at a youth group meeting such as 4-H or Scouts
- Provide a booth at a mutt strut or other pet-related event

4.6 Veterinarians

The veterinarian is the team leader. It is very important that they have a strong belief in the importance of dentistry. They should set proficiency goals, schedule dental training meetings, work with their team to develop a highly trained and efficient working group, and understand the importance of providing the best-quality care possible. Veterinarians are the only team members who can diagnose disease. They should evaluate the data provided by the veterinary technician/nurse, follow up in areas of concern, and combine the information they obtain with the dental X-rays to determine a diagnosis and treatment plan. The veterinarian should perform all dental treatments and

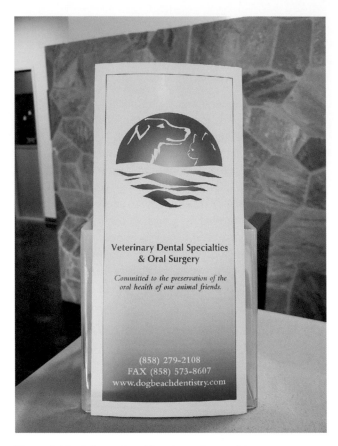

Figure 4.13 Informational brochures in a waiting room.

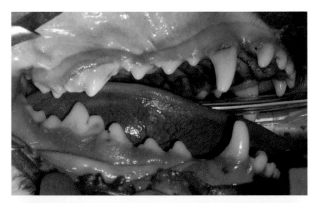

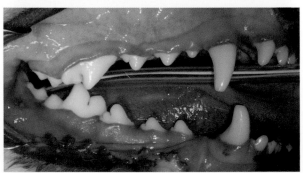

Figure 4.14 Before and after smile book examples.

surgical procedures, including dental extractions. They should be comfortable with the procedures they perform and know the limitations of their training: if a treatment is outside its scope, they should readily refer the patient to a veterinary dental specialist.

4.7 Pet Owners

The pet owner or client plays a large role in the veterinary practice. As a customer, they make the decisions on who will care for their beloved pet. They should feel comfortable and work closely with the veterinary team to determine the best options for their oral health. They are the home care provider for oral care and must have buy-in to the best home care options available. Not all options work for everyone, so the team must work to determine the best one for them.

4.8 Conclusion

The success of the dental aspect of a veterinary practice is dependent upon all members of the team working together toward one common goal. Each role is vital. With a well-educated and well-trained team, there is no limit to the success a practice can achieve. Clients may be influenced by many factors, but often they will stay with a practice where they receive stellar service and care.

References

Bellows, J. (1999). *The Practice of Veterinary Dentistry: A Team Effort*. Ames, IA: Iowa State Press.

Bellows, J. (2004). Periodontal equipment, materials, and techniques. In: *Small Animal Dental Equipment, Materials, and Techniques, a Primer* (ed. J. Bellows), 115–173. Hoboken, NJ: Wiley-Blackwell.

Holmstrom, S.E., Frost, P., and Eisner, E.R. (1998). Dental prophylaxis. In: *Veterinary Dental Techniques*, 2e (eds. S.E. Holmstrom, P. Frost and E.R. Eisner), 133–166. Philadelphia, PA: W.B. Saunders.

Holmstrom SE. (2013) *Veterinary Dentistry A Team approach*. 2nd Ed. Elsevier St Louis

Lobprise, H.B. and Wiggs, R.B. (2000). *The Veterinarian's Companion for Common Dental Procedures*. Lakewood, CO: AAHA Press.

Niemiec, B.A. (2010). *A Color Handbook Small Animal Dental, Oral & Maxillofacial Disease*. London: Manson.

Perrone, J. (2012). *Small Animal Dental Procedures for Veterinary Technicians and Nurses*. Hoboken, NJ: Wiley-Blackwell.

Westfelt, E., Rylander, H., Dahlen, G. et al. (1998). The effect of supragingival plaque control on the progression of advanced periodontal disease. *J. Clin. Periodontol.* 25 (7): 536–541.

5

Prophylactic Program for Oral Health

Brook Niemiec

Veterinary Dental Specialties and Oral Surgery, San Diego, CA, USA

5.1 Introduction

Periodontal disease is the most common disease process in small-animal patients. Proper therapy for periodontal disease consists of four components, based on the level of disease (Niemiec 2008):

- Professional dental cleaning
- Periodontal surgery
- Extractions
- Home care

These various procedures are covered in detail in other chapters; this chapter will focus on the client's role in controlling periodontal (gum) disease.

The prophylactic oral health program includes two major parts: regular dental examinations and established regular oral home care.

5.2 Regular Dental Examinations (and cleanings)

The protocol of regular dental examinations should take approximately 10 minutes and consists of three parts: 3 minutes of history taking and the client completing a questionnaire, 3 minutes of dental/periodontal examination of the conscious patient, and 3 minutes of presentation of diagnosis to the client, instruction on home oral hygiene methods, and recommendation of professional treatment. Parameters are recorded and scored utilizing standardized charts, and should include:

- Age of the patient
- Type of diet fed (dry, mixed [dry and soft], or soft food; home-made foods are classified as soft)

- Extent of home oral hygiene (active or passive):
  - Regular home care
  - Irregular home care
  - A complete lack of home care

The basic oral clinical exam should include an assessment of the size of the mandibular lymph nodes on palpation, the presence and amount of dental deposits, and the presence and degree of periodontal disease.

The size of the mandibular lymph nodes is classified as:

- Normal
- Slightly enlarged
- Moderately to severely enlarged

The presence of dental deposits is determined visually on the most severely affected tooth and is recorded as:

- Absent
- Up to 50% of the crown affected
- More than 50% of the crown affected

The presence of periodontal disease features is also determined visually on the most severely affected tooth. Gingivitis is recorded when there is inflammation of gingival tissue, which is determined as abnormal redness, swelling, or bleeding of the gums. Periodontitis is recorded when a tooth has gingival recession or is mobile on digital palpation (Gawor et al. 2006).

Scores are presented in Table 5.1.

The summation of scores obtained for the preceding three parameters plus the patient's diet and their level of home care provides the oral health index (OHI), where 0 points indicates optimal oral health and 10 points indicates the worst possible oral health (Gawor et al. 2006). Patients scoring 0–2 receive prophylactic advice. For patients scoring 3–6, significant improvements to the

The Veterinary Dental Patient: A Multidisciplinary Approach, First Edition. Edited by Jerzy Gawor and Brook Niemiec.
© 2021 John Wiley & Sons Ltd. Published 2021 by John Wiley & Sons Ltd.
Companion website: www.wiley.com/go/gawor/veterinary-dental-patient

home prophylactic program are required, and a professional dental cleaning may be recommended. Patients scoring 7–10 require immediate exam and treatment under general anesthesia.

This simplified method of oral assessment is useful for public campaigns such as the "Pet Smile" campaign and "National Pet Dental Health Month," and for inclusion in leaflets and brochures offering free dental exams. It can be easily performed by first-contact veterinarians, students, and nurses after brief training. Smartphone apps are being prepared to help pet owners know when they should make an appointment with a veterinarian or dental specialist. Apps focused on at-home oral cavity assessment are also available (e.g. Dental Index, offered by Hill's Pet Nutrition) (Figure 5.1).

Table 5.1 Oral health parameters assessed during patient examination and interview.

Score parameter	0	1	2
Size of mandibular lymph nodes on palpation	Normal	Slightly enlarged	Moderately to severely enlarged
Presence of dental deposits (plaque, calculus, and stain)	Absent	Up to 50% of the dental crown affected	More than 50% of the dental crown affected
Presence of periodontal disease	Absent	Gingivitis	Periodontitis
Diet fed	Home-prepared, soft diet	Mixed (soft/dry)	Dry
Home care	None	Irregular	Regular

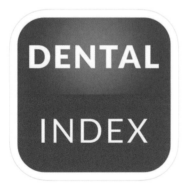

Dental Index 4+

Colgate-Palmolive Company

Free

iPhone Screenshots

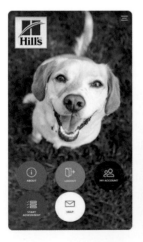
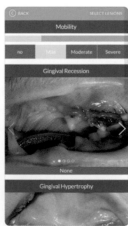
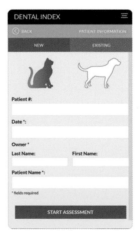
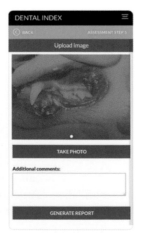

Figure 5.1 Dental Index app.

5.3 Established Regular Oral Home Care

5.3.1 Importance of Home Dental Care

Home care is an essential component of effective periodontal therapy. Bacterial plaque forms on tooth surfaces within 24 hours of cleaning (Boyce et al. 1995; Wiggs and Lobprise 1997) and will begin to calcify into calculus within one day (Tibbitts and Kashiwa 1998) (Figure 5.2). Without regular home care, therefore, gingival infection and inflammation quickly recurs (within two weeks) (Payne et al. 1975; Corba et al. 1986a,b; Fiorellini et al. 2006; Rober 2007; Debowes 2010). A human study found that professional cleanings were of little value without home care (Needleman et al. 2005).

In cases of established periodontal disease, home care is even more important. A human study found that periodontal pockets become reinfected within two weeks of a prophylaxis and that pocket depth returns to pretreatment depths within six weeks of therapy if home care is not performed (Rober 2007).

5.3.2 Client Discussion/Instruction

The benefits of routine home care should be conveyed to each client on a regular basis. Homecare should ideally be discussed on their **first visit** to the practice, which is often the well puppy/kitten or vaccination visit (Wiggs and Lobprise 1997) (Figure 5.2). Early institution of dental home care provides the greatest benefit, as the frequency of care can be lessened if it is started before periodontal disease (even gingivitis) begins (Tromp et al. 1986a,b). More importantly, early institution of home care increases acceptance by the patient and makes training easier. The importance of home care should also be discussed following each dental cleaning. Compliance may be increased by providing detailed instructions and demonstrations. Ideally, such

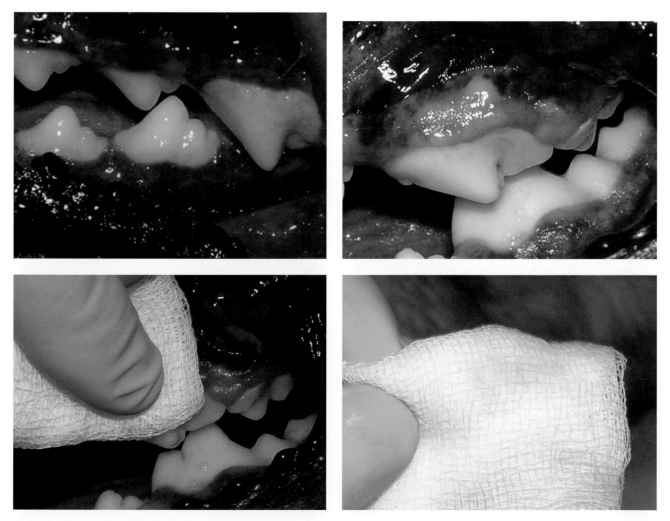

Figure 5.2 Dental plaque identification is part of pet owner education, and should be discussed ideally on the first visit to the practice.

instruction should be offered and respected by the entire staff (Wiggs and Lobprise 1997).

5.3.3 Goals of Home Plaque Control

The primary goal of home plaque control is to limit or reduce the amount of plaque on the teeth (Perry 2006). This in turn should decrease the level of gingival inflammation and, ultimately, of periodontal disease. However, it will not eliminate the need for professional cleanings (Hale 2003).

It is important to note that supragingival plaque and calculus has little to no effect on periodontal disease. It is the plaque at *and below* the gingival margin that creates inflammation and initiates periodontal disease (Harvey and Emily 1993; Westfelt et al. 1998; Niemiec 2008). Therefore, controlling marginal and subgingival plaque is the key to maintaining periodontal health. Keep this in mind when reviewing various home care options. Information on the suitability of different methods of plaque control is covered later.

Brushing is the most effective means of mechanically removing plaque (Hale 2003). Chew-based products may be effective, but only if properly formulated. However, oral sprays, rinses, and water additives are in this authors opinion an insufficient means of plaque control, due to the tenacity with which plaque adheres to the teeth and the high resistance of the plaque biofilm to antiseptics (reported to be up to 500 000 times that of singular bacteria: Williams 1995; Quirynen et al. 2006).

5.3.4 Types of Home Care

There are two major types of home plaque control: active and passive. Both can be effective if performed correctly and consistently, but active home care is the "gold standard" (Hale 2003). Typical methods of active home care are brushing and rinsing. Passive methods are typically based on chewing behaviors via treats or specially formulated diets, though recently water additives have been introduced. It has been shown that active home care is most effective on the rostral teeth (incisors and canines) while passive home care is more effective on the distal teeth (premolars and molars) (Bjone et al. 2007; Capik 2007).

5.3.4.1 Active Home Care

Active home care is defined as the client actively participating in the removal of plaque. This can be achieved either by brushing or by rinsing/applying antiseptic/antiplaque solutions.

5.3.4.1.1 Tooth Brushing When properly performed, tooth brushing is the most effective means of plaque control (Hale 2003). Therefore, while compliance is rare, all veterinarians should still promote tooth brushing for all patients.

5.3.4.1.2 Materials and Methods The only critical piece of equipment is a toothbrush. There are numerous veterinary brushes available,[1] which should be selected based on patient size. Double- and triple-sided[2,3] and circular feline brushes[4] are effective products and should be considered along with the standard veterinary brushes (Figure 5.3). This author does not recommend "finger brushes" as they do not generally address the subgingival areas of the teeth; additionally, they significantly increase the chances of the owner being bitten. Gauzes and washcloths are not recommended for the same reasons (Holmstrom et al. 1998).

Human toothbrushes may be substituted, with soft-bristled brushes typically being recommended. A child's toothbrush is often the correct size for small patients and may be more effective than the larger veterinary version. An infant brush may work best for toy-breed dogs, cats, or juvenile patients.

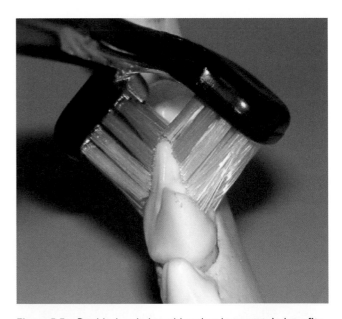

Figure 5.3 Double-headed toothbrushes have certain benefits in plaque control.

---

1 CET Dual-Ended Toothbrush, Virbac Animal Health, Fort Worth TX.

2 Triple-Pet EZ Dog Toothbrush.

3 Quadbrush Cat Toothbrush.

4 CET Cat Toothbrush, Virbac Animal Health, Fort Worth, TX.

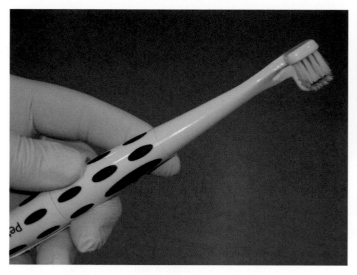 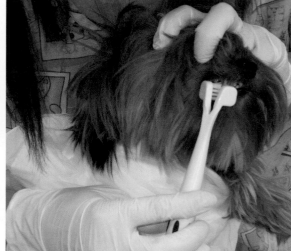

Figure 5.4 Mechanized toothbrush used in dogs.

Mechanized (sonic[5] and rotary[6]) brushes are superior to standard brushes for humans (Deery et al. 2004; Moritis et al. 2008) (Figure 5.4). These products are also likely superior for use in veterinary patients, and may make the process more time efficient, which is important in animal patients for acceptance reasons. In addition to the numerous human product options, there is currently a mechanized veterinary brush on the market.[7] One concern with these brushes is that the movement/vibration can feel strange and may scare the patient (Holmstrom et al. 1998). Secondly, one has to be careful and avoid situation when hair around the mouth becomes entangled in a mechanical brush. This author recommends initiating brushing very slowly with a standard toothbrush, and then progressing to a mechanical type after acceptance is achieved.

There are a number of veterinary toothpastes available,[8] which may increase acceptance by the patient (Figure 5.5). They often contain a calcium chelator[9] in order to decrease the accumulation of dental calculus (Liu et al. 2002; White et al. 2002; Hennet et al. 2007). However, remember that calculus is largely nonpathogenic (Wiggs and Lobprise 1997), so the paste is not a significant player in the reduction of plaque and gingivitis. Consequently, palatability can be increased by using alternative flavorings (Wiggs and Lobprise 1997; Niemiec 2008), such as tuna juice (especially for cats), garlic powder (in small amounts), and beef broth. Dipping the brush in a canned food that the pet enjoys may also be considered on initiation of home brushing.

Antimicrobial products[10] are also available (see later). They improve plaque and gingivitis control when used in combination with brushing, and should be considered especially in high-risk patients or in cases of established periodontal disease (Overholser et al. 1990; Maruniak et al. 1992; Eaton et al. 1997; Hase et al. 1998; Hennet 2002; Stratul et al. 2010). Human toothpastes and products that contain baking soda should be avoided as they typically contain detergents and fluoride, which may cause gastric upset or other issues if swallowed (Wiggs and Lobprise 1997; Niemiec 2008).

5.3.4.1.3 Brushing Technique Note that the ideal technique may only be possible in the most tractable patients. Clients should be encouraged to work toward this level of care, but to accept any degree of brushing as successful (Figure 5.6). Forcing home care on a patient is counterproductive and may decrease the client–animal bond (Holmstrom et al. 1998). Furthermore, coercing clients may drive them away from your practice (Holmstrom et al. 1998). Therefore, it is important to understand your clients and patients and tailor your recommendation based on the situation.

The keys to achieving success with home tooth brushing are as follows (Niemiec 2013):

- **Start Early:** Young patients are more amenable to training (Holmstrom et al. 1998).
- **Go Slow:** Start with just holding the mouth, then progress to a finger, and finally start brushing slowly.
- **Be Consistent:** Make tooth brushing a routine.
- **Make it a Positive Experience:** Using food, treats, hair brushing, or playtime as a reward will greatly increase the likelihood of acceptance.

---

5 Sonicare toothbrush, Phillips.

6 Oral B Vitality toothbrush, Braun.

7 Sonic Canine Premium Pet toothbrush.

8 CET Enzymatic Toothpaste, Virbac Animal Health, Fort Worth, TX.

9 Sodium hexametaphosphate.

---

10 CET Oral Hygiene Rinse, Virbac Animal Health, Fort Worth, TX.

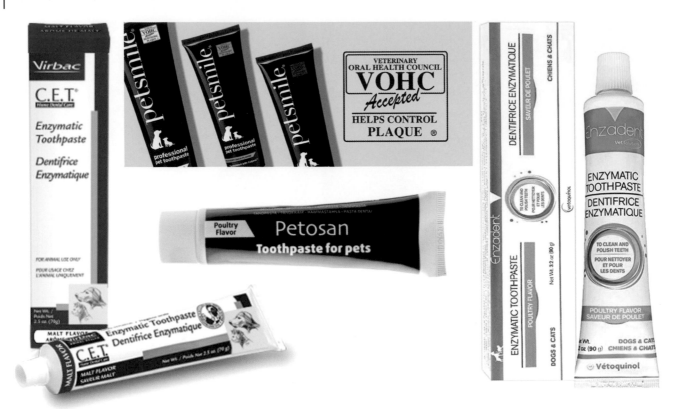

Figure 5.5   Selection of toothpastes.

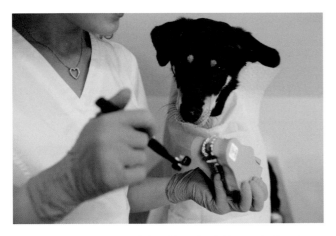

Figure 5.6   Teaching tooth brushing should be gradual and gentle. *Source:* Emilia Klim.

However, it is important to ensure that the patient's temperament is amenable for this process. Advise your clients that getting bitten is not worth it (Holmstrom et al. 1998).

The ideal tooth brushing technique begins with the brush at a 45° angle to the long axis of the tooth. The brush should be placed at the gingival margin and moved along the arches utilizing a rotary motion. The buccal/ labial surfaces of the teeth are the most accessible, and fortunately are the most important, as they generally have more calculus accumulation and gingival inflammation (Niemiec 2013). Pet owners should not attempt to open their pet's mouth, especially early on (Figure 5.7). Most animals greatly dislike their mouth being opened, and it will likely decrease the chances of their accepting the procedure. Clients should be instructed to begin by working toward effectively brushing the buccal surfaces of the teeth with the mouth closed. The distal teeth may be cleaned by gently inserting the brush inside the cheek, relying on tactile feel to achieve proper positioning.

If the patient is amenable, the client may progress to caring for the palatal/lingual surfaces of the teeth. This is critical if periodontal therapy/surgery has been performed on them, which is most common in cases of deep pockets on the palatal surfaces of the maxillary canine teeth. The best and safest way to open the mouth is to place the thumb of the nondominant hand just behind the mandibular canines. This allows for some leverage, and is also the safest place in the mouth for the finger to rest.

Frequency of brushing is a controversial subject. Once a day is the gold standard, as this level of care is required to stay ahead of plaque formation (Wiggs and Lobprise 1997; Niemiec 2008; Harvey et al. 2015). Furthermore,

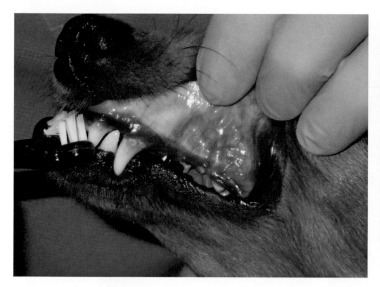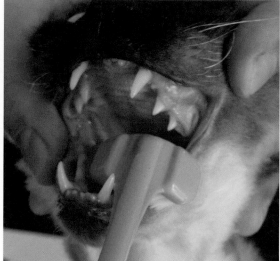

Figure 5.7 Avoid wide opening of the mouth when teaching tooth brushing.

every-other-day brushing has been shown to be ineffective at gingivitis control (Gorrel and Rawlings 1996; Harvey et al. 2015). Three days a week is considered the *minimum* frequency for patients in good oral health (Tromp et al. 1986a,b). Brushing once a week is not considered sufficient to maintain good oral health (Niemiec 2013; Harvey et al. 2015). For patients with established periodontal disease (even gingivitis), daily brushing is required to maintain oral health, and twice daily may be recommended (Corba et al. 1986a,b; Tromp et al. 1986a,b; Gorrel and Rawlings 1996; Wiggs and Lobprise 1997; Niemiec 2008; Harvey et al. 2015). Finally, consistency with home care is critical. If brushing is suspended for as little as 30 days, gingival inflammation will return to the same level as in patients who have never had home care (Ingham and Gorrel 2001).

5.3.4.1.4 *Antiseptic Rinses* The other option for active home care is the application of antiseptic/antiplaque solutions. The traditional antiseptic of choice is chlorhexidine (CHX).[11,12] CHX disrupts the bacterial cell walls and penetrates the cells, creating a precipitation of the cytoplasm (Jenkins et al. 1988). It is an excellent product for oral disinfection, for several reasons:

- There is no known method of bacterial resistance (Robinson 1995; Roudebush et al. 2005)
- It has a quick onset and minimal systemic uptake (Salas Campos et al. 2000)
- It is very safe (Robinson 1995)

- It maintains antiseptic effects for up to seven hours after application (substantivity) (Bonesvoll 1977; Cousido 2009; Tomás 2009)
- It has been shown in numerous studies to decrease gingivitis if applied correctly and consistently (Hull and Davies 1972; Hamp and Emilson 1973; Hamp et al. 1973; Tepe et al. 1983; Overholser 1990; Maruniak 1992; Eaton et al. 1997; Hase et al. 1998; Hennet 2002; Kantmann 2005; Stratul 2010).

There are two minor concerns with the use of CHX. First, it lacks palatability, which may hinder home care efforts (Holmstrom et al. 1998). Second, chronic use has been shown to cause dental staining (Holmstrom et al. 1998; Olympio et al. 2006). However, this staining is reversible, can be polished off, and has not been reported in an animal patient.

Proper application requires only a small amount of the solution. Ideally, the rinse should be directly applied to the surface of the teeth and gingiva, but getting it between the cheek and teeth is often the best that can be done in practice.

An additional option for home plaque control is the use of soluble zinc salts, which have been shown to decrease viable plaque biomass (Wolinsky et al. 2000). One veterinary-labeled oral zinc ascorbate gel[13] has been proven to decrease plaque and gingivitis (Clarke 2001) (Figure 5.8). It is also tasteless, which should improve acceptance, especially in cats. Finally, it contains ascorbic acid, which supports/induces collagen synthesis (Booth and Uitto 1981;

11 Nolvadent, Fort Dodge Animal Health, Fort Dodge, IA.
12 Ceva.

13 Maxiguard oral hygiene gel, Addison Biological Laboratory, Fayette, MO.

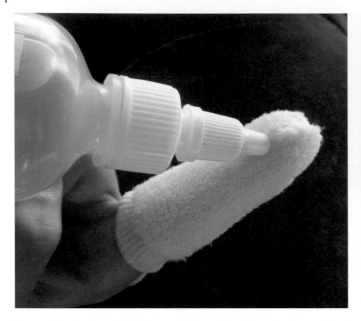
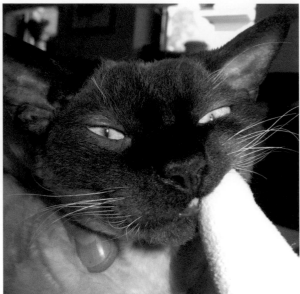

Figure 5.8   Indirect (with the use of fingerbrush) application of Maxiguard in a cat's mouth.

Murad 1981; Pinnel et al. 1987; Holmstrom et al. 1998), potentially improving healing following dental scaling and oral surgery.

5.3.4.1.5 *Barrier Sealant*   A final option for active home care is the application of a barrier sealant[14] (Figure 5.9). This product works by changing the electrostatic charge of the teeth and so creating a hydrophobic surface that prevents plaque attachment (Homola and Dunton 1999), decreasing the accumulation of plaque and calculus (Gengler et al. 2005). A review of this product using evidence-based means supports the use of its professional application, but not its home care version (Roudebush et al. 2005). Therefore, this product may be most effective in the postoperative phase, until the mouth is healed, inflammation resolves, and a more established means of home care (such as brushing) can be instituted.

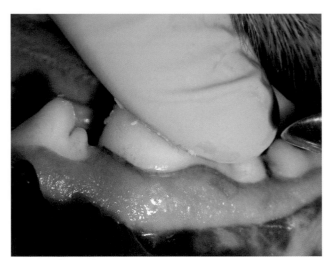

Figure 5.9   Application of the waxy barrier sealant.

5.3.4.2 Passive Home Care

Passive home care is a popular alternative means of decreasing periodontal disease. It consists of the use of specially formulated diets, chews, and treats, as well as water additives. There are numerous products available, but only a few have *any* scientific evidence that they produce a health benefit. Therefore, it is recommended that veterinary professionals review the literature to determine for themselves whether or not to recommend a particular product (Roudebush et al. 2005). It is always best to evaluate

the research behind product claims, and not simply read the marketing hype.

An invaluable resource for the busy practitioner is the Veterinary Oral Health Council (VOHC), a group of veterinary dentists who evaluate product claims and give a seal of approval to worthy products. A list of such products can be found on the group's website: www.vohc.org.

However, most studies, along with the VOHC, only give an overall plaque and calculus reduction score and do not tell us where the plaque was reduced. Therefore, results may not correlate with decreased periodontal disease. Look for softer-texture products that maintain contact with the tooth all the way to the gingival margin.

------

14 Oravet, Merial, Deluth, GA.

Since passive home care requires no real effort by the owner, compliance and regular application are far more likely than with active care. This is very important, as long-term consistency is the key factor in effective home dental care (Ingham and Gorrel 2001). It has been shown that the compliance rate for tooth brushing among *highly motivated* pet owners is only around 50% after six months (Miller and Harvey 1994). In fact, one study showed that passive home care may therefore be superior to active home care, simply due to the fact that it is actually performed (Vrieling et al. 2005). This does not mean that it is more effective, just that the average client is not compliant with active care.

This section provides recommendations for several products based on a review of the current literature combined with the authors professional experience. This list is not comprehensive, and new information and new products are continually available. The particular position on the list of homecare means, have products branded by HealthyMouth LLC which are classified in several groups like: water additives, toothpastes, edible treats, sprays and gels.

5.3.4.2.1 Tartar-Control Diets

It has long been believed that traditional dry dog food is good for oral health, and one study appeared to support this (Gawor et al. 2006). However, other studies show that dry food is *not* superior to moist foods in this regard (Harvey et al. 1996). There are several specially formulated diets available that have been shown to decrease plaque and tartar build-up (Jensen et al. 1995). These products simply employ abrasives to scrape the teeth. The individual kibbles in these therapeutic diets tend to be larger than those in standard pet food (Vrieling et al. 2005; Hennet et al. 2007), which increases the amount of chewing performed and the efficacy of the abrasive aspects (Larsen 2010) (Figure 5.10). Many products also contain a calcium chelator[15] to further reduce dental calculus (Lage et al. 1990; Liu 2002; White et al. 2002; Stookey and Warrick 2005; Hennet et al. 2007).

Numerous products in this segment have received the VOHC seal as effective in tartar (and in some cases, plaque) reduction.[16,17,18,19,20] However, even though these products may decrease plaque and calculus, many are only effective on the cusp tips, not at the gingival margin (Stookey and Warrick 2005). This is an important point as supragingival

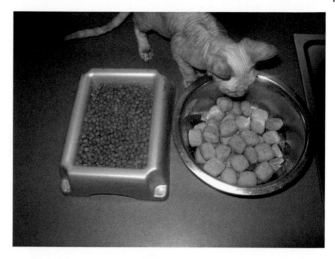

Figure 5.10 Kibbles intended for oral hygiene (right) are larger than normal pet food kibbles (left).

plaque and calculus are nonpathogenic, so minimal control of gingivitis may be obtained via this method of calculus control (Roudebush et al. 2005). Of the available diets, only one[21] has been scientifically proven to decrease gingivitis (Logan et al. 1999, 2002; Logan 2001). The main reason for this product's effectiveness is the fiber arrangement within the kibble, which requires the tooth to fully enter the kibble prior to its breaking apart, allowing the entire tooth (including the marginal area) to be cleaned (Figure 5.11a,b).

5.3.4.2.2 Dental Treats and Chews

There are numerous treats/chews available for passive home care. The original and most common are the biscuit-style treats. Plain biscuits have not been shown to aid in the reduction of periodontal disease (Roudebush et al. 2005). A better choice appears to be biscuits coated with hexametphosphate (HMP), though there are studies that support as well as question their efficacy (Stookey et al. 1996; Logan et al. 2000).

Over the last few years, several new edible treats have been brought to market, with varying efficacies. Many of the relevant studies are unpublished, but there are several products with VOHC approval in this class.[22,23,24]

The most prevalent and proven products of this type are the rask and rawhide chews (Lage et al. 1990; Hennet et al. 2006) (Figure 5.12). These work like tartar-control diets, with the abrasives cleaning the tooth surface, but additionally may include calcium chelators or other substances

---

15 Sodium hexametaphosphate.

16 Oral Care canine and feline, Hills Pet Nutrition Inc., Topeka, KS.

17 Chunk Dental Defense Diet for Dogs, Iams, Dayton, OH.

18 Eukanuba Adult Maintenance Diet for Dogs, Iams, Dayton, OH.

19 Purina Veterinary Diets DH Dental Health brand canine and feline formulas, Nestlé Purina PetCare Company, St. Louis, MO.

20 Friskies Feline Dental Diet, Nestlé Purina PetCare Company, St. Louis, MO.

---

21 Prescription Diet Canine and Feline t/d, Hills Pet Nutrition Inc., Topeka, KS.

22 BlueChews, Vetradent Inc., Ft. Lauderdale, FL.

23 Canine Greenies all sizes and formulations (lite, senior), Franklin, TN.

24 Bright Bites and Checkups Chews for Dogs, Diamond Foods Inc., Stockton, CA.

(a)   (b)

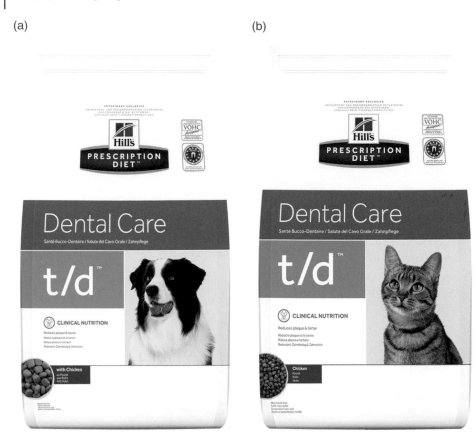

Figure 5.11   Hill's Dental Care T/D diet for dogs and cats.

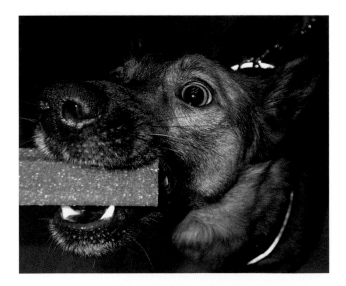

Figure 5.12   Dental treats/chews must be attractive for pets.

to further increase their antiplaque efficacy (Warrick 2001). The addition of CHX to rawhide chews was found to further decrease plaque accumulation, but not gingivitis level (Rawlings et al. 1998; Brown and McGenity 2005). Of the

products available, only a handful[25,26,27,28,29] have been shown to decrease periodontal disease markers (Gorrel et al. 1999; Gorrel and Bierer 1999; Warrick et al. 2001; Brown and McGenity 2005; Mariani et al. 2009; Stookey 2009; Clarke et al. 2011; Quest 2013). A new chew-based treat[30] has data to support plaque and calculus control and has been shown to decrease halitosis. This same product contains an antiplaque agent,[31] which may provide some protective effect on the canine and incisor teeth.

One important point to remember is that many chew treats that claim to help control dental disease are very hard in texture. The chewing of these products may (and often does) result in tooth fracture. A good rule of thumb is that if you cannot make an indentation into the product with your fingernail, it is too hard (Niemiec 2013). Also,

25 CET hexachews, Virbac Animal Health, Fort Worth, TX.

26 Pedigree Rask/Dentabone, Mars, McLean, VA.

27 Tartar Shield Soft Rawhide Chews for Dogs, Therametric Technologies Inc., Noblesville, IN.

28 Greenies Dental Treats, Mars, McLean, VA.

29 Veggiedent, Virbac Animal Health, Fort Worth, TX.

30 Oravet dental hygiene chew, Merial, Deluth, GA.

31 Delmopinol.

(a)

(b)

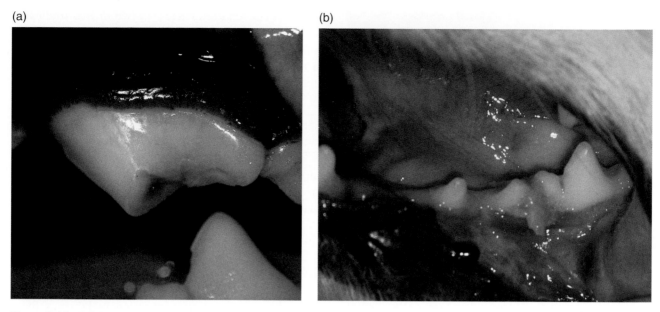

Figure 5.13 With bones or very hard chews, there is danger of (a) breaking the teeth or (b) trapping pieces of bone between them.

just because a product is effective for dental disease does not necessarily mean it is safe. For this reason, VOHC describes the risk of tooth fracture caused by chew treats, and recommends that companies provide mechanical testing results (Figure 5.13).

5.3.4.2.3 Water Additives This is a relatively new area of home dental care, with several products available (Figure 5.14). While there are some studies on the human side that show the active ingredients have some efficacy (Hamp and Emilson 1973; Chapek et al. 1995), there is currently minimal to no peer-reviewed evidence to support their use in controlling periodontal disease in veterinary patients. One product with xylitol[32] was shown to decrease plaque and calculus (Clarke 2006); there were concerns about its potential negative systemic effects (possible hypoglycemia and liver derangement) (Dunayer 2004, 2006; Xia et al. 2009), but it has been shown to be safe at the prescribed concentration (Anthony et al. 2011). Note that water additives will not work when the animal prefers tap water (Figure 5.15).

5.3.4.2.4 Probiotics Nitric oxide (NO) is an important inflammatory mediator that is seen in increased levels in human periodontitis (Matejka et al. 1998; Lappin et al. 2000). Products that decrease its production or effects may be helpful in the control of periodontal disease (Paquette and Williams 2000). *Lactobacillus brevis* is a probiotic bacteria containing high levels of arginine

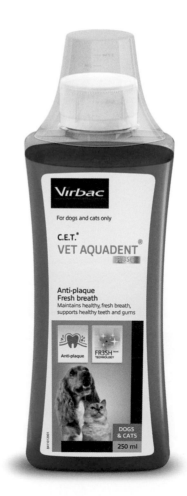

Figure 5.14 The new version of Vet Aquadent without xylitol.

---

32 Aquadent, Virbac Animal Health, Fort Worth, TX.

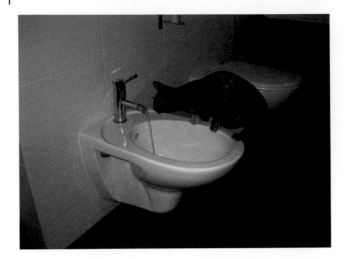

Figure 5.15 Water additives will not work when the animal prefers tap water.

deiminase, which when applied topically decreases inflammatory mediators involved in periodontitis (Maekawa and Hajishengallis 2014).

5.3.4.2.5 Fatty Acids 1-Tetradecanol complex (1-TDC) B is an esterified monounsaturated fatty acid (MUFA)

mixture of several fatty acids. In two *in vivo* studies on New Zealand rabbits, 1-TDC stopped the progression of periodontal disease and caused a significant reduction in macroscopic periodontal inflammation, attachment, and bone loss (Hasturk et al. 2007, 2009).

5.3.4.2.6 Other Supplements Plaque Off products containing seaweed (Ascophyllum nodosum) are available as 'dental bites' and powder to be added to the diet, and have systemic action possibly associated with stimulating the oral defense system and changing saliva content (Gawor et al. 2018) (Figure 5.16).

5.4 Conclusion

Home care is a critical aspect of periodontal therapy, but it is often ignored. Early and consistent client education is the key to obtaining compliance. There are numerous options, but tooth brushing remains the gold standard. Of the products available for passive home care, only a few are truly effective, and the reader is urged to critically review the clinical studies when deciding which to recommend to their clients.

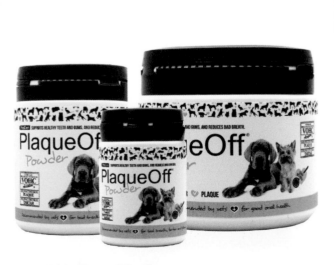
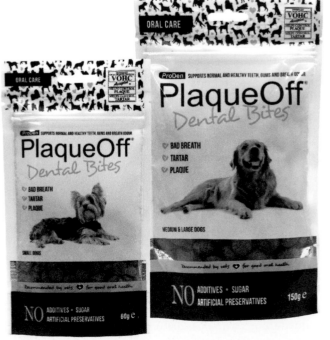

Figure 5.16 Plaque Off series.

References

Anthony, J.M.G., Weber, L.P., and Alkemade, S. (2011). Blood glucose and liver function in dogs administered a xylitol drinking water additive at zero, one and five times dosage rates. *Vet. Sci. Dev.* 1: e2.

Bjone, S., Brown, W., and Harris, A. (2007). Influence of chewing on dental health in dogs. Proceedings of the 16th European Congress of Veterinary Dentistry, pp. 45–46.

Bonesvoll, P. (1977). Oral pharmacology of chlorhexidine. *J. Clin. Periodontol.* 4: 49–65.

Booth, B.A. and Uitto, J. (1981). Collagen biosynthesis by human skin fibroblasts. III. The effects of ascorbic acid on procollagen production and prolyl hydroxylase activity. *Biochim. Biophys. Acta.* 675 (1): 117–122.

Boyce, E.N., Ching, R.J., Logan, E.I. et al. (1995). Occurrence of gram-negative black-pigmented anaerobes in subgingival plaque during the development of canine periodontal disease. *Clin. Infect. Dis.* 20 (Suppl. 2): S317–S319.

Brown, W.Y. and McGenity, P. (2005). Effective periodontal disease control using dental hygiene chews. *J. Vet. Dent.* 22 (1): 16–19.

Capik, I. (2007). Periodontal health vs. different preventative means in toy breeds – clinical study. Proceedings of the 16th European Congress of Veterinary Dentistry, pp. 31–34.

Chapek, C.W., Reed, O.K., and Ratcliff, P.A. (1995). Reduction of bleeding on probing with oral-care products. *Compend. Contin. Educ. Dent.* 16 (2): 188–192.

Clarke, D.E. (2001). Clinical and microbiological effects of oral zinc ascorbate gel in cats. *J. Vet. Dent.* 18 (4): 177–183.

Clarke, D.E. (2006). Drinking water additive decreases plaque and calculus accumulation in cats. *J. Vet. Dent.* 23: 79–82.

Clarke, D.E., Kelman, M., and Perkins, N. (2011). Effectiveness of a vegetable dental chew on periodontal disease parameters in toy breed dogs. *J. Vet. Dent.* Winter 28 (4): 230–235.

Corba, N.H., Jansen, J., and Pilot, T. (1986a). Artificial periodontal defects and frequency of tooth brushing in beagle dogs (I). Clinical findings after creation of the defects. *J. Clin. Periodontol.* 13 (3): 158–163.

Corba, N.H., Jansen, J., and Pilot, T. (1986b). Artificial periodontal defects and frequency of tooth brushing in beagle dogs (II). Clinical findings after a period of healing. *J. Clin. Periodontol.* 13 (3): 186–189.

Cousido, M.C. (2009). *In vivo* substantivity of 0.12% and 0.2% chlorhexidine mouthrinses on salivary bacteria. *Clin. Oral Investig.* 14: 397–402.

Debowes, L.J. (2010). Problems with the gingiva. In: *Small Animal Dental, Oral and Maxillofacial Disease, a Color Handbook* (ed. B.A. Niemiec), 159–181. London: Manson.

Deery, C., Heanue, M., Deacon, S. et al. (2004). The effectiveness of manual versus powered toothbrushes for dental health: a systematic review. *J. Dent.* 32 (3): 197–211.

Dunayer, E.K. (2004). Hypoglycemia following canine ingestion of xylitol-containing gum. *Vet. Hum. Toxicol.* 46 (2): 87–88.

Dunayer, E.K. (2006). New findings on the effects of xylitol ingestion in dogs. *Vet. Med.* 101 (12): 791–797.

Eaton, K.A., Rimini, F.M., Zak, E. et al. (1997). The effects of a 0.12% chlorhexidine-digluconate containing mouthrinse versus a placebo on plauq and gingival inflammation over a 3-month period. A multicentre study carried out in general dental practices. *J. Clin. Periodontol.* 24 (3): 189–197.

Fiorellini, J.P., Ishikawa, S.O., and Kim, D.M. (2006). Clinical features of gingivitis. In: *Carranza's Clinical Periodontology* (eds. F.A. Carranza, M.G. Newman, H.H. Takei and P.R. Klokkevold), 362–372. St. Louis, MO: W.B. Saunders.

Gawor, J., Jank, M., Jodkowska, K. et al. (2018). Effects of edible treats containing *Ascophyllum nodosum* on the oral health of dogs: a double-blind, randomized, placebo-controlled single-center study. *Front. Vet. Sci.* 5: 168.

Gawor, J.P., Reiter, A.M., Jodkowska, K. et al. (2006). Influence of diet on oral health in cats and dogs. *J. Nutr.* 136: 2021S–2023S.

Gengler, W.R., Kunkle, B.N., Romano, D. et al. (2005). Evaluation of a barrier sealant in dogs. *J. Vet. Dent.* 22 (3): 157–159.

Gorrel, C. and Bierer, T.L. (1999). Long-term effects of a dental hygiene chew on the periodontal health of dogs. *J. Vet. Dent.* 16 (3): 109–113.

Gorrel, C. and Rawlings, J.M. (1996). The role of tooth-brushing and diet in the maintenance of periodontal health in dogs. *J. Vet. Dent.* 13 (4): 139–143.

Gorrel, C., Warrick, J., and Bierer, T.L. (1999). Effect of a new dental hygiene chew on periodontal health in dogs. *J. Vet. Dent.* 16 (2): 77–81.

Hale, F.A. (2003). Home care for the veterinary dental patient. *J. Vet. Dent.* 20 (1): 52–54.

Hamp, S.E. and Emilson, C.G. (1973). Some effects of chlorhexidine on the plaque flora of the beagle dog. *J. Periodontol. Res.* 12: 28–35.

Hamp, S.E., Lindhe, J., and Loe, H. (1973). Long term effects of chlorhexidine on developing gingivitis in the beagle dog. *J. Periodontol. Res.* 8: 63–70.

Harvey, C.E. and Emily, P.P. (1993). Periodontal disease. In: *Small Animal Dentistry* (eds. C.E. Harvey and P. Emily), 89–144. St. Louis, MO: Mosby.

Harvey, C.E., Shofer, F.S., and Laster, L. (1996). Correlation of diet, other chewing activities, and periodontal disease in North American client-owned dogs. *J. Vet. Dent.* 13: 101–105.

Harvey C, Serfilippi L, Barnvos D. Effect of Frequency of Brushing Teeth on Plaque and Calculus Accumulation, and Gingivitis in Dogs. Journal of Veterinary Dentistry. 2015;32(1):16-21. doi:10.1177/089875641503200102

Hase, J.C., Attström, R., Edwardsson, S. et al. (1998). 6-month use of 0.2% delmopinol hydrochloride in comparison to 0.2% chlorhexidine digluconate and placebo, effect on plaque formation and gingivitis. *J. Clin. Periodontol.* 25 (9): 746–753.

Hasturk, H., Goguet-Surmenian, E., Blackwood, A. et al. (2009). 1-Tetradecanol complex: therapeutic actions in experimental periodontitis. *J. Periodontol.* 80 (7): 1103–1113.

Hasturk, H., Jones, V.L., Andry, C. et al. (2007). 1-Tetradecanol complex reduces progression of *Porphyromonas gingivalis*-induced experimental periodontitis in rabbits. *J. Periodontol.* 78 (5): 924–932.

Hennet, P. (2002). Effectiveness of a dental gel to reduce plaque in beagle dogs. *J. Vet. Dent.* 19 (1): 11–14.

Hennet, P., Servet, E., and Venet, C. (2006). Effectiveness of an oral hygiene chew to reduce dental deposits in small breed dogs. *J. Vet. Dent.* 23 (1): 6–12.

Hennet, P., Servet, E., Soulard, Y. et al. (2007). Effect of pellet food size and polyphosphates in preventing calculus accumulation in dogs. *J. Vet. Dent.* 24 (4): 236–239.

Holmstrom, S.E., Frost, P., and Eisner, E.R. (1998). Dental prophylaxis. In: *Veterinary Dental Techniques*, 2e (ed. S.E. Holmstrom), 133–166. Philadelphia, PA: W.B. Saunders.

Homola, A.M. and Dunton, R.K. (1999). Methods, compisitions, and dental delivery systems for the protection of the surfaces of teeth. U.S. Patent Nos. 5665333 and 5961958.

Hull, P.S. and Davies, R.M. (1972). The effect of a chlorhexidine gel on tooth deposits in beagle dogs. *J. Small Anim. Pract.* 13: 207–212.

Ingham, K.E. and Gorrel, C. (2001). Effect of long-term intermittent periodontal care on canine periodontal disease. *J. Small Anim. Pract.* 42 (2): 67–70.

Jenkins, S., Addey, M., and Wade, W. (1988). The mechanism of action of chlorhexidine. A study of plaque growth on enamel inserts in vivo. *J. Clin. Periodontol.* 15: 415–424.

Jensen, L., Logan, E., Finney, O. et al. (1995). Reduction in accumulation of plaque, stain, and calculus in dogs by dietary means. *J. Vet. Dent.* 12 (4): 161–163.

Kantmann, C.L. (2005). The evaluation of the rate of gingivitis and plaque formation in cats treated with different antimicrobial solutions. Proceedings of the 19th Annual American Veterinary Dental Forum, Orlando, FL.

Lage, A., Lausen, N., Tracy, R. et al. (1990). Effect of chewing rawhide and cereal biscuit on removal of dental calculus in dogs. *JAVMA* 197 (2): 213–219.

Lappin, D.F., Kjeldsen, M., Sander, L. et al. (2000). Inducible nitric oxide synthase expression in periodontitis. *J. Periodontal. Res.* 35: 369–373.

Larsen, J. (2010). Oral products and dental disease. Compendium: Continuing Education for Veterinarians, pp. E1–E3.

Liu, H. (2002). Anticalculus efficacy and safety of a novel whitening dentifrice containing sodium hexametaphosphate: a controlled six-month clinical trial. *J. Clin. Dent.* 13 (1): 25–28.

Liu, H., Segreto, V.A., Baker, R.A. et al. (2002). Anticalculus efficacy and safety of a novel whitening dentifrice containing sodium hexametaphosphate: a controlled six-month clinical trial. *J Clin Dent.* 13 (1): 25–28.

Logan, E.I. (2001) Dietary effect on tooth surface debris and gingival health in cats. Proceedings of the 15th Annual American Veterinary Dental Forum, San Antonio, TX, p. 377.

Logan, E.I., Berg, M.L., and Coffman, L. et al. (1999). Dietary control of feline gingivitis: results of a six month study. Proceedings of the 13th Veterinary Dental Forum, p. 54.

Logan, E.I., Finney, O., and Hefferren, J.J. (2002). Effects of a dental food on plaque accumulation and gingival health in dogs. *J. Vet. Dent.* 19 (1): 15–18.

Logan, E.I., Wiggs, R.B., Zetner, K. et al. (2000). Dental disease. In: *Small Animal Clinical Nutrition*, 4e (eds. M.S. Hand, C.D. Thacher, R.L. Remillard and P. Roudebush), 475–492. Topeka, KS: Mark Morris Institute.

Maekawa, T. and Hajishengallis, G. (2014). Topical treatment with probiotic *Lactobacillus brevis* CD2 inhibits experimental periodontal inflammation and bone loss. *J. Periodontal. Res.* 49 (6): 785–791.

Mariani, C., Douhain, J., Servet, E. et al. (2009). Effect of toothbrushing and chew distribution on halitosis in dogs. Proceedings of the 18th Congress of Veterinary Dentistry, Zurich, pp. 13–15.

Maruniak, J. (1992). The effect of 3 mouthrinses on plaque and gingivitis development. *J. Clin. Periodontol.* 19 (1): 19–23.

Maruniak, J., Clark, W.B., Walker, C.B. et al. (1992). The effect of 3 mouthrinses on plaque and gingivitis development. *J. Clin. Periodontol.* 19 (1): 19–23.

Matejka, M., Partyka, L., Ulm, C. et al. (1998). Nitric oxide synthesis is increased in periodontal disease. *J. Periodontal. Res.* 33: 517–518.

Miller, B.R. and Harvey, C.E. (1994). Compliance with oral hygiene recommendations following periodontal treatment in client-owned dogs. *J. Vet. Dent.* 11 (1): 18–19.

Moritis, K., Jenkins, W., Hefti, A. et al. (2008). A randomized, parallel design study to evaluate the effects of a Sonicare and a manual toothbrush on plaque and gingivitis. *J Clin Dent.* 19 (2): 64–68.

Murad, S. (1981). Regulation of collagen synthesis by ascorbic acid. *Proc. Natl. Acad. Sci. U. S. A.* 78 (5): 2879–2882.

Needleman, I., Suvan, J., Moles, D.R. et al. (2005). A systematic review of professional mechanical plaque removal for prevention of periodontal diseases. *J. Clin. Periodontol.* 32 (Suppl. 6): 229–282.

Niemiec, B.A. (2008). Periodontal therapy. *Top Companion Anim. Med.* 23 (2): 81–90.

Niemiec, B.A. (2008). Periodontal disease. *Top. Companion Anim. Med.* 23 (2): 72–80.

Niemiec, B.A. (2013). Home plaque control. In: *Veterinary Periodontology* (ed. B.A. Niemiec). Ames, IA: Wiley-Blackwell.

Olympio, K.P., Bardal, P.A., de M Bastos, J.R. et al. (2006). Effectiveness of a chlorhexidine dentifrice in orthodontic patients: a randomized-controlled trial. *J. Clin. Periodontol.* 33 (6): 421–426.

Overholser, C.D. (1990). Comparative effects of 2 chemotherapeutic mouthrinses on the development of supragingival dental plaque and gingivitis. *J. Clin. Periodontol.* 17 (8): 575–579.

Overholser, C.D., Meiller, T.F., DePaola, L.G. et al. (1990). Comparative effects of 2 chemotherapeutic mouthrinses on the development of supragingival dental plaque and gingivitis. *J. Clin. Periodontol.* 17 (8): 575–579.

Paquette, D.W. and Williams, R.C. (2000). Modulation of host inflammatory mediators as a treatment strategy for periodontal diseases. *Periodontol.* 24: 239–252.

Payne, W.A., Page, R.C., Olgolvie, A.L. et al. (1975). Histopathologic features of the initial and early stages of experimental gingivitis in man. *J. Periodontal Res.* 10: 51.

Perry, D.A. (2006). Plaque control for the periodontal patient. In: *Carranza's Clinical Periodontology* (eds. F.A. Carranza, M.G. Newman, H.H. Takei and P.R. Klokkevold), 728–748. St. Louis, MO: W.B. Saunders.

Pinnel, S.R., Murad, S., and Darr, D. (1987). Induction of collagen synthesis by ascorbic acid. A possible mechanism. *Arch. Dermatol.* 123 (12): 1684–1686.

Quest, B.W. (2013). Oral health benefits of a daily dental chew in dogs. *J. Vet. Dent.* 30 (2): 84–87.

Quirynen, M., Teughels, W., Kinder Haake, S. et al. (2006). Microbiology of periodontal diseases. In: *Carranza's Clinical Periodontology* (eds. F.A. Carranza, M.G. Newman, H.H. Takei and P.R. Klokkevold), 134–169. St. Louis, MO: W.B. Saunders.

Rawlings, J.M., Gorrel, C., and Markwell, P.J. (1998). Effect on canine oral health of adding chlorhexidine to a dental hygiene chew. *J. Vet. Dent.* 15 (3): 129–134.

Rober, M. (2007). Effect of scaling and root planing without dental homecare on the subgingival microbiota. Proceedings of the 16th European Congress of Veterinary Dentistry, pp. 28–30.

Robinson, J.G. (1995). Chlorhexidine gluconate – the solution to dental problems. *J. Vet. Dent.* 12 (1): 29–31.

Roudebush, P., Logan, E., and Hale, F.A. (2005). Evidence-based veterinary dentistry: a systematic review of

homecare for prevention of periodontal disease in dogs and cats. *J. Vet. Dent.* 22 (1): 6–15.

Salas Campos, L., Gómez Ferrero, O., Villar Miranda, H. et al. (2000). Antiseptic agents: chlorhexidine. *Rev. Enferm.* 23 (9): 637–640.

Stookey, G.K. (2009). Soft rawhide reduces calculus formation in dogs. *J. Vet. Dent.* 26 (2): 82–85.

Stookey, G.K., and Warrick, J.M. (2005). Calculus prevention in dogs provided diets coated with HMP. Proceedings of the 19th Annual American Veterinary Dental Forum, Orlando, FL, pp. 417–421.

Stookey, G.K., Warrick, J.M., Miller, L.L. et al. (1996). Hexametphosphate-coated snack biscuits significantly reduce calculus formation in dogs. *J. Vet. Dent.* 13 (1): 27039.

Stratul, S.I. (2010). Prospective clinical study evaluating the long-time adjunctive use of chlorhexidine after one-stage full-mouth SRP. *Int. J. Dent. Hyg.* 8 (1): 35–40.

Stratul, S.I., Rusu, D., Didilescu, A. et al. (2010). Prospective clinical study evaluating the long-time adjunctive use of chlorhexidine after one-stage full-mouth SRP. *Int. J. Dent. Hyg.* 8 (1): 35–40.

Tepe, J.H., Leonard, G.J., Singer, R.E. et al. (1983). The long term effect of chlorhexidine on plaque, gingivitis, sulcus depth, gingival recession, and loss of attachment in beagle dogs. *J. Periodontal. Res.* 18: 452–458.

Tibbitts, L. and Kashiwa, H. (1998). A histochemical study of early plaque mineralization. Abstract #616. *J. Dent. Res.* 19 (202): 170–171.

Tomás, I. (2009). Evaluation of chlorhexidine substantivity on salivary flora by epifluorescence microscopy. *Oral Dis.* 15 (6): 428–433.

Tromp, J.A., Jansen, J., and Pilot, T. (1986a). Gingival health and frequency of tooth brushing in the beagle dog model. Clinical findings. *J. Clin. Periodontol.* 13 (2): 164–168

Tromp, J.A., van Rijn, L.J., and Jansen, J. (1986b). Experimental gingivitis and frequency of tooth brushing in the beagle dog model. Clinical findings. *J. Clin. Periodontol.* 13 (3): 190–194

Vrieling, H.E., Theyse, L.F., van Winkelhoff, A.J. et al. (2005). Effectiveness of feeding large kibbles with mechanical cleaning properties in cats with gingivitis. *Tijdschr. Diergeneeskd.* 130 (5): 136–140.

Warrick, J.M. (2001). Reducing caclculus accumulation in dogs using an innovative rawhide treat system coated with hexametaphosphate. Proceedings of the 15th Annual American Veterinary Dental Forum, San Antonio, TX, pp. 379–382.

Warrick, J.M., Stookey, G.K., Inskeep, G.A. et al. (2001). Reducing caclculus accumulation in dogs using an innovative rawhide treat system coated with hexametaphosphate. Proceedings of the 15th Annual American Veterinary Dental Forum, San Antonio, TX, pp. 379–382.

Westfelt, E., Rylander, H., Dahlen, G. et al. (1998). The effect of supragingival plaque control on the progression of advanced periodontal disease. *J. Clin. Periodontol.* 25 (7): 536–541.

White, D.J., Cox, E.R., Suszcynskymeister, E.M. et al. (2002). *In vitro* studies of the anticalculus efficacy of a sodium hexametaphosphate whitening dentifrice. *J Clin Dent.* 13 (1): 33–37.

Wiggs, R.B. and Lobprise, H.B. (1997). Periodontology. In: *Veterinary Dentistry, Principals and Practice* (eds. R.B. Wiggs and H.B. Lobprise), 186–231. Philadelphia, PA: Lippincott-Raven.

Williams, J.E. (1995). Microbial contamination of dental lines. Current and Future Trends in Veterinary Dentistry: Proceedings of the Upjohn Worldwide Companion Animal Veterinary Dental Forum, pp. 8–11.

Wolinsky, L.E., Cuomo, J., Quesada, K. et al. (2000). A comparative pilot study of the effects of a dentifrice containing green tea bioflavonids, sanguinarine, or triclosan on oral bacterial biofilm formation. *J. Clin. Dent.* 11: 535–559.

Xia, Z., He, Y., and Yu, J. (2009). Experimental acute toxicity of xylitol in dogs. *J. Vet. Pharmacol. Ther.* 32 (5): 465–469.

6

Nutrition, Oral Health, and Feeding Dental Patients
Michał Jank

Division of Pharmacology and Toxicology, Department of Preclinical Sciences, Institute of Veterinary Medicine, Warsaw University of Life Sciences (WULS-SGGW), Warsaw, Poland

6.1   Introduction

Nutrition is one of the key elements of the treatment of dental patients since all pathological disorders occurring in the oral cavity may directly influence food intake. In addition, all nutrients get into our patients via the mouth and the first part of digestion happens there. Disorders of the oral cavity are most common in small-animal veterinary patients, but they often remain underestimated or undiagnosed. The most common oral cavity disorder is periodontal disease; however, as with other systems and organs, we can divide oral health problems into developmental, infectious and inflammatory, immune-mediated, trauma, and neoplasia. Regarding developmental disorders, trauma, and neoplasia of the oral cavity, the appropriate selection of nutrition is the key element of patient management. For infectious, inflammatory, and immune-based oral pathologies, the type and composition of the food can directly influence the course of the disease and the risk of its recurrence. Food can deliver both causative and preventive ingredients. Feeding is a basic element of home care, and as such the aim must be to control the oral cavity environment and prevent recurrence of the problem. These changes may target the oral cavity microbiome, pH, mineral content, and immune status. Since the majority of oral/dental problems have a complex etiology, it is hypothesized that a change in just one of the elements of the oral cavity environment could positively influence disease outcome.

As previously stated, the most frequently diagnosed oral cavity disorder is periodontal disease. Its occurrence is directly related to the presence of selected clinical features such as dental plaque, calculus (tartar), gingivitis, and halitosis (malodor). Since the etiologic agent of periodontal disease is bacterial plaque accumulation, it is not surprising that the main goal of home care in dental patients is plaque control. Without plaque accumulation on the teeth surfaces, there will be no gingivitis. Evidence-based medicine (EBM) which is followed by the VOHC submission and review system, shows that the most effective means of plaque and gingivitis control are tooth brushing, chlorhexidine (CHX)-containing products, dental diets with adequate texture, some dental treats/chews, and short-term use of dental sealants. For calculus (tartar) control, the order is slightly different: tooth brushing, dental foods with textural characteristics, dental foods or treats with polyphosphates, and rawhide chews (dogs only) (Roudebush et al. 2005). Some of these elements are directly related to nutrition: dental food with textural characteristics, dental foods with polyphosphates (or other ingredients of this type), and selected chews. They all play a significant role in both plaque and calculus reduction, but to be effective they must be given consistently. Periodic professional dental cleanings without home care will not provide oral health, since plaque forms within hours after a cleaning (Boyce 1995; Wiggs and Lobprise 1997). When calculus or established periodontitis is present, home care procedures are simply not sufficient.

6.2   Modifications of the Oral Cavity Microbiome

Periodontal disease development is strictly related to the presence of different bacteria in the oral cavity, and therefore nutritional interventions related to the prevention and treatment of periodontal disease are focused on two areas. The first is modification (or elimination) of oral microflora that participates in dental plaque formation. These bacteria are responsible for local, regional, and distant infections. They form a structured biofilm on the tooth surface, create

The Veterinary Dental Patient: A Multidisciplinary Approach, First Edition. Edited by Jerzy Gawor and Brook Niemiec.
© 2021 John Wiley & Sons Ltd. Published 2021 by John Wiley & Sons Ltd.
Companion website: www.wiley.com/go/gawor/veterinary-dental-patient

gingivitis, and can extend into the gingival sulcus where they may initiate inflammation of deeper tissues, leading to periodontitis. Modification of the oral microflora aims to selectively eliminate potentially pathogenic bacteria. This can be achieved by targeting specific bacteria through the use of antimicrobial substances or by mechanical removal of bacteria from tooth surfaces (elimination of dental plaque). The second aspect of nutritional intervention in the case of inflammatory and infectious disease of the oral cavity is independent of microbiome modification and focuses instead on prevention of the transformation of dental plaque into tartar. In this case, the aim of an intervention is to eliminate from the oral cavity specific microelements that contribute to calculus formation. These microelements react with various substances present in dental plaque to form insoluble salts deposited on the tooth surface.

6.2.1 Canine Oral Cavity Microbiome

The alimentary tract of dogs contains thousands of different microbes. The majority live within the large intestine, but the small intestine, stomach, and oral cavity also have their own specific ecosystems. Though the content of the intestinal microbiome has been the subject of intensive investigations for some time, that of the oral cavity has only become a focus of study quite recently. Currently, we know that the oral cavity microbiome contains over 400 different bacterial species, though we do not know the exact role of the majority of them. These bacteria do not stimulate the host's natural defense mechanisms, so it could be presumed they remain unnoticed by the mucosal immune system. Recent studies suggest, however, that an imbalance between the endogenous microflora and local immunity could favor development of opportunistic bacteria, which might be responsible for the majority of oral cavity diseases, including periodontal disease and mucosal and dental lesions.

Recent studies on identification of the oral microbiome show at least 353 canine bacterial taxa, placed in 14 bacterial phyla, 23 classes, 37 orders, 66 families, and 148 genera (Dewhirst et al. 2012). The identified phyla are *Firmicutes*, *Proteobacteria*, *Bacteroidetes*, *Spirochaetes*, *Synergistetes*, *Actinobacteria*, *Fusobateria*, *TM7*, *Tenericutes*, *GNO2*, *SR1*, *Chlorobi*, *Chloroflexi*, and *WPS-2*. Interestingly, 80% of bacterial taxa in the canine oral microbiome are still unnamed. The same studies show that there is little similarity between the oral bacteria in dogs and humans; in one of the largest, similarity is found only in 16% of taxa. This suggests that attempts to transfer strategies of oral microbiome modification from one species to another are of little value.

Also important is that disease development causes significant changes in the oral microbiome. One study conducted on 223 dogs with different stages of periodontal disease compared the oral microbiomes of healthy dogs, dogs with gingivitis, and dogs with mild periodontitis (<25% attachment loss) (Davis et al. 2013). Each group contained more than 70 individual animals. The study identified a total of 274 taxonomic bacterial units, showing that regardless of disease status, the most frequently occurring bacterial genus remained *Porphyromonas* spp. In healthy dogs, two other frequently occurring genera were *Moraxella* and *Bergeyella*. In mild periodontitis, the most abundant genera were *Peptostreptococcus*, *Actinomyces*, and *Peptostreptococcaceae*. As in previous studies, a significant difference between the oral microbiomes of dogs and humans was confirmed. The clinically important result of this study is that healthy canine plaque is predominantly created by Gram-negative bacteria, whereas plaque in diseased animals is dominated by Gram-positive anaerobes. This is particularly important because it stands in contrast to the situation in humans, where the dental plaque in diseased individuals is dominated by Gram-negative anaerobes. An earlier study showed the main periodontal pathogen is *Porphyromonas gingivalis*, identified in periodontitis cases in humans, mice, and rats (Shofiqur et al. 2011). Its virulence is associated with the production and secretion of the proteolytic enzyme gingipain (Genco 1999), which can degrade key components of the immune system and plays a key role in bacterial proliferation and survival in periodontal pockets.

A recent study conducted on 52 miniature schnauzers over 60 weeks showed that in the course of periodontal disease development, some changes occurred in the oral microbiome, namely a decrease in *Bergeyella zoohelcum* COT-186, *Moraxella* sp. COT-017, *Pasteurellaceae* sp. COT-080, and *Neisseria shayeganii* COT-090 (Wallis et al. 2015). On the other hand, increased severity of gingivitis has been connected with increased abundance of *Firmicutes*. This study showed that periodontitis could be related to a reduction of previously abundant, health-associated taxa.

In summary, recent observations are of real interest in two aspects: our understanding of disease development and potential treatment strategies. The critical observation is that the development of periodontal disease is related to changes in existing bacterial microflora and not the appearance of new bacteria previously not present in the oral cavity. The question is whether the switch from Gram-negative to Gram-positive bacteria is a cause or a consequence of periodontal disease, and whether a change in the oral cavity environment favoring the survival of Gram-negative bacteria could help restore health.

6.2.2 Feline Oral Cavity Microbiome

Recent research has provided new and extensive insights into the feline oral cavity microbiome. Perez-Salcedo et al. (2013) isolated and identified some bacterial pathogens involved in development of periodontal disease in cats. The most common were *Porphyromonas gulae* (86% of cases), *Porphyromonas circumdentaria* (70%), and *Fusobacterium nucleatum* (90%). The authors also pointed to a significant role for *P. gulae*, which occurred in high proportion across all microbiota (32.5%). The same study confirmed the previously described role of *Porphyromonas* sp. in periodontal disease in cats (Norris and Love 1999).

Studies of the feline oral cavity microbiome have revealed many new bacterial taxa involved in both healthy and diseased microflora. The first studies conducted using new genomic techniques revealed bacteria belonging to 171 feline oral taxa in 11 phyla: *Firmicutes* (72), *Proteobacteria* (38), *Bacteroidetes* (26), *Spirochaetes* (16), *Actinobacteria* (10), *Synergistetes* (4), *Chlorobi* (1), *Chloroflexi* (1), *Fusobacteria* (1), *SR1* (1), and TM7 (1) (Dewhirst et al. 2015).

In the most recent comprehensive study, subgingival plaque bacteria were sampled from a total of 92 cats: 20 with healthy gingiva, 50 with gingivitis, and 22 with mild periodontitis (PD1) (Harris et al. 2015). A total of 267 different bacterial taxa were identified, but unlike in canine oral microbiomes, there were no differences in bacterial species diversity among cats with different oral health statuses. The only difference was in the proportions of aerobes, anaerobes, and facultative anaerobes. In all groups investigated, the anaerobic species dominated, being present in 50% of healthy cats and more than 80% of cats with mild periodontitis. In the latter group, extremely low amounts of aerobic bacteria were noted (between 2 and 8% of all identified species). Similar to dogs, and in contrast to humans, cats affected by mild periodontitis had a higher number of Gram-positive species. In healthy cats, dental plaque was dominated by Gram-negative species. The same study identified a bacterial strain that could be a potential marker of mild periodontitis: *Peptostreptococcaceae* XIII [G-2] bacterium FOT-027. The homolog of this bacterium was also involved in periodontitis in dogs.

6.3 Current Nutritional Strategies for Oral Microflora Modification

6.3.1 Targeting Specific Bacteria

Based on recent studies, no straightforward analogies can be made between dogs, cats, and humans regarding oral microflora composition. In addition, there are still no evidence-based data on the effective manipulation of specific oral bacterial strains aimed at the improvement of periodontal disease in dogs. It seems clear that the composition of the oral microbiome is influenced at least by type of diet and salivary pH. Since these two factors are completely different in humans than in dogs and cats, one can expect modifications in bacterial strains due to changes in diet or saliva pH. In humans, an important factor in modifying the oral microbiome is dietary sugar content, as a diet that contains a lot of sugar leads to an increase in *Streptococcal* species, along with species that depend on them, such as *Veillonella*. In humans, reduction of sugar intake in the diet leads to a decrease in *Streptococcus* sp. and *Actinobacteria*; thus, in dogs and cats, diet could significantly modify the oral microflora. Commercial dry food contains at least 30–40% of starch (in dry matter), so a switch from dry pet food to a homemade diet based on natural ingredients could completely change the types of dominating bacteria. Of course, starch is not a simple carbohydrate, and both dogs and cats lack oral amylase, which is present in humans, so conclusions from studies conducted in humans cannot be directly used in them. Regardless, this is an avenue worth exploring.

There is a very interesting possibility of modifying the oral microbiome using probiotic bacterial strains in humans. For this purpose, *Lactobacilli* were used, even though *Lactobacillus* sp. make up only 1% of the total oral bacteria. However, *L. acidophilus*, *L. casei*, *L. fermentum*, *L. plantarum*, *L. rhamnosus*, and *L. salivarius* were identified in human saliva, which provided the rationale for their potential use in the modification of oral microflora (Teanpaisan 2006). Moreover, it was shown that *L. casei* subsp. *paracasei* and *L. rhamnosus* have significant antagonistic effects on human oral cavity pathogenic bacteria, including *Streptococcus mutans* and *P. gingivalis* (Sookkhee et al. 2001). It was also shown that *Porphyromonas intermedia* requires vitamin K for growth, and *Lactobacilli* may provide a positive competitive role (Wang et al. 1990). Since *Porphorymonas* spp. have been identified as the most frequently occurring pathogenic bacterial genus in dogs and cats, perhaps a similar approach could be of value in animals. Some species of *Lactobacillus* and *Bifidobacterium* occur naturally in dairy products and have the ability to adhere to the mucosa of the oral cavity and teeth (Haukioja et al. 2006). Based on the concept of replacing the opportunistic bacteria in the oral cavity niche with probiotic strains, theoretically one could modify the microfloral composition and control the development of potential pathogens. One such a probiotic strain could be *Streptococcus salivarius*, though its beneficial role has been described only in cases of dental caries, which is not a significant problem in small-animal dentistry (Wescombe et al. 2012).

Probiotic bacteria can influence the oral cavity microflora both directly and indirectly. Direct action occurs via competition within specific niches, and through competition for nutrients. In addition, they can influence biofilm formation by modifying bacterial attachments to the biofilm. *Streptococcus* sp. prevents colonization of the oral cavity with bacteria involved in periodontal disease (i.e., by production of a special biosurfactant, which inhibits adhesion of pathogenic *S. mutans*). Additionally, it changes the molecular structure of protein-binding sites and binds some salivary agglutinins necessary for *S. mutans* adhesion (Zambori 2014). Probiotic bacteria also produce antibacterial substances such as hydrogen peroxide and bacteriocins. *Streptococcus salivarius* produces two salivaricins, one of which prevents caries in humans, while the other is used in treatment of halitosis caused by *Prevotella* spp. and *Micromona micra* (Balakrishnan et al. 2000).

One potential indirect action of bacterial strains on the oral microflora relates to the interaction between probiotic bacteria and the local oral cavity immune system. Studies conducted *in vitro* show that *Lactobacillus brevis* is able to exert some anti-inflammatory effect on periodontal disease, mainly by decreasing the levels of metalloproteinase, prostaglandin E2 (PGE2), and interferon- gamma (INF-γ) (Della Riccia et al. 2007). On the other hand, several bacteria are capable of producing substances enhancing the development of periodontal disease, and the tools of novel immunotherapy can be used to inhibit their activity. For example, in the case of *Porphorymonas gingivitis*, which produces gingipain, the use of anti-gingipain IgY (IgY-GP) produced from egg yolk, known as hyperimmune γ-livetin, has been described. This substance contains anti-gingipain antibodies obtained from chicken embryos. In experimental studies, it was used either in the form of a powder mixed with dry food pellets or as an ingredient of a neutral ointment, administered topically on the gums. In both cases, the anti-gingipain IgY decreased inflammation in the oral cavity of dogs, but an effect on periodontal pocket depth was achieved only with the ointment (after four weeks of use). This provides evidence that oral immunomodulation based on IgY-GP could become part of the preventive or therapeutic plan for periodontal disease management in dogs. Also of interest is that the action of IgY against gingipain released by *P. gingivalis* cross-reacted with the same enzyme produced by *P. gulae*, which also produces other proteases potentially involved in periodontal disease development in dogs. Unfortunately, in cats and dogs, there is no clear association between the presence of *P. gulae* and the occurrence of periodontitis, even though the genomes of *P. gulae* strains occurring in dogs contain the vast majority of the known *P. gingivalis* genes. In both dogs and cats, *P. gulae* is also highly prevalent in healthy dental plaque, so it cannot be related to periodontitis as it is in humans.

6.3.2 Modification of Saliva Composition

One of the key factors contributing to plaque and calculus formation is saliva. It is believed that the mineral composition and pH of saliva could influence the speed of mineral deposition in calculus formation. Dog and cat saliva is naturally more alkaline than that of humans. In a study of 37 dogs belonging to three different breeds (dachshund, Labrador retriever, and Jack Russel terrier), Lavy et al. (2012) found that the average salivary pH was 8.53, with no statistical differences between breeds (the pH of human saliva is 6.5–7.5). These values seem quite high, since other sources show that dog saliva has pH 7.34–7.80 and cat saliva pH 7.50 (Altman and Dittmer 1968). Nonetheless, dog and cat salivary pH is more alkaline than that of humans, which could explain the lack of caries as an important disorder of the oral cavity in these species. It is also known that in alkaline pH, the saturation of calcium and phosphorus increases, so that these chemicals can precipitate more readily, becoming nuclei for calculus formation. It was found that the level of calcium and phosphorus in the saliva of Labrador retrievers was higher (Ca by 40%, P by 150%) than that in dachshunds and Jack Russel terriers. Since the difference is statistically insignificant, it could be that the higher occurrence of dental calculus in this breed is a combined result of this and of a higher salivary pH. These studies led to attempts to decrease salivary pH and calcium (and phosphorus) levels in the oral cavity. It was shown that a 5% solution of glucose given orally could decrease salivary pH, whereas a urea solution could increase it (Loux et al. 1972). However, it is not clear whether such a decrease would lead to caries formation in dogs.

Saliva contains many different substances with antibacterial features, namely specific antibodies, salivary peroxidase, free radicals, lysozyme, lactoferrin, and glycoproteins agglutinating streptococci (Dardzińska and Dworecka-Kaszak 2014). That is why the modification of saliva content became a very attractive approach to modifying the oral cavity microbiome and reducing the risk of dental calculus formation. This mode of action is postulated as the basis for using a supplement containing seaweed (*Ascophyllum nodosum*), which has been claimed to reduce both calculus and plaque accumulation after oral administration. A study conducted on both dogs and cats showed that when the supplement containing *A. nodosum* was given for 42 days following an oral hygienic procedure, oral health index (OHI) values were reduced by more than 50% in both species when compared to control animals (Gawor et al. 2013). The results are interesting, but the single active substance responsible for this effect has not been identified. More recent studies show a significant reduction of both dental plaque and calculus after 90 days of supplementation of edible treats with *A. nodosum*. Dogs treated with

A. nodosum also exhibited significantly lower concentrations of volatile sulfur compounds (VSC) and better oral health status (e.g., gingival bleeding index [GBI] and OHI) compared to controls (Gawor et al. 2018).

According to the manufacturer, *A. nodosum* is rich in natural iodine- and fucose-containing sulfated polysaccharides, which interfere with bacterial growth and accumulation. These and other ingredients are absorbed from the intestines and return to the oral cavity via the saliva, which is why they slow biofilm and calculus build-up in beagles and reduce plaque by up to 87% and tartar by up to 68% in humans (Winker et al. unpublished). It is important to note that saliva itself, being a very rich medium for many oral microorganisms, plays an important role in plaque deposition.

6.3.3 Antibacterial Ingredients in Nutritional Products

There are numerous nutritional products currently available that contain specific ingredients intended to modify the oral cavity microflora. This modification is aimed not only at prevention of dental plaque formation but also at halitosis reduction. These ingredients include: zinc salts (both organic and inorganic), which exert some bacteriostatic properties; essential oils (eucalyptus); and tea polyphenols (Girard and Servet 2008). Eucalyptus oil helps to reduce the number of amino acids containing sulfur in the oral cavity and in this way inhibits the growth of bacteria in humans (Pan et al. 2000). It was proven that it can inhibit the growth of *P. gingivalis*, *Fusobacterium nucleatum*, and *Streptococcus sorbinus*. It may also reduce the intensity of oral malodor. Copaiba oil (from *Copaifera officinalis*) was applied topically in dogs and the results were equal to those obtained with CHX (Pieri et al. 2012). Additionally, some *in vitro* tests were performed to analyze the antimicrobial activity of copaiba oil against plaque-forming bacteria (Valdevite et al. 2007) and assess the adherence inhibition in *Streptococcus* sp. in glass capillaries using the same phytotherapy. Other researchers have looked for other natural antibacterial ingredients, such as propolis, *Camellia sinensis* (Chang et al. 2009), *Mimosa tenuiflora* (Macêdo-Costa et al. 2009), *Vitisa murensis* (Yim 2010), *Rhinacanthus nasutus* (Puttarak et al. 2010), *Murraya koenigii*, *Allium sativum*, and *Melaleuca alternifolia* (Prabhakar et al. 2009). They all used different formulations, but all focused on periodontal disease prevention by plaque formation control.

An inhibitory effect on bacterial growth in the oral cavity can be also achieved by the use of zinc salts. These salts exert bacteriostatic activity both *in vitro* and *in vivo*, but their effectiveness has been verified mainly through the use of an oral gel containing zinc salts in cats (Clarke 2001).

Based on this, many attempts have been made to prepare food or chews containing zinc salts that will be effective in the reduction of bacterial activity in the oral cavity. The only concern with the use of zinc salts in dogs is the potential toxicity of zinc. A recent recommendation from the Fédération Européenne de l'Industrie des Aliments pour Aminaux Familiers (FEDIAF) sets the legal safety limit of zinc for both adult dogs and adult cats at 227 mg/kg of dry matter of food. The exact amount of zinc in a dental treat or chew must be given on the label.

The antibacterial activities of polyphenols of different origins (e.g., green tea) have been described. Catechin has been postulated to exert the strongest effect, with published data showing it reducing the amount of *Porphyromonas* bacteria in dental plaque in dogs after two months of administration, as well as the capacity of these bacteria to adhere to the surfaces of epithelial cells. These data came from studies on the action of polyphenols versus *P. gingivalis*, which, based on recent data, is not the key oral pathogenic bacteria in dogs and cats (unlike in humans). It appears that the previous result should be verified against *P. gulae*. On the other hand, polyphenols were also effective against *Prevotella* spp., *Streptococcus slaivarius*, *Streptococcus mutans*, *Streptococcus salivarius*, and *Streptococcus sanguis*. Therefore, one could expect positive results from the application of polyphenols in dogs and cats with periodontal disease (Hennet 2006).

6.4 Elimination of Dental Plaque by Nutritional Products

Bearing in mind the important role of dental plaque in the development of periodontal disease in dogs and cats, it is not surprising that many products claiming to remove plaque have been created, with trials conducted on a variety of specific mechanical and other properties.

The effect of the consistency (texture) of food on plaque formation or elimination is quite well studied. Several studies show that soft (i.e., minced) food leads to greater accumulation of dental plaque, perhaps due to mechanical action, reduction of saliva flow, reduction in enzyme secretion, and functional atrophy. It is logical, then, to assume that dry food will reduce the formation of dental plaque, but the results of clinical studies in this area are conflicting. In one study conducted on 1350 dogs, no significant difference in dental plaque deposition between those fed dry food and those fed other food types was found (Harvey et al. 1996). On the other hand, in a study conducted in Poland on almost 30 000 dogs and over 9000 cats, it was shown that feeding of solely dry food was related to an at least two times lower OHI when compared to feeding with soft food only (the OHI in animals fed with mixed food fell in the middle, and the difference was a little more evident in cats than in dogs) (Gawor et al. 2006). But this study also showed that even dogs fed dry food could accumulate plaque and develop periodontal disease and gingivitis, so the protection from dental diseases afforded by dry food is not complete. There is agreement that the beneficial role of dry commercial food results not from its low moisture content but from its fibrosity. The role of fibrosity is also evident when soft (wet) food is fed to animals: when dogs receive wet food in a minced formula, the accumulation of dental plaque is greater than when the same ingredients are given in their natural shape (as a raw meat). Thus, the tearing of pieces of food may reduce the development of dental deposits. This observation has been used in the development of commercial dental pet diets.

Commercial dry dental diets have been developed based on the concept that during chewing, the kibble should not crumble. The crumbling of dry food results in contact with only the incisional edge of the tooth surface, providing no mechanical cleaning. The specific fibrous structure of the dental pet diet, however, causes the kibble to stay almost entirely uncrushed during chewing and so maintains contact with the whole surface of tooth, resulting in mechanical cleaning. This fibrous structure has been considered a "natural toothbrush." It requires certain types of fiber combined with a special manufacturing process in which the fibers are oriented properly within the kibble matrix. Thus, the food is no longer just a "food" but possesses some beneficial cleaning properties, slowing the deposition of plaque. After 25 weeks of feeding, the plaque index was reduced by 39% and the gingivitis index by 36% when compared to dogs receiving regular pet food (Logan et al. 2002). Similar positive results were observed when cats were fed with larger, rectangular kibbles of dry food with a higher penetration index (+25%) as compared to small triangular kibbles (Servet et al. 2003), with a reduction of dental plaque deposition of 41%.

In one recent study, it was shown that it was possible to significantly reduce plaque accumulation by coating dry food with an antiplaque agent belonging to the sodium ascorbic phosphate group, which is related to ascorbic acid (vitamin C). The exact action of this ingredient in patients with periodontal disease is unclear, but a relationship between ascorbic acid and gingival health has been identified. The data suggest that it is possible to reduce dental plaque accumulation not only through the special consistency of dry-food kibbles but also by the action of specific ingredients added to the food (Clarke et al. 2010).

The mechanical action of pet food is not limited to dental diets, as many chews and treats with beneficial oral hygiene properties have been developed, with numerous products that claim to have antiplaque and anticalculus features. Most have a specific shape (bars), length (around 9 cm for small-breed dogs), and texture (elastic), since they require a dog to use its teeth to chew them before swallowing. One of the most important characteristics of these products is the chewing time before complete swallowing. Chewing stimulates excretion of saliva, which contains antibacterial agents that promote oral health (Gorrel and Bierer 1999). Thus, both the initial physical abrasion of chewing and the resulting salivary flow help keep the mouth clean (Figure 6.1). There are many studies describing the actions of different dental bars, chews, and treats, and their results are quite variable. One chew was found to reduce dental plaque by 17% after four months of use (Hennet et al. 2005), while another (containing sodium tripolyphosphate and zinc sulfate) reduced plaque by 38% (Brown and McGenity 2005). In both cases, the key factor was the mechanical action of the bar and not the phosphate salts content, since it has been shown that food containing sodium tripolyphosphate given for 28 days did not reduce dental plaque in cats (Clarke et al. 2010). Thus, if a vehicle (kibble, bar, or chew) of phosphate salt delivery has no direct mechanical dental action, it will be effective in calculus reduction but not in reduction of plaque.

Clarke et al. (2007) evaluated a vegetable chew with a unique Z-shaped design and found a 37% reduction in mean plaque scores.

There is evidence that even dental bars can differ significantly in their action, with a number of different parameters describing their usefulness. In one study, two dental bars were compared: chew A, a regular starch-based extruded dental bar, and chew B, a chew containing additional fiber to increase its toughness. Chew A required more than 50 gnaws and around 180 bites to consume, while chew B required 130 gnaws and around 330 bites. It thus took significantly more time for chew B to be consumed by dogs, but the final effects in terms of reduction of dental plaque and calculus were similar (Bjone 2005).

6.5 Inhibition of Calculus Formation

One strategy of oral health maintenance in both dogs and cats is the prevention of the formation of dental calculus. Calculus is a mineralized form of dental plaque that is deposited on the tooth surface, favoring accumulation of new dental plaque due to its porous character. Since it is formed mainly of inorganic salts, the main strategy for its prevention is to eliminate the free ions that could create insoluble salts from the oral cavity. The most important element in this regard, occurring in high amounts in saliva and participating in calculus development, is calcium. Thus, one of the main strategies for controlling dental calculus formation is to chelate calcium with polyphosphate salts. These salts will also chelate other cations (like magnesium),

(a) (b)

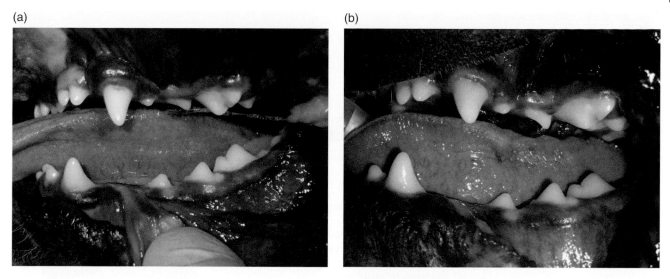

Figure 6.1 Comparison of the dentition of a dog that regularly received a dental chew for 30 days: (a) T0, (b) T30.

preventing their incorporation in calculus. Diets containing polyphosphate salts can reduce calculus formation in cats by 32%. When they were used in commercial pet foods formulated with larger triangular kibbles, plaque was reduced by 30% and calculus by 45% (Girard and Servet 2008). The type of chelating agent is also important to preventive action. Sodium hexametaphosphate reduced calculus deposit by 36% and sodium tripolyphosphate by 55% after one month's administration. Still, when a chelating agent is added to the kibble, its effectiveness is slightly less when compared with agents that are coated on to it. Sodium hexametaphosphate when added to kibble reduced calculus formation by 34.2% after three months of administration, but when coated on the kibble it reduced it by 47.6% (Pinto et al. 2008). Cation-chelating ingredients are used not only in diets but also in other nutritional products for dogs and cats, such as toothpastes, snacks, and treats. Addition of 0.6% sodium pyrophosphate to biscuits given once a day reduced dental calculus by 18.9% after four weeks of administration (Carciofi et al. 2007). However, when sodium hexametaphosphate was used as a coating, the reduction of calculus was 46% in one study (Stookey et al. 1996) and almost 80% in another (Stookey et al. 1995).

For many years, it has been postulated that the lower amount of dental deposits in feral cats/dogs is a result of "natural" food eating, with a special focus on rawhide and raw bones as an element related to natural diets. While this seems to be reasonable, there are no evidence-based data published to prove this, especially where the matter of raw bones is concerned. However, in one very recent study, the authors investigated the role of bovine raw cortical or "compact" bone (CB) from femur diaphysis and bovine raw "spongy" bone (SB) from the femoral epiphysis to see if they reduced calculus build-up in beagles (Marx et al. 2016).

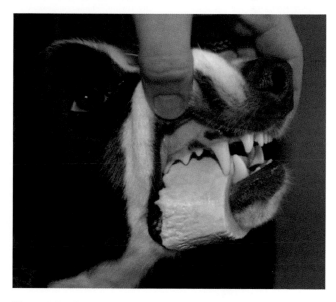

Figure 6.2 Entrapment of a large piece of bone in a dog's mandible. *Source:* Courtesy of Dr. Jan Schreyer.

One bone was given per day, with the CB bones provided for 12 days and the SB bones for 20 days. In dogs receiving CB bones, a reduction of dental calculus of 70.6% was seen on day 12, with the remaining calculus covering only 12.3% of the tooth area. In dogs receiving SB bones, the reduction of dental calculus on day 12 was 81%, with the remaining calculus covering only 7.1% of the tooth area; on day 20, it covered just 4.2%. Even though the results were similar at day 12, it seems that SB results in faster action and significantly greater reduction of dental calculus in the first few days after initiation of administration (Figure 6.2). Rawhide chews were evaluated more precisely than raw bones and the results suggest that they reduce dental calculus significantly better (by 19.4%) than dental biscuits (Lage

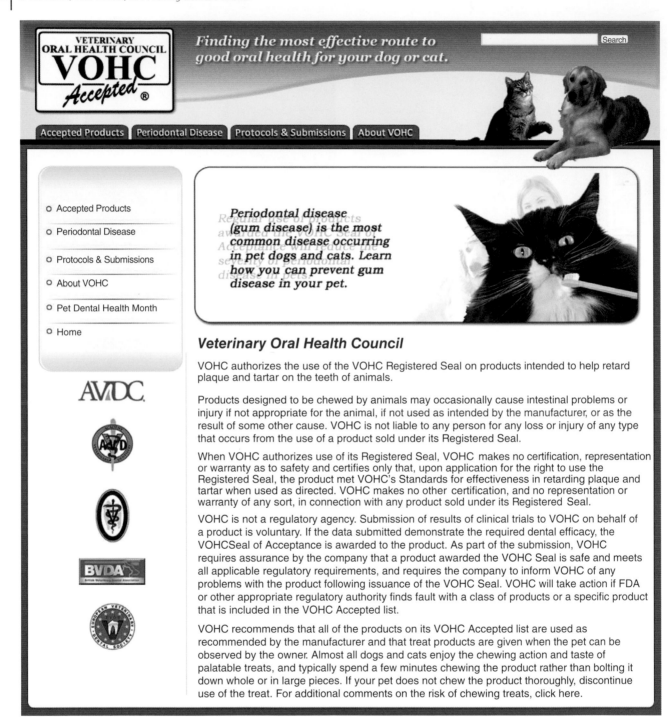

Veterinary Oral Health Council

VOHC authorizes the use of the VOHC Registered Seal on products intended to help retard plaque and tartar on the teeth of animals.

Products designed to be chewed by animals may occasionally cause intestinal problems or injury if not appropriate for the animal, if not used as intended by the manufacturer, or as the result of some other cause. VOHC is not liable to any person for any loss or injury of any type that occurs from the use of a product sold under its Registered Seal.

When VOHC authorizes use of its Registered Seal, VOHC makes no certification, representation or warranty as to safety and certifies only that, upon application for the right to use the Registered Seal, the product met VOHC's Standards for effectiveness in retarding plaque and tartar when used as directed. VOHC makes no other certification, and no representation or warranty of any sort, in connection with any product sold under its Registered Seal.

VOHC is not a regulatory agency. Submission of results of clinical trials to VOHC on behalf of a product is voluntary. If the data submitted demonstrate the required dental efficacy, the VOHCSeal of Acceptance is awarded to the product. As part of the submission, VOHC requires assurance by the company that a product awarded the VOHC Seal is safe and meets all applicable regulatory requirements, and requires the company to inform VOHC of any problems with the product following issuance of the VOHC Seal. VOHC will take action if FDA or other appropriate regulatory authority finds fault with a class of products or a specific product that is included in the VOHC Accepted list.

VOHC recommends that all of the products on its VOHC Accepted list are used as recommended by the manufacturer and that treat products are given when the pet can be observed by the owner. Almost all dogs and cats enjoy the chewing action and taste of palatable treats, and typically spend a few minutes chewing the product rather than bolting it down whole or in large pieces. If your pet does not chew the product thoroughly, discontinue use of the treat. For additional comments on the risk of chewing treats, click here.

Home | Accepted Products | Periodontal Disease | Protocols & Submissions | About VOHC | Contact VOHC

The Veterinary Oral Health Council VOHC accepted certification mark is a registered certification mark of the Veterinary Oral Health Council.

Figure 6.3   VOHC website.

et al. 1990). When the effectiveness of soft rawhide given once daily four hours after feeding dry diet was compared to control animals receiving no treat, dental calculus scores were found to be reduced by 28.2% (Stookey 2009).

6.6 Veterinary Oral Heath Council Seal of Acceptance

In 1997, the American Veterinary Dental College (AVDC) launched the Veterinary Oral Health Council (VOHC) as a platform for the recognition of products that meet pre-set standards of plaque and calculus (tartar) retardation in dogs and cats. The VOHC sets standard protocols for the evaluation of any type of product aimed at exerting some dental activity. Each product that receives its Seal of Acceptance is evaluated in controlled studies, the results of which are frequently published. The required minimum difference in "mouth mean scores" (the mean of all scored teeth for all animals in a group) between a test group and negative control group is a 15% reduction in the plaque or tartar score in each of two trials, and **20% in the mean of the two**, with a statistically significant difference ($p < 0.05$) in both.

The VOHC Seal of Acceptance is accepted by several national and international veterinary dental societies in North America, Asia, and Europe. Should you wish to check whether a product you would like to recommend has received the Seal of Acceptance, just visit the council website (www.vohc.org) (Figure 6.3).

6.7 Role of Chewing in Passive Hygiene

Mastication is a result of the interaction of dentition, tongue movement, and jaw motion steered by the temporomandibular joint and muscles of mastication. All these aspects contribute to the first part of digestion, and thus the quality of digestion is related to the correct function of occlusion, which is the relationship between the **maxillary** (upper) and **mandibular** (lower) teeth when they approach each other, as occurs during chewing or at rest. The caudal teeth (premolars and molars) are responsible for chewing. When the relationship between maxillary and mandibular dentition is optimal in terms of correct number of teeth (no missing or supernumerary teeth) and correct alignment (interdigitation), this is termed a "scissors bite." To provide the appropriate strength of mastication, all teeth and their associated periodontium must be healthy (Figure 6.4). Any discrepancies in occlusion, periodontium, or tooth condition affect the functions of mastication and thus compromise the self-cleaning process.

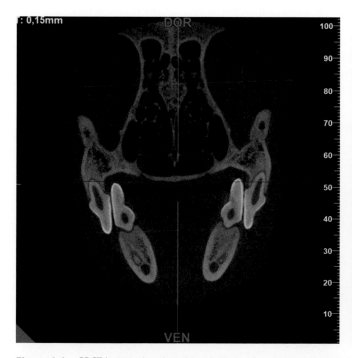 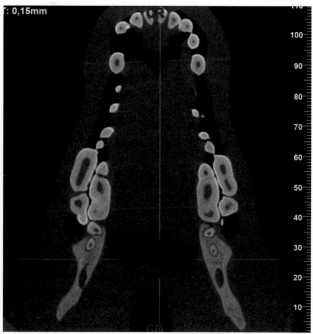

Figure 6.4 CBCT image showing the relations of occlusion of teeth in different planes.

6.8 Conclusion

The nutrition of the canine or feline dental patient is mainly focused on disease prevention. Control of plaque and calculus accumulation and prevention of recurrence after descaling may decrease the risk of negative consequences of plaque (i.e., periodontal disease). Dental diets are one of the most important elements of the oral prophylactic program and of home care in dogs or cats. This nutrition has several goals: modification of the oral cavity microflora, reduction of oral pathogenic bacteria, reduction of the level of free calcium in the oral cavity, reduction of volatile sulfur compound activity in the oral cavity, and control of dental plaque formation and its calcification into calculus. Based on this list, one could assume that food given to dental patients should contain probiotics (modification of oral microflora), antibacterial agents (i.e., essential oils, polyphenols, zinc, plant extracts), and chelating agents (polyphosphates), as well as possessing some textural characteristics (fibrosity in both wet and dry food, shape in dental bars and chews). In most cases, these features refer to the diets of dentulous animals without significant systemic diseases, not to those affected by advanced periodontal disease.

The appendix dedicated to Assisted feeding in dental patients is available at www.wiley.com/go/gawor/veterinary-dental-patient

References

Altman, P.L. and Dittmer, D.S. (1968). *Biological Handbooks: Metabolism*. Bethesda, MD: Federation of American Societies for Experimental Biology.

Balakrishnan, M., Simmonds, R.S., and Tagg, J.R. (2000). Dental caries is a preventable infectious disease. *Aust. Dent. J.* 45: 235–245.

Bjone, S. (2005). Influence of chewing on dental health in dogs. Proceedings of the Australian Veterinary Association Annual Conference, Gold Coast, Australia, May 16–19.

Boyce, E.N. (1995). Occurrence of Gram-negative black-pigmented anaerobes in subgingival plaque during the development of canine periodontal disease. *Clin. Infect. Dis.* 20 ((Suppl. 2)): S317–S319.

Brown, W.Y. and McGenity, P. (2005). Effective periodontal disease control using dental hygiene chews. *J. Vet. Dent.* 22 (1): 15–19.

Carciofi, A.C., Bazolli, R.S., Barbudo, G.R. et al. (2007). Evaluation of the effect of extruded biscuit coated with sodium pyrophosphate on the pre-existing plaque and dental calculus in dogs. *Ars Vet.* 23: 47–53.

Chang, H., Hwang, H., Kang, E. et al. (2009). The effect of green tea bag in dogs with periodontal disease. *J. Vet. Clin.* 26: 41–47.

Clarke, D.E. (2001). Clinical and microbiological effects of oral zinc ascorbate gel in cats. *J. Vet. Dent.* 18 (4): 177–181.

Clarke, D.E., Kelman, M., and Perlins, N. (2007). Effectiveness of vegetable dental chew on periodontal disease parameters in toy breed dogs. *J. Vet. Dental* 28 (4): 230–235.

Clarke, D.E., Servet, E., Hendriks, W. et al. (2010). Effect of kibble size, shape, and additives on plaque in cats. *J. Vet. Dent.* 27: 84–89.

Dardzińska, W. and Dworecka-Kaszak, B. (2014). Biofilm bakteryjny płytki nazębnej i jego znaczenie w chorobach jamy ustnej psów i kotów [Biofilm of dental plaque and its involvement in dogs and cats oral cavity diseases]. *Życie Weterynaryjne.* 89 (3): 216–221.

Davis, I.J., Wallis, C., Deusch, O. et al. (2013). A cross-sectional survey of bacterial species in plaque from client owned dogs with healthy gingiva, gingivitis or mild periodontitis. *PLoS One* 8 (12): e83158.

Della Riccia, D.N., Bizzini, F., Perilli, M.G. et al. (2007). Anti-inflammatory effects of lactobacillus brevis (CD2) on periodontal disease. *Oral Dis.* 13: 376–385.

Dewhirst, F.E., Klein, E.A., Bennett, M.L. et al. (2015). The feline oral microbiome: a provisional 16S rRNA gene based taxonomy with full-length reference sequences. *Vet. Microbiol.* 175: 294–303.

Dewhirst, F.E., Klein, E.A., Thompson, E.C. et al. (2012). The canine oral microbiome. *PLoS One* 7 (4): e36067.

Gawor, J., Jank, M., Jodkowska, K., Klim, E., Svensson, U.K. et al. (2018). Effects of edible treats containing *Ascophyllum nodosum* on the oral health of dogs: a double-blind, randomized, placebo-controlled single-center study. *Front. Vet. Sci.* 5: 168.

Gawor, J., Jodkowska, K., and Jank, M. (2013). Effect of an *Ascophyllum nodosum* contained in supplement on oral health index in dogs and cats. *Weterynaria W Praktyce* 10: 74–79.

Gawor, J.P., Reiter, A.M., Jodkowska, K. et al. (2006). Influence of diet on oral health in cats and dogs. *J. Nutr.* 136: 2021S–2023S.

Genco, C.A. (1999). Role of gingipains R in the pathogenesis of *Porphyromonas gingivalis*-mediated periodontal disease. *Clin. Infect. Dis.* 28: 456–465.

Girard, N. and Servet, E. (2008). Nutrition and oral health in cats. In: P. Pibot, V. Biourge, and D. Elliott (eds.), *Encyclopedia of Feline Clinical Nutrition*. Aimargues: Royal Canin.

Gorrel, B. and Bierer, T.L. (1999). Long term effects of dental hygienic chew on the periodontal health of dogs. *J. Vet. Dent.* 16 (3): 109–113.

Harris, S., Croft, J., O'Flynn, C. et al. (2015). A pyrosequencing investigation of differences in the feline subgingival microbiota in health, gingivitis and mild periodontitis. *PLoS One* 10 (11): e0136986.

Harvey, C.E., Shofer, F.S., and Laster, L. (1996). Correlation of diet, other chewing activities and periodontal disease in north-Americal client-owned dogs. *J. Vet. Dent.* 13 (3): 101–105.

Haukioja, A., Yli-Knuuttila, H., Loimaranta, V. et al. (2006). Oral adhesion and survival of probiotic and other lactobacilli and bifidobacteria *in vitro*. *Oral Microbiol. Immunol.* 21: 326–332.

Hennet, P. (2006). Canine nutrition and oral health. In: *Encyclopedia of Feline Clinical Nutrition* (eds. P. Pibot, V. Biourge and D. Elliott). Aimargues: Royal Canin.

Hennet, P., Servet, E., and Venet, C. (2005). Effects of feeding a daily oral hygiene chew on dental deposits in small breed dogs: a 4-month trial. Proceedings of the 13th European Congress of Veterinary Dentistry, Krakow, pp. 47–48.

Lage, A., Lausen, N., Tracy, R. et al. (1990). Effect of chewing rawhide and cereal biscuit on removal of dental calculus in dogs. *J. Am. Vet. Med. Assoc.* 197: 213–219.

Lavy, E., Goldberger, D., Friedman, M. et al. (2012). pH values and mineral content of saliva in different breeds of dogs. *Israel J. Vet. Med.* 67: 244–248.

Logan, E.I., Finney, O., and Hefferren, J.J. (2002). Effects of dental food on plaque accumulation and gingival health in dogs. *J. Vet. Dent.* 9 (10): 15–18.

Loux, J.J., Alioto, R., and Yankell, S.L. (1972). Effects of glucose and urea on dental deposit pH in dogs. *J. Dent. Res.* 51: 1610–1613.

Macêdo-Costa, M., Pereira, M., Pereira, L. et al. (2009). Atividade Antimicrobiana do Extrato da mimosa tenuiflora. *Pesquisa Brasileira de Odontopediatria Clínica Integrada* 9: 161–165.

Marx, F.R., Machado, G.S., Pezzali, J.G. et al. (2016). Raw beef bones as chewing items to reduce dental calculus in beagle dogs. *Aust. Vet. J.* 94: 18–23.

Norris, J.M. and Love, D.N. (1999). Associations among three feline *Porphyromonas* species from the gingival margin of cats during periodontal disease and health. *Vet. Microbiol.* 65: 195–207.

Pan, P., Barnett, M.L., and Coelho, J. (2000). Determination of the in situ bactericidal activity of essential oil mouth rinse using vital stain method. *J. Clin. Periodontol.* 27: 256–261.

Perez-Salcedo, L., Herrera, D., Esteban-Saltiveri, D. et al. (2013). Isolation and identification of Porphyromonas spp. and other putative pathogens from cats ith periodontal disease. *J. Vet. Dent.* 30 (4): 208–213.

Pieri, F.A., Daibert, A.P.F., Bourguignon, E. et al. (2012). Periodontal disease in dogs. In: C.C. Perez-Marin (ed.), *A Bird's-Eye View of Veterinary Medicine*, print on demand.

Pinto, A.B.F., Saad, F.M.O.B., Leite, C.A.L. et al. (2008). Sodium tripolyphosphate and sodium hexametaphosphate in preventing dental calculus accumulation in dogs. *Arq. Bras Med. Vet. Zoo* 60: 1426–1431.

Prabhakar, A.R., Vipin, A., and Basappa, N. (2009). Effect of curry leaves, garlic and tea tree oil on Streptococcus mutans and lactobacilli in children. *Pesquisa Brasileira de Odontopediatria Clínica Integrada* 9: 259–263.

Puttarak, P., Charoonratana, T., and Panichayupakaranant, P. (2010). Antimicrobial activity and stability of rhinacanthins-rich Rhinacanthus nasutus extract. *Phytomedicine* 17: 323–327.

Roudebush, P., Logan, E., and Hale, F.A. (2005). vidence-based veterinary dentistry: a systematic review of homecare for prevention of periodontal disease in dogs and cats. *J. Vet. Dent.* 22 (1): 6–15.

Servet, E., Hendriks, W., and Clarke, D. (2003). Kibbles can be a useful means in the prevention of feline periodontal disease. *Waltham Focus* 13: 32–35.

Shofiqur, R.A.K.M., Ibrahim, E.S.M., Isoda, R. et al. (2011). Effect of passive immunization by anti-gingipain IgY on periodontal health of dogs. *Vet. Sci. Dev.* 1 (e8): 35–39.

Sookkhee, S., Chulasiri, M., and Prachyabrued, W. (2001). Lactic acid bacteria from healthy oral cavity of Thai volunteers: inhibition of oral pathogens. *J. Appl. Microbiol.* 90 (2): 172–179.

Stookey, G.K. (2009). Soft rawhide reduces calculus formation in dogs. *J. Vet. Dent.* 26: 82–85.

Stookey, G.K., Warrick, J.M., and Miller, L.L. (1995). Effect of sodium hexametaphosphate on dental calculus formation in dogs. *Am. J. Vet. Res.* 56: 913–918.

Stookey, G.K., Warrick, J.M., Miller, L.L. et al. (1996). Hexametaphosphate-coated snack biscuits significantly reduce calculus formation in dogs. *J. Vet. Dent.* 13: 27–30.

Teanpaisan, R. and Dahlen, G. (2006). Use of polymerase chain reaction techniques and sodium dodecyl sulfate-polyacrylamide gel electrophoresis for differentiation of oral *Lactobacillus* species. *Oral Microbiol. Immunol.* 21: 79–83.

Valdevite, L.M., Leitão, D.P., Leite, M.F. et al. (2007). Study of the *in vitro* effect of copaíba oil upon virulence factors of the cariogenic bacterium *Streptococcus mutans*. Annals of 10th IUBMB Conference e 36a Reunião Anual da SBBq, Salvador, Brazil.

Wallis, C., Marshall, M., Colyer, A. et al. (2015). A longitudinal assessment of changes in bacterial community composition associated with the development of periodontal disease in dogs. *Vet. Microbiol.* 181: 271–282.

Wang, H.L., Greenwell, H., and Bissada, N.F. (1990). Crevicular fluid iron changes in treated and untreated periodontally diseased sites. *Oral Surg. Oral Med. Oral Pathol. Oral Radiol. Endod.* 69: 450–456.

Wescombe, P.A., Hale, J.D.F., Heng, N.C.K. et al. (2012). Developing oral probiotics from *Streptococcus salivarius*. *Disclosures Future Microbiol.* 7 (12): 1355–1371.

Wiggs, R.B. and Lobprise, H.B. (1997). Periodontology. In: *Veterinary Dentistry: Principles and Practice* (eds. H.B. Lobprise and J.R. Dodd), 186–231. Philadelphia, PA: Lippincott-Raven.

Winker, S, Timander, S, and Bergstorm, J. (unpublished) The systemic effect of food additive on dental plaque and calculus.

Yim, N. (2010). The antimicrobial activity of compounds from the leaf and stem of *Vitis amurensis* against two oral pathogens. *Bioorg. Med. Chem. Lett.* 20: 1165–1168.

Zambori, C. (2014). The antimicrobial role of probiotics in the oral cavity in humans and dogs. *Scientific Papers: Anim. Sci. Biotechnol.* 47: 126–130.

7

Antimicrobials in Veterinary Dentistry

J. Scott Weese

Ontario Veterinary College, University of Guelph, Guelph, ON, Canada

7.1   Introduction

Antimicrobials have revolutionized the practice of veterinary medicine. Without access to effective and affordable antimicrobials, veterinary medicine would be much different than it is today. Antimicrobials play an important role in the prevention and treatment of oral disease, as well as extraoral disease associated with dental procedures. Yet, they can also be both over- and misused, leading to suboptimal patient care and potential impacts on antimicrobial resistance. The general approach to antimicrobial use in veterinary dentistry is no different than that in other areas of medicine; however, specific data are very sparse. Factors such as expected bacteria, antimicrobial susceptibility (based on culture or reasonable expectations), drug spectrum, drug pharmacokinetics and pharmacodynamics, drug safety, and owner compliance must all be considered when choosing an antimicrobial. Yet, even determination of when to use an antimicrobial and optimal duration can be a challenge. Further, the complex, polymicrobial nature of the canine and feline oral microbiota and the fastidious nature of many potential pathogens create further challenges. Thus, understanding the pathophysiology and optimal methods for preventing and treating disease may be much more complicated than with infections of otherwise sterile body sites.

7.2   Oral Microbiota of Dogs and Cats

The mouth harbors a complex microbial population (the "microbiota") that is increasingly recognized as playing a critical role in many oral and extraoral diseases. An understanding of the "normal" microbiota is important for understanding disease and treatment. Because of the polymicrobial nature of the oral microbiota and the commonness of fastidious organisms that are difficult or impossible to grow using conventional culture methods, it is only in recent years – with broader access to next-generation sequencing – that the oral microbiota has begun to be better understood.

The composition of the microbiota has been described in both dogs and cats (Sturgeon et al. 2014; Costa et al. 2015; Harris et al. 2015; Wallis et al. 2015; Weese et al. 2015), providing important insight. Still, our understanding of specific components of the microbiota that influence the development of plaque, periodontitis, and other conditions is still rather superficial. It must be remembered that the "oral microbiota" is not one specific population. Rather, there are different ecological niches within the oral cavity that presumably foster different microbiota populations. Thus, a composite oral swab might provide interesting information about the general oral environment but little insight into the composition of plaque. Subgingival populations might also be different from supragingival populations, because of the different local environments (e.g., oxygen tension). It must be realized that while developing information about the microbiota may be interesting, application in a clinical context is currently difficult, if not impossible. This will likely change, and it is possible that in the near future, study of the microbiota of different oral niches will provide important guidance for treatment or prevention of disease, or for identification of individuals at high risk for certain diseases.

In both dogs and cats, a wide range of bacterial species are present in highly diverse populations that include a range of dental and opportunistic pathogens, as well as various zoonotic pathogens. The results of studies have varied somewhat based on sampling techniques and laboratory methods, but some general trends can be noted.

The Veterinary Dental Patient: A Multidisciplinary Approach, First Edition. Edited by Jerzy Gawor and Brook Niemiec.
© 2021 John Wiley & Sons Ltd. Published 2021 by John Wiley & Sons Ltd.
Companion website: www.wiley.com/go/gawor/veterinary-dental-patient

In healthy dogs, genera such as *Porphyromonas*, *Bergeyella*, *Actinomyces*, *Peptostreptococcus*, *Pseudomonas*, *Capnocytophaga*, *Pasteurella*, and *Derxia* tend to be predominant (Riggio et al. 2011; Dewhirst et al. 2012; Davis et al. 2013; Sturgeon et al. 2013), while in cats we see *Porphyromonas*, *Moraxella*, *Fusobacterium*, *Pasteurella*, *Neisseria*, *Acinetobacter*, *Pseudomonas*, *Moraxella*, and *Peptostreptococcaceae* (Sturgeon et al. 2014; Harris et al. 2015; Weese et al. 2015). Members of many of these genera are recognized oral or extraoral pathogens. It must be noted that all members of a given genus do not necessarily behave in the same way. The pathogenicity of different species or even strains of the same species may vary – something that is not detected with most current microbiota studies.

Confident association of specific members of the microbiota with health or disease is currently a challenge based on limited study and the complex nature of the microbiota. Associations between certain bacterial taxa and dental disease can be made, but whether these are true causal associations is unclear. It also remains to be determined whether disease is dependent on the presence or absence of certain species versus either their relative abundance (proportion) or absolute abundance, or whether disease effects are due to the effects of single organisms versus combinations of microbes or broader modification of the microbiota. The progression from plaque to gingivitis and periodontitis may also involve different "waves" of inciting microbes, further compounding identification of key components. It is likely that organism abundance and the overall microbiota at different times in the pathophysiology of oral pathology are key determinants of oral cavity disease. This would help reconcile the commonness of taxa typically assumed to be oral pathogens (e.g., *Porphyromonas*, *Treponema*) in healthy animals with results from recent sequence-based studies. Despite these limitations, interesting associations have been identified. Decreases in populations of a variety of Gram-negative bacteria, such as *Bergeyella zoohelcum*, *Moraxella*, *Neisseria shayeganii*, and *Pasteurellaceae*, in plaque were noted during progression to mild periodontitis in one longitudinal study (Wallis et al. 2015). Overrepresentation of *Peptostreptococcus*, *Actinomyces*, *Peptostreptococcaceae*, *Lachnospiraceae*, and *Corynebacterium canis* was noted in dogs with mild periodontitis in another (Davis et al. 2013). In cats, increased relative abundances of *Chlorobi*, *Capnocytophaga*, *Porphyromonas circumdentaria*, and *Bacteroides* sp. in the subgingivial microbiota were associated with health, compared to gingivitis and periodontitis (Harris et al. 2015). *Filifactor villosus* and *Treponema* were positively associated with mild periodontitis in the same study. These results are not entirely consistent with previous assumptions regarding

dental pathogens in dogs and cats, such as a proposed list of putative canine and feline periodontal pathogens that focused on *Bacteroides*, *Porphyromonas* spp., *Peptostreptococcus* spp., *Campylobacter rectus*, and *Treponema denticola* (Harvey 2013). As further research is performed – particularly next-generation sequence-based studies – it is likely that the list of putative canine and feline periodontal pathogens will evolve. Clearly, many questions remain to be answered regarding the microbial pathogenesis of periodontitis, gingivitis, and other conditions of the oral cavity.

7.3 Antimicrobial Use in Human Dentistry

While the oral microbiota, risk of disease, and pathophysiology of disease in humans are not always directly comparable to those in animals, consideration of approaches in human dentistry is warranted, particularly given the relative paucity of data in veterinary medicine. Reasons for antimicrobial administration can generally be divided into four groups: prevention of infective endocarditis, prevention of extraoral implant infections, prevention of oral infections, and treatment of oral infections.

7.3.1 Prevention of Infective Endocarditis

Any procedure that penetrates or traumatizes a mucosal surface creates the potential for translocation of bacteria into tissues and the bloodstream. Transient bacteremia is likely a common (e.g., daily) event in most individuals' lives from minor insults to the oral, gastrointestinal, or reproductive mucosae. Yet, for adverse clinical consequence to occur, there must be an adequate dose of a pathogenic organism that overwhelms the ability of the immune system to contain the event. In humans, bacteremia rates of 7–96% have been reported after dental extraction or dental implant surgery (Lockhart et al. 2008; Piñeiro et al. 2010; Bölükbaşı et al. 2012; Maharaj et al. 2012). Duration of bacteremia tends to be low – typically, less than 15 minutes (Roberts et al. 2006; Maharaj et al. 2012). Even minimally invasive procedures can trigger bacterial translocation, as evidenced by bacteremia rates of 3–46% following tooth brushing (Bhanji et al. 2002; Maharaj et al. 2012). Thus, bacteremia should be considered an expected event following manipulation of the oral mucosa. However, the low dose and duration and the body's immune system typically prevent any adverse consequences.

Despite the rare overall occurrence of infectious sequelae after dental procedures, there are subsets of the population that are known to be at increased risk of infectious

Table 7.1 American Heart Association recommendations for antimicrobial prophylaxis in humans for the prevention of infective endocarditis (Wilson et al. 2007).

Procedures[a]	Patients[a]
All dental procedures that involve manipulation of gingival tissue or the periapical region of teeth or perforation of the oral mucosa	Prosthetic heart valve
	Previously diagnosed infective endocarditis
	Unrepaired cyanotic congenital heart disease, including palliative shunts and conduits
	Completely repeated heart defect with prosthetic material or device during the first six months after the procedure
	Repaired congenital heart disease with residual defects at or adjacent to the site of a prosthetic patch or prosthetic devices
	Heart transplant recipients with developed valvulopathy

[a] At least one criterion from each column must be fulfilled for antimicrobial prophylaxis to be indicated.

complications following bacterial translocation, and antimicrobial prophylaxis is used in human dentistry to reduce the risk of disease in these situations. However, while it can be agreed that there are procedural and patient factors that indicate an elevated risk of complications, actual clinical recommendations are somewhat variable and controversial.

The most strongly supported recommendation for antimicrobial prophylaxis is for individuals with heart diseases that predispose them to infective endocarditis (ADA 2015). American Heart Association (AHA) guidelines, endorsed by the American Dental Association (ADA), Infectious Diseases Society of America (IDSA), and Pediatric Infectious Diseases Society (PIDS), recommend prophylaxis of a relatively small population of patients (Table 7.1) (Wilson et al. 2007). In such individuals, dosing is consistent with perioperative prophylaxis (Bratzler et al. 2013), with the goal of having therapeutic drug levels throughout the period of risk – typically consisting of a single dose of antimicrobial prior to surgery (Wilson et al. 2007). If preoperative dosing is missed, the antimicrobial can be given up to two hours after the procedure (Wilson et al. 2007), after which point there is little use. Amoxicillin is the main recommendation, based on streptococci being the main concern; alternatively, cephalosporins (particularly first- or second-generation drugs), clindamycin, or macrolides are recommended for individuals with drug allergies or intolerances (Wilson et al. 2007).

While the concept that prophylaxis should be reserved for specific high-risk patients is clearly accepted, there is not universal agreement about what that means. The United Kingdom's 2008 National Institute for Health and Care Excellence (NICE) guidelines are somewhat different from AHA recommendations and list individuals with acquired valvular heart disease with stenosis or regurgitation, valve replacement, structural congenital disease,

previous infective endocarditis, and hypertrophic cardiomyopathy as predisposed (NICE 2008). Other guidelines have other differences in patient populations, in large part as a reflection of the limited information about risk for specific cardiac conditions. Regardless, the common focus of these guidelines is the lack of indication for antimicrobial prophylaxis for healthy individuals and those with less profound cardiac disease.

Because of widespread overuse of antimicrobial prophylaxis, antimicrobial stewardship efforts have involved investigation and education regarding prescribing practices. However, a British study reported a significant decrease in antimicrobial prophylaxis for prevention of infective endocarditis after introduction of the NICE guidelines, along with a significant increase in infective endocarditis (Dayer et al. 2015). While this does not indicate a causal relationship, it has raised concerns that current guidelines might be too restrictive or that efforts to curb unnecessary use have inadvertently led to decreased treatment of patients who truly have an indication for prophylaxis. Guidelines for infective endocarditis prevention therefore remain somewhat controversial and will likely continue to evolve.

7.3.2 Prevention of Extra-Oral Implant Infections

Implant-associated infections are a concern because treatment can be difficult and expensive. This is particularly true with total joint infections, where there can be significant patient and economic impacts. In 2009, guidelines developed by the American Academy of Orthopedic Surgeons (AAOS) recommended consideration of antimicrobial prophylaxis for all individuals with total joint replacements prior to any procedure that could cause bacteremia (Little and Jacobson 2010). However, the evidence behind the recommendation for prophylaxis in these individuals was quickly challenged (Brondani 2013), and no association between dental procedures and development of prosthetic joint implant infection has been found (Skaar et al. 2011). In 2012, a revised AAOS guideline (developed in conjunction with the ADA) recommended discontinuing routine prescription of antimicrobials for individuals with total joint implants undergoing dental procedures (AAOS 2012). Similarly, a 2014 panel convened by the ADA Council on Scientific Affairs concluded that prophylactic antibiotics are not recommended for patients with prosthetic joint implants prior to dental procedures (Sollecito et al. 2015).

7.3.3 Prevention of Oral Infections

As with surgical procedures at other body sites, antimicrobial prophylaxis can be used for dental procedures to reduce the risk of local, procedure-associated infections. For oral procedures, this is approached similarly to well-established surgical-site prophylaxis guidelines (Bratzler et al. 2013), with the goal of maintaining therapeutic drug levels at the surgical site throughout the duration of the procedure. This involves administration of an appropriate antimicrobial prior to (usually within 30–60 minutes) of the procedure, with intraoperative redosing every two half-lives of the drug (e.g., ~90 minutes for cefazolin).

Patient and procedure factors dictate when there is a need for prophylaxis. Antimicrobial prophylaxis of all types is coming under increased scrutiny because of concerns about exposing patients unnecessarily to potential adverse effects of antimicrobials and increasing the likelihood of the emergence of antimicrobial resistance.

Antimicrobial prophylaxis has been studied for different dental procedures in humans, with different results. This may be because of differences in efficacy, study rigor, drug regimens, and outcomes. For example, a single preoperative dose of amoxicillin significantly reduced dental implant failure in one study (Veitz-Keenan and Keenan 2015). Yet, in a systematic review, while antimicrobial prophylaxis reduced implant loss by 2%, subgroup analysis identified no benefit in uncomplicated surgery in healthy patients (Lund et al. 2015). Another systemic review concluded that antimicrobial administration was associated with a reduction in implant failure but had no impact on postoperative infection risk (Keenan and Veitz-Keenan 2015). Adverse effects that can be associated with antimicrobial use must also be considered. A systematic review of antimicrobial therapy during third molar extractions identified moderate-quality evidence that the limited benefits obtained (decreased infection risk, alveolar osteitis, and pain) might not justify the adverse effects that

could be encountered (Marghalani 2014). Therefore, even disregarding antimicrobial resistance concerns, adverse effects may negate any advantage in some populations.

7.4 Antimicrobials in Veterinary Dentistry

Issues pertaining to antimicrobial use in veterinary dentistry are analogous to those encountered in human medicine, though there is a paucity of veterinary-specific data. The first and perhaps most important consideration is why an antimicrobial might be needed. This is critical for the identification of patients who need (or, more commonly, do not need) antimicrobials and for the selection of appropriate drugs and dosing regimens.

7.4.1 Treatment of Oral and Dental Infections

The oral cavity is a complex polymicrobial site inhabited by a wide range of potential opportunistic pathogens, as well as bacterial species that contribute to plaque formation. Oral and dental infections are also often complex and would be poorly responsive to antimicrobials as the sole approach, even if the causative agent were identified and susceptibility testing performed. Therefore, the approach to these infections often differs from that toward infections of other body sites.

The American Veterinary Dental College (AVDC) recommends that "Antibiotics should never be considered a monotherapy for treatment of oral infections" (AVDC 2005), a reasonable recommendation given the types of disease that occur. The need to address any underlying causes or factors that would inhibit response to antimicrobials, such as the presence of an abscess or foreign body or of an infection in an avascular site (e.g., a nonvital tooth), is critical for successful treatment and cannot be overemphasized.

Antimicrobials may be indicated as an adjunctive treatment measure in cases where there is infection of normally noninfected sites, where those sites are adequately vascularized and other measures are not adequate to address the infection (e.g., removal of an abscessed tooth). The presence of an infection at an otherwise sterile site does not necessarily mean antimicrobials are indicated. In some situations, other measures can adequately control the infection, such as drainage of an abscess where there is limited evidence of infection of associated tissues (e.g., no cellulitis in the adjacent areas, no systemic signs not attributable to the pain of the abscess). When antimicrobials are used, culture and susceptibility results should be considered. This can be problematic in situations where collecting an uncontaminated sample is difficult. Aspiration of potentially infected sites through aseptically prepared skin rather than through oral mucosal surfaces may be an option in some cases, and when sampling must be done through a polymicrobial site where contamination in unavoidable, it is reasonable to question whether culture will provide much guidance. Another potential limitation of culture is the commonness of anaerobic infections. The ability of diagnostic laboratories to isolate, identify, and perform antimicrobial susceptibility testing on anaerobes and other fastidious organisms is variable. Anaerobes are often also fastidious and can die between sampling and the laboratory. Collecting samples into anaerobic transport media and ensuring prompt transportation to the laboratory can increase the yield (Figure 7.1). The transport medium must be exactly the one recommended by the referring laboratory. Samples for anaerobic culture are best kept at room temperature for short storage, rather than refrigeration temperature, because oxygen diffuses into them more readily at lower temperatures. Regardless of what is done, it is important to remember that a negative culture does not necessarily mean that an infection was not present. If clinical signs and understanding of the disease process are supportive of an infection, cases should be managed as if an infection were present, typically ensuring that adequate anaerobic coverage is provided.

The choice of antimicrobials is dictated in part by culture results, where available. However, whether based on culture or empirical decisions, a small number of drugs are commonly used in dental infections, particularly clindamycin and amoxicillin/clavulanic acid (Table 7.2). These provide excellent antianaerobic activity and are active against the main pathogens that are typically encountered, but they may not be optimal in all situations.

Osteomyelitis can be difficult to treat because of poor vascularity and associated difficulties delivering therapeutic drug levels to the infected site (Figure 7.2).

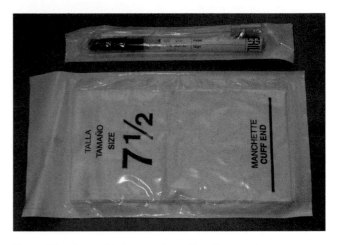

Figure 7.1 Anaerobic transport medium for sample collection (top). Sterile gloves should be used when obtaining samples (bottom).

Table 7.2 Common dental antimicrobials.

Antimicrobial	Dose	Comments
Clindamycin	Dogs: 11–22 mg/kg (q 12–24 h) Cats: 11–33 mg/kg (q 24 h)	Excellent anaerobic spectrum. Reasonable penetration into bone (Zetner et al. 2003).
Amoxicillin/clavulanic acid	12.5–20 mg/kg (q 12 h)	Broad spectrum, including aerobes and anaerobes. Excellent oral option for anaerobes and Gram-positives. Less effective against beta-lactamase-producing *E. coli* than Gram-positives. Injectable formulation available in some regions.
Doxycycline	5 mg/kg PO (q 12 h)	Broad-spectrum bacteriostatic drug. Has many good properties but is difficult to justify over beta-lactams.
Cefovecin	8 mg/kg SC	Tissue levels and duration of activity in oral infections are not known. Duration of activity is usually beyond what is needed.
Cefazolin	20–22 mg/kg IV preoperatively	First-generation cephalosporin. Good Gram-positive and anaerobic activity. Reasonable Gram-negative activity. Good for periprocedural administration.
Cefoxitin	20–30 mg/kg IV preoperatively	Second-generation cephalosporin, with broader Gram-negative activity compared to cefazolin. Good for periprocedural administration.
Metronidazole	Dogs: 15 mg/kg PO (q 12 h) Cats: 10–25 mg/kg PO (q 24 h)	Excellent anaerobic spectrum. No activity against aerobes.
Amoxicillin	22 mg/kg PO (q 8 h)	Good activity against Gram-negatives, Gram-positives, aerobes, and anaerobes. Ineffective against beta-lactamase-producing bacteria.
Ampicillin	20–40 mg/kg IV	As for amoxicillin. Good for periprocedural prophylaxis, especially for streptococci.

(a)

(b)

(c)

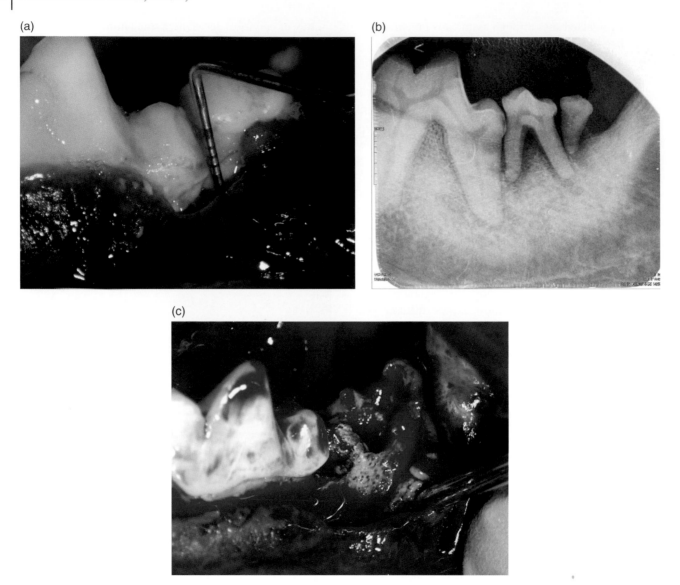

Figure 7.2 (a) Deep periodontal pocket in the left mandibular molar area of a German Shepherd. (b) Radiograph showing features of periodontal disease, osteomyelitis and bone necrosis. (c) Debridement of necrotic bone during the surgical procedure.

The potential for biofilm involvement and the presence of sequestra further complicate treatment. Treatment of osteomyelitis is best guided by culture and susceptibility data from properly (aseptically) collected samples. This can be difficult with some infected sites but should be performed whenever possible to allow for optimal antimicrobial selection. Antimicrobials that achieve good levels in bone should be chosen. This can be complicated because of limited veterinary data. In humans, injectable antimicrobials are preferred because of the typically greater bone penetration. Long-term (e.g., four to six weeks) injectable therapy is often unrealistic in veterinary patients. Clindamycin, metronidazole, fluoroquinolones, and doxycycline penetrate bone reasonably well in humans (Spellberg and Lipsky 2012) and are reasonable considerations in dogs and cats, depending on the known or suspected pathogens.

Dental abscesses are common, and while they are typically the result of bacterial infections, antimicrobials are rarely indicated (Figure 7.3). Elimination of bacteria within abscesses is difficult because of poor vascularity (and therefore limited drug delivery) and inhibition of antimicrobials by organic debris or local conditions (e.g., pH). Incision and draining is the hallmark approach to treatment of any abscess that can be drained. In most situations, opening of the abscess and removal of any inciting cause (e.g., tooth) is adequate for complete resolution of disease. Antimicrobials should be reserved for situations where there is evidence of local tissue involvement (e.g., cellulitis, osteomyelitis) or systemic disease.

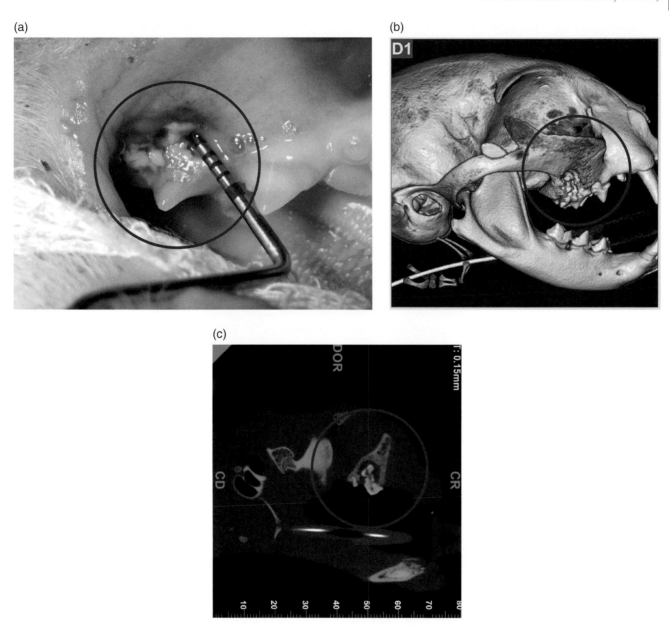

Figure 7.3 Odontogenic abscess in a cat: (a) deep periodontal pocket (circles) in the area of 108; (b) 3D reconstruction of the affected maxilla; and (c) CBCT scan showing features of 108 abscess and tooth resorption.

7.4.2 Prevention of Oral Infections Associated with Dental Procedures

The principles of antimicrobial prophylaxis for surgical-site infections can be applied to dental procedures, though the range of procedures for which prophylaxis is indicated is essentially unknown. It presumably is for any procedure involving an implant, because of the difficulty in eliminating implant-associated infections, as well as any procedure with extensive involvement or compromise of bone. Otherwise, despite the fact that oral surgery involves a site contaminated with the oral microbiota, the extent is unclear. Extrapolation from humans is reasonable when no corresponding veterinary data are available, so recommendations such as a single perioperative antimicrobial dose of a beta-lactam (e.g., cafazolin, cefoxitin) would be reasonable. Clindamycin is widely used in veterinary dentistry because of its efficacy against anaerobes; however, it has a limited Gram-negative spectrum – something that could be of concern given the potential role of bacteria such as *Pasteurella* in oral infections. Intravenous administration is preferred whenever possible. Intramuscular administration tends to result in relatively rapid systemic drug levels, but is less predictable than intravenous administration. Oral antimicrobials should not be used for pre-procedure antimicrobial prophylaxis. Duration of therapy has been poorly studied. In human medicine, post-procedure antimicrobials are rarely indicated: something that probably also applies to most veterinary procedures in the absence of pre-existing infection or other complicating factors.

7.4.3 Prevention of Bacteremia and Infective Endocarditis

Probably the area with the most use – and overuse (Figure 7.4) – of antimicrobials in veterinary dentistry is peri-dental-procedure prophylaxis. As in human dentistry, it is an area of increasing discussion and concern, but also one that is sorely lacking in data. Bacteremia rates associated with dental procedures are undoubtedly high in dogs and cats, though objective data are limited. A small study reported bacteremia in 85% of dogs (17/20) within 20 minutes of the start of dental procedures, with a mean duration of detectable bacteremia of 47 minutes (Nieves et al. 1997).

Study of the association between dental procedures and infective endocarditis has been limited. While complications such as endocarditis and pericardial effusion have been reported after dental prophylaxis (Tou et al. 2005; Lobetti 2007), the high frequency of dental procedures must be considered when evaluating reports that simply describe single cases or series of cases without an indication of proportions or relative risk. If a procedure is performed on many animals, there will invariably be those that develop disease afterward, whether as a result of the procedure or due to an unrelated event. A retrospective case-control study did not identify a history of dental or

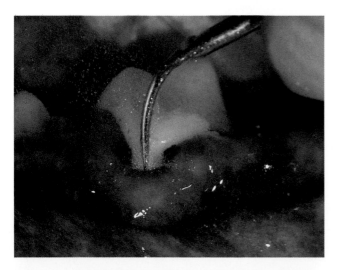

Figure 7.4 Antimicrobial prophylaxis for routine descaling is the most common overuse of antibiotics in veterinary dentistry.

oral procedures in the three months preceding diagnosis of endocarditis in any of 76 affected dogs (Peddle et al. 2009). This would suggest that routine antimicrobial prophylaxis is not needed for all dogs undergoing dental procedures, but the study did not look at dogs that would plausibly be deemed at higher risk (e.g., those with cardiac disease), where an association might be present. A historical-observational study evaluating dogs with a history of periodontal disease identified a sixfold increase in the incidence of endocarditis in those with severe periodontal disease compared to those with no or mild disease (Glickman et al. 2009). A study such as this cannot prove causation, however, and provides only limited guidance, because of a lack of information about factors that might drive the risk (e.g., is it higher for all dogs or just those with specific risk factors such as mitral valve abnormalities?).

Accordingly, limitations in veterinary data preclude good evidence-based decision making regarding antimicrobial prophylaxis. In the absence of species-specific data, it is reasonable to assume that the same general concepts and risks should apply to animals as to humans. A 2005 policy statement by the AVDC recommends the use of antimicrobials to reduce bacteremia for "animals that are immune compromised, have underlying systemic disease (such as clinically-evident cardiac, hepatic, and renal diseases) and/or when severe oral infection is present" (AVDC 2005). However, what constitutes "immune compromised" is not explained, and "clinically evident cardiac, hepatic and renal disease" could encompass a wide range of high- and low-risk patients. Therefore, this statement provides little specific guidance and will probably lead to unnecessary treatment.

More specific guidance is required for effective and prudent perioperative antimicrobial therapy. Ideally, this would be based on veterinary-specific evidence – including high-level evidence (i.e., randomized controlled trials). However, prospective trials are difficult, given the low incidence of infectious complications and the corresponding need for massive sample sizes. While that should not be taken as a reason not to try to get good evidence, it must be understood that from a practical standpoint, current guidance will be based on human data, limited (and typically lower-level) veterinary data, and principles of antimicrobial prophylaxis, infectious diseases, and infection control. A key aspect is determining which patients and which procedures constitute enough risk to justify antimicrobial prophylaxis. As with the AVDC position statement, some recommendations have been quite broad, such as that for antimicrobial prophylaxis in patients with immunocompromise, feline immunodeficiency virus infection, surgical implants, or a wide range of metabolic, hepatic, cardiac, pancreatic, and renal disorders (Peak 2013). Similarly, it has

Table 7.3 Potential criteria for identification of veterinary patients that require antimicrobial prophylaxis prior to dental procedures (Soukup 2015).

Patient factors[a]	Procedures[a]
Patent ductus arteriosis	Dental cleaning that is expected to cause hemorrhage
Unrepaired cyanotic congenital heart disease	Any oral or periodontal surgery
Subaortic or aortic stenosis	Endodontic surgery
Previous infective endocarditis	
Imbedded pacemaker leads	

[a] At least one factor from *each* column must be present.

been recommended that geriatric or debilitated animals, animals with pre-existing heart or system disease, and animals with immunocompromise receive prophylactic antimicrobials (Gorrel 2013). Both of these recommendations would potentially result in treatment of a relatively large percentage of patients and would be inconsistent with current recommendations for human dentistry. Further, clarity regarding what constitutes "immunocompromise" or a relevant comorbidity is lacking. A more restrictive set of criteria has been suggested (Table 7.3). While subjective, these would constitute a reasonable approach to identifying patient and procedure combinations that represent a high risk. Under them, a very small subject of patients would quality for antimicrobial prophylaxis.

When prophylactic therapy is used, the goal is to have therapeutic drug levels at the site of the procedure throughout its duration. While there is little objective guidance for veterinary dentistry, surgical-site prophylaxis and human dentistry guidelines can reasonably be applied. For time-dependent antimicrobials (e.g., beta-lactams), the goal is to administer them within one hour of the start of the procedure. Because of the short half-life of most beta-lactams, administration prior to that can result in subtherapeutic levels throughout the duration of the procedure, necessitating redosing every two half-lives of the drug.

Drug choices should be focused on the most likely causes of infective endocarditis, not necessarily the most common inhabitants of the oral microbiota or what is used to treat dental infections. In humans, amoxicillin and ampicillin are the main recommendations for prevention of infective endocarditis or prosthetic device-associated infection (Wilson et al. 2007), with clindamycin recommended for penicillin-allergic patients. If patients are at particularly high risk (i.e., individuals with previous infective endocarditis or an artificial heart valve), amoxicillin/ampicillin plus gentamicin is recommended.

Gram-positive cocci, particularly *Streptococcus canis*, tend to be the most commonly reported causes of infective

endocarditis in dogs and cats (Sykes et al. 2006), so prophylactic therapy should be targeted toward these groups. Enterobacteriaceae and other Gram-negative bacteria are not uncommon and must be considered, particularly given the commonness of some members (e.g., *Pasteurella*) in the oral microbiota. Ampicillin is highly effective against streptococci and is a reasonable consideration. In regions where injectable amoxicillin/clavulanic acid or ampicillin/sulbactam is available, this would be a good choice to provide broader coverage against beta-lactamase-producing organisms (especially staphylococci and Enterobacteriaceae). Amoxicillin/clavulanic acid is widely available as an oral preparation, but this is suboptimal for peri-procedure prophylaxis as it is harder to predict the onset and duration of therapeutic levels, and intraoperative redosing is not possible. Clindamycin provides excellent anaerobic and streptococcal coverage, and it can be considered, but it is ineffective against Gram-negatives. Cephalosporins are also good options because of their efficacy against streptococci and most beta-lactamase-producing bacteria (Figure 7.5).

Treatment before a dental procedure outside of the peri-procedure prophylaxis window (e.g., more than one hour before the procedure) is often performed in veterinary patients, but this approach has not been evaluated. The general concept is to use antimicrobials a few days to a week before a procedure to reduce the bacterial burden and therefore bacterial translocation. Whether pretreatment actually reduces overall bacterial burden or decreases translocation risk (since an abundant microbiota will remain, regardless of treatment) is unclear. It is possible that a clinically relevant reduction in bacterial load could occur. It is also possible that pretreatment would select for more of a resistant oral population that would increase the chance of a resistant bacterial infection. No reasonable conclusion can be made with current evidence about whether pretreatment is effective, neutral, or harmful if there is no underlying disease that is being treated.

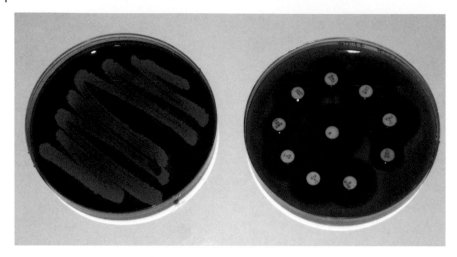

Figure 7.5   Cultured bacteria from a periodontal abscess with antibiotic susceptibility.

7.5   Prophylaxis for Patients with Orthopedic Implants

While there is fairly widespread (albeit not universal) support for prophylaxis for prevention of infective endocarditis in certain situations, the risk associated with surgical implants or prosthetic joints is very unclear. This author is aware of no evidence or anecdotal information suggesting that dogs with prosthetic joints or other surgical implants (e.g., tibial-plateau-leveling osteotomy, TPLO) are at increased risk of infection. Delayed-onset infections – those that occur months to years after the surgery – are rare in animals, but they do occur. While these might be the result of transient bacteremia well after the time of surgery, data suggesting that dental procedures have been an inciting cause are lacking. Given the lack of any evidence from veterinary medicine, and with human guidelines that do not support prophylactic treatment, prophylaxis for patients with a surgical implant cannot be recommended.

7.6   Periodontal Disease Control

While periodontitis is incited by the effects of bacteria, systemic antimicrobials are not recommended for routine periodontal disease prevention or treatment (Gorrel 2013). In humans, systemic antimicrobials are sometimes used for generalized aggressive and necrotizing periodontal disease, in conjunction with other treatments (Purucker et al. 2001; Casarin et al. 2012; Teughels et al. 2014). Amoxicillin plus metronidazole, clindamycin, or amoxicillin/clavulanic acid are commonly used. However, this is applicable to only a small percentage of individuals with severe and specific types of periodontal disease. The complex microbial nature of the oral environment, limited tissue penetration of bacteria involved in the pathophysiology of disease, reduced efficacy of antimicrobials in organic debris-laden environments, and limited antimicrobial efficacy in plaque, among other factors, limit the potential efficacy of systemic antimicrobials for most types of periodontal disease, particularly when scaling and root planing is highly efficacious.

As in humans, there may be specific veterinary patients with periodontal disease that benefit from systemic antimicrobials as an adjunct to other treatments. Which patients this group encompasses is not well defined, but it probably includes those with severely affected tissues that antimicrobials are capable of penetrating. Antimicrobials may help reduce inflammation, improve the rate of recovery, and reduce the likelihood of extension of infection into bone or other structures. They should be reserved for those patients with particularly severe disease in whom proper adjunctive treatment is performed. They should not be used in lieu of appropriate dental therapy, regardless of the severity of disease. To the degree that antimicrobials are indicated, proper concurrent dental treatment is an absolute necessity.

A broader range of patients with periodontal disease would likely benefit from local therapy. Local application of antimicrobials into periodontal pockets has been used to provide a high-dose local effect with limited systemic exposure. In humans, various effects such as decreased inflammation, improved wound healing, and reduced osteoclast function have been identified (Garrett et al. 1999, 2000; Wennström et al. 2001; Paquette et al. 2004). Doxycycline and clindamycin local-delivery systems have been studied and used in veterinary patients as adjunctive treatments to scaling and root planing. Application of a clindamycin hydrochloride gel reduced periodontal pocket depth, gingival index, and gingival bleeding in dogs (Johnston et al. 2011). A biodegradable doxycycline delivery system reduced bleeding on probing and probe depths in beagles with severe periodontal disease (Polson et al. 1996), while reduced gingival index and increased attachment were achieved with a doxycycline polymer (Zetner and Rothmueller 2002). The amount of exposure of the oral microbiota and potential impacts on resistance are not well understood. However, local administration of small volumes of antimicrobial gel within periodontal pockets presumably results in minimal exposure of the microbiota and poses limited risk of antimicrobial resistance or other adverse effects.

Use of doxycycline for its anti-inflammatory properties has been reported. A reduction in periodontal disease score was identified in research beagles following administration of an eight-week course of low-dose (2 mg/kg PO q 24 h) doxycycline (Kim et al. 2015). However, it has been recommended that antimicrobials not be used in animals for any non-antimicrobial effects (Weese et al. 2015), because of the typically limited clinical efficacy and concerns about antimicrobial resistance. While one study reported no emergence of resistance during doxycycline treatment, the design was inadequate to make any reasonable assessment; accordingly, the use of doxycycline – a drug ranked "highly important" by the World Health Organization (WHO 2005) – in this manner should be discouraged.

Pulse therapy involving periodic (e.g., one week a month) systemic antimicrobial treatment has been used by some clinicians as a means of controlling disease. It has not been shown to be effective, and approaches such as this should be avoided in the absence of evidence of efficacy (Weese et al. 2015).

7.7 Plaque Control

Plaque is a bacterial biofilm: a complex structure containing a sessile community of bacteria embedded in a matrix of carbohydrates, protein, and DNA (Figure 7.6).

Since plaque accumulation is a precursor to gingivitis and periodontal disease (Lindhe et al. 1975), plaque reduction is a critical aspect of care. While plaque is produced by bacteria, antimicrobial approaches to plaque control are limited based on a poor understanding of plaque development (e.g., which species contribute), the omnipresent potential for plaque formation in the oral cavity, limitations in the efficacy of antimicrobials against biofilm-embedded bacteria, and the efficacy of physical removal. Within a biofilm, bacteria typically have decreased susceptibility to antimicrobials and the immune system. Plaque possesses a physical protective barrier that hampers penetration of antimicrobials and immune-system activity. Further, biofilm-embedded bacteria typically have an altered (down-regulated) metabolism that decreases susceptibility to antimicrobials, particularly those that target actively dividing cells. The minimum inhibitory concentrations of most antimicrobials can be profoundly elevated in biofilms, rendering susceptibility data of limited clinical value. Most systemically delivered antimicrobials would be expected to have limited impact on the complex and abundant biofilm-associated microbiota. Eradication of plaque-producing bacteria – species that have evolved with the dog – is impractical and simply creates increased opportunities for antimicrobial resistance.

Oral administration of biocides such as chlorhexidine (CHX), amine fluoride/stannous fluoride/zinc lactate, triclosan, cetylpyridinium, and sodium hypochlorite can reduce plaque and associated dental diseases in humans (Galván et al. 2014; Ayad et al. 2015; Elias-Boneta

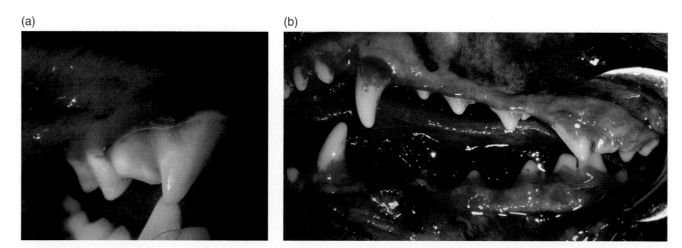

(a) (b)

Figure 7.6 Presence of dental plaque demonstrated with the use of (a) ultraviolet light and (b) disclosing solution.

(a)

(b)

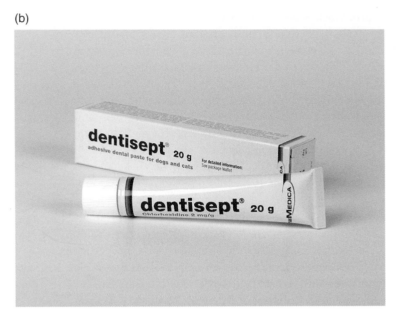

(c)

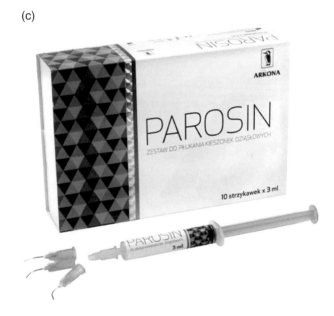

Figure 7.7 Antiseptics used in veterinary dentistry: (a) Vet aquadent, containing Xylitol; (b) Dentisept, containing chlorhexidine (CHX); and (c) Parosin, containing nanocolloid silver.

et al. 2015a,b; Marchetti et al. 2017). Numerous commercial products are available (Figure 7.7). Use of mouthwashes is not feasible in animals, but other local plaque-control approaches such as dental chews may be applied. Whether biocides can be added to chews is an open question, since non-biocide chews have been associated with reduced plaque, gingivitis, and calculus (Gorrel and Rawlings 1996; Rawlings et al. 1998; Gorrel and Bierer 1999; Ingham et al. 2002; Brown and McGenity 2005;

Hennet et al. 2006; Clarke et al. 2011; Quest 2013), without side effect (Rawlings et al. 1998; Hennet 2001; Brown and McGenity 2005).

Direct topical application is another approach, though of lesser practicality. A CHX-containing dental gel that was applied following teeth cleaning had a short-term impact on plaque formation (Hennet 2002). Whether the effort required versus regular tooth brushing is justified is unclear.

7.8 Infection Control

While infection control is an emerging field in veterinary hospitals, there has been virtually no study of it as it relates to veterinary dentistry. This is in stark contrast with human dentistry, where profound advances have occurred over the past few decades, driven by the potential for transmission of serious bloodborne (e.g., human immunodeficiency virus [HIV] and hepatitis B virus [HBV]) and respiratory (e.g., influenza virus, tuberculosis) pathogens between patients on equipment. Transmission can occur through various routes, including direct contact with blood and body fluids and indirect contact via contaminated objects (e.g., equipment, environment), as well as mucous membrane exposure to infectious droplets, aerosols (small particles transmitted over short distances), and airborne pathogens (microbes that remain suspended in air for prolonged periods and distances). Because most, if not all, of the relevant pathogens can be transmitted from clinically normal individuals, routine infection-control practices are designed to reduce the risk of exposure in the event that any given individual possesses an infectious disease risk (Kohn et al. 2004). Enhanced precautions may be applied in situations where increased risk is present, but the main focus is on the routine use of good hygiene practices.

Fortunately, veterinary dentistry is not associated with exposure to the same spectrum of human pathogens. However, every veterinary patient harbors multiple zoonotic pathogens, and the close contact with the oral cavity, close proximity of the operator's eyes and mucous membranes to the patient, and high frequency of aerosolization create an inherent risk. Meanwhile, cross-contamination of various pathogens on equipment and environmental surfaces could be associated with transmission of pathogens between patients. Therefore, infection control is an important but often overlooked area, and one that is necessary for optimal patient care and protection of veterinary personnel.

Extensive infection-control guidelines are available for human dentistry, such as the US Centers for Disease Control and Prevention's (CDC) "Guidelines for Infection Control in Dental Health-care Settings" (Kohn et al. 2004). This comprehensive document, along with general veterinary infection-control resources (NASPHV 2006; Anderson et al. 2008), could form the foundation of a veterinary dental infection control program. A comprehensive overview of infection control in veterinary dental settings is beyond the scope of this chapter, but some selected areas will be examined here.

7.8.1 Personal Protective Equipment

Personal protective equipment (PPE) is designed to reduce contamination of the skin, mucous membranes, and clothing.

Basic PPE consists of dedicated clinic outerwear, which is typically a lab coat over street clothes. Surgical scrubs are widely used in veterinary facilities as a combination of clothing and protective outerwear, but they are a suboptimal choice. In human dentistry, scrubs (or any other type of uniform) are not considered PPE and must still be covered by a laboratory coat or gown (Kohn et al. 2004). Lab coats can be easily and quickly changed when contaminated and provide more body protection (e.g., full arms). Scrubs can be part of in-clinic clothing, but they should be covered by another item during any patient care activities. Outerwear should be worn only in the clinic, to avoid transmission of pathogens to the community. It should be changed whenever visibly soiled, and on a regular basis otherwise (even when outwardly clean), since contamination is not always readily apparent. Additional PPE may be required depending on the patient and the activities to be performed. This could include gowns, gloves, masks, eye protection, or a face shield (Figure 7.8).

For routine examination, a lab coat is adequate. In contrast, dental procedures are somewhat unique in the potential for aerosolization of microbes and the close proximity of personnel to the aerosolized "cloud." Ocular infections are a recognized occupational risk in human dentistry (Al Wazzan et al. 2001; Farrier et al. 2006); similar risks are likely present in veterinary dentistry, because any activity that involves the use of forced air and/or water or high-speed instruments can aerosolize potential pathogens over short distances. The distance of aerosolization depends on the velocity (which will vary greatly) and the particle size generated, but the main risk is probably over a few meters or less. Nonetheless, the oral, nasal, and ocular mucous membranes of personnel involved in dental procedures can easily be exposed to infectious aerosols. This typically

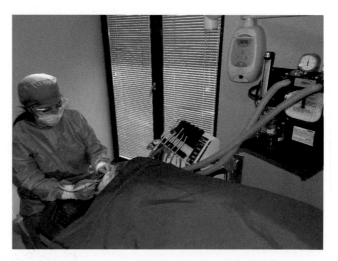

Figure 7.8 Personal protective equipment: gown, gloves, mask, and eye protection.

includes assistants and individuals monitoring anesthesia. For these reasons, a face shield or a mask and eye protection should be used for any procedure that has a reasonable likelihood of generating aerosols. Reusable outerwear (e.g., glasses/goggles, face shield) should be disinfected (usually by spraying or wiping with a good environmental disinfectant) after removal. Anecdotally, contact lens-associated ocular infections have occurred in veterinarians performing dental procedures, probably through a combination of inadequate eye protection and the increased risk of infection in contact lens wearers (Lin et al. 2015). This population should be particularly diligent about eye protection when performing any dental procedures (Figure 7.9).

Gloves provide a useful barrier and are standard-use in human dentistry, but are less commonly used during examinations in animals. Bare-hand examination of the mouth is probably of limited risk to most individuals, but this risk can nonetheless be reasonably assumed to be higher than when wearing gloves. Gloves should be mandatory when there are breaks in an individual's skin or where the individual is at increased risk of opportunistic infection (e.g., immunocompromised, pregnant). However, while gloves can be useful, they are not an absolute barrier and must be used properly. Micropunctures are not uncommon, even with surgical gloves (Na'aya et al. 2009; Harnoss et al. 2010; Hübner et al. 2010), and can lead to contamination. Contamination of the hands during glove removal is

also common. Therefore, hand hygiene must be performed after removal – something that is often overlooked (Anderson et al. 2014).

7.8.2 Hand Hygiene

One of the simplest and least expensive infection-control practices, hand hygiene is often poorly performed in veterinary hospitals (Anderson et al. 2014). It can involve hand washing or the use of alcohol-based hand sanitizers, and can significantly reduce bacterial burden on the hands and presumably the risk of transmission of pathogens to patients, the environment, and personnel. Hand washing and the use of hand sanitizers are largely interchangeable, but the former is indicated when there has been gross contamination of the hands or where an alcohol-resistant organism is of concern (e.g., clostridial spores, a nonenveloped virus, dermatophytes). Hand sanitizers are increasingly used because of their convenience and lesser tendency to irritate the skin. When hand washing is performed in a clinical setting, antibacterial soap should be used. Common problems with hand hygiene include failing to do anything, inadequate duration of washing, inadequate volume of sanitizer, and recontamination immediately after washing (Anderson et al. 2014).

7.8.3 Facility Design

Proper facility design is necessary to reduce the risk of infection to dental patients, clients, and personnel. A properly designed facility helps personnel follow standard infection-control practices and reduces the risk of direct or indirect transmission of pathogens, while poorly designed facilities can hamper (or preclude) the use of good practices and contribute to risk.

Common problems include:

- Performing dental procedures in an open area where aerosol exposure of other patients may occur (e.g. bandage changing, pre-operative preparation).
- Locating sinks in areas not conducive to good hand hygiene.
- Storing consumable items (e.g. bandage material) in open cabinets or on countertops in the vicinity of aerosol-generating procedures.

7.8.4 Sharps Handling

Among all the areas that differ between veterinary and human medicine, one of the more striking is the approach to sharps handling and sharp injuries (Figure 7.10). In human medicine, bloodborne pathogens such as HIV and hepatitis viruses have prompted intensive efforts to reduce

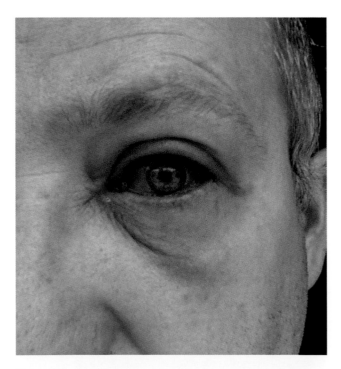

Figure 7.9 Conjunctivitis as a result of wearing contact lenses during a dental procedure without sufficient eye protection. Source: Maciej Gawor

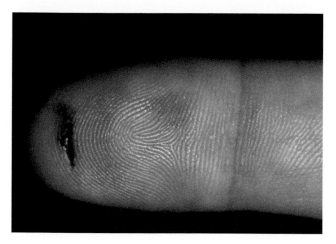

Figure 7.10 Skin wound caused by lack of protection of sharp working tips.

Table 7.4 Basic measures to reduce the incidence of needlestick injuries.

Dispose of needles and scalpel blades directly into an approved sharps container

Have sharps containers located everywhere sharps are used

Never recap a needle by hand: use a scoop method, forceps, or some other hands-free approach

Never leave needles (capped or uncapped) on counters or in pockets

Ensure proper technique is used when passing sharp objects

Record needlestick injuries so that rates can be known and patterns detected

Ensure proper restraint of the patient (physical or chemical) is used whenever sharps are employed

sharps injuries, encompassing training, surveillance of sharps injuries, and the use of safety-engineered devices (e.g., syringes with retractable needles). Sharps injuries are considered significant events. In veterinary medicine, by contrast, there is much less attention to sharps injuries, to the point where they are often considered an inherent and unremarkable "part of the job." Needlestick injury rates are very high in veterinary personnel (Poole et al. 1998; Leggat et al. 2009; Weese and Faires 2009), and while most do not cause problems, complications ranging from local pain to drug reactions, severe infections, and even death can occur (Jones 1996; Wilkins and Bowman 1997; Poole et al. 1998; O'Neill et al. 2005; Veenhuizen et al. 2006; Weese and Faires 2009). The author is unaware of any specific study of sharps injuries associated with dental procedures, but it is likely that injuries from needles, scalpel blades, and other sharp instruments are far from uncommon.

Two main approaches can be made to reducing sharps injuries: physical and behavioral. Physical approaches involve the use of sharps that pose a lower risk of injury, such as retractable needles. These are uncommonly used in veterinary medicine, in part because of cost but probably mainly because of lack of recognition of the problem. The advantage of safety-engineered devices is that they reduce reliance on behaviors, and behaviors are usually the weakest link in any infection-control program. Yet, optimizing how people handle sharps remains the most important approach in veterinary medicine (Table 7.4).

7.8.5 Environmental Cleaning and Disinfection

Cleaning and disinfection are routine practices for veterinary facilities, but often limited thought goes into the development of regimens. Cleaning and disinfection are

two separate steps, both of which must be performed properly for effective reduction in environmental pathogen burdens. The goal of environmental cleaning and disinfection is to reduce the environmental microbial burden, not to sterilize the environment. A wide range of microorganisms, including opportunistic pathogens, zoonotic pathogens, and multidrug-resistant bacteria, will remain in the clinic environment even after a thorough cleaning and disinfection (Weese et al. 2000; Weese 2007; Hamilton et al. 2012). Cleaning and disinfection should help reduce these burdens and decrease the likelihood of infection of patients and personnel.

The first and most important step is cleaning. Physical removal of debris through cleaning with water and detergent removes the majority of pathogens. It also renders the environment amenable to disinfection, since organic debris can inactive disinfectants. After a surface has been adequately cleaned, an appropriate disinfectant should be applied at the correct concentration and for the indicated amount of time. Spectrum of activity, concentration, contact time, and other factors vary between disinfectants, and the choice among them should be made based on these and on cost, safety, and risk aversion. Quaternary ammonium disinfectants are widely used in veterinary facilities and are generally low-cost, reasonably effective products. Newer approaches – particularly accelerated hydrogen peroxide – offer benefits in terms of enhanced spectrum of activity, safety, contact time, and effectiveness in organic debris.

7.8.6 Pre-Procedure Biocide Mouth Rinse

Oral rinsing with biocides such as CHX can effectively reduce bacterial numbers in some species. This may be desirable in patients undergoing dental procedures, particularly ones involving penetration into deeper, sterile sites or patients with advanced oral disease. In humans,

CHX mouth washing has been shown to reduce post-extraction bacteremia (Barbosa et al. 2015). It is unclear whether reduction of oral bacterial bioburden through peri-procedural biocide rinsing can confer a clinical benefit in dogs and cats, since an abundant microbiota would remain. Another potential benefit of pre-procedure mouth rinsing is a reduction in bacterial aerosolization, something that has been demonstrated in humans (Kaur et al. 2014).

7.8.7 Equipment Cleaning, Disinfection, and Sterilization

A comprehensive discussion of cleaning, disinfection, and sterilization is beyond the scope of this section, but it is important to understand some general concepts (Table 7.5). Cleaning involves the removal of gross contamination, and with it, the majority of contaminants. Disinfection is designed to reduce the contaminant burden, and is classified into three categories: low-, intermediate-, and high-level. Sterilization involves elimination of all viable microorganisms.

Spaulding's classification (Spaulding 1968) (Table 7.6) is the most widely recognized system for identifying disinfection and sterilization needs, and is applicable to most veterinary situations. Differentiating between dental instruments that contact mucous membranes and those that enter sterile tissue can be difficult. Since most pieces

of dental equipment tolerate steam sterilization, all dental tools that can be autoclaved, should be autoclaved (Figure 7.11).

"Cold sterilization" is a misnomer, but the procedure is still widely used in some regions. It is better referred to as chemical disinfection, as that is more descriptive and reinforces that fact that disinfection – not sterilization – is typically the goal. Chemical disinfection involves immersion of instruments in a disinfectant solution, but it is fraught with potential problems, including those caused by the use of a poor disinfectant, contamination of the disinfectant solution, inadequate cleaning prior to immersion, inadequate disinfectant concentration, and inadequate contact time. Contact times vary between products, but typically are many hours, and every time an instrument (or finger) enters the solution, the contact time must restart, even for items that were not directly handled. These issues probably account for the ability to isolate viable bacteria from a reasonable percentage of cold-sterile solutions in veterinary clinics (Murphy et al. 2010). Because of the simple effectiveness of steam sterilization, cold sterilization should not be used for items that can be steam sterilized and that are used for surgical or dental procedures.

Some items cannot tolerate steam sterilization, and for these, clear instructions must be made available – ideally from the manufacturer – about appropriate decontamination methods. This can be problematic for items that are marketed for single-use in the human medical field but are

Table 7.5 Basic goals of cleaning, disinfection, and sterilization.

Method	Targeted effect
Cleaning	Removal of visible contamination and reduction in invisible contamination (e.g. biofilm)
Low-level disinfection	Inactivation of vegetative bacteria, non-enveloped viruses, and some fungi
Intermediate-level disinfection	Inactivation of vegetative bacteria and most viruses and fungi. Does not necessarily eliminate bacterial spores, mycobacteria, or hardy (non-enveloped) viruses
High-level disinfection	Inactivation of all microorganisms except bacterial spores
Sterilization	Inactivation of all microorganisms

Table 7.6 Required cleaning and disinfection practices for different types of equipment.

Classification	Patient use	Examples	Decontamination method[a]
Noncritical	Contacts intact skin	Stethoscopes	Low- or intermediate-level disinfection
Semicritical	Contacts mucous membranes and non-intact skin	Dental equipment that is used in the mouth but does not penetrate mucosal surfaces	High-level disinfection or sterilization
Critical	Enters sterile tissue	Surgical items; dental equipment that penetrates mucosal surfaces	Sterilization

[a] Initial cleaning is required for all.

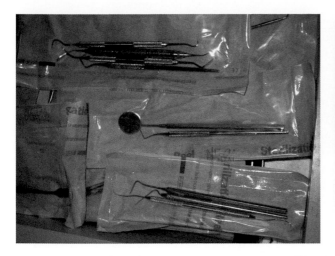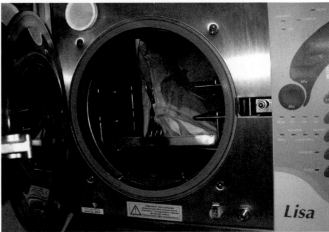

Figure 7.11   Autoclaved instruments are a necessary condition for performing safe operatory dentistry.

reused in veterinary medicine (e.g. endotracheal tubes). However, through either manufacturer's recommendations or veterinary guidance (Crawford and Weese 2015), specific protocols should be put in place for their proper management. This could include chemical disinfection, ethylene oxide gas, or hydrogen peroxide vapor.

Occasionally, rapid sterilization of an instrument is needed, such as when the only available instrument is contaminated during a procedure or when poor planning has resulted in intraoperative discovery of a needed item. Flash sterilization is a rapid sterilization cycle that is used in such situations, and typically involves a short autoclave cycle (e.g. 132 °C for three minutes at 27–28 pounds of pressure) with the item unwrapped (DHQP 2008; Rutala et al. 2008). This method should never be used for implants.

7.8.8   Instrument Pack Handling

Autoclaved instruments should be opened using an aseptic technique after the patient is in the dental suite and properly positioned, to avoid inadvertent aerosol contamination. The entire pack should be reprocessed after each procedure, even if some instruments were not used. The same pack should never be used for multiple patients, even if there is no cross-use of instruments, because of the potential for cross-contamination.

7.8.9   Intraoperative Patient Management

A variety of factors can potentially influence infection risk, as well as other complications. Patients should be properly positioned, using active or passive methods employed to maintain body temperature. Close monitoring of anesthesia is required to detect and intervene should problems develop. Patients with comorbidities that could influence

anesthesia, the procedure, or infection risk should be managed with a predetermined plan (e.g. pre- and intraoperative glucose monitoring in diabetic patients). They should ideally be covered, when possible, both to maintain heat and to reduce contamination of the haircoat from infectious aerosols generated during the procedure.

7.8.10   Surgical Antisepsis

While standard guidelines are available for human and veterinary surgery, their application in dental surgery can be problematic, and at times illogical. In comparison with most surgical procedures, where an incision is made through a clean, prepared site and into a sterile area, dental procedures are typically performed in the microbiological milieu of the oral cavity. This can create added risk and essentially negate the benefits of some otherwise routine infection-control practices. Some data from human medicine do not indicate a difference in infection rate when using sterile versus nonsterile gloves (Cheung et al. 2001; Giglio et al. 1993). However, sterile gloves are still widely recommended because of the potential that there could be an unproven effect, along with the more rigorous standards that are used for manufacturing sterile surgical gloves versus nonsterile examination gloves (Kohn et al. 2004). They also likely provide a better barrier because of their greater durability over the duration of potentially prolonged dental procedures. Use of sterile surgical gloves is a reasonable recommendation for procedures that are anticipated to result in major breaches of mucosal barriers, even though it is recognized that they will almost immediately become contaminated. As with human dentistry, nonsterile examination gloves should be adequate for routine dental cleaning and minimally invasive procedures.

7.8.11 Surveillance

A significant limitation of infection prevention and control in veterinary medicine is the lack of comprehensive data. Whether at the population or the in-clinic level, data about complications such as procedure-associated infections are needed in order to allow us to understand the risks, and to design and test infection-control practices.

7.8.12 Zoonotic Infections

A wide range of opportunists inhabit the mouths of healthy animals, some of which can cause severe infections in certain individuals. These include some, such as *Pasteurella*, that pose some degree of risk to all individuals, and others, such as *Capnocytophaga canimorsus*, that pose little to no risk to most individuals but can cause fatal infections in certain high-risk groups (particularly individuals without a functional spleen). Veterinary personnel need to be aware of the routine dangers and preventive measures, as well as situations that put them at increased risk. A reasonably large percentage of veterinary personnel may have some degree of immunocompromise because of age (>65 years of age), disease, treatment (e.g., immunosuppressive therapy), or pregnancy. Understanding one's own risk is important to help ensure compliance with standard practices in higher-risk situations and to identify scenarios where alterative procedures are indicated or where complete withdrawal is necessary.

References

Al Wazzan, K.A., Almas, K., Al Qahtani, M.Q. et al. (2001). Prevalence of ocular injuries, conjunctivitis and use of eye protection among dental personnel in Riyadh, Saudi Arabia. *Int. Dent. J.* 51: 89–94.

AAOS. (2012). Prevention of Orthopedic Implant Infection in Patients Undergoing Dental Procedures. Available from https://pubmed.ncbi.nlm.nih.gov/23457068/ (accessed July 5, 2020).

ADA. (2015). Antibiotic Prophylaxis Prior to Dental Procedures. Available from https://www.ada.org/en/member-center/oral-health-topics/antibiotic-prophylaxis (accessed July 5, 2020).

Anderson, M.E.C., Montgomery, J., Weese, J.S., and Prescott, J.R. (2008). *Infection Prevention and Control Best Practices for Small Animal Veterinary Clinics*. Guelph, ON: Canadian Committee on Antibiotic Resistance.

Anderson, M.E.C., Sargeant, J.M., and Weese, J.S. (2014). Video observation of hand hygiene practices during routine companion animal appointments and the effect of a poster intervention on hand hygiene compliance. *BMC Vet. Res.* 10: 106.

AVDC. (2005). Policy Statement: The Use of Antibiotics in Veterinary Dentistry. Available from https://avdc.org/download/30/position-statements/2873/antibiotic-use-april-2019.pdf (accessed July 5, 2020).

Ayad, F., Mateo, L.R., Dillon, R. et al. (2015). Randomized clinical trial of two oral care regimens in reducing and controlling established dental plaque and gingivitis. *Am. J. Dent.* 28 (A): 27A–32A.

Barbosa, M., Prada-López, I., Álvarez, M. et al. (2015). Post-tooth extraction bacteraemia: a randomized clinical trial on the efficacy of chlorhexidine prophylaxis. *PLoS One* 10: e0124249.

Bhanji, S., Williams, B., Sheller, B. et al. (2002). Transient bacteremia induced by toothbrushing a comparison of the Sonicare toothbrush with a conventional toothbrush. *Ped. Dent.* 24: 295–299.

Bölükbaşı, N., Özdemir, T., Öksüz, L., and Gürler, N. (2012). Bacteremia following dental implant surgery: preliminary results. *Medicina Oral, Patología Oral y Cirugía Bucal* 17: e69–e75.

Bratzler, D.W., Dellinger, E.P., Olsen, K.M. et al. (2013). Clinical practice guidelines for antimicrobial prophylaxis in surgery. *Surg. Infect.* 14: 73–156.

Brondani, M.A. (2013). Evidence does not support antibiotics for dental patients with joint replacements. *J. Cal. Dent. Assoc.*: 169.

Brown, W.Y. and McGenity, P. (2005). Effective periodontal disease control using dental hygiene chews. *J. Vet. Dent.* 22: 16–19.

Casarin, R.C.V., Peloso Ribeiro, E.D., Sallum, E.A. et al. (2012). The combination of amoxicillin and metronidazole improves clinical and microbiologic results of one-stage, full-mouth, ultrasonic debridement in aggressive periodontitis treatment. *J. Periodontol.* 83: 988–998.

Cheung, L.K., Chow, L.K., Tsang, M.H., and Tung, L.K. (2001). An evaluation of complications following dental extractions using either sterile or clean gloves. *Int. J. Oral Maxillofac. Surg.* 30: 550–554.

Clarke, D.E., Kelman, M., and Perkins, N. (2011). Effectiveness of a vegetable dental chew on periodontal disease parameters in toy breed dogs. *J. Vet. Dent.* 28: 230–235.

Costa, M.C., Stämpfli, H.R., Arroyo, L.G. et al. (2015). Changes in the equine fecal microbiota associated with the use of systemic antimicrobial drugs. *BMC Vet. Res.* 11: 19.

Crawford, S. and Weese, J.S. (2015). Efficacy of endotracheal tube disinfection strategies for elimination of *Streptococcus zooepidemicus* and *Bordetella bronchiseptica*. *J. Am. Vet. Med. Assoc.* 247: 1033–1036.

Davis, I.J., Wallis, C., Deusch, O. et al. (2013). A cross-sectional survey of bacterial species in plaque from client owned dogs with healthy gingiva, gingivitis or mild periodontitis. *PLoS One* 8: e83158.

Dayer, M.J., Jones, S., Prendergast, B. et al. (2015). Incidence of infective endocarditis in England, 2000-13: a secular trend, interrupted time-series analysis. *Lancet* 385: 1219–1228.

Dewhirst, F.E., Klein, E.A., Thompson, E.C. et al. (2012). The canine oral microbiome. *PLoS One* 7: e36067.

DHQP Guideline for Disinfection and Sterilization in Healthcare Facilities, 2008. 2008.

Elias-Boneta, A.R., Toro, M.J., Mateo, L.R. et al. (2015a). Efficacy of two fluoride-free, alcohol-free mouthwashes containing 0.075% or 0.07% CPC in controlling established dental plaque and gingivitis over a 6-week period on adults in Puerto Rico. *Am. J. Dent.* 28 (A): 14A–20A.

Elias-Boneta, A.R., Toro, M.J., Noboa, J. et al. (2015b). Efficacy of CPC and essential oils mouthwashes compared to a negative control mouthwash in controlling established dental plaque and gingivitis: a 6-week, randomized clinical trial. *Am. J. Dent.* 28 (A): 21A–26A.

Farrier, S.L., Farrier, J.N., and Gilmour, A.S.M. (2006). Eye safety in operative dentistry – a study in general dental practice. *Brit. Dent. J.* 200: 218–223.

Galván, M., Gonzalez, S., Cohen, C.L. et al. (2014). Periodontal effects of 0.25% sodium hypochlorite twice-weekly oral rinse. A pilot study. *J. Periodontol. Res.* 49: 696–702.

Garrett, S., Johnson, L., Drisko, C.H. et al. (1999). Two multi-center studies evaluating locally delivered doxycycline hyclate, placebo control, oral hygiene, and scaling and root planing in the treatment of periodontitis. *J. Periodontol.* 70: 490–503.

Garrett, S., Adams, D.F., Bogle, G. et al. (2000). The effect of locally delivered controlled-release doxycycline or scaling and root planing on periodontal maintenance patients over 9 months. *J. Periodontol.* 71: 22–30.

Giglio, J.A., Rowland, R.W., Laskin, D.M. et al. (1993). The use of sterile versus nonsterile gloves during out-patient exodontia. *Quintessence Int.* 24: 543–545.

Glickman, L.T., Glickman, N.W., Moore, G.E. et al. (2009). Evaluation of the risk of endocarditis and other cardiovascular events on the basis of the severity of periodontal disease in dogs. *J. Am. Vet. Med. Assoc.* 234: 486–494.

Gorrel, C. (2013). *Veterinary Dentistry for the General Practitioner*. Amsterdam: Elsevier.

Gorrel, C. and Bierer, T.L. (1999). Long-term effects of a dental hygiene chew on the periodontal health of dogs. *J. Vet. Dent.* 16: 109–113.

Gorrel, C. and Rawlings, J.M. (1996). The role of tooth-brushing and diet in the maintenance of periodontal health in dogs. *J. Vet. Dent.* 13: 139–143.

Hamilton, E., Kaneene, J.B., May, K.J. et al. (2012). Prevalence and antimicrobial resistance of *Enterococcus* spp and *Staphylococcus* spp isolated from surfaces in a veterinary teaching hospital. *J. Am. Vet. Med. Assoc.* 240: 1463–1473.

Harnoss, J.-C., Partecke, L.-I., Heidecke, C.-D. et al. (2010). Concentration of bacteria passing through puncture holes in surgical gloves. *Am. J. Infect. Control* 38: 154–158.

Harris, S., Croft, J., O'Flynn, C. et al. (2015). A pyrosequencing investigation of differences in the feline subgingival microbiota in health, gingivitis and mild periodontitis. *PLoS One* 10: e0136986.

Harvey, C.E. (2013). Bacteriology of periodontal disease. In: *Veterinary periodontology* (ed. B.A. Niemiec), 35–37. Ames, IA: Wiley.

Hennet, P. (2001). Effectiveness of an enzymatic rawhide dental chew to reduce plaque in beagle dogs. *J. Vet. Dent.* 18: 61–64.

Hennet, P. (2002). Effectiveness of a dental gel to reduce plaque in beagle dogs. *J. Vet. Dent.* 19: 11–14.

Hennet, P., Servet, E., and Venct, C. (2006). Effectiveness of an oral hygiene chew to reduce dental deposits in small breed dogs. *J. Vet. Dent.* 23: 6–12.

Hübner, N.-O., Goerdt, A.-M., Stanislawski, N. et al. (2010). Bacterial migration through punctured surgical gloves under real surgical conditions. *BMC Infect. Dis.* 10: 192.

Ingham, K.E., Gorrel, C., and Bierer, T.L. (2002). Effect of a dental chew on dental substrates and gingivitis in cats. *J. Vet. Dent.* 19: 201–204.

Johnston, T.P., Mondal, P., Pal, D. et al. (2011). Canine periodontal disease control using a clindamycin hydrochloride gel. *J. Vet. Dent.* 28: 224–229.

Jones, D.P. (1996). Accidental self inoculation with oil based veterinary vaccines. *NZ Med. J.* 109: 363–365.

Kaur, R., Singh, I., Vandana, K.L., and Desai, R. (2014). Effect of chlorhexidine, povidone iodine, and ozone on microorganisms in dental aerosols: randomized double-blind clinical trial. *Ind. J. Dent. Res.* 25: 160–165.

Keenan, J.R. and Veitz-Keenan, A. (2015). Antibiotic prophylaxis for dental implant placement? *Evid. Based Dent.* 16: 52–53.

Kim, S.E., Hwang, S.Y., Jeong, M. et al. (2015). Clinical and microbiological effects of a subantimicrobial dose of oral doxycycline on periodontitis in dogs. *Vet. J.*

Kohn, W.G., Collins, A.S., Cleveland, J.L. et al. (2004). Guidelines for infection control in dental health-care settings – 2003. *J. Am. Dent. Assoc.* 135: 33–47.

Leggat, P.A., Smith, D.R., and Speare, R. (2009). Exposure rate of needlestick and sharps injuries among Australian veterinarians. *J. Occu. Med. Toxicol.* 4: 25.

Lin, T.-Y., Yeh, L.-K., Ma, D.H.K. et al. (2015). Risk factors and microbiological features of patients hospitalized for microbial keratitis: a 10-year study in a referral center in Taiwan. *Med.* 94: e1905.

Lindhe, J., Hamp, S.E., and Löe, H. (1975). Plaque induced periodontal disease in beagle dogs. A 4-year clinical, roentgenographical and histometrical study. *J. Periodontol. Res.* 10: 243–255.

Little, J.W., Jacobson, J.J., Lockhart, P.B., and AAOM (2010). The dental treatment of patients with joint replacements: a position paper from the American Academy of Oral Medicine. *J. Am. Dent. Assoc.* 141: 667–671.

Lobetti, R.G. (2007). Anaerobic bacterial pericardial effusion in a cat. *JSAVA* 78: 175–177.

Lockhart, P.B., Brennan, M.T., Sasser, H.C. et al. (2008). Bacteremia associated with toothbrushing and dental extraction. *Circulation* 117: 3118–3125.

Lund, B., Hultin, M., Tranaeus, S. et al. (2015). Complex systematic review - perioperative antibiotics in conjunction with dental implant placement. *Clin. Oral Implant. Res.* 26 (Suppl. 11): 1–14.

Maharaj, B., Coovadia, Y., and Vayej, A.C. (2012). An investigation of the frequency of bacteraemia following dental extraction, tooth brushing and chewing. *Card. J. Afr.* 23: 340–344.

Marchetti, E., Casalena, F., Capestro, A. et al. (2017). Efficacy of two mouthwashes on 3-day supragingival plaque regrowth: a randomized crossover clinical trial. *Int. J. Dent. Hyg.* 15: 73–80.

Marghalani, A. (2014). Antibiotic prophylaxis reduces infectious complications but increases adverse effects after third-molar extraction in healthy patients. *J. Am. Dent. Assoc.* 145: 476–478.

Murphy, C.P., Weese, J.S., Reid-Smith, R.J., and McEwen, S.A. (2010). The prevalence of bacterial contamination of surgical cold sterile solutions from community companion animal veterinary practices in southern Ontario. *Can. Vet. J.* 51: 634–636.

Na'aya, H.U., Madziga, A.G., and Eni, U.E. (2009). Prospective randomized assessment of single versus double-gloving for general surgical procedures. *Niger. J. Med.* 18: 73–74.

NASPHV. (2006). Compendium of Veterinary Standard Precautions. Available from http://www.nasphv.org/Documents/VeterinaryStandardPrecautions.pdf (accessed July 5, 2020).

NICE. (2008). Prophylaxis Against Infective Endocarditis. Available from https://www.nice.org.uk/guidance/cg64 (accessed July 5, 2020).

Nieves, M.A., Hartwig, P., Kinyon, J.M., and Riedesel, D.H. (1997). Bacterial isolates from plaque and from blood during and after routine dental procedures in dogs. *Vet. Surg.* 26: 26–32.

O'Neill, J.K., Richards, S.W., Ricketts, D.M., and Patterson, M.H. (2005). The effects of injection of bovine vaccine into a human digit: a case report. *Environ. Health* 4: 21.

Paquette, D.W., Hanlon, A., Lessem, J., and Williams, R.C. (2004). Clinical relevance of adjunctive minocycline microspheres in patients with chronic periodontitis: secondary analysis of a phase 3 trial. *J. Periodontol.* 75: 531–536.

Peak, R.M. (2013). Antibiotics in periodontal disease. In: *Veterinary Periodontology* (ed. B.A. Niemiec), 186–189. Ames, IA: Wiley.

Peddle, G.D., Drobatz, K.J., Harvey, C.E. et al. (2009). Association of periodontal disease, oral procedures, and other clinical findings with bacterial endocarditis in dogs. *J. Am. Vet. Med. Assoc.* 234: 100–107.

Piñeiro, A., Tomás, I., Blanco, J. et al. (2010). Bacteraemia following dental implant placement. *Clin. Oral Implant. Res.* 21: 913–918.

Polson, A.M., Southard, G.L., Dunn, R.L. et al. (1996). Periodontal pocket treatment in beagle dogs using subgingival doxycycline from a biodegradable system. I. Initial clinical responses. *J. Periodontol.* 67: 1176–1184.

Poole, A.G., Shane, S.M., Kearney, M.T., and Rehn, W. (1998). Survey of occupational hazards in companion animal practices. *J. Am. Vet. Med. Assoc.* 212: 1386–1388.

Purucker, P., Mertes, H., Goodson, J.M., and Bernimoulin, J.P. (2001). Local versus systemic adjunctive antibiotic therapy in 28 patients with generalized aggressive periodontitis. *J. Periodontol.* 72: 1241–1245.

Quest, B.W. (2013). Oral health benefits of a daily dental chew in dogs. *J. Vet. Dent.* 30: 84–87.

Rawlings, J.M., Gorrel, C., and Markwell, P.J. (1998). Effect on canine oral health of adding chlorhexidine to a dental hygiene chew. *J. Vet. Dent.* 15: 129–134.

Riggio, M.P., Lennon, A., Taylor, D.J., and Bennett, D. (2011). Molecular identification of bacteria associated with canine periodontal disease. *Vet. Microbiol.*: 1–23.

Roberts, G.J., Jaffray, E.C., Spratt, D.A. et al. (2006). Duration, prevalence and intensity of bacteraemia after dental extractions in children. *Heart* 92: 1274–1277.

Rutala WA, Weber DJ and HICPAC. (2008). Guideline for Disinfection and Sterilization in Healthcare Facilities, 2008. Available from https://www.cdc.gov/infectioncontrol/pdf/guidelines/disinfection-guidelines-H.pdf (accessed July 5, 2020).

Skaar, D.D., O'Connor, H., Hodges, J.S., and Michalowicz, B.S. (2011). Dental procedures and subsequent prosthetic joint infections: findings from the Medicare Current Beneficiary Survey. *J. Am. Dent. Assoc.* 142: 1343–1351.

Sollecito, T.P., Abt, E., Lockhart, P.B. et al. (2015). The use of prophylactic antibiotics prior to dental procedures in patients with prosthetic joints: evidence-based clinical practice guideline for dental practitioners – a report of the American Dental Association Council on Scientific Affairs. *J. Am. Dent. Assoc.* 146: 11–16.e8.

Soukup, J.W. (2015). Judicious use of prophylactic antibiotics in dentistry and oral procedures. 13th World Veterinary Dental Congress, Monterey, CA.

Spaulding, E.H. (1968). Chemical disinfection of medical and surgical materials. In: *Disinfection, Sterilization and Preservation* (eds. C. Lawrence and S.S. Block), 517–531. Philadelphia, PA: Lea & Febiger.

Spellberg, B. and Lipsky, B.A. (2012). Systemic antibiotic therapy for chronic osteomyelitis in adults. *Clin. Infect. Dis.* 54: 393–407.

Sturgeon, A., Stull, J.W., Costa, M.C., and Weese, J.S. (2013). Metagenomic analysis of the canine oral cavity as revealed by high-throughput pyrosequencing of the 16S rRNA gene. *Vet. Microbiol.* 162: 891–898.

Sturgeon, A., Pinder, S.L., Costa, M.C., and Weese, J.S. (2014). Characterization of the oral microbiota of healthy cats using next-generation sequencing. *Vet. J.* 201: 223–229.

Sykes, J.E., Kittleson, M.D., Pesavento, P.A. et al. (2006). Evaluation of the relationship between causative organisms and clinical characteristics of infective endocarditis in dogs: 71 cases (1992-2005). *J. Am. Vet. Med. Assoc.* 228: 1723–1734.

Teughels, W., Dhondt, R., Dekeyser, C., and Quirynen, M. (2014). Treatment of aggressive periodontitis. *Periodontol. 2000* 65: 107–133.

Tou, S.P., Adin, D.B., and Castleman, W.L. (2005). Mitral valve endocarditis after dental prophylaxis in a dog. *J. Vet. Intern. Med.* 19: 268–270.

Veenhuizen, M.F., Wright, T.J., McManus, R.F., and Owens, J.G. (2006). Analysis of reports of human exposure to Micotil 300 (tilmicosin injection). *J. Am. Vet. Med. Assoc.* 229: 1737–1742.

Veitz-Keenan, A. and Keenan, J.R. (2015). Antibiotic use at dental implant placement. *Evid. Based Dent.* 16: 50–51.

Wallis, C., Marshall, M., Colyer, A. et al. (2015). A longitudinal assessment of changes in bacterial community composition associated with the development of periodontal disease in dogs. *Vet. Microbiol* 181: 271–282.

Weese, J.S. (2007). Environmental surveillance for MRSA. *Methods Mol. Biol.* 391: 201–208.

Weese, J.S. and Faires, M. (2009). A survey of needle handling practices and needlestick injuries in veterinary technicians. *Can. Vet. J.* 50: 1278–1282.

Weese, J.S., Staempfli, H.R., and Prescott, J.F. (2000). Isolation of environmental *Clostridium difficile* from a veterinary teaching hospital. *J. Vet. Diagn. Invest.* 12: 449–452.

Weese, J.S., Nichols, J.B., Jalali, M., and Litster, A. (2015). The oral and conjunctival microbiotas in cats with and without feline immunodeficiency virus infection. *Vet. Res.* 46: 21.

Weese, J.S., Giguère, S., Guardabassi, L. et al. (2015). ACVIM consensus statement on therapeutic antimicrobial use in animals and antimicrobial resistance. *J. Vet. Intern. Med.* 29: 487–498.

Wennström, J.L., Newman, H.N., MacNeill, S.R. et al. (2001). Utilisation of locally delivered doxycycline in non-surgical treatment of chronic periodontitis. A comparative multi-centre trial of 2 treatment approaches. *J. Clin. Periodontol.* 28: 753–761.

WHO. (2005). Critically Important Antibacterial Agents for Human Medicine for Risk Management Strategies of Non-Human Use: Report of a WHO Working Group Consultation, 15–18 February 2005, Canberra, Australia. Geneva: World Health Organization. Available from https://apps.who.int/iris/handle/10665/43330 (accessed July 5, 2020).

Wilkins, J.R. and Bowman, M.E. (1997). Needlestick injuries among female veterinarians: frequency, syringe contents and side-effects. *Occup. Med. (Lond.)* 47: 451–457.

Wilson, W., Taubert, K.A., Gewitz, M. et al. (2007). Prevention of infective endocarditis. Guidelines from the American Heart Association. A guideline from the American Heart Association Rheumatic Fever, Endocarditis, and Kawasaki Disease Committee, Council on Cardiovascular Disease in the Young, and the Council on Clinical Cardiology, Council on Cardiovascular Surgery and Anesthesia, and the Quality of Care and Outcomes Research Interdisciplinary Working Group. *Circulation* 116: 1736–1754.

Zetner, K. and Rothmueller, G. (2002). Treatment of periodontal pockets with doxycycline in beagles. *Vet. Ther.* 3: 441–452.

Zetner, K., Schmidt, H., and Pfeiffer, S. (2003). Concentrations of clindamycin in the mandibular bone of companion animals. *Vet. Ther.* 4: 166–171.

8

Dental Patient Welfare

Kymberley C. McLeod

Conundrum Consulting, Toronto, ON, Canada

8.1   Introduction

Routine high-quality dental care is necessary to provide optimum health and quality of life (QOL) for our patients. Untreated dental and oral issues may lead to unrelenting pain, contribute to other serious local or systemic diseases, and interfere in the natural expression of oral and facial behaviors, due to a lack of appropriate physiological coping mechanisms (Niemiec 2008a,b, 2013; Palmeira et al. 2017).

Due to their severity, frequency, and chronicity, dental disorders have been found to have the most significant impact on overall health-related welfare, compared with other common disorders (Summers et al. 2019). While a concerted focus on the welfare of our patients is considered a critical aspect of veterinary medicine (Paul and Podberscek 2000), many veterinarians find incorporating animal-welfare conversations into their daily practice a challenge, especially when what is in the best interest of the pet may contradict the client's preferences or willingness to treat.

Dental conditions present a unique client communication challenge for both general practitioners and specialists, as knowledge and understanding of the negative impact on quality and potentially QOL that dental disease creates is lacking in many who own or care for animals. While negative welfare outcomes such as pain and infection are occasionally recognized by owners, more commonly animals suffer chronically from the effects of their dental disease in virtual silence, with the owner completely unaware of the issues their pet is facing. Un- and undertreated dental disease have a serious impact on the welfare of the patient, and as such are unacceptable conditions for any veterinarian to leave purposefully unaddressed.

Using the central tenets of the "Five Freedoms" (Brambell 1965) and the more current "Five Animal Welfare Needs" (UK Government 2006), the welfare challenges of dental conditions may be more easily evaluated, and can be discussed with clients in a language they understand and embrace. Only when an owner understands, accepts, and incorporates the changes they must make do our patients truly benefit from our knowledge.

8.2   What Is Animal Welfare?

Animal welfare has many definitions, but at its most basic level it encompasses the physical, psychological, social, and environmental well-being of animals (Ryan et al. 2018). The terms "animal welfare" and "animal well-being" are often used interchangeably. It should be noted that in some countries, welfare is synonymous with prevention of animal abuse; that is not the definition utilized in this chapter. Humans are increasingly concerned with the treatment of animals within society and with allowing them to live a life of good welfare (Siegford et al. 2010). How to decide on what good animal welfare is and what it looks like, however, can be a complex thing.

At the root of animal welfare assessment lies the desire to evaluate how well an animal can cope with its environment and the challenges it faces in its daily life. These challenges historically have been evaluated with a focus on health needs, resource or environmental needs, and cognitive and emotional needs. Ultimately, the science of animal welfare encompasses all of these needs under its umbrella.

It is important to separate animal welfare science from the subject of the ethical use of animals. Animal ethics focuses on what we, as humans, think about an animal's situation, based on our own morals/viewpoint. This varies greatly according to cultural and geographical norms. Dental diseases have a wide variety of effects on individual animals, and as such may be seen to pose animal welfare concerns in many areas.

The Veterinary Dental Patient: A Multidisciplinary Approach, First Edition. Edited by Jerzy Gawor and Brook Niemiec.
© 2021 John Wiley & Sons Ltd. Published 2021 by John Wiley & Sons Ltd.
Companion website: www.wiley.com/go/gawor/veterinary-dental-patient

8.3 Modern Animal Welfare Needs Assessment

When developing measures of welfare to create viable animal welfare needs assessment (AWNA) options in companion animal clinical practice, we must consider three things (Ryan et al. 2018):

1) Objective scientific factors, to assist us in evaluating what animals need
2) Ethical considerations of what animals should be provided in any given society
3) Legal requirements concerning how animals must be treated in any given region or country

   Many welfare assessment methods have been developed for lab animals, zoo animals, and farm animals, such as the European Commission's Severity Assessment Framework (for research colonies) and the Royal Society for the Prevention of Cruelty to Animals' (RSPCA) Freedom Food Scheme (for production animals). It can be challenging for the practicing small-animal veterinarian to find applicability for these assessment strategies in companion animal practice. However, veterinarians by nature are excellent at assimilating information from a variety of observable sources in order to create a holistic conclusion on the health of a patient. Like disease states, welfare assessment exists on a spectrum. With disease, the spectrum travels from non-existent (patient has no evidence of disease) to severe (the patient is moribund). Similarly, welfare states exist from optimal (the patient's body and mental needs exist in an optimal state, with natural behaviors satisfied) to minimal (no aspect of the animals' welfare is being met) (Hewson 2003a, b).

8.4 Five Freedoms and Five Animal Welfare Needs

The Five Freedoms are one option for guiding practicing veterinarians in conversations regarding AWNAs for un- or undertreated dental disease. They were first formally published by the UK Farm Animal Welfare Council, and have been refined over the years by various groups and committees. They have been adopted and endorsed by organizations including the World Organization for Animal Health (OIE), the American Society for the Prevention of Cruelty to Animals (ASPCA), and the RSPCA. They represent an ideal situation that should be strived for with each animal under care.

Currently, the Five Freedoms encompass:

- Freedom from hunger, thirst, and malnutrition
- Freedom from pain and injury
- Freedom from infection and disease
- Freedom from fear and distress
- Freedom to express natural behaviors

While the Five Freedoms are a wonderful basis from which to begin this discussion, it is apparent that they are likely unpractical and perhaps even evolutionarily illogical. All sentient beings experience some stress in the process of existing in the world as we know it. Without feeling thirst, an animal wouldn't drink. As well, the Five Freedoms focus on the types of problems that at the time of their creation were the focus of animal welfare. While their practicality was immediately obvious for farm animals, zoological species, and laboratory/research animals, practitioners and welfare advocates found them harder to apply to companion animals in their wide variety of roles. As such, a more meaningful and applicable approach to verbalizing these "Freedoms" was developed in 2006, and rewritten as the Five Animal Welfare Needs.

The Five Animal Welfare Needs are a practitioner-friendly way of promoting and thinking about the many facets of animals' requirements in a companion animal setting. They encompass:

- The need for a suitable environment
- The need for a suitable diet
- The need to be able to exhibit normal behavior patterns
- The need to be housed with, or apart from, other animals
- The need to be protected from pain, suffering, injury, and disease

While acknowledging the strengths of what the Five Freedoms achieved – creating a much-needed discourse on the importance of understanding, identifying, and minimizing negative welfare states – the Five Animal Welfare Needs are worded in a more proactive way, and help both veterinarians and owners see the practical implications for companion animals' daily lives. By ensuring our clients understand what it means to provide good nutrition, a good environment, good health, opportunities for appropriate behavioral expression, and positive mental experiences, we can positively guide how they care for their animals – and potentially how they choose future breeding stock.

In the context of a veterinary hospital, AWNA utilizing the Five Animal Welfare Needs can be performed through appropriate client communication and information gathering, clinical assessment, and behavioral observations. Maintaining and improving companion animal welfare in veterinary clinics requires factual and regular recording of AWNA, including of a patient's physical and psychological welfare. Already in use in the United Kingdom to provide information to pet owners and to benchmark owner knowledge and protection of animal welfare (PDSA 2018), the Five Animal Welfare Needs allow practitioners to approach and evaluate physical and psychological well-being in a practical manner (Ryan et al. 2018).

8.5 Measuring Quality of Life

QOL measurement tools are often used in managing end-stage chronic diseases. Their applicability in assessing QOL for dental-disease patients has merit, especially with growing client understanding of the concept in the human world. Belshaw et al. (2015) found a distinct lack of well-validated general methods for measuring QOL, with the majority of QOL measures available for companion animal use being disease-specific. There is currently no dentally specific QOL assessment available. However, two novel assessments for companion animals, the Canine Symptom Assessment Scale (PennCHART 2016) and the Pet Problem Severity Scale (Spitznagel et al. 2018), may prove useful.

When evaluating the overall impact of dental disorders on health-related welfare in dogs in the United Kingdom, Summers et al. (2019) utilized criteria including chronicity of condition, prevalence, and severity. As many owners underestimate the welfare impacts that chronic dental disease may have on an animal, discussing dental disease and the ability to appropriately address it must be a part of any QOL assessment.

8.6 Prevalence of Dental Disease

Historically, it was a commonly held belief that companion animals required little if any dental care. We now know that dental disease is one of the most common medical conditions in this population. Studies show that over 80% of dogs (some papers report 90%) and 70% of cats have evidence of periodontitis by two years of age (Lund et al. 1999; Kortegaard et al. 2008; Marshall et al. 2014). Further, 10% of dogs have a fractured tooth with painful direct pulp exposure, also known as a complicated crown fractures (Golden et al. 1982), while 20–75% of mature cats are clinically affected by oral resorptive lesions, depending on the population examined (Bellows 2010). It is estimated that 50% of large-breed dogs have smaller or uncomplicated crown fractures with painful dentin exposure (Hirvonen et al. 1992). A large majority of veterinary patients are thus dealing with significant pain or infection, or both, on a daily basis.

8.7 Dental Disease Associations with Compromised Animal Welfare Needs

When generating assessments of dental patient welfare utilizing the Five Animal Welfare Needs framework, the majority of the focus is placed on the need to be protected from pain, suffering, injury, and disease and the need to be able to exhibit normal behavior patterns.

The International Association for the Study of Pain (ISAP) defines pain as "an unpleasant sensory and emotional experience associated with actual or potential tissue damage or described in terms of such damage" (Merskey and Bogduk 1994). It is well documented in humans that dental pain can be extreme (Bender 2000; Hargreaves and Kaiser 2004). Multiple published articles link dental pain to decreased productivity sleep disturbance and significant social and psychological impacts (Anil et al. 2002; Heaivilin et al. 2011; Choi et al. 2019). However, pain is an experience unique to each individual and behavioral demonstrations of pain are incredibly species-specific (Chidiac et al. 2002; Paul-Murphy et al. 2004; Seksel 2007), in part due to variations in the number, distribution, and morphology of opioid receptors (Landau 2006). In comparison to their human counterparts, companion animals show few behaviors one can directly link to oral pain. It is important to note that despite the apparent lack of behavioral indicators, an animal's experience of dental pain and infection is likely to be equally present (Holmstrom et al. 1998; Chidiac et al. 2002; Cohen and Brown 2002), given that the pain thresholds of people and animals are quite similar (Bennett and Xie 1988; Rollin 1989).

To illustrate this more definitively, non-human mammals have been found to be excellent models for dental pain in the human world (Ahlberg 1978; Le Bars et al. 2001; Chidiac et al. 2002) and have been prolifically utilized in nociception and therapeutic research. Small rodents are an excellent model for pulpitis, a condition reported to create extreme pain responses in humans. Notable and repeatable behavioral changes from pulpal pain include weight loss and decreased growth rate, increased time to complete meals, shaking, open-mouthed facial grimace, freezing, and overall decreased activity (Chidiac et al. 2002; Chudler and Byers 2005). Dogs and cats have also been utilized to show behavioral changes with pulpal and nonpulpal pain (Ahlberg 1978). It is interesting to note that despite the common belief among veterinary professionals and owners alike that dental pain will lead to a dramatic decrease or total cessation of appetite, this has rarely been noted in the published research. Additional work is strongly recommended in order to better understand oral pain and how it should best be assessed in common companion animal species (Evangelista et al. 2019).

There is substantive belief within the profession that despite not always being able to prove an animal is in pain, we should seek to relieve any pain we suspect it is in, in all circumstances. When oral pain can be reasonably suspected, effective therapy is justified to alleviate it. While temporary measures may be possible with pharmaceuticals, the only way to remove pain more definitively is to address the issue with appropriate dental therapy.

8.8 Physiological Signs of Stress

In the context of AWNA, stressors are defined as events that alter homeostatic equilibrium and therefore require adaptation to reestablish natural homeostasis. Physiological disturbance from such stressors create a state of physiological stress, which may create suffering and mental distress (Moberg 2000). Infectious etiologies such as endodontic and periodontal disease impose a significant bacterial disease burden on the body (DeBowes 1996; Niemiec 2013). Unchecked pain and infection can lead to potentially deleterious consequences as the body's natural stress responses are activated (Broom 2006). Stimulation of the sympathetic nervous system (SNS) and hypothalamic–pituitary–adrenal (HPA) axis leads to the release of adrenalin, noradrenalin, and cortisol. Dentally, stimulation in a conscious animal of a severe tooth resorption lesion may create observable responses, such as increased heart rate, trembling, vocalization, attempts to escape stimulation, and release of glucose in preparation to fight or flee. Longer-term daily stimulation of such a lesion from salivating and eating may lead to more chronic stimulation of the HPA axis. Chronic stressors, as such, have the opportunity to negatively affect multiple body systems. Immune-function impacts may first be noted with the development of an acute stress leukogram, progressing to leukopenia and immunosuppressive inflammatory cytokine changes with chronicity (Hekman et al. 2014). Several publications have linked chronic stress responses to decreased ability to eliminate bacterial infection and increased susceptibility to disease in humans and mice (Biondi and Zannino 1997; Karin et al. 2006; Kiank et al. 2006). Untreated dental disease can lead to chronic inflammation and infection of the oral tissues (Rawlinson et al. 2011; Nemec et al. 2013). As in other areas of the body, unchecked infection is an ethically unacceptable condition to leave without appropriate therapy (Broom 2006).

8.9 Behavior Changes

Behavioral scores for the evaluation of pain exist for a variety of systems and species. However, it is important to note that dental pain indicators are often vague and nonspecific.

Conditions that may cause oral pain for our patients include periodontal disease, tooth and jaw fractures, tooth resorption, caries, traumatic malocclusions, feline oralfacial pain syndrome, and some oral neoplasias. It is important for practitioners to understand that the absence of a notable behavioral change does not mean that the pain is not there, nor does it imply any lack of severity. Many dogs and cats simply do not show the pain they are forced to endure daily to their owners and veterinarians in an easily observable or understandable way (Merola and Mills 2016). Pain behaviors that have been well attributed to dental pain include pawing, rubbing, drooling, mutation of the mouth, and slightly decreased appetite (Rusbridge and Heath 2015).

Interpreting behavioral signals of oral pain can be a complex matter, but it is a simple fact that animals will continue to eat despite debilitating and extreme dental pain. Animals require nourishment to survive, and the instinct to survive is stronger than the desire to avoid pain. It is important to remember that while many animals will demonstrate normal oral behaviors despite experiencing dental pain, such as playing with toys, marking with facial glands, or using their mouth to explore their environment, others may be prevented from doing so. Additionally, clients report that they are happier to know their pets are not in pain (McElhenny 2005). Regardless of any change in behavior, or lack of it, underlying pain should not be a condition that an animal is expected to endure, either by its veterinarian or by its owner.

8.10 Client Education Matters

As veterinarians, it is our responsibility to proactively diagnose, treat, and relieve pain and suffering for our animal patients. When resistance to our treatment plan is met, additional client education may allow for increased understanding of the decreased welfare associated with the animal's condition.

At the practitioner level, a simple questionnaire or discussion with the owner regarding current oral and facial behaviors should be conducted during regular health exams, and the results should be recorded in the patient's medical record. While anecdotally it appears that most owners and many veterinarians feel oral pain will decrease appetite (and therefore, in its absence, lead to misreported changes), we encourage practitioners to consider a more universal view of the wide variety of changes that may be noted as sequelae to oral disease. When taking a history from an owner, it is important for the veterinarian to not ask leading or closed-ended questions, but to appeal to the owner to evaluate any changes they may or may not have noticed. Equally important is to follow up on the information

Table 8.1   Comparison of selected parameters characterizing pet oral care in Poland in two different periods.

Parameter	2003–04		2010–11	
	Dogs	Cats	Dogs	Cats
Number examined	29 702 (76.6%)	9074 (23.4%)	3250 (72%)	1265 (28%)
Fed dry food (%)	22.5	33.7	45.0	44.5
Daily oral hygiene (%)	5.2	4.4	10.3	6.1
No hygiene at all (%)	60.1	71.4	33.9	70.4

provided. Follow-up at two weeks and two months is commonly advised, in order to get a full picture of the situation following therapy.

A country's economic status may have an impact on oral care compliance. Poland has recently been recognized as showing incredible economic growth compared to its peers within the European Union. As such, Polish pet owners are experiencing improved economic status overall. Surveys on compliance conducted in 2003–04 and 2010–11 highlight the differences in this area, as presented in Table 8.1 (Gawor et al. 2012).

8.11 Welfare Issues Surrounding the Veterinary Visit, Handling Techniques, and Procedural Design

The welfare needs of the patient during a veterinary visit begin from the time they leave their home to visit the practice. While standards of care, educational and socioeconomic levels, resource availability, and societal demands may vary around the world, the welfare needs of veterinary patients are constant, and must be considered with each interaction we have with them. As sentient beings, our companion animals have the ability to experience both positive (pleasure, comfort, stimulatory) and negative (fear, anxiety) emotions (Mellor 2016).

Dental assessment and treatment should be conducted by properly trained veterinary professionals. Ethically, the veterinary healthcare team makes a principal commitment to "do no harm." Handling must be gentle and humane at all times. Low-stress and feline-friendly handling techniques are recommended during initial examination and the introduction of anesthetic agents; commonly accepted recommendations are outlined in the American Academy of Family Physicians (AAFP) guidelines (Rodan et al. 2011). The use of therapeutics to reduce stress and anxiety is highly encouraged, where appropriate.

After a thorough conscious evaluation of the oral cavity has been performed, any and all pathology must be communicated to the client, and an appropriate treatment plan

must be recommended to resolve the issues noted. Lack of intervention in the face of dental disease contributes to continued negative welfare implications for our patients, and thus a decreased level of well-being. When appropriate therapy is available, it must be recommended and advocated for, as without advocacy through excellent communication, clients may not understand the urgency or importance of addressing the dental source of negative welfare.

Patients experiencing stress during veterinary preoperative care may require higher doses of anesthesia and analgesia, with potentially increased adverse anesthetic outcomes (See more in Chapter 11). Careful consideration of pre- and postoperative handling techniques, along with conscientious hospital design to allow for appropriate patient housing while awaiting surgery, can greatly reduce the amount of stress a patient experiences during dental procedures. Stressors during time spent at the veterinary hospital surrounding procedures can sensitize the central nervous system with repeated stimulation of C-fiber nociceptors, leading to central spinal neuron sensitization. The resulting increase in intensity of perceived pain and the subsequent physiological and physical responses from the animal are known as "wind-up pain." Along with reducing preoperative sources of wind-up pain, gentle, efficient, and thoughtful tissue handling (minimally invasive surgery) is recommended to prevent excessive pain and swelling postprocedure. Appropriate choice of mouth gag, or avoidance of its use altogether, may help prevent trauma, especially in cats (Stiles et al. 2012; de Miguel Garcia et al. 2013). Local and regional anesthetic blocks and adequate pre- and postoperative pain management are absolutely necessary for controlling the pain that may be experienced during dental therapeutic procedures and preventing excessive suffering after anesthetic recovery. Continued pursuit of education into minimally invasive techniques is essential to reducing the negative well-being associated with traumatic surgery and postoperative pain and inflammation.

The human–animal bond is tenuous, and fear experienced during handling as part of a veterinary procedure can disrupt it quickly (Knesl et al. 2016). Anxiety, pain, and fear can lead to stimulation of the SNS and HPA, leading to aggressive behavior during handling, decreased immune function, extended healing times, and breakdown of surgical closure (Moberg 2000; Hong et al. 2018). Education on and commitment to reducing the stress involved with handling for oral exams and procedures is essential when addressing dental disease in our patients. If reasonable, gentle attempts are unsuccessful, suitable sedation or antianxiety medications must be considered. Punishment, rough handling, and dominant handling techniques have no place in the veterinary hospital and should be wholly avoided.

8.12 Welfare Implications of Anesthesia-Free Dentistry

Performing dental procedures without anesthesia – commonly known as anesthesia-free dentistry (AFD) or nonanesthetic dentistry (NAD) – holds no medical benefit for the animal (Nemec et al. 2013). Animal welfare scientists maintain that preventable and predictable pain, stress, and anxiety should be avoided during veterinary care for both moral and ethical reasons. There are multiple aspects of a complete professional dental cleaning and oral assessment that, if conducted without adequate pain and anxiety relief, would create significant negative animal welfare outcomes and concern for overall patient well-being.

Periodontal probing is essential to determining the health of gingival tissues. Performing a thorough and accurate probing on all surfaces of the tooth – especially the caudal teeth and all lingual/palatal surfaces – is exceedingly challenging in a typical awake animal, and therefore likely to be inaccurate (Bauer et al. 2018). Challenges include animal head movement, tongue interference, and difficulty in visualization. While this may be a procedure that creates minimal pain and stress in healthy individuals, probing diseased tissues such as resorptive lesions elicits a significant and predictable pain response. Determining which animals will experience pain on probing is rarely possible based upon visual cues, and as such, a practitioner has little way of ensuring the process will not be painful or stressful to the patient before beginning (Niemiec 2013).

The positioning required to accurately assess all areas of the mouth and perform a thorough scaling and polishing of the teeth demands extended time in potentially stressful and compromising body positions for the patient. The use of water and physical removal of infectious debris within the oral cavity while in these positions, without protection of the airways with a physical barrier (e.g., gauze or a well-cuffed tube), increases the potential for aspiration pneumonia. Scaling and polishing teeth with gingival recession,

tooth resorption, or fractures may cause unnecessary pain to the animal.

Dental procedures performed without anesthesia cannot include radiological examination of the subgingival anatomy. Without effective evaluation of the supra- and subgingival areas, meaningful treatment may not be delivered to the patient. This increases the likelihood that painful, infectious disease will remain in the mouth after a cosmetic procedure has been performed.

Removal of tartar and polishing of the visible surfaces of the teeth may lead to an oral cavity with persistent infection, inflammation, and pain under the gumline. Therefore, not only is this procedure potentially ineffective for removing pain and infection, but it often results in a false sense of security for the owner (and practitioner), which may lead to delays in appropriate care for the animal (McFadden and Marretta 2013) (Figure 8.1). The stress and discomfort incurred are wholly avoidable when a reasonable alternative is utilized (appropriate anesthesia), and indefensible from a medical and ethical standpoint.

All of the proceeding directly opposes the welfare benefits and improvements to patient well-being and QOL that are at the center of humane dental care. As such, the practice of veterinary dental procedures without appropriate anesthesia is not recommended. It is inadequate and provides a substandard level of care that may be misleading to the pet owner. This conclusion has been echoed by multiple local, national, and international veterinary medical organizations and specialty colleges of veterinary dentistry (Niemiec et al. 2020).

8.13 Economic Consequences of Improved Welfare Outcomes

In addition to professional satisfaction, protecting the welfare of animals may provide positive economic benefits for the veterinary clinic. Owners will prefer a clinical setting where their pet is well cared for and not distressed during a visit. Dogs and cats may become agitated by any procedure, including manual restraint, possibly creating lasting impact on their emotional state. This can predispose to a negative conditioned emotional response, leading to increased difficulty during future visits. Gentle handling and appropriate sedation, where required, can help avoid stressful encounters and improve welfare outcome for both cats and dogs. Owners who appreciate these improved outcomes are more likely to remain loyal clients and to help introduce new ones through word of mouth. Economic benefits to the clinic can then follow (Niemiec et al. 2020).

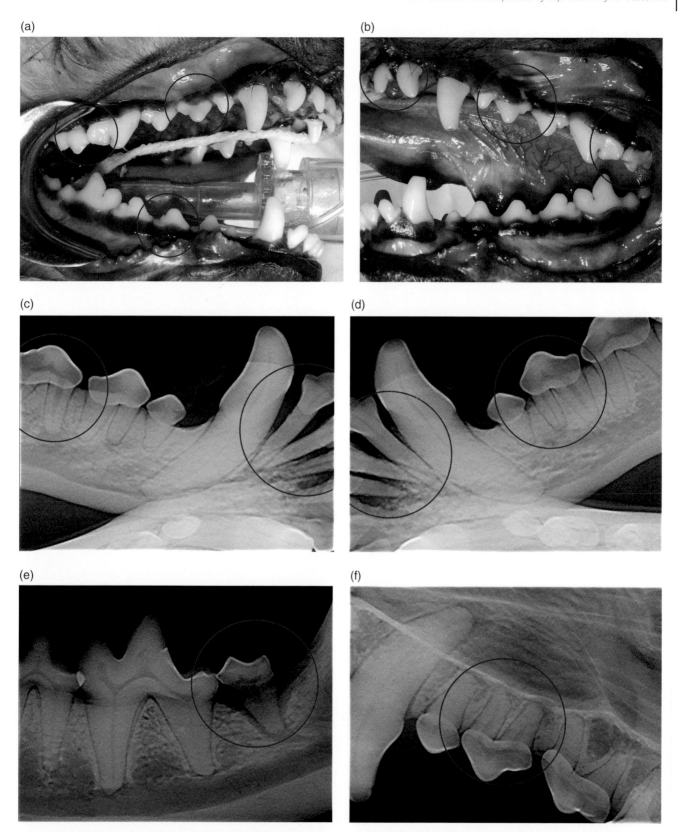

Figure 8.1 (a, b) One week before these images were taken, this seven-year-old miniature Schnauzer underwent a teeth cleaning without anesthesia and the most of the teeth seemed to be very clean. However, the owner noted the dog still showed signs of oral discomfort. Clinical assessment under general anesthesia (a–b) allowed the identification of numerous additional problems, and radiographic assessment revealed pathologies that required action and which could not be diagnosed without thorough clinical and radiographic evaluation. Circled are additional problems revealed in clinical and radiographic evaluation.

(g) (h)

(i) (j)

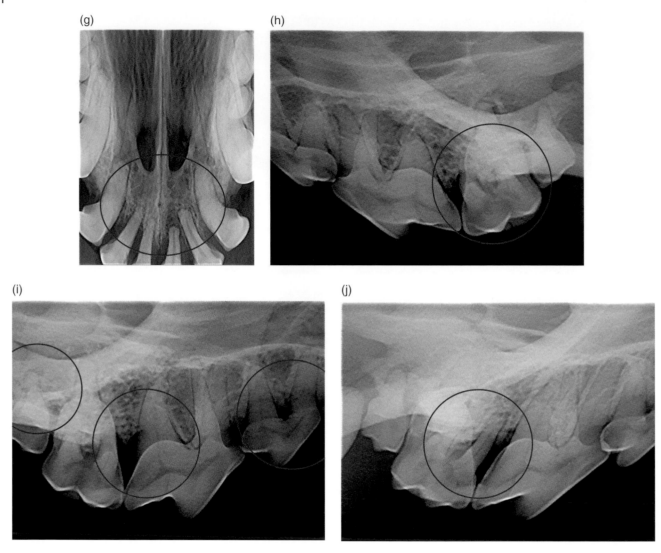

Figure 8.1   (Continued)

8.14   Conclusion

As advocates of humane animal husbandry and veterinary care, we as veterinarians are called to continuously improve in the ways we safeguard the welfare needs of our animal patients. As a profession, we must continue to voice the need for optimal oral health for companion animals, to advocate for their proper dental care, and to educate our clients on the importance of dental health to the daily welfare of their pets. By utilizing the Five Animal Welfare Needs as our guide, we can use regular dental examination and proper therapy to help address infection, control pain, relieve suffering, and allow return to regular behavior.

References

Ahlberg, K.F. (1978). Dose-dependent inhibition of sensory nerve activity in the feline dental pulp by anti-inflammatory drugs. *Acta Physiol. Scand.* 102: 434–440.

Anil, S., Anil, L., and Deen, J. (2002). Challenges of pain assessment in domestic animals. *J. Am. Vet. Med. Assoc.* 220: 313–319.

Bauer AE, Stella J, Lemmons M, Croney CC. Evaluating the validity and reliability of a visual dental scale for detection of periodontal disease (PD) in non-anesthetized dogs (Canis familiaris). PLoS One. 2018 Sep 26;13(9):e0203930. doi: 10.1371/journal.pone.0203930. PMID: 30256813; PMCID: PMC6157863.

Bellows, J. (2010). Treatment of tooth resorption. In: *Feline Dentistry: Oral Assessment, Treatment, and Preventative Care* (ed. J. Bellows), 222–241. Ames, IA: Wiley-Blackwell.

Belshaw, Z., Asher, L., Harvey, N., and Dean, R. (2015). Quality of life assessment in domestic dogs: an evidence-based rapid review. *Vet. J.* 206 (2): 203–212.

Bender, I.B. (2000). Pulpal pain diagnosis: a review. *J. Endodont.* 26: 175–179.

Bennett, G.J. and Xie, Y.K. (1988). A peripheral mononeuropathy in rat that produces disorders of pain sensation like those seen in man. *Pain* 33 (1): 87–107.

Biondi, M. and Zannino, L.G. (1997). Psychological stress, neuroimmunomodulation, and susceptibility to infectious diseases in animals and man: a review. *Psychother. Psychosom.* 66 (1): 3–26.

Brambell, R. (1965). Report of the Technical Committee to Enquire Into the Welfare of Animals Kept Under Intensive Livestock Husbandry Systems. HM Stationery Office, pp. 1–84.

Broom, D.M. (2006). Behaviour and welfare in relation to pathology. *Appl. Anim. Behav. Sci.* 97: 73–83.

Chidiac, J.J., Rifai, K., Hawwa, N.N. et al. (2002). Nociceptive behaviour induced by dental application of irritants to rat incisors: a new model for tooth inflammatory pain. *Eur. J. Pain* 6: 55–67.

Choi, J.W., Choi, Y., Lee, T. et al. (2019). Employment status and unmet dental care needs in South Korea: a population-based panel study. *BMJ Open* 9: e022436.

Chudler, E.H. and Byers, M.R. (2005). Behavioural responses following tooth injury in rats. *Arch. Oral Biol.* 50: 333–340.

Cohen, A.S. and Brown, D.C. (2002). Orofacial dental pain emergencies: endodontic diagnosis and management. In: *Pathways of the Pulp*, 8ee (eds. A.S. Cohen and R.C. Burns), 31–76. St. Louis, MO: Mosby.

DeBowes, L.J. (1996). The effects of dental disease on systemic disease. *Vet. Clin. N. Am. Small* 28 (5): 1057–1062.

de Miguel Garcia, C., Whiting, M., and Alibhai, H. (2013). Cerebral hypoxia in a cat following pharyngoscopy involving use of a mouth gag. *Vet. Anaesth. Analg.* 40 (1): 106–108.

Evangelista MC, Watanabe R, Leung VSY, Monteiro BP, O'Toole E, Pang DSJ, Steagall PV. Facial expressions of pain in cats: the development and validation of a Feline Grimace Scale. Sci Rep. 2019 Dec 13;9(1):19128. doi: 10.1038/s41598-019-55693-8. PMID: 31836868; PMCID:

Gawor, J., Jodkowska, K., Kurski, G., and Polkowska, I. (2012) Oral health status and level of oral hygiene in dogs and cats in Poland. Comparison of results collected in 2003–2004 and 2010–2011. Handbook of Proceedings, 21st ECVD, Lisbon, Portugal.

Golden, A.L., Stoller, N., and Harvey, C.E. (1982). A survey of oral and dental diseases in dogs anaesthetised at a veterinary hospital. *J. Am. Anim. Hosp. Assoc.* 18: 891–899.

Hargreaves, K.M. and Kaiser, K. (2004). New advances in the management of endodontic pain emergencies. *J. Calif. Dent. Assoc.* 32: 469–473.

Heaivilin, N., Gerbert, B., Page, J.E., and Gibbs, J.L. (2011). Public health surveillance of dental pain via Twitter. *J. Dent. Res.* 90 (9): 1047–1051.

Hekman, J.P., Karas, A.Z., and Sharp, C.R. (2014). Psychogenic stress in hospitalized dogs: cross species comparisons, implications for health care, and the challenges of evaluation. *Animals (Basel)* 4 (2): 331–347.

Hewson, C.J. (2003a). Focus on animal welfare. *Can. Vet. J.* 44: 335–336.

Hewson, C.J. (2003b). What is animal welfare? Common definitions and their practical consequences. *Can. Vet. J.* 44: 496–499.

Hirvonen, T., Ngassapa, D., and Narhi, M. (1992). Relation of dentin sensitivity to histological changes in dog teeth with exposed and stimulated dentin. *Proc. Finn. Dent. Soc.* 88 (Suppl. 1): 133–141.

Holmstrom, S.E., Frost, P., and Eisner, E.R. (1998). Dental prophylaxis. In: *Veterinary Dental Techniques*, 2ee (eds. S.E. Holmstrom, P. Frost and E.R. Eisner), 133–166. St. Louis, MO: W.B. Saunders.

Hong B, Bulsara Y, Gorecki P, Dietrich T. Minimally invasive vertical versus conventional tooth extraction: An interrupted time series study. J Am Dent Assoc. 2018 Aug;149(8):688–695. doi: 10.1016/j.adaj.2018.03.022. Epub 2018 May 24. PMID: 29803427.

Karin, M., Lawrence, T., and Nizet, V. (2006). Innate immunity gone awry: linking microbial infections to chronic inflammation and cancer. *Cell* 124 (4): 823–835.

Kiank, C., Holtfreter, B., Starke, A. et al. (2006). Stress susceptibility predicts the severity of immune depression and the failure to combat bacterial infections in chronically stressed mice. *Brain Behav. Immun.* 20 (4): 359–368.

Knesl, O., Hart, B.L., Fine, A.H. et al. (2016). Opportunities for incorporating the human-animal bond in companion animal practice. *J. Am. Vet. Med. Assoc.* 249 (1): 42–44.

Kortegaard, H.E., Eriksen, T., and Baelum, V. (2008). Periodontal disease in research beagle dogs – an epidemiological study. *J. Small Anim. Pract.* 49 (12): 610–616.

Landau, R. (2006). One size does not fit all: genetic variability of mu-opioid receptor and postoperative morphine consumption. *Anesthesiology* 105 (2): 235–237.

Le Bars, D., Gozariu, M., and Cadden, S.W. (2001). Animal models of nociception. *Pharmacol. Rev.* 53 (4): 597–652.

Lund, E.M., Armstrong, P.J., Kirk, C.A. et al. (1999). Health status and population characteristics of dogs and cats examined at private veterinary practices in the United States. *J. Am. Vet. Med. Assoc.* 214: 1336–1341.

Marshall, M.D., Wallis, C.V., Milella, L. et al. (2014). A longitudinal assessment of periodontal disease in 52 miniature Schnauzers. *BMC Veterinary Research* 10: 166.

McElhenny, J. (2005). Taking away the pain. *Vet. Med.* 100 (Suppl): 61–64.

McFadden, T. and Marretta, S.M. (2013). Consequences of untreated periodontal disease in dogs and cats. *J. Vet. Dent.* 30 (4): 266–275.

Mellor, D. (2016). Updating animal welfare thinking: moving beyond the "Five Freedoms" towards "a life worth living.". *Animals* 6 (3): 21.

Merola, I. and Mills, D.S. (2016). Behavioural signs of pain in cats: an expert consensus. *PLoS One* 1: e0150040.

Merskey, H. and Bogduk, N. (1994). *Classification of Chronic Pain: Descriptions of Chronic Pain Syndromes and Definitions of Pain Terms.* Seattle, WA: International Association for the Study of Pain Press.

Moberg, G. (2000). Biological response to stress: implications for animal welfare. In: *The Biology of Animal Stress: Basic Principles and Implications for Animal Welfare* (ed. G. Moberg), 1–21. Wallingford: CABI.

Nemec, A., Verstraete, F.J., Jerin, A. et al. (2013). Periodontal disease, periodontal treatment and systemic nitric oxide in dogs. *Res. Vet. Sci.* 94: 542–544.

Niemiec, B.A. (2008a). Oral pathology. *Top. Companion Anim. M.* 23: 59–71.

Niemiec, B.A. (2008b). Periodontal disease. *Top. Companion Anim. M.* 23: 72–80.

Niemiec, B.A. (2013). Understanding the disease process. In: *Veterinary Periodontology* (ed. B.A. Niemiec), 18–34. Ames, IA: Wiley-Blackwell.

Niemiec, B.A., Gawor, J., Nemec, A., et al. (2020). WSAVA Global Dental Guidelines. Available from https://www.wsava.org/WSAVA/media/Documents/Guidelines/Dental-Guidleines-for-endorsement_0.pdf (accessed July 5, 2020).

Palmeira, M.I., de Oliveira, J.T., and Requicha, J.F. (2017). Dental diseases and pain in cats (Felis catus). Proceedings of the European Congress of Veterinary Dentistry.

Paul, E. and Podberscek, A. (2000). Veterinary education and students' attitudes towards animal welfare. *Veterinary Record* 146 (10): 269–272.

Paul-Murphy, J., Ludders, J., Robertson, S. et al. (2004). The need for a cross-species approach to the study of pain in animals. *J. Am. Vet. Med. Assoc.* 224 (5): 692–697.

PDSA. (2018). Your Pet's 5 Welfare Needs. Available from http://www.pdsa.org.uk/taking-care-of-your-pet/looking-after-your-pet/all-pets/5-welfare-needs (accessed July 5, 2020).

PennCHART. (2016). The Canine Symptom Assessment Scale. Available from http://www.vet.upenn.edu/research/clinical-trials/vcic/pennchart (accessed July 5, 2020).

Rawlinson, J.E., Goldstein, R.E., Reiter, A.M. et al. (2011). Association of periodontal disease with systemic health indices in dogs and the systemic response to treatment of periodontal disease. *J. Am. Vet. Med. Assoc.* 238: 601–609.

Rodan, I., Sundahl, E., Carney, H. et al. (2011). AAFP and ISFM feline-friendly handling guidelines. *J. Feline Med. Surg.* 13: 364–375.

Rollin, B. (1989). *The Unheeded Cry: Animal Consciousness, Animal Pain, and Science*, 117–118. New York: Oxford University Press.

Rusbridge, C. and Heath, S. (2015). Feline orofacial pain syndrome. In: *Feline Behavioural Health and Welfare* (eds. I. Rodan and S. Heath), 213–226. St. Louis, MO: Elsevier.

Ryan, S., Bacon, H., Edenburg, N., et al. (2018). WSAVA Animal Welfare Guidelines. Available from https://www.wsava.org/WSAVA/media/resources/Guidelines/WSAVA-Animal-Welfare-Guidelines-(2018).pdf (accessed July 5, 2020).

Seksel, K. (2007). How pain affects animals. Proceedings of the Australian Animal Welfare Strategy Science Summit on Pain and Pain Management, Melbourne, Australia.

Siegford, J., Cottee, S., and Widowski, T. (2010). Opportunities for learning about animal welfare from online courses to graduate degrees. *J. Vet. Med. Educ.* 37 (1): 49–55.

Spitznagel, M., Jacobson, D., Cox, M., and Carlson, M. (2018). Predicting caregiver burden in general veterinary clients: contribution of companion animal clinical signs and problem behaviors. *Vet. J.* 236: 23–30.

Stiles, J., Weil, A.B., and Packer, R.A. (2012). Post-anesthetic cortical blindness in cats: twenty cases. *Vet. J.* 193 (2): 367–373.

Summers, J.F., O'Neill, D.G., Church, D. et al. (2019). Health-related welfare prioritisation of canine disorders using electronic health records in primary care practice in the UK. *BMC Vet. Res.* 15: 163.

UK Government. (2006) Animal Welfare Act. Available from http://www.legislation.gov.uk/ukpga/2006/45/contents (accessed July 5, 2020).

Part II

The Dental Patient

9

Local, Regional, and Systemic Complications of Dental Diseases

Jerzy Gawor[1] and Brook Niemiec[2]

[1] Veterinary Clinic Arka, Kraków, Poland
[2] Veterinary Dental Specialties and Oral Surgery, San Diego, CA, USA

9.1 Introduction

Dental disease is the number one problem in small animal patients, and thus oral pathology is exceedingly common. In addition, there is a very wide variety of pathologies that are encountered within the oral cavity. These conditions often cause significant pain and localized, regional, and systemic infection. Since oral health is critical for all other body systems, including the other vital assessments (nutrition, pain, etc.), it should be evaluated in every patient on every visit.

9.2 Oral Health Impacts General Health

Pets with poor oral health often have other health problems, and oral disease can result in systemic issues. Dental professionals have long suspected that oral infections can lead to problems elsewhere in the body. Heart, liver, kidney, and other diseases have been associated with bacteria from periodontal disease (Debowes et al. 1996; Pavlica et al. 2008). For a long time, it was thought that bacteria were the primary factor that linked periodontal disease to other infections in the body. More recent research demonstrates that inflammation and the host immune response are significant and may link periodontal disease to other chronic conditions (Scannapieco 2004).

Experts in human medicine agree that there is an association between periodontal diseases and other chronic inflammatory conditions, such as diabetes and heart disease. Therefore, treating inflammation as well as bacteria may not only help control periodontal disease, but may also facilitate the management of other chronic inflammatory conditions.

The oral cavity plays a key role in getting nutrients to the remainder of the gastrointestinal (GI) tract. Pets with painful teeth/mouth may experience partial to complete anorexia.

They – and those without teeth – may not chew properly, which is known to decrease proper digestion and assimilation of nutrients regardless of a proper diet.

Oral disease has numerous local/regional and systemic ramifications. There are several mechanisms by which this occurs. Quite often, the infection is spread through surrounding tissues or via the lymph/blood circulation system. Destruction of the natural host barriers when the oral defense system is weakened allows the infection to progress significantly faster. Progressing disease further damages the area and enables local and regional transfer of abscessation or damage of adjacent organs and compartments.

The local group of complications include: abscesses, pathologic mandibular fracture, ocular damage/eye loss, increased incidence of oral cancer, osteomyelitis/osteonecrosis, oronasal communication, and nasal infection of dental origin, which may further decrease eating and compromise functions of the nasal senses (Niemiec 2008).

Systemic diseases that may be associated with dental infections include: renal, liver, and heart disease, increased risk of certain cancers, increased incidence and worsened complications of diabetes mellitus, risk of early mortality, and general lethargy (Finch et al. 2016; Glickman et al. 2009; Niemiec 2013a; Trevejo et al. 2018).

Chronic inflammation associated with infection is the basic characteristic of periodontal diseases. Such a process undoubtedly negatively affects the immune system, causes production of immune complexes (antigen/antibody), and thus influences overall systemic balance and health (Takai 2005; Rawlinson et al. 2011).

Most oral conditions are associated with pain. Pain in and of itself, as a very destructive sensation, should be considered a distinct disease process that negatively affects patient welfare and behavior. Chronic pain can be responsible for the development of feline orofacial pain syndrome (FOPS) in cats (McFadyen et al. 2010). Stress from oral pain and dysfunction of the digestive apparatus can be a causative factor for other oral problems (Koch and Imsirovic 2014).

Taking into account that the oral cavity participates in sensory perception of the surrounding environment, it is obvious that diseased structures of the oral cavity affect an animal's functions not only in digestion, but also in grooming, playing, and self-hygiene.

All of these factors show that oral/dental health is critical to patient health and quality of life (QOL).

9.3   Oronasal Communication/Fistulas

Oronasal fistulas (ONFs) are the most common local consequence of periodontal disease (Niemiec 2010). They are generally seen in older, small-breed dogs (especially chondrodystrophic and dolichocephalic breeds), but they can occur in any breed, as well as felines. This breed predisposition is caused by the unfavorable ratio of the relatively large size of the teeth to the relatively small amount of the alveolar bone in their periodontium, maxillary teeth crowding and the deficit of alveolar bone in the palatal aspect of the canine tooth alveolus. ONFs are created by the apical progression of periodontal disease on the palatal surface of the maxillary canines (however, any maxillary tooth is a candidate). This will eventually result in the destruction of the maxillary bone, causing a communication between the oral and nasal cavities and leading to a chronic infection (rhinitis, sinusitis) (Marretta and Smith 2005).

Clinical signs of an ONF include chronic nasal discharge, sneezing, and occasionally anorexia and halitosis (Figure 9.1). It is possible to provoke sneezing by gently touching the canine teeth through the cheeks.

Occasionally, a fistula may be noted on conscious exam (Figure 9.2) – especially one that has resulted from an extraction – but definitive diagnosis of an ONF typically requires a thorough examination under general anesthesia (Figure 9.2). The diagnosis is made by introducing a periodontal probe into the periodontal space on the palatal surface of the tooth (Figure 9.3). Interestingly, ONFs may occur despite the fact that the remainder of the patient's periodontal tissues are healthy, including other surfaces of the affected tooth (Niemiec 2013b). Appropriate treatment of an ONF requires extraction of the tooth and closure of the defect with a mucogingival flap. However, if a deep periodontal pocket is discovered prior to development of a fistula, periodontal surgery with guided tissue regeneration may be performed to save the tooth (Niemiec 2013b).

Patients with chronic, long-term untreated oronasal communication suffer significantly from decreased nasal senses and

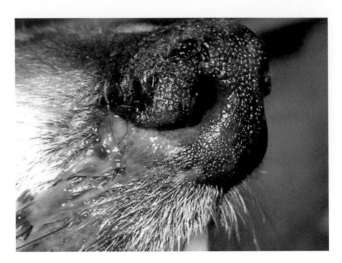

Figure 9.1   Oronasal fistula (ONF) signalments: nasal discharge.

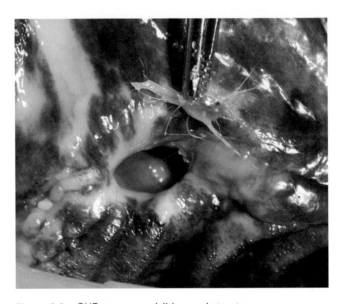

Figure 9.2   ONF presence: visible nasal structures.

food accumulation in the nasal cavity (Figure 9.4). Infection and progressive destruction of turbinates is often irreversible, as once the nasal structures are destroyed, they will not recover. Despite closing the ONF, the normal functions of the rostral respiratory tract quite often will not return. Additionally, leftover purulent discharge, as well as food remnants, may contaminate the respiratory tract with every breath.

9.4   Periapical Lesions

There are two major types of periapical lesions endo-perio lesions (type 1) and perio-endo lesions (type 2).

The perio-endo lesions are another potential consequence of periodontal disease. They can be seen mostly in multirooted teeth, but also in canine teeth and incisors

(Figure 9.5). They occur when the alveolar bone loss caused by periodontitis progresses apically and gains access to the endodontic system through the blood supply (apical delta), creating endodontic disease via bacterial contamination. Such infection typically occurs via the apex, but it may also happen due to non-apical ramifications (blood supply other than at the apex). The deep vertical bone loss in a single-rooted tooth can also deliver infection to pulp and cause its necrosis, gangrene (anaerobic infection), and accelerated pathologic processes (Figure 9.6).

The endodontic infection subsequently spreads though the tooth via the common pulp chamber and causes periapical ramifications on the other root(s). However, the

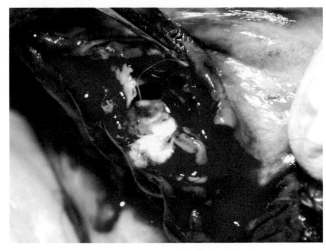

Figure 9.4 Picture during ONF repair: nasal cavity filled with debris.

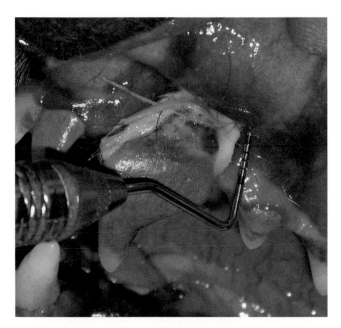

Figure 9.3 ONF diagnosis with the use of a periodontal probe.

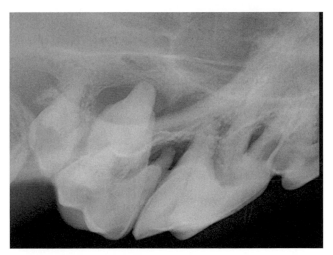

Figure 9.5 Perio-endo lesions in 109. Note the furcation involvement in 109 and 108.

(a)

(b)

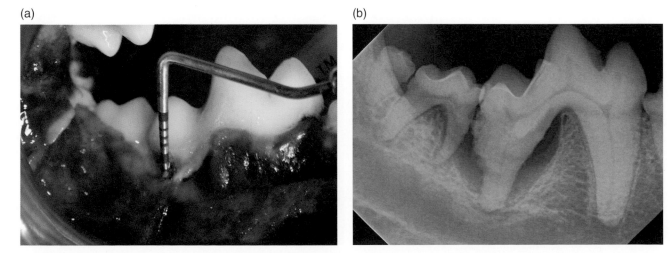

Figure 9.6 Deep vertical bone loss in the distal root of 409: (a) clinical appearance; (b) radiograph.

infected tooth may be held in position by the large surface area of these other roots.

The most common site for class II perio-endo lesions in small-animal patients is the distal root of the mandibular first molar, but they can occur in any multirooted tooth (Figure 9.7). They are seen most commonly in older small- and toy-breed dogs, but any dogs of any age and size can be affected.

Periapical abscesses not only cause pain and disfunction, but are also a means of access for toxins, which go on to create local and systemic negative effects. Each time pressure is applied (i.e., during mastication), toxins and bacteria gain access to the vascular system and spread throughout the patient.

So-called facial infraorbital or "carnassial" abscess are local infectious odontogenic complications associated with

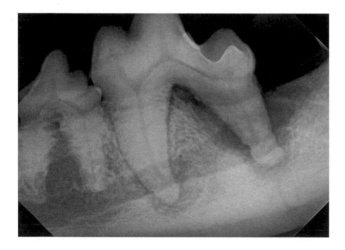

Figure 9.7 Distal root of mandibular firts molar is very common site for class II perio endo lesions. Note the periapical lesion in mesial root of 309, missing 310 and ankylosis affecting both roots of 308.

drainage of an abscess through the skin following facial swelling (Figure 9.8). Any facial swelling should be investigated via an orodental consultation and diagnostic imaging.

Dental abscesses can also drain into the oral cavity and create a parulis (opening of the drainage canal to the oral vestibule or to the mouth proper) (Figure 9.9). This kind of complication can be difficult to diagnose and is often incidentally revealed during routine dental check-up (Figure 9.10).

9.5 Pathologic Fracture

One of the most severe common consequences of periodontal disease is a pathologic jaw fracture (Figure 9.11). Such fractures typically occur in the mandible (especially at the area of the canines and first molars) due to chronic periodontal loss, which weakens the bone in affected areas. This condition is most common in small- and toy-breed dogs, as their teeth (especially the mandibular first molar) are larger in proportion to their mandible as compared to large-breed dogs (Figure 9.12). Thus, small-breed dogs have minimal bone apical to the tooth root, putting this area at high risk of fracture when significant bone loss occurs (Gioso et al. 2001). In addition, they tend to have more severe periodontal disease than medium- to large-breed dogs. Finally, small- and toy-breed dogs tend to live longer than larger breeds, allowing for more advanced periodontal disease in their geriatric years.

Pathologic jaw fractures typically occur as a result of mild trauma (dog fights are common), but they can often also occur during a dental extraction. Some dogs have

(a)

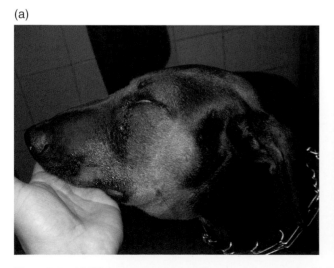

(b)

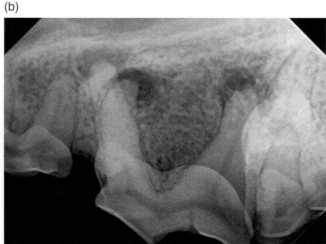

Figure 9.8 (a) Clinical appearance of the Carnassial abscess. (b) Periapical radiolucencies in all roots of the 208 (b) in the patient illustrated with carnassial abscess (a).

(a)

(b)

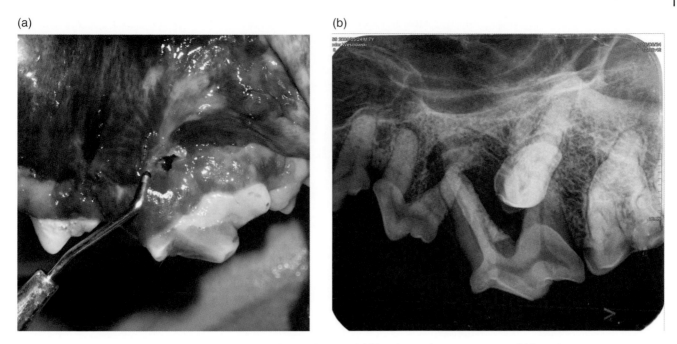

Figure 9.9   (a) Intraoral dental sinus drainage (parulis). (b) Infection of 208 and ectopic supernumerary 208 tooth.

(a)

(b)

(c)

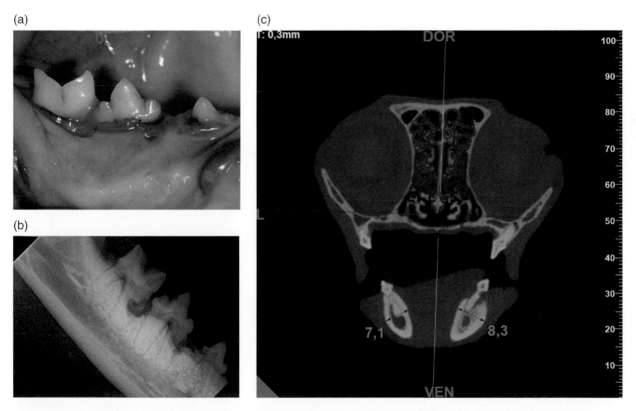

Figure 9.10   Incidentally revealed pathology: Right mandibular teeth : 407, 408, 409 present signs of periodontal disease (a) radiographically all these teeth shows presence of teeth resorption (b), in 3dimensional imaging right mandible is thickened and (c) biopsy confirmed osteomyelitis.

(a)

(b)

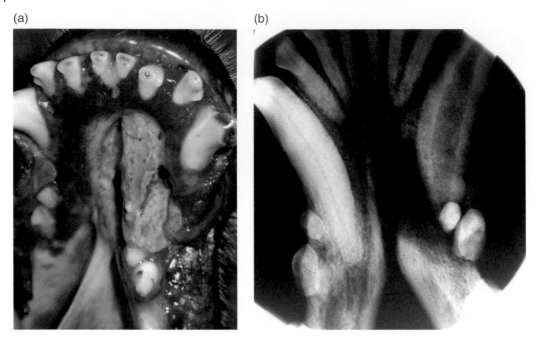

Figure 9.11   Pathologic mandibular fracture as a sequela of 304 pulp necrosis, periapical inflammation, osteomyelitis, and osteonecrosis; (a) clinical and (b) radiographic picture. Note the presence of 305 and 306 in the fracture line.

(a)

(b)

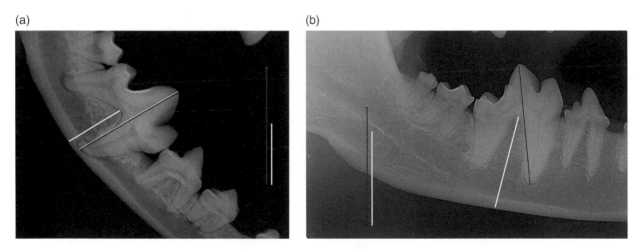

Figure 9.12   Relation of bone/tooth in (a) small- and (b) large-breed dogs.

suffered fractures while simply eating or playing. This is typically considered a disease of older patients, but there are reports of young animals being affected.

Pathologic fractures carry a guarded prognosis, for several reasons. Adequate healing is difficult to obtain due to lack of remaining bone, low oxygen tension, and difficulty in rigidly fixating the caudal portion of mandible. (Niemiec 2001, Taney and Smith, 2010) There are numerous options for fixation, but the use of advanced surgical methods like microplates or wires is generally required. Regardless of the method chosen, the periodontally diseased root(s) *must* be extracted for healing to occur (Figure 9.13).

Awareness of the risk of pathologic fracture can help practitioners avoid complications in at-risk patients during dental procedures. If one root of a multirooted tooth is periodontally healthy, there is a greater chance of mandibular fracture due to the increased force needed to extract it. An alternative form of treatment for these cases is to section the tooth, extract the periodontally diseased root, and perform root canal therapy on the periodontally healthy root. In cases where severe alveolar bone loss is noted (especially if the mandibular canine or first molar is affected), it is recommended that the owners be informed of the possibility of an iatrogenic jaw fracture prior to attempting extraction.

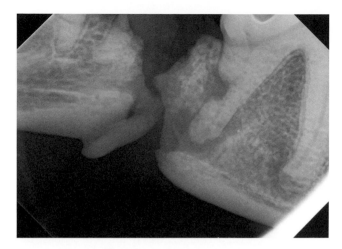

Figure 9.13 Infection at the area of fracture requires extraction of the diseased tooth or root prior to fracture fixation.

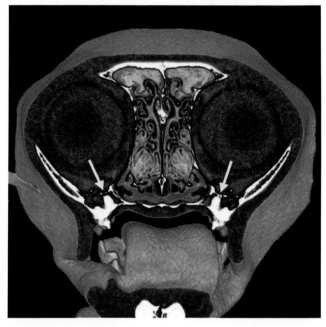

Figure 9.15 Proximity of maxillary teeth roots and their apices (arrows) and orbitum in a cat.

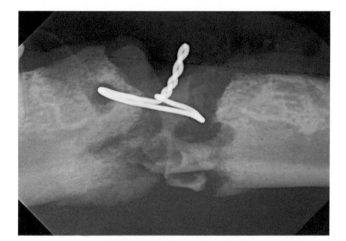

Figure 9.14 Damaged area of bone surrounding a fracture due to an unsuccessful fixation attempt.

A reasonable option in such a case is to refer the patient to a specialist. Unsuccessful attempts to treat pathologic fractures may lead to progressing bone loss and significant deficits of the jaw structure (Figure 9.14). This further lowers the chance of healing. In cases of non-union or difficulty in stabilization of the pathologic fracture (or any fracture), referral to a specialist is recommended. (See Part IV for more on when to call a specialist).

Abnormally weakened bone at the area of fracture should also be biopsied to rule out the possibility of neoplasia.

9.6 Ocular Damage

Another local consequence of severe periodontal disease results from inflammation close to the orbit, which can potentially lead to ocular inflammation, naso-lacrimal disease,

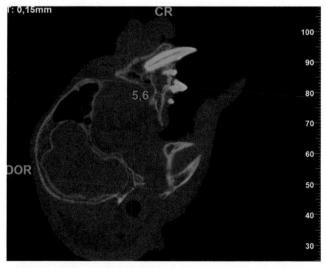

Figure 9.16 In brachycephalic cats, the apex of the canine tooth is very close to the orbitum.

and possibly blindness. (Ramsey et al, 1996) The proximity of the tooth root apices of the maxillary molars and fourth premolars places the delicate optic tissues in jeopardy (Figure 9.15). In cats (especially brachycephalic breeds), the apices of the maxillary canine teeth lie in this area and can create similar issues (Figure 9.16).

Chronic conjunctivitis or ocular discharge should always be investigated with an accurate oral assessment and dental radiographs (see Chapter 14).

9.7 Oral Cancer

Recent studies in human dentistry have linked chronic periodontal disease to an increased risk of oral cancer (Wen et al. 2014). The association in this case is likely due to the chronic inflammatory state that exists with periodontitis. The rough surface of tartar creates long-term mechanical irritation, causing erosion and ulceration and potentially acting as a cancerogenic factor (Figure 9.17).

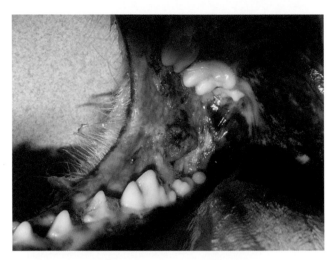

Figure 9.17 Chronic irritation of the oral mucosa in plaque-associated contact ulceration can act as a cancerogenic factor.

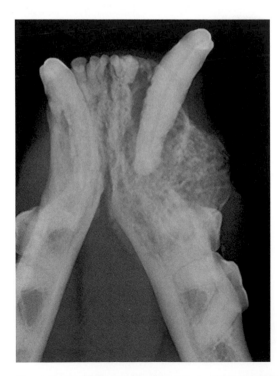

Figure 9.18 Radiographic appearance of osteomyelitis in the rostal mandible of a cat.

Since neoplasia typically requires a promoter to propagate, it is generally controlled in patients with healthy gingival tissues. The significant inflammation associated with periodontal disease acts as a co-founder to the body's defenders, much in the same way that smoking increases the incidence of lung cancer. In fact, in cats, one of the reported etiologic factors for the development of oral squamous-cell carcinoma (SCC) is passive smoking (Bertone et al. 2003).

9.8 Osteomyelitis

Alveolar osteomyelitis is defined as an area of inflamed infected bone with partial necrosis in forms of sequestrum (Figure 9.18) (Bell and Soukup., 2015).

Periodontal disease and other dental diseases (e.g., tooth resorption) are the most common causes of oral osteomyelitis. In addition, improper use of power equipment in the mouth can create it iatrogenically (see Chapter 17). Furthermore, once an area of bone is necrotic, it does not respond effectively to antibiotic therapy, as the dead bone does not have a blood supply and thus the associated microorganisms are protected from the antibiotics. Therefore, definitive therapy generally requires aggressive surgical debridement of all necrotic tissue, followed by adequately long medical treatment (Figure 9.19). In most cases, the antibiotic treatment of osteomyelitis should last 6–12 weeks, and therefore selection of the correct antibiotic is important and should be based on culture of the infected bone.

Radiographically, osteomyelitis can resemble other bone pathologies such as cancer; therefore, histopathologic assessment is always recommended (Figure 9.20).

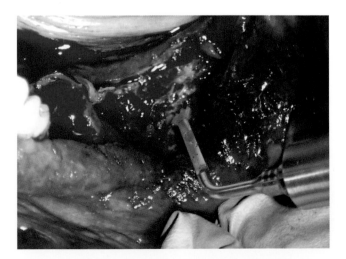

Figure 9.19 Debridement of the necrotic part of a bone affected by osteomyelitis through the use of piezosurgery.

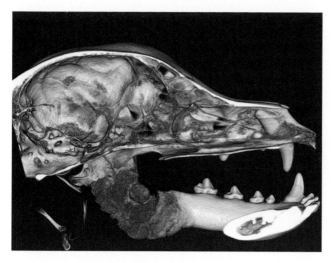

Figure 9.20 CBCT appearance of osteomyelitis resembling cancer.

Empiric treatment without surgical debridement can result in recurrence of the disease after discontinuation of the antibiotic regime following temporary improvement when the treatment is applied. Unfortunately, such an approach may lead to antibiotic resistance and must be avoided. (See more in Chapter 7) In some cases, the bacterial infection may also result in sepsis, which is a life-threatening condition.

Patients typically present with pain and halitosis, and quite often the bone is thickened and regional lymph nodes are enlarged.

Intraoral dental radiographs will reveal proliferation of the bone and other signs of bone destruction. Within the affected area, one should expect to find a diseased tooth causing this condition (Figure 9.21).

9.9 Systemic Complications of Oral Diseases

The most common chronic infection of an organism is the complex of periodontal diseases. Pathogenesis of systemic complications of periodontal diseases comes from the fact that bacteria disperse from the oral cavity, through the alimentary tract (with every swallow), the respiratory tract (with every breath), and an inflamed and compromised gingival epithelium, into the cardiovascular system, causing bacteriemia and provoking the immune system to alert local defenses.

Stress accompanying oral pain dysfunctions of oral structures and infection decrease general and local immunity levels and predispose to the development of opportunistic diseases.

Blood distribution of bacteria delivers infection to organs and affects their functions. Studies show effects on the liver and kidneys (Pavlica et al. 2008; Rawlinson

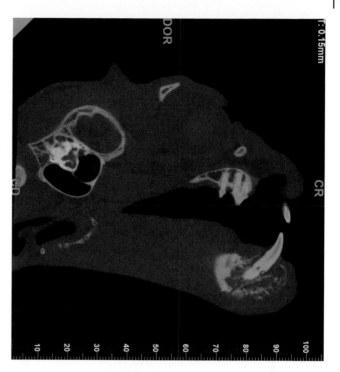

Figure 9.21 Tooth resorption of a canine tooth as a possible origin of osteomyelitis.

et al. 2011), association of bacteriemia with cholestasis (Taboada and Meyer 1989), and bacterial infection of the liver with portal fibrosis and parenchymal inflammation (Debowes 2008) (Figure 9.22).

The risk of endocarditis is approximately sixfold higher for dogs with stage 3 periodontal disease compared with those without such disease (Glickman et al. 2009). Periodontal disease may affect the hypertrophic cardiomyopathy in cats, as it has been shown to be associated with left-ventricular hypertrophy (Franek et al. 2005). One veterinary study has revealed a possible link between periodontal disease and cardiomyopathies in dogs (Glickman et al. 2009). Increased C-reactive protein in periodontally affected veterinary patients has been also reported (Debowes 2008; Kouki et al. 2013). (Nemec et al. (2013) noted a transitory increase in nitric oxide following appropriate periodontal therapy.

The lungs, brain, and spleen have been shown to become the target of infection in human studies (Mealey 1999; Bui et al. 2019). Long-term infection and massive production of immune complexes may occur in polyarthritis etiopathogenesis, though this needs to be confirmed (Cheng et al. 2017). Oral bacteriemia can cross the placental membrane and affect development of the fetus, birth weight, and the moment of birth, as well as causing preeclampsia (Vamos et al. 2015). A large retrospective study (Trevejo *et al.* 2018) showed increased risk of renal diseases and and cystitis incidence with increased stages of periodontal diseases.

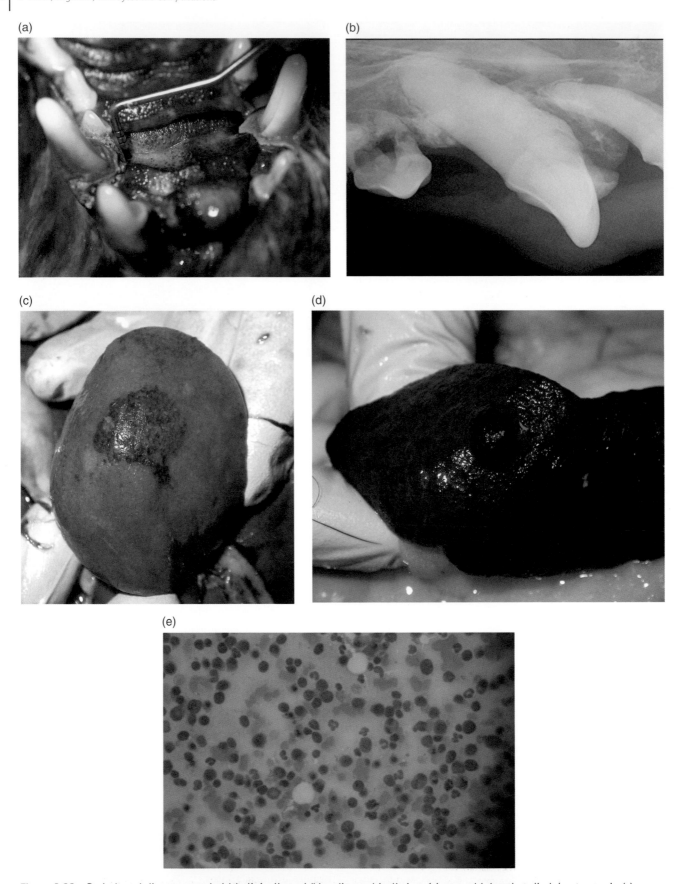

Figure 9.22 Periodontal disease revealed (a) clinically and (b) radiographically in a 14-year-old dog that died due to sepsis. (c) Necropsy-diagnosed spleen and (d) liver abscesses. (e) Onsite cytologic assessment of the spleen showed an abnormal presence of neutrophiles in a slide impression of the abscess area.

Some insurance companies require dental treatment prior to planned prosthetic surgery like joint replacement or cardiosurgery (Field et al. 2000). Periodontal diseases, as immune-related diseases, can affect the treatment and course of other chronic immune-mediated problems like diabetes mellitus and renal failure. Many links between stabilization of diabetes and periodontal diseases are reported in human medicine (Grossi and Genco 1998; Mealey and Ocampo 2006).

9.10 Conclusion

Chronic periodontal disease in veterinary patients can have disastrous consequences within the oral cavity. Furthermore, many of these disease processes will not have obvious clinical signs until very late in the disease course, if ever. Obtaining a definitive diagnosis often requires careful evaluation under general anesthesia. It is important to note that all such conditions can be prevented with standard, routine oral care that includes daily hygiene and veterinary oral check-ups.

We know that periodontal disease is an infectious process that requires affected patients to deal with dangerous bacteria on a daily basis, leading to a state of chronic disease (Harvey and Emily 1993; Holmstrom et al. 1998). Therefore, we must learn to view it not merely as a dental problem that causes bad breath and tooth loss, but as an initiator of more severe systemic consequences (Niemiec 2013a).

These subjects should be discussed with *all* clients, especially owners of small- and toy-breed dogs. In fact, a discussion of home care should take place at the initial visit to the practice (e.g., at well-puppy exam) don't wait until periodontal disease is established. Appropriate client education should increase compliance with oral health-care recommendations and help avoid these disastrous consequences.

References

Bell CM, Soukup JW. Histologic, Clinical, and Radiologic Findings of Alveolar Bone Expansion and Osteomyelitis of the Jaws in Cats. Vet Pathol. 2015 Sep;52(5):910-8. doi: 10.1177/0300985815591079. Epub 2015 Jun 25. PMID: 26113612.

Bertone, E.R., Snyder, L.A., and Moore, A.S. (2003). Environmental and lifestyle risk factors for oral squamous cell carcinoma in domestic cats. *J. Vet. Intern. Med.* 17: 557–562.

Bui, F.Q., Almeida-da-Silva, C.L.C., Huynhet, B. et al. (2019). Association between periodontal pathogens and systemic disease. *Biomed. J.* 42: 27–35.

Cheng, Z., Meade, J., Mankia, K. et al. (2017). Periodontal disease and periodontal bacteria as triggers for rheumatoid arthritis. *Best Pract. Res. Clin. Rheumatol.* 31 (1): 19–30.

Debowes, L.J. (2008) C-reactive protein and periodontal disease. Proceedings of the 22nd Annual Dental Forum.

Debowes, L.J., Mosier, D., Logan, E. et al. (1996). Association of periodontal disease and histologic lesions in multiple organs from 45 dogs. *J. Vet. Dent.* 13: 57–60.

Field, M.J., Lawrence, R.L., and Zwanziger, L. (2000). Medically necessary dental services. In: *Extending Medicare Coverage for Preventive and Other Services* (eds. M.J. Field, R.L. Lawrence and L. Zwanziger), 63–98. Washington, DC: National Academies Press.

Finch, N. C., Syme, H. M. & Elliott, J. (2016) Risk Factors for Development of Chronic Kidney Disease in Cats. *Journal of Veterinary Internal Medicine* 30, 602–610.

Franek, E., Blach, A. et al. (2005). Association between chronic periodontal disease and left ventricular hypertrophy in kidney transplant recipients. *Transplantation* 80: 3–5.

Gioso, M., Shofer, P., Barros, P., and Harvey, C.E. (2001). Mandible and mandibular first molar tooth measurements in dogs: relationship of radiographic height to body weight. *J. Vet. Dent.* 18 (2): 65–68.

Glickman, L.T., Glickman, N.W., Moore, G.E. et al. (2009). Evaluation of the risk of endocarditis and other cardiovascular events on the basis of the severity of periodontal disease in dogs. *J. Am. Vet. Med. Assoc.* 234 (4): 486–494.

Grossi, S.G. and Genco, R.J. (1998). Periodontal disease and diabetes mellitus: a two way relationship. *Ann. Periodontal.* 3: 51–61.

Harvey, C.E. and Emily, P.P. (1993). Periodontal disease. In: *Small Animal Dentistry* (eds. C.E. Harvey and P.P. Emily), 89–144. St. Louis, MO: Mosby.

Holmstrom, S.E., Frost, P., and Eisner, E.R. (1998). Dental Prophylaxis. In: *Veterinary Dental Techniques*, 2ee (eds. S.E. Holmstrom, P. Frost and E. Eisner), 133–166. Philadelphia, PA: W.B. Saunders.

Koch, D.A. and Imsirovic, A.A. (2014). What is the role of stress in the pathophysiology of feline chronic gingivostomatitis and resorptive lesions? Proceedings of the 23rd EVCD.

Kouki, M., Papadimitriou, S., Kazakos, G. et al. (2013). Periodontal disease as a potential factor for systemic inflammatory response in the dog. *J. Vet. Dent* 30 (1): 26–29.

Mealey, B.L. (1999). Influence of periodontal infections on systemic health. *Periodontol. 2000* 21: 197–209.

Mealey, B.L. and Ocampo, G.L. (2006). Diabetes mellitus and periodontal disease. *J. Periodontol.* 77 (8): 1289–1303.

Marretta, S.M. and Smith, M.M. (2005). Single mucoperiosteal flap for oronasal fistula repair. *J. Vet. Dent.* 22: 200–205.

McFadyen, K., Rusbridge, C., Heath, S. et al. (2010). Feline orofacial pain syndrome (FOPS): a retrospective study of 113 cases. *J. Feline Med. Surg.* 12: 498.

Niemiec, B.A. (2001) Treatment of mandibular first molar teeth with endodontic-periodontal lesions in a dog. *Journal of Veterinary Dentistry* 18, 21–25.

Niemiec, B.A. (2008). Periodontal disease. *Top. Companion Anim. Med.* 23: 72–80.

Niemiec, B.A. (2010). *Small Animal Dental, Oral & Maxillofacial Disease*, 9–38. Boca Raton, FL: CRC Press.

Niemiec, B.A. (2013a). Systemic manifestations of periodontal disease. In: *Veterinary Periodontology* (ed. B.A. Niemiec), 81–90. Ames, IA: Wiley-Blackwell.

Nicmiec, B.A. (2013b). *Veterinary Periodontology*. Ames, IA: Wiley-Blackwell.

Nemec, A., Verstraete, F. J., Jerin, A., et al. (2013) Periodontal disease, periodontal treatment and systemic nitric oxide in dogs. *Research in Veterinary Science* **94**, 542–544.

Pavlica, Z., Petelin, M., Juntes, P. et al. (2008). Periodontal disease burden and pathological changes in the organs of dogs. *J. Vet. Dent.* 25: 97–108.

Ramsey, D. T., Marretta, S. M., Hamor, R. E., *et al.* (1996). Ophthalmic manifestations and complications of dental disease in dogs and cats. *Journal of the American Animal Hospital Association* 32, 215–224.

Rawlinson, J.E., Goldstein, R.E., Reiter, A.M. et al. (2011). Association of periodontal disease with systemic health indices in dogs and the systemic response to treatment of periodontal disease. *J. Am. Vet. Med. Assoc.* 238: 601–609.

Scannapieco, F.A. (2004). Periodontal inflammation: from gingivitis to systemic disease? *Compend. Contin. Educ. Dent.* 25: 16–25.

Taboada, J. and Meyer, D.J. (1989). Cholestasis in associated with extrahepatic bacterial infection in five dogs. *J. Vet. Intern. Med.* 3: 216–220.

Takai, T. (2005). Fc receptors and their role in immune regulation and autoimmunity. *J. Clin. Immunol.* 25: 1–18.

Taney, K.G. & Smith, M. M. (2010) Problems with muscles, bones, and joints. In; Small animal dental, oral, and maxillofacial disease, a color handbook. Ed B. A. Niemiec Manson, London. pp 199–204.

Trevejo, R. T., Lefebvre, S. L., Yang, M., *et al.* (2018) Survival analysis to evaluate associations between periodontal disease and the risk of development of chronic azotemic kidney disease in cats evaluated at primary care veterinary hospitals. Journal of American Veterinary Medical Association 252, 710–720.

Vamos, C.A., Thompson, E.L., Avendano, M. et al. (2015). Oral health promotion interventions during pregnancy: a systematic review. *Community Dent. Oral Epidemiol.* 43 (5): 385–396.

Wen, B. W., Tsai, C. S., Lin, C. L., et al. (2014) Cancer risk among gingivitis and periodontitis patients: a nationwide cohort study. *QJM* **107**, 283–290.

10

Hereditary Oral Disorders in Purebred Dogs and Cats
Jerzy Gawor

Veterinary Clinic Arka, Kraków, Poland

Approximately 900 hereditary diseases and 200 genetic predispositions are currently recognized in dogs and cats. Inherited diseases such as hip dysplasia, brachycephalic airway syndrome, cardiomyopathies, endocrine dysfunctions, blood disorders, and many more affect the quality of life (QOL) and lifespan of dogs (Koharik 2007). Sterile feline lower urinary tract disease (FLUTD) is the number one hereditary feline predisposition, followed by diabetes and lymphocytic or plasmacytic inflammatory disease, which most frequently manifest as either gingivostomatitis (Harley et al. 2011) or inflammatory bowel disease (IBD) (Jergens 2012).

Some hereditary diseases are associated with a single pair of genes, while others have a more complicated method of transfer down the generations. There are also those in which their putative heritability is based on observation only and the mechanism of inheritance is not known, which are given the description "of family nature" (Meyers-Wallen 2003).

The Feline Advisory Bureau (FAB) proposes dividing hereditary conditions in cats (confirmed and suspected) into three groups (FAB n.d.):

- The genetics of the condition has been confirmed and/or a genetic test is available.
- A breed predisposition is recognized and the condition is strongly suspected to be inherited.
- A potential breed predisposition is recognized but it is not currently known if the condition is inherited or not, as only single case reports are available or evidence is anecdotal.

Localization of the exact genes responsible for specific conditions may be easier in dogs as a canine genome map is currently available (Mellersh 2008).

Diagnostic methods are presented in Table 10.1, a ranking of the negative influences of different diseases on QOL is given in Table 10.2, and 49 breeds that may have genetic oral disorders are listed in Appendix D, along with suggestions on how to evaluate and record their respective diseases.

Advances in diagnostic techniques have provided dozens of tests that may confirm the genetic basis of any disease. The number of such tests will likely increase annually going forward, and thus they will play an increasingly important role in the future. Nonetheless, the first part of any procedure is always a thorough examination of the patient, with particular attention to the specific symptoms and proper diagnostic testing.

The selection process for breeding has long been based on particular characteristics of the appearance of breeding animals. However, the effects on their health were not considered. This type of breeding can consolidate the presence of certain diseases in the population of purebred dogs (Sampson 2004). Specific breeds often appear drastically different from their ancestors, and many metabolic characteristics differ between different breeds. These facts undoubtedly have an impact on the appearance of clinical problems recognized as hereditary syndromes or diseases associated with metabolic or immune-mediated defects (Ackerman 1999).

The diagnosis of a particular disease is based on precise criteria, including clinical assessment, imaging, and laboratory tests (histopathologic or genetic). Documentation of a registered disease is either photographic or radiographic. Each case is evaluated in terms of its negative influence on health and vital functions. Scores are given on a scale of 1–3, with 1 being the lowest and 3 the highest level of disturbance (see Table 10.2).

The Veterinary Dental Patient: A Multidisciplinary Approach, First Edition. Edited by Jerzy Gawor and Brook Niemiec.
© 2021 John Wiley & Sons Ltd. Published 2021 by John Wiley & Sons Ltd.
Companion website: www.wiley.com/go/gawor/veterinary-dental-patient

Table 10.1   Description of the tests required to diagnose hereditary diseases and provide certification.

Examination and recording method	Requirements
Photography (Ph)	Requires photographic documentation of the disease, with characteristic signalments
Laboratory	
Genetic (G)	Test must be performed in a referral laboratory
Histopathologic (H)	Test must be performed in a referral laboratory
Other (L)	Test must be performed in a referral laboratory
Clinical ©	Clinical examination according to AVD, EVDC, and AVDC standards a) Conscious examination b) Anesthetized examination
Radiography (X)	Projection and positioning appropriate to the condition

AVD, Academy of Veterinary Dentistry; EVDC, European Veterinary Dental College; AVDC, American Veterinary Dental College.

Table 10.2   Scale for the negative influence of hereditary disease on patient comfort and health

Ranking	Clinical importance
1	Low to moderate influence on life comfort. Treatment not always necessary.
2	Significant influence on life comfort. Treatment mandatory.
3	Critical influence on health. Treatment mandatory. In severe cases, likely consideration of euthanasia.

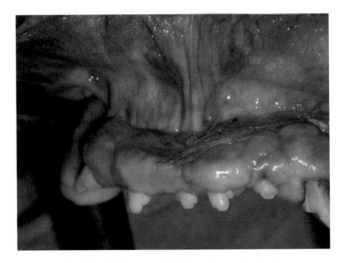

Figure 10.1   Gingival hyperplasia in a Dogue de Bordeaux.

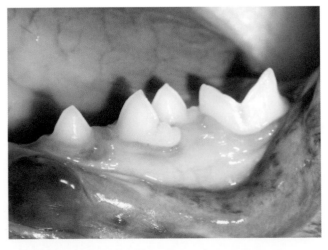

Figure 10.2   Supernumerary teeth in a Russian blue cat.

Some hereditary oral conditions are not located exclusively in the mouth (e.g., craniomandibular osteopathy [CMO], uveodermatologic [UV] syndrome, plasmacytic inflammatory disease in cats) (Kern et al. 1985; Gawor 2006), but they all affect oral health and functionality. Other problems are "just dental" (e.g., gingival hyperplasia, supernumerary teeth) but still influence general health (Wiggs and Lobprise 1997a; Lewis and Reiter 2005) (Figures 10.1 and 10.2). There are also a few systemic problems that have a strong influence on the oral cavity, particularly when oral surgery or other dental procedures are performed (e.g., von Willebrand's disease) (Brooks et al. 2001). Selected anatomical anomalies have shown a tendency to inheritance and more frequent occurrence in certain breeds (e.g., gingival hyperplasia in boxers, retrogenia associated with class II malocclusion in long-haired dachshunds) (Gruneberg and Lea 1940; Gawor 2005).

Some of the conditions listed in Appendix D may be controversial, as there is no "proof" for their hereditary origin, but clinical observations in the population of a particular breed indicate their strong tendency to inheritance, such as persistent primary dentition in Yorkshire terriers

(Gawor 2008) (Figure 10.3). Historically, an anomaly that was considered hereditary and existed as a selective factor in breeding was a cleft palate (Edmonds et al. 1972).

Among oral problems, there are diseases that only slightly affect QOL but which carry a potential risk of significant negative consequences if neglected, or treated improperly. These include retained, impacted, and missing teeth. Disorders of tooth eruption may have features of a generalized disorder, such as delayed eruption in Tibetan terrier (Stapleton and Clarke 1999), or of a local problem, such as impaction of the first mandibular premolar followed by formation of odontogenic cysts in shi-tzu and other brachycephalic dogs (Okuda 2003) (Figure 10.4).

This chapter provides no specific clinical descriptions of the disease entities, only images showing the most important symptoms.

The Polish Small Animal Veterinary Association (PSAVA) has created a proposal aimed at meeting the growing problem of the presence of genetic defects in pedigreed animals (Gawor 2013). Veterinarians and pet owners are often misled by the impression that purchasing a pedigree dog provides a warranty that the animal is free from defects and serious diseases. In fact, such a warranty cannot be provided even in the best situations. The current selection criteria leave a lot of room for the transfer of negative traits into the reproductive pool, affecting animals' offspring.

(a) (b)

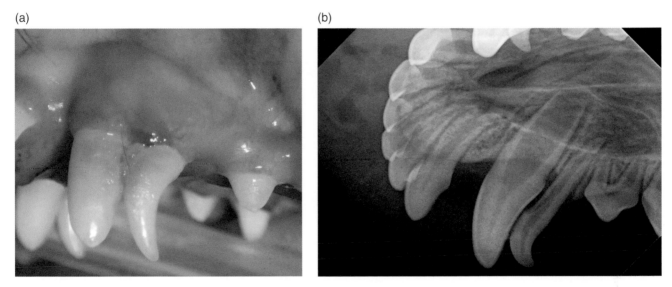

Figure 10.3 Persistent deciduous left maxillary canine tooth (604) in a Yorkshire terrier: (a) clinical picture; (b) radiographic assessment.

(a) (b)

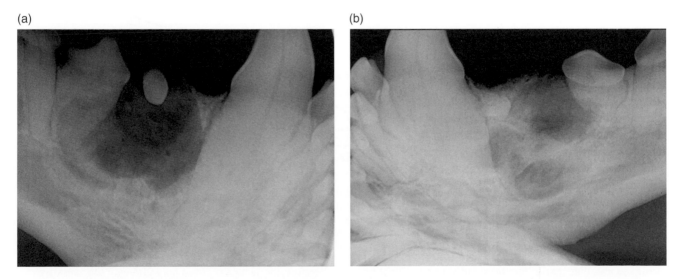

Figure 10.4 Dentigerous cyst (DTC) in the area of (a) 405/406, and (b) 305/306, in a brachycephalic breed (boxer) aged six years.

Current knowledge allows us to determine which defects are indisputably dangerous to life and compromise the health of the patient, and which seem to be less important for QOL (McGreevy and Nicholas 1999; Gough and Thomas 2006; Surgeon 2007). It is important to add to the list conditions that seem to be just "cosmetic" but in fact may seriously affect health or create severe consequences (Giger 2003).

For many years, veterinarians have attempted to decrease the incidence of hereditary diseases in pedigreed

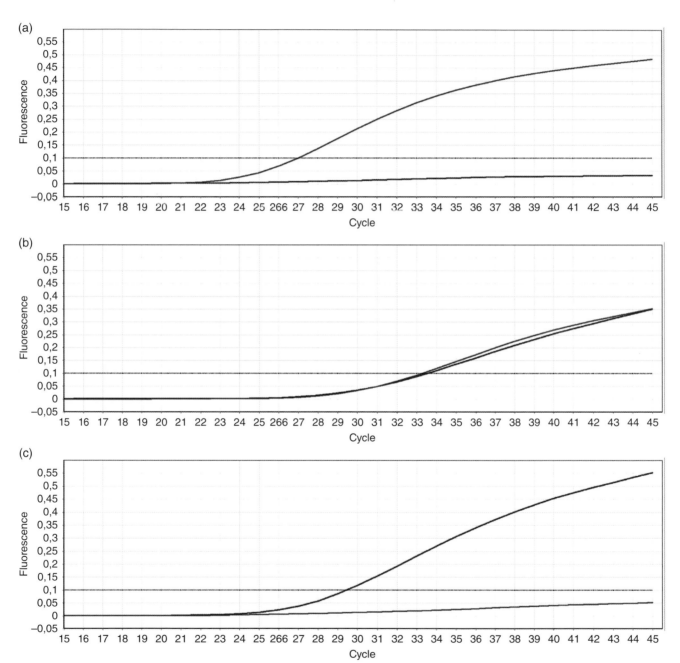

Figure 10.5 Results of genetic test for craniomandibular osteopathy (CMO). (a) A fluorescent signal is only detected for the fluorescent marker of the wildtype probe. This signal is represented by the green line, that crosses the threshold at cycle 27 of the PCR. Therefore, the sample contains only wildtype DNA. Genotype N/N (free) (b) Fluorescent signals are detected for the fluorescent markers of both probes (wildtype and variant). These signals are represented by the green and red line correspondingly and cross the threshold after cycle 33 of the PCR. Therefore, the sample contains wildtype DNA and DNA with the causative variant. Genotype N/MUT (carrier) (c) A fluorescent signal is only detected for the fluorescent marker of the variants probe. This signal is represented by the red line, that crosses the threshold after cycle 29 of the PCR. Therefore, the sample contains only DNA with the causative variant. Genotype MUT/MUT (affected). *Source:* courtesy of LABOKLIN GmbH & CO.KG.

dogs (Mullan and Main 2001; Hernandez 2003; Evans et al. 2007). These efforts are articulated in the recommendations for kennel clubs and the professional media. Specific recommendations can be found in Finland, Norway, Canada, and the Netherlands (Leppänen et al. 2000; Indrebo 2004; van Hagen et al. 2004; Koharik 2007). Additionally, in 2004, the Federation of European Companion Animals Veterinary Associations (FECAVA) symposium was dedicated to congenital defects and diseases (Hedhammar 2004; Indrebo 2004; Sampson 2004).

A range of methods are available for the diagnosis of hereditary diseases (see Table 10.1; the proper means of recording the results are described in Appendix D.

Photographic documentation (Ph) is performed to record symptoms considered pathognomic or typical for a particular disease.

Genetic testing (G) currently does not apply to certain diseases simply because there is no commercial test available (though it is likely that a test for CMO will be available shortly). If there is no test available, another criterion of the diagnosis must be fulfilled (e.g., for CMO: radiological and histopathological examination) (Giger 2003) (Figure 10.5).

Histopathological examination (H) should be performed at referral laboratories, with evaluation by a qualified veterinary pathologist (Gawor 2004).

Laboratory testing (L) is not genetic in nature. It can apply to a number of diseases listed in Appendix D.

Clinical assessment (C) follows the standards of the European Veterinary Dental College (EVDC) or American Veterinary Dental College (AVDC). This includes physical assessment of the oral cavity, occlusion, periodontium, dentition, and mucous membranes. Documentation of such is the protocol of oral examination and photographs. Photographs are taken of specific features of a problem, with the correct position, quality, and magnification (Wiggs and Lobprise 1997b).

Radiographic examination (X) must be carried out properly, using appropriate imaging equipment and projection. The diagnostic value of an image is based on its resolution, contrast, and projection (DuPont and DeBowes 2009). Three-dimensional imaging may be superior in revealing problems associated with temporomandibular joint (TMJ) dysplasia.

To date, very few health problems have had a significant impact on the decision to allow an individual to reproduce. Among the dental problems considered are number of teeth and, to a certain extent, occlusal assessment (FCI n.d.). Many other important anatomical and metabolic disorders or abnormalities are unfortunately ignored. This situation favors an increased number of dental disorders among purebred dogs.

Appendix D examines the breeds that predominate among dental patients. All of the conditions listed should be treated or palliated. The majority can be successfully treated, though it requires financial investment and may be time-consuming. The goal is to limit the ability of affected animals to propagate a problem within the breed.

Problems not related to specific breeds but with a certain degree of genetic background include plasmacytic lymphocytic stomatitis, microdontia, microglossia, skull asymmetry, and soft-palate hypoplasia.

References

Ackerman, L. (1999). *The Genetic Connection: A Guide to Health Problems in Purebred Dogs*, 1–28. Lakewood, CO: AAHA Press.

Brooks, M.B., Erb, H.N., Foureman, P.A., and Ray, K. (2001). von Willebrand disease phenotype and von Willebrand factor marker genotype in Doberman pinschers. *Am. J. Vet. Res.* 62 (3): 364–369.

DuPont, G. and DeBowes, L. (2009). *Atlas of Dental Radiography*, 5–122. Philadelphia, PA: Saunders-Elsevier.

Edmonds, L., Stewart, R.W., and Selby, L. (1972). Cleft lip and palate in dogs (Boxer breed): a preliminary report. *Carnivore Genetics Newsletter* 9: 204–209.

Evans, R.I., Herbold, J.R., Bradshaw, B.S., and Moore, G.E. (2007). Causes for discharge of military working dogs from service: 268 cases (2000–2004). *J. Am. Vet. Med. Assoc.* 231 (8): 1215–1220.

FAB. (n.d.). Inherited disorders in cats – confirmed and suspected. Available from www.fabcats.org (accessed July 5, 2020).

FCI. (n.d.). FCI breeds nomenclature. Available from http://www.fci.be/en/nomenclature/ (accessed July 5, 2020).

Gawor, J. (2004). Szczenię jako pacjent stomatologiczny. *Mag. Wet.* 13 (87): 9–12.

Gawor, J. (2005). Nadziąślaki – aktualne informacje na temat rozpoznawania I leczenia u psów i kotów Magazyn Wet. Nr 5, 12.

Gawor, J. (2006). Craniomandibular osteopathy in dogs. Proceedingds of the BVDA 18th Scientific Meeting, April 19, Birmingham, UK.

Gawor, J. (2008). Kliniczna I radiologiczna ocena uzębienia u szczenięcia w trakcie wyrzynania. Przypadek kliniczny. Zycie Wet.

Gawor, J. (2013). Hereditary oral disorders in pedigree dogs. Proposals for their evidence and assessment. *EJCAP Online* 23 (3).

Giger, U. (2003). Hereditary & genetic diseases modern diagnostics for hereditary disorders in dogs and cats. Proceedings of the XXVIII WSAVA Congress, Bangkok, Thailand.

Gough A. and Thomas A. (2006). Predyspozycje rasowe do chorób u psów i kotów SIMA WLW. Warsaw, Poland.

Gruneberg, H. and Lea, A.J. (1940). An inherited jaw anomaly in long haired dachshunds. *J. Genet.* 39: 285–296.

Harley, R., Gruffydd-Jones, T.J., and Day, M.J. (2011). Immunohistochemical characterization of oral mucosal lesions in cats with chronic gingivostomatitis. *J. Comp. Pathol.* 144 (4): 239–250.

Hedhammar, I. (2004). FCI approach to health dog breeding. FECAVA Symposium, WSAVA/FECAVA Congress, October 8, Rhodes, Greece.

Hernandez, M. (2003). Breed predisposition to oral pathology. Proceedings of the 8th WCVD, July 11–13, Kyoto, Japan.

Indrebo, A. (2004).Breeding of healthy dogs – a breeder's perspective. FECAVA Symposium, WSAVA/FECAVA Congress, October 8, Rhodes, Greece.

Jergens, A.E. (2012). Feline idiopathic inflammatory bowel disease: what we know and what remains to be unraveled. *J. Feline Med. Surg.* 14 (7): 445–458.

Kern, T.J., Walton, D.K., Riis, R.C. et al. (1985). Uveitis associated with poliosis and vitiligo in six dogs. *J. Am. Vet. Med. Assoc.* 187 (4): 408–414.

Koharik, A. (2007). A new direction for kennel club regulations and breed standards. *Can. Vet. J.* 48: 953–965.

Leppänen, M., Paloheimo, A., and Saloniemi, H. (2000). Attitudes of Finnish dog-owners about programs to control canine genetic diseases. *Prev. Vet. Med.* 43 (3): 145–158.

Lewis, J.R. and Reiter, A.A. (2005). Management of generalized gingival enlargement in a dog – case report and literature review. *J. Vet. Dent.* 22 (3): 160–169.

McGreevy, P.D. and Nicholas, F.W. (1999). Some practical solutions to welfare problems in dog breeding. *Animal Welfare* 8: 329–341.

Mellersh, C. (2008). Give a dog a genome. *Vet. J.* 178 (1): 46–52.

Meyers-Wallen, V.N. (2003). Ethics and genetic selection in purebred dogs. *Reprod. Domest. Anima.* 38 (1): 73–76.

Mullan, S. and Main, D. (2001). Principles of ethical decision-making in veterinary practice. *Practice*: 396–401.

Okuda, A. (2003). Dentigerous cysts in brachycephalic breed dogs and diagnostic findings and treatment with bone augmentation. WSAVA 2003 Congress Proceedings, October 24–27, Bangkok Thailand.

Sampson, J. (2004). The geneticist's view on dog breeding: How can improved health be achieved? FECAVA Symposium, WSAVA/FECAVA Congress, October 8, Rhodes, Greece.

Stapleton, B.L. and Clarke, L.L. (1999). Mandibular canine tooth impaction in a young dog – treatment and subsequent eruption: a case report. *J. Vet. Dent.* 16 (3): 105–108.

Surgeon, T.W. (2007). Indications planning and ethical considerations for orthodontic treatment. *Pesquisa Veterinária Brasileira* 27 (Suppl): 78–79.

van Hagen, M.A., Janss, L.L., van den Broek, J., and Knol, B.W. (2004). The use of a genetic-counseling program by Dutch breeders for four hereditary health problems in boxer dogs. *Prev. Vet. Med.* 63 (1–2): 39–50.

Wiggs, R.B. and Lobprise, H.B. (1997a). Clinical oral pathology. In: *Veterinary Dentistry Principles and Practice*, 104–139. Philadelphia, PA: Lippincott-Raven.

Wiggs, R.B. and Lobprise, H.B. (1997b). Oral examination and diagnosis. In: *Veterinary Dentistry Principles and Practice*, 87–104. Philadelphia, PA: Lippincott-Raven.

11

Pain Management in the Dental Patient

Paulo Steagall[1] and Peter Pascoe[2]

[1] *Department of Clinical Sciences, Faculty of Veterinary Medicine, Université of Montréal, Saint-Hyacinthe, QC, Canada*
[2] *Department of Surgical and Radiological Sciences, School of Veterinary Medicine, University of California, Davis, CA, USA*

11.1 Introduction

According to the International Association for the Study of Pain (IASP), pain is a multidimensional and complex phenomenon that requires comprehensive and ongoing assessment and effective management. Pain has also been defined as "an aversive, sensory experience which represents awareness (by the animal) of damage or threat to the integrity of tissues; it changes the animal's physiology and behaviour to reduce or avoid the damage, to reduce the likelihood of recurrence and to promote recovery; nonfunctional pain occurs when the intensity or duration of the experience is not appropriate for the damage sustained (especially if none exists) and when physiological and behavioral responses are unsuccessful in alleviating it" (Molony 1997; Molony and Kent 1997). This type of pain can produce long-term distress with significant deleterious physiological effects, affecting quality of life (QOL) in both humans and animals (Sheiham 2006; Ferreira et al. 2017). Oral disease and its associated pain are serious welfare issues for veterinary patients and should be addressed accordingly (Niemiec et al. 2017). Indeed, dental disease is considered as one of the most important causes of chronic pain in dogs (Bell et al. 2014) and cats.

The multidimensional nature of dental and orofacial pain requires *an interdisciplinary approach* to its assessment and management (http://www.iasp-pain.org/Education/). Human dentists often work in collaboration with neurologists and anesthesiologists on major procedures and the treatment of complex painful cases, given the plethora of conditions presented. The same trend has been observed in veterinary medicine. The World Small Animal Veterinary Association (WSAVA) Dental Standardization Committee, which is made up of specialists in dentistry, anesthesiology and pain management, and animal welfare and nutrition, has recently published its Global Dental Guidelines, providing an in-depth review of the subject (Niemiec et al. 2020). Most dogs and cats have some form of oral disease (e.g., periodontal disease, fractured teeth, stomatitis, malocclusions, neoplasia), often at an early age, whcih can produce pain and inflammation (Lund et al. 1999; Niemiec 2008). Therefore, pain relief is an important issue in the practice of veterinary dentistry. This is a matter of ethics and welfare, but it should be also seen as a strategy to reestablish organ function and accelerate hospital discharge. This chapter provides an overview of different aspects of pain management in the small-animal dental patient, including pathophysiology, dental nociception, assessment and treatment.

11.2 Impact of Oral Disease and Pain on Nutrition/Food Intake and Quality of Life

Recent systematic reviews in humans show a significant association between periodontal disease, pain, and poor QOL (Buset et al. 2016). Patients with gingivitis and dental pain show mild to severe discomfort and physical and psychological impairment (Yang et al. 2016). Periodontal disease and oral pain have a significant negative effect on the nutritional status of children (Sheiham 2006). A high prevalence of dental caries (74%) and oral pain (47%) exists, and both caries and pain are associated with decreased body weight (Khanh et al. 2015). Another study revealed that three-year-old children with caries weighed approximately 1 kg less than those without caries (Acs et al. 1992). People with orofacial pain have issues eating, drinking, speaking, and sleeping, with strong psychological impairment and disability (Kiyak et al. 1990).

The Veterinary Dental Patient: A Multidisciplinary Approach, First Edition. Edited by Jerzy Gawor and Brook Niemiec.
© 2021 John Wiley & Sons Ltd. Published 2021 by John Wiley & Sons Ltd.
Companion website: www.wiley.com/go/gawor/veterinary-dental-patient

Similar studies are lacking in veterinary medicine and it is difficult to extrapolate these findings to canine and feline patients. However, animals with oral and dental disease may experience oral/dental pain, which will impact their nutritional status and QOL (Harvey 2005; Holmstrom et al. 2013). For example, cats with severe oral disease, including gingivitis-stomatitis complex, have dysphagia with dry food, intense oral discomfort, weight loss, sialorrhea and poor grooming (De Vries and Putter 2015; Winer et al. 2016; Rolim et al. 2017). Cats with severe oral disease have decreased food intake before and up to six days after dental extractions when compared with those with minimal oral disease (Watanabe et al. 2019). These cats present specific pain behaviours (Watanabe et al. 2020). In some cases of chronic dental pain, the owner–pet bond can be affected due to the unpleasantness of halitosis and sialorrhea, and the animal may become isolated. Future studies should elucidate the specific impact of dental pain on QOL in veterinary patients.

11.3 Present and Future Challenges in Pain Management for the Veterinary Dental Patient

Recognition of pain-induced behaviors is crucial for appropriate treatment and provision of analgesics, and this can be considered one of the main challenges in veterinary dentistry. Difficulties with pain assessment are one of the major barriers to adequate treatment of pain (Bell et al. 2014). Behavioral signs of oral disease-induced pain have not been systematically investigated in veterinary medicine and current knowledge on the subject is mostly based on anecdotal evidence, textbooks, and review articles by experts (Lommer 2013; Frank 2014; Watanabe et al. 2020a). Additionally, veterinarians receive minimal to no training in pain management associated with oral disease and pain, and dental pain is underrecognized and undertreated in small-animal practice. If signs of pain are not recognized, treatment of dental disease may be delayed until pain is severe or there is a substantial impact on the animal's nutritional/welfare status. Knowledge of pain behaviors in oral disease could increase veterinary visits, improving canine and feline healthcare.

Most studies on pain management for the dental patient have only reported the use of local anesthetic techniques to reduce anesthetic requirements and provide intraoperative analgesia in dogs and cats (Woodward 2008; Snyder and Snyder 2013; Aguiar et al. 2015; Snyder et al. 2016). The WSAVA Global Pain Council has published an open-access article on the prevention, assessment, and treatment of pain in companion animals (Mathews et al. 2014). It describes the use of local anesthetics, opioids, and nonsteroidal anti-inflammatory drugs (NSAIDs) as a first-line treatment of acute pain. However, it provides only limited information on oral pain and its assessment and treatment, mostly due to the lack of information in the literature on this subject. Ultimately, there is a clear need for better continuing education in pain management in veterinary medicine. Studies addressing evidence-based analgesic therapies in this field are warranted.

11.4 Physiology of Pain

A basic knowledge of the physiology of pain and potential changes associated with inflammation and maladaptive changes in chronic pain are important to understanding disease mechanisms and identifying appropriate analgesic therapeutic interventions. The nociceptive input occurs via *transduction, transmission, modulation and perception* of noxious stimuli. Nociceptors are specialized, free-ending peripheral sensory neurons that are present in the skin, gingiva, tooth roots and bone. Briefly, nociceptor activation by noxious (mechanical, chemical, electrical, or thermal) stimuli induces ion-channel changes, membrane depolarization and the generation of an action potential in the periphery (**transduction**). This signal is relayed to the dorsal horn of the spinal cord by a first-order neuron via Aδ and C fibers (**transmission**) in normal states. The medium-diameter lightly myelinated Aδ fibers are fast-conducting afferents responsible for the instant sharp pain. The small unmyelinated C fibers are high-threshold afferents with slow conduction velocities responsible for the dull aching sensation. The involvement of Aβ fibers (touch and proprioception) in nociception may be observed in pathological states such as central sensitization and allodynia. At the spinal cord, stimuli will be either amplified or inhibited (**modulation**) depending on the release of neurotransmitters and the nature of the stimulus. The neurotransmitters can be excitatory (e.g., glutamate, substance P, calcitonin gene-related peptide [CGRP]), inhibitory (e.g., GABA) or modulatory (e.g., noradrenaline, serotonin, opioids, etc.). The nociceptive signal can be inhibited at the level of the spinal cord and by the *descending inhibitory system*, which is located in the supraspinal areas. Finally, the second-order neuron will relay the information to the cerebral cortex, where the nociceptive stimulus is conveyed and integrated. This final step results in the actual painful sensation (**perception**; "ouch"). Autonomic and emotional responses, as well as nocifensive behaviors including reflexes (e.g., jumping, withdrawing, etc.) and conditioned motor responses (e.g., escape, avoidance, aggressiveness), will occur at this point (Dubin and Patapoutian 2010; Meintjes 2012). General anesthetics (e.g., isoflurane, propofol, alfaxalone, etc.) do not inhibit the nociceptive process. Therefore, the administration of analgesics (e.g., local anesthetics, opioids, NSAIDs, etc.) with antinociceptive properties is mandatory during general anesthesia for the treatment of oral disease and surgery.

Sustained noxious stimuli (e.g., persistent postoperative surgical pain, severe inflammation, neuropathic and chronic pain, etc.) alter nociception . This can lead to neuroplasticity, a dynamic modulation of nociceptive signaling with changes in the central nervous system and the formation of "new connections". This pathological change may affect the inhibitory and excitatory modulation of pain, compromising/reducing inhibitory mechanisms and enhancing/amplifying excitatory ones, leading to the facilitation and amplification of the nociceptive stimuli. For example, the descending inhibitory system and endogenous pain modulation do not function properly in some patients with neuropathic pain. In other words, a longterm *maladaptive process* is established in chronic conditions (i.e., trigeminal neuralgia and chronic periodontal disease), making pain much more difficult to treat with classic analgesics such as NSAIDs (Figure 11.1). Nociceptive

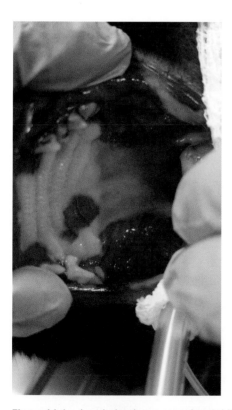

Figure 11.1 A maladaptive process is established in chronic conditions such as gingivostomatitis in cats. Pain becomes more difficult to treat with classic analgesics alone and may require long-term treatment with multimodal analgesia. Nociceptive transmission is altered and can be generated within the central nervous system (i.e., central sensitization). *Source:* Courtesy of Dr. Paulo Steagall.

transmission is altered and can be generated within the CNS. Pain is perpetuated even after healing of the original primary cause and becomes a disease on its own. The small animal patient can thus be affected by widespread central sensitization (i.e., changes in spinal dorsal horn neurons that increase the perception of pain, especially in regions adjacent to the primary site of the injury). Central sensitization results in **hyperalgesia** (an increase in the perception of pain elicited by a noxious stimulus in the area of injury [primary] or the region of injury [secondary]) and **allodynia** (pain evoked by a normally innocuous stimulus). Appropriate perioperative pain management will prevent and sometimes reverse central sensitization. This highlights the importance of analgesic administration in the management of the veterinary dental patient. Analgesics will act on different parts of the nociceptive process (transduction, transmission, modulation, and perception; see earlier). The administration of different classes of analgesic drugs and the application of nonpharmacological therapies constitute the basis of **multimodal analgesia** (see later).

11.5 Dental Nociception, Inflammation, and Hypersensitivity

Specific differences exist between the mechanisms of dental nociception and other tissues of the body. Indeed, the underlying dental nociceptive process is less known than other somatic signaling mechanisms. The tooth pulp is densely innervated and surrounded by mineralized dentin and enamel. The latter is avascular, noninnervated, and nonporous, offering a protective layer to the tooth. However, in this low-compliant environment and during inflammation, minimal swelling of the pulp will lead to severe pain. The exact mechanism of nociceptive transmission across the tooth structure is not well elucidated. Experimental studies using the cat lower canine tooth pulp show fast A, Aδ, and C fibers, with the majority being fast A and the other two types appearing in about equal numbers (Ikeda et al. 1995, 1997). The thresholds to electrical stimulation are lower for the larger ones. About half the Aδ and C fibers respond to slow elevations in temperature, whereas only the A fibers respond to rapid changes in temperature and negative hydrostatic pressure. Bradykinin directly applied to the exposed pulp stimulates all the C fibers and most of the Aδ fibers but none of the fast A fibers; however, this may be due to the nerve endings for these fibers being deeper in the pulp. In other studies, the C fibers have been shown not to respond to drilling scratching, air blast, or hypertonic saline applied to the dentinal surface (Narhi et al. 1982; Hirvonen et al. 1984; Narhi and Hirvonen 1987). Based on comparisons of human experience with recordings from cats, it is thought that the sharp and shooting pain sensations of short onset are evoked by Aδ fibers, whereas C fiber activity is associated with a dull, burning pain of late onset that is difficult to localize (Mengel et al. 1993).

In contrast to the skin, heat and cold do not elicit pain when applied to a healthy tooth because of the thermal insulating properties of enamel, unless extreme temperatures are applied. However, in the inflamed tooth or when the enamel is missing, the dentin is exposed and stinging pain can be easily provoked. Therefore, dental nociception is mostly observed in inflammation but not in healthy states with intact enamel. It is fairly reasonable to think that veterinary patients feel dental pain and discomfort with periodontal disease similar to toothache in humans even when our means of pain assessment are limited and we cannot easily identify their suffering.

It is generally accepted that inflammatory tooth pain occurs via activation of the ion-channel receptors transient receptor potential vanniloid 1 (TRPV1) and transient receptor potential ankyrin 1 (TRPA1), which are present in the dentinal tubules. These receptors respond to external stimuli and different ranges of noxious temperatures. They are commonly upregulated and overexpressed in inflammation, even in adjacent teeth. Overall, inflammatory tooth pain responds well to the administration of NSAIDs.

The same does not hold for intense pain produced by normally innocuous stimuli, or **dental hypersensitivity** (Chung et al. 2013). Three theories have been proposed to explain this form of pain. The **neural theory** suggest the nociceptive trigeminal ganglion neurons are actually dental nociceptors that are present in the pulp and are densely populated with thermo-TRPV1 and -TRPA1 receptors. They thus contribute to the detection of cold- and hot-induced hypersensitivity. Alternatively, according to the **odontoblastic transduction theory**, odontoblasts (ciliated cells lying at the border of the pulp that secrete calcium matrix to form dentin) have mechano- and thermosensitive channels and thus act as *key sensory transducers* of noxious dental stimuli, transmitting action potentials to other peripheral nerve endings (Magloire et al. 2010; Chung et al. 2013). Finally, according to the **hydrodynamic theory**, inward and outward fluid movement and changes in the pulpal microvasculature (i.e., vasoconstriction or vasodilation) in the dentinal tubules activate nociceptors mostly via recruitment of Aδ fibers, leading to dentin hypersensitivity and dull pain. This has been demonstrated in exposed dentine of cats (Vongsavan and Matthews 1992; Matthews and Vongsavan 1994).

The local release of potent vasoactive peptides (i.e., substance P and CGRP) and growth factors may induce the release of chemical mediators and inflammatory cytokines.

This is important because the pulp has a denser nerve supply to CGRP and substance P when compared with periodontal issues (Heyeraas et al. 1993). The concentration of substance P is markedly elevated in tooth inflammation and irreversible pulpitis when compared with healthy conditions. Substance P can activate TRPV1 receptors and proinflammatory mediators. Serotonin is involved in the sensitization of intradental nerves, as shown by experimental studies in canine nerves (Ngassapa et al. 1992). These substances reduce the nociceptive threshold and contribute to central and peripheral sensitization and to the allodynia observed in dental pain. They play an active role in the maintenance of local neurogenic inflammation and can change the vascular permeability responsible for pulsating inflammatory pain leading to migraine in humans (Sacerdote and Levrini 2012).

An understanding of the physiology of pain and dental nociception may aid in finding the origin of pain, facilitating diagnosis and treatment. This is a definite challenge when dealing with nonverbal patients as in veterinary medicine. Appropriate diagnosis of dental pain requires oral examination and radiographs under general anesthesia.

11.6 Causes of Dental and Orofacial Pain

Periodontal disease is common in small animal practice (allodynia), and a significant cause of pain. Periodontal pain is usually localized and can be persistent (Figure 11.2). Inflammation of the gingiva or periodontal tissues can also become a source of chronic pain, which is likely underdiagnosed and undertreated (Perry and Tutt 2015). Periodontal/gingival abscesses can produce deep pain. The insulating capacity of the enamel prevents thermal sensitivity in a healthy tooth; however, this may not hold true in the face of chronic inflammation, as previously discussed (Le Fur-Bonnabesse et al. 2017). Feline chronic gingivostomatitis is commonly observed in clinical practice and is characterized by bilateral, multifocal, or diffuse, friable, proliferative ulcerative lesions around the tongue base and palatoglossal fold, with intense oral discomfort. It leads to anorexia, dysphagia, sialorrhea, halitosis, and weight loss. It can also produce oral hemorrhage.

Acute pain can persist after surgery and become maladaptive (i.e., chronic) and is a significant concern in human medicine, where chronic pain associated with some surgical procedures can occur in up to 50% of patients (Reddi and Curran 2014). This **persistent postsurgical pain** is produced by activation of N-methyl D-aspartate (NMDA) receptors, central sensitization and neuroplasticity following nerve injury, extensive tissue injury, excessive

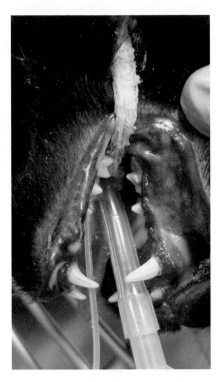

Figure 11.2 Periodontal disease is common in small-animal practice. It causes pain and discomfort, and animals tend to suffer without outward clinical signs. Inflammation of the gingiva or periodontal tissues can become a source of chronic pain, which is underdiagnosed and undertreated in companion animals. *Source:* Courtesy of Dr. Paulo Steagall).

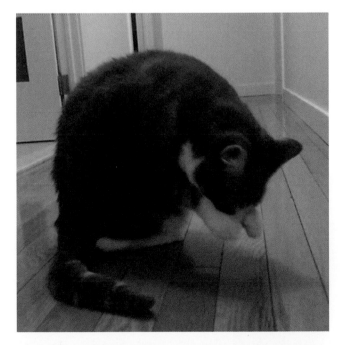

Figure 11.3 A cat with suspected feline orofacial pain syndrome. Clinical signs can be triggered by mouth movement or spontaneously, and include pawing at the mouth, vocalization, exaggerated licking, and escape behavior. Dental treatment is always recommended for these cases. *Source:* Courtesy of Dr. Paulo Steagall.

inflammation, and inadequate treatment of perioperative pain. This type of pain may be a concern after invasive oral procedures such as full-mouth extractions in patients with feline stomatitis, maxillectomies and mandibulectomies. The severity of acute postoperative pain correlates with the risk of developing chronic postoperative pain in humans. This highlights the importance of long-term and aggressive multimodal analgesic management with gentle tissue handling to minimize nerve/tissue injury during oral surgery.

In humans, the origin of orofacial pain is commonly associated with a pathological condition or disorder related to somatic and neurological structures. The resulting orofacial pain involves musculoligamentous, dentoalveolar and neurovascular mechanisms, which are often different than in dental pain. The presentation is frequently not easy to diagnose, rendering treatment difficult. Human dentists can differentiate the presence of abnormal sensory responses to touch (paresthesia, an abnormal tingling sensation; dysesthesia, an abnormal unpleasant sensation; and allodynia), which is difficult in nonverbal species. The most common causes of chronic orofacial pain in humans are temporomandibular joint disorders and trigeminal neuralgia, but these are rarely diagnosed as a cause of pain in dogs and cats. However, a similar condition to trigeminal neuralgia has been observed in cats, known as **feline orofacial pain syndrome**. This is a chronic condition with acute unilateral episodes and a suspected hereditary component that may be triggered by stress (Figure 11.3). Any cat can be affected, but it seems that Burmese cats are overrepresented (Rusbridge et al. 2010). Clinical signs can be triggered by *mouth movement or spontaneously* and include *pawing at the mouth, exaggerated licking and chewing movements, spontaneous vocalization with escape behavior and decreased appetite.* Mutilation has been anecdotally reported in severe cases. The diagnosis is usually performed by exclusion once dental and oral disease have been ruled out as part of the diagnosis.

Other common causes of dental pain include trauma, infection of the dental pulp (pulpitis: involvement of nerves and vessels) or pulp disease, neoplasia, occlusal trauma, abscesses, cracked-tooth syndrome, fractures, invasive oral surgical procedures (i.e., maxillectomies, mandibulectomies, etc.) and oral cancer (Figure 11.4).

11.7 Assessment and Recognition

The assessment and recognition of pain in small animals is an extensive topic that goes beyond the scope of this chapter. The information provided here is thus focused on specific canine and feline pain assessment for the dental patient, taking into consideration changes related to oral disease and treatment.

Pain management and nutrition are the fourth and fifth vital signs, respectively, and should be assessed as part of the temperature, pulse, and respiratory rate (TPR) in every veterinary patient. A lack of pain assessment lessens analgesic administration and contributes to inadequate treatment (Simon et al. 2017). Pain assessment is generally subjective and based on the veterinarian's interpretation of pain-induced behaviors, since it is well accepted that physiological indicators are not sensitive or reliable for this purpose. Postoperative pain leads to peripheral inflammation and sensitization that can be detected by decreases in mechanical nociceptive thresholds when measured objectively by algometry or subjectively by palpation. Adequate

treatment of pain should increase these thresholds back or at least close to normal values (i.e., before oral surgery), but algometry has been difficult to apply to dental patients because an animal with a sore mouth is likely to move before the algometer is applied (Figure 11.5). Acute postoperative pain may be indicated by restlessness, pawing at the mouth, frequent licking and swallowing, ptyalism, avoidance behaviors when the sore area is approached, increased aggression associated with handling, fractiousness, and, with extreme pain, increases in heart and respiratory rates and blood pressure. Facial expression has long been recognized as indicative of pain intensity in humans, and this area has been thoroughly investigated in cats (see the Feline Grimace Scale) (Steagall and Monteiro 2018; Evangelista et al. 2019). Facial changes have been specifically used for dental pain in cats (Figures 11.6) (Watanabe et al. 2020b). A standard form for the evaluation of these behaviors

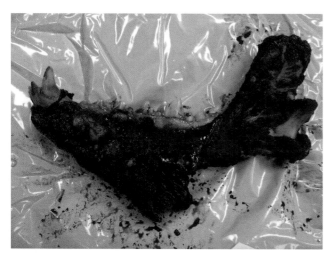

Figure 11.4 Oral cancer can be a significant source of severe pain. It may produce an impact on quality of life and the nutritional status of the patient. Central sensitization may be present and pain can be difficult to treat. A multidisciplinary approach to treatment, including dentistry, surgery, oncology, nutrition and anesthesia is ideal. *Source:* Courtesy of Dr. Paulo Steagall.

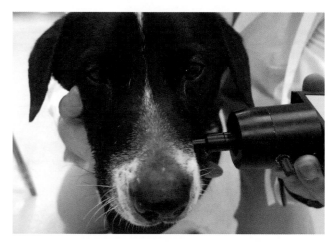

Figure 11.5 Application of an algometer to the lateral aspect of the maxilla in order to measure the mechanical nociceptive threshold of a dog after dental extractions. *Source:* Courtesy of Dr. Paulo Steagall.

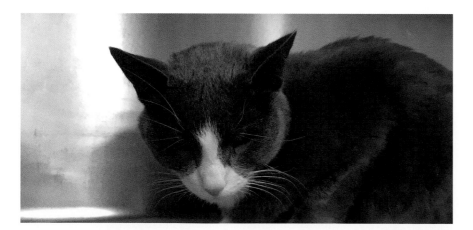

Figure 11.6 Changes in facial expressions can be great indicators of pain in cats. The Feline Grimace Scale (www.felinegrimacescale.com) may add better means of acute pain assessment. In this example, the distance between the tips of the ears is increased, the eyes are partially closed and the muzzle is retracted backwards. *Source:* Courtesy of Dr. Paulo Steagall.

provides the clinician with a way to document and track the effectiveness of therapy and can improve patient management. Examples of pain scoring systems include the short form of the Glasgow canine and feline pain scales (Reid et al. 2007, 2017), the UNESP-Botucatu multidimensional composite scale (cats) (Brondani et al. 2011), the University of Melbourne pain scale (dogs) (Firth and Haldane 1999), and the Colorado canine and feline acute pain scales (Epstein et al. 2015). The clinician should recognize that older animals may show signs of pain unrelated to the dental procedure; if an old arthritic animal is placed in dorsal recumbency for several hours without support for the joints, for example, it may be very painful. Beyond the immediate perioperative period, the development of new behaviors or the absence of old ones may be indicative of pain. This can be particularly true for feeding (e.g., changes in appetite, dysphagia) and playing (e.g., refusing to play anymore after dental surgery) behaviors, changes in demeanor, and reluctance to play with toys and grooming (e.g., where the fur looks greasy, lackluster and frail; Rolim et al. 2017) in cats. Many dogs and cats have been anecdotally reported to regain some old normal behaviors following dental treatment, so a further assessment of pain may simply be the response to analgesics. If the clinician is uncertain about a particular behavior, it is best to treat the animal with a rapidly acting potent analgesic and see if pain goes away. It is important that the animal is reassessed shortly after administration to ensure that analgesia is effective.

In the clinical setting, pain can be assessed and scored using one of the previously mentioned scales, such as the Glasgow pain scoring tools for dogs (Reid et al. 2007) and cats (Reid et al. 2017). These two instruments have not been specifically validated for patients with oral disease, but they provide an idea of the "overall" picture and can be used for any medical/surgical condition. The assessment takes into account posture, comfort, activity, attitude, response to palpation and demeanor. However, it is not known if all or just some of these are specifically altered in dental pain. Pain assessment also depends on disease severity, breed, sedation, the observer, anesthetic drugs, drug-induced changes in behavior (e.g., dysphoria, emergence delirium) and demeanor, among other things. The truth is that our means of dental pain assessment are still limited.

Pain should be assessed every hour in the first few hours postoperatively, and it is especially important that the assessor takes time to observe the animal prior to opening the cage/run. It may take several minutes to recognize that an animal is not settling in one place because it is in too much pain to get comfortable. The animal may not need to be disturbed if it appears to be resting in one location with normal posture. Frequency and duration of assessment will be dependent on patient status, type of surgery, and prognosis. For example, if the patient is eating and drinking normally with normal behaviors and analgesic administration is continued, assessments can be sparse. If an animal continues to demonstrate signs of pain, assessment should continue until the pain has subsided or the prognosis has improved. The animal care staff and nursing team should always be involved in the recognition of pain so that everyone is "part of the change" in clinical practice. For chronic pain, the health-related quality of life (HRQL) instruments can be useful, since pain and QOL are considered together (Reid et al. 2018). Here, the owner is involved in the assessment. This approach could be useful in future studies related to veterinary dentistry.

11.8 Treatment

Treatment of dental and orofacial pain is complex, due to the variety and number of conditions that may be presented. This section provides an overview of the analgesic strategies and classes of drugs used for pain relief of the dental patient. Analgesic administration is required in all patients where surgery and inflammation are present. For minor procedures, a single analgesic may be sufficient, but in most instances the use of more than one will provide better pain control as different drugs act at different points in the nociceptive pathway (transduction, transmission, modulation, and perception; see earlier). This approach is known as multimodal or balanced analgesia and uses the additive or synergistic properties of several therapies to allow for lower doses of each individual drug to provide adequate analgesia. The only downside is that it increases the odds of an adverse reaction to one or more of the drugs used. In general, perioperative pain is best treated with the administration of NSAIDs, opioids and local anesthetics. Chronic oral conditions might require the administration of drug infusions, including ketamine for the prevention or treatment of central sensitization. Oral administration of NSAIDs, gabapentin, and tramadol is commonly used after hospital discharge (see later). Nonpharmacological therapies should not be underestimated and are used as adjuvants to complement the treatment of pain. For example, a clean, dry and calm environment with appropriate nursing and positioning and separated areas for dogs and cats is important in reducing stress and anxiety and promoting patient comfort (Figure 11.7). Icing can be beneficial and reduces inflammation, edema, muscle spasm and tissue damage after invasive oral surgery; this might be applied for 15–20 minutes immediately after surgery and during anesthetic recovery, and it is thought to inhibit nociceptive input while modulating the descending inhibitory system with the release of endogenous opioids.

(a)

(b)

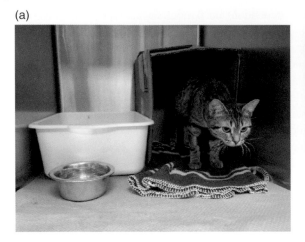

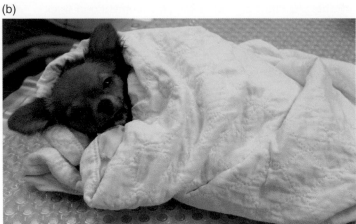

Figure 11.7 (a) Cat following recovery from anesthesia. It is located in an elevated cage in a cat-only ward with environmental enrichment for sleeping and hiding and has access to the top of the box. Pain management is not only about giving analgesic drugs, but also reducing stress, nausea and anxiety during hospitalization while using nonpharmacological therapies. (b) Dog on a warm water-circulating blanket while recovering from anesthesia with hypothermia. The principle of tender, loving, care can be applied at low cost in any clinic. *Source:* Courtesy of Dr. Paulo Steagall.

Cats and dogs have species-specific differences in terms of drug metabolism, pharmacokinetics and pharmacodynamics and volatile-anesthetic sparing effect (i.e., changes in minimum alveolar concentration), among other things. However, they should receive analgesics in a similar manner: if a surgical procedure is painful for a dog, it will be painful for a cat. The same approach is used for outpatients after hospital discharge, but the doses and intervals of administration should be tailored to the individual animal. Experience in both human and veterinary medicine has demonstrated that there are huge variations in analgesic requirements, and the clinician should try to design the best approach for each animal. Historically, cats have received fewer analgesics than dogs for the same surgical procedure, due to fear of analgesic-induced adverse effects, lack of training in pain assessment, and misconceptions regarding analgesic therapy (Dohoo and Dohoo 1998). A common one is that an otherwise healthy cat can develop NSAID-induced adverse effects after a single dose; another is that cats may develop manic behavior after the administration of morphine. In fact, pain can be treated adequately in cats, especially with the availability of approved analgesic drugs for this species. Indeed, the challenges in feline pain management are similar to those in dogs, and an analgesic therapeutic plan should be developed on an individual basis. A recent study showed that cats with severe oral disease undergoing full-mouth dental extractions required the administration of NSAIDs and opioids for up to 96 hours after surgery even when local anesthetic blocks had been administered during the procedure (Watanabe et al. 2019). Clinical experience shows that some cats may require long-term treatment with NSAIDs for weeks.

A further issue in pain management is when to administer the analgesics. Preemptive analgesia (administering treatment prior to the onset of pain) has been shown to be effective in many laboratory studies, but it does not appear to translate well to the clinical setting. This has led to the concept of **preventive analgesia**, where the aim is to prevent pain as much as possible regardless of when analgesics are administered.

The administration of agonists of α_2-adrenoreceptors for the dental patient and in balanced anesthesia is discussed in Chapter 11 and 12.

11.8.1 Opioids

Opioids are drugs that bind to opioid receptors in the central and peripheral nervous system. They hyperpolarize neuronal membranes, inhibiting the action potential associated with nociceptive input, and so reduce the release of excitatory neurotransmitters. Different opioids have different receptor affinities, potencies and efficacies. In general, full μ-opioid agonists (i.e., morphine, methadone, hydromorphone, fentanyl, etc.) produce dose-dependent analgesia and should be chosen for invasive procedures and severe pain. Partial μ-agonists such as buprenorphine and κ-agonists/μ-antagonists such as butorphanol and nalbuphine can be used for mild to moderate pain. Opioids are commonly administered as part of premedication alone or in combination with sedatives such as acepromazine and agonists of α_2-receptors. Indeed, they are the cornerstone of acute pain management and full μ-opioid agonists produce dose-dependent analgesic effects. Adverse effects include bradycardia due to increased vagal tone, urinary retention, changes in behavior (i.e., dysphoria or euphoria) and respiratory depression. These effects are mild and can be avoided by dose titration, the administration of opioid antagonists (i.e., naloxone), or appropriate therapy (e.g., administration of anticholinergics for opioid-induced bradycardia). Opioids can also be given to ill patients via different routes of administration, including infusions. They produce variable sedation that is patient-dependent while decreasing the requirements for volatile and injectable anesthetics.

Morphine is a μ-agonist and an effective analgesic that produces moderate sedation. When given to a dog that is not in pain, with no other drugs, it is common to see panting, bradycardia, and vomiting. The panting appears to be due to the action of the drug at the thermoregulatory center, causing the animal to cool itself down. When used postoperatively, when the patient's thermoregulatory center may be depressed, respiratory depression is more common (Campbell et al. 2003). Bradycardia is seen with high doses but is generally not a problem in the postoperative period and can be easily treated with the administration of anticholinergics. Vomiting is a common side effect in the awake dog but is not commonly seen when morphine is given as a postoperative analgesic. Urine production is decreased for several hours after morphine administration (Robertson et al. 2001). Morphine can produce a significant release of histamine when given intravenously (Robinson et al. 1988). The amount of histamine released is related to the rate and quantity of morphine injected, so it is safe to use the drug intravenously as long as small quantities are injected slowly. Infusion of morphine at 0.34 mg/kg/hour increased plasma histamine concentrations, though there was no effect on cardiovascular parameters (Guedes et al. 2006). The dose for the dog is 0.2–1.0 mg/kg IM or SC. The duration of action is two to four hours. In one study, morphine (0.3–0.8 mg/kg) provided good analgesia in about 70% of dogs for at least four hours after a variety of orthopedic surgeries (Taylor and Houlton 1984). In another, it gave adequate analgesia (0.3 mg/kg IM) in most cases over a seven-hour assessment period following arthrotomy in dogs (Brodbelt et al. 1997). At 0.15 mg/kg IV, morphine gave less than four hours' analgesia in six dogs after left lateral thoracotomy; five of the six had received additional doses by this time (Popilskis et al. 1993). Morphine has also been used as a continuous intravenous infusion in dogs at a rate of 0.1–1.0 mg/kg/hour (0.2 mg/kg/hour is a good dose to start at) following a 0.3–0.5 mg/kg dose IM or IV for moderate to severe pain (Lucas et al. 2001). Cats can be given 0.05–0.3 mg/kg IM; if given intravenously, morphine should be diluted and given slowly to avoid excitement. The pharmacokinetics of morphine in cats suggest that it has a relatively short duration

of action (elimination half-life ~1.5 hours) (Taylor et al. 2001), but clinically it seems to have a similar duration of action to that in dogs.

Hydromorphone is a μ-agonist with a potency approximately five to seven times that of morphine and a slightly longer duration of action. It does not appear to cause histamine release when given intravenously (Smith et al. 2001). It may result in greater side effects such as panting or dysphoria if a more than adequate dose is administered. There are two reports of postoperative hyperthermia in cats following hydromorphone administration (Niedfeldt and Robertson 2006; Posner et al. 2007), and in one experimental study the skin temperature of cats increased over time (Lascelles and Robertson 2004). The dose range is 0.05–0.2 mg/kg IV, IM in both cats and dogs.

Fentanyl is a potent agonist with a relatively short duration of action. For this reason, it has not been used widely for the management of pain in dogs or cats. However, because it has a relatively rapid onset of action (five to seven minutes), an intravenous bolus may be used to control severe pain (up to 10 μg/kg). It is commonly used as an infusion to provide a continuous level of analgesia. Since respiratory depression with opioids can be profound, an animal on such an infusion should be monitored at all times. Assisted or mechanical ventilation may be required. In dogs, an infusion could start with a 3–5 μg/kg bolus followed by an infusion of 3–6 μg/kg/hour. In cats, about half of this is used: a bolus of 2–3 μg/kg with an infusion of 2–3 μg/kg/hour. Intraoperatively, a bolus of 5–10 μg/kg and a constant-rate infusion (CRI) at 0.3–1 μg/kg/minute is used in dogs, while the lower end of these doses is used in cats. A transdermal patch used in humans is often applied to dogs and cats. This is an adhesive patch that is placed on the skin after shaving and cleaning to deliver a specific dose of drug (12.5, 25, 50, 75, or 100 μg/hour; the dose calculated is 2–3 μg/kg/hour) through the skin and into the plasma. The patch provides a controlled release of the drug from the adhesive matrix. The onset of action is at about 6 and 12 hours in dogs and cats, respectively. Analgesic effects can be observed up to 72–96 hours. In this case, patients are hospitalized and pain is continuously monitored (Hofmeister and Egger 2004).

Methadone is 1–1.5 times as potent as morphine and has similar analgesic properties. There are two optical isomers (d- and l- forms), and l-methadone is the one with opioid activity. Both isoforms bind to NMDA receptors and act as antagonists (Gorman et al. 1997). In Europe, methadone is usually sold as just the l-isomer (i.e., levomethadone), but solutions in the United States and Canada contain a racemic mixture. This effect on the NMDA receptor may give it a slightly broader spectrum of activity and helps to explain its use in addicted patients.

In humans, methadone is used because of its great duration of effect, but this has not been demonstrated in dogs and cats. It is also used because it rarely causes emesis in dogs and cats. Clinically, it appears to give good analgesia for moderate pain for at least four hours. It does not cause histamine release and can be given intravenously if a more rapid onset is needed. An initial dose of methadone at 1 mg/kg IV given before the start of surgery, followed by subsequent doses of 0.25–0.5 mg/kg, produced profound analgesia lasting for 120–180 minutes (Dobromylskyj 1993b). In cats, analgesia lasted from 1.5 to 6.5 hours following doses of 0.1–0.5 mg/kg (Dobromylskyj 1993a; Steagall et al. 2006b). The recommended dose range is 0.1–0.5 mg/kg IM in cats and up to 1 mg/kg in dogs.

Meperidine is less potent than morphine and produces less sedation but has similar adverse effects. Panting is rare following meperidine, but this drug is even more likely to cause histamine release than the other opioids and should not be used intravenously. It has a short duration of action and will provide 0.5–2 hours of pain relief in dogs, though it may have a longer duration of action in cats (elimination half-life is >3 hours) (Taylor et al. 2001). This short duration of action can be an advantage when it is necessary to reassess the degree of pain within a short period in order to understand the progression of a condition (e.g., abdominal pain), but it limits its potential as a long-term analgesic. In one clinical trial, about 70% of dogs had no analgesia at 90 minutes after receiving meperidine (3.5 mg/kg) just before or just after the end of anesthesia (Waterman and Kalthum 1992). In another study, dogs receiving meperidine (5 mg/kg IM) at the end of surgery had lower pain scores than controls at one hour but not at two hours (Lascelles et al. 1997). In this study, the dogs receiving the same treatment before the beginning of surgery had similar pain scores to the controls until four hours after the procedure (ovariohysterectomy). From 8 to 20 hours, these dogs had lower scores, supporting the concept of preemptive analgesia (Lascelles et al. 1997). In cats following ovariohysterectomy, there appeared to be no difference in pain scores or further analgesic requirements between meperidine (5 mg/kg IM) and control (Slingsby and Watermanpearson 1998). The dose in both dogs and cats is 3–5 mg/kg IM.

Tramadol binds weakly to μ-opioid receptors (1/600th the potency of morphine) but also inhibits serotonin and noradrenaline reuptake. It has a bioavailability in dogs of 65%, which is much higher than that of traditional opioids. The analgesic effects of tramadol in humans are mostly due to the production of its active metabolite (*O*-desmethyltramadol), which is also responsible for opioid-induced analgesic and adverse effects. Dogs do not produce much of this metabolite, but cats do, so current evidence suggests that it is a better analgesic in the latter species. This metabolite is formed more rapidly in cats (3.9-fold), where it has a longer elimination half-life and a higher concentration (Perez Jimenez et al. 2016). The half-life in dogs of both tramadol and the active metabolite is considerably shorter than in humans (two vs. seven hours), so doses probably need to be given four to six times a day (Wu et al. 2001; Kukanich and Papich 2004). Its effects in acute and chronic pain have been shown to be minimal in dogs (Budsberg et al. 2018; Schutter et al. 2017), but it may be a useful drug for acute pain in cats (Steagall et al. 2008; Pypendop et al. 2009).

Tramadol is widely available, though it is a controlled substance in some countries; for example, it is a schedule IV drug in the United States. The injectable formulation is used in perioperative pain management in Southern Europe and Latin America, whereas the oral formulation is mostly prescribed in North America, Oceania, and other countries in Europe. Tramadol has high bioavailability after oral administration in cats (Pypendop and Ilkiw 2008). In dogs there is high individual variability in bioavailability with it often being very low such that plasma concentrations do not reach therapeutic values (Kukanich et al. 2017, Benitez et al. 2015). The oral formulation is often prescribed for the control of postoperative pain in dogs and cats after dental extractions even if there is little evidence for a benefit in dogs. Most oral formulations are not palatable, which can easily become an issue with long-term administration every 8 or 12 hours, especially in cats and after dental procedures. Cats may salivate profusely after drug administration (Figure 11.8). Tramadol medications can be mixed with soft/canned food in this species (Figure 11.9).

Tramadol can induce adverse effects such as sedation and constipation. Contraindications include concomitant administration of other drugs that impact serotonin reuptake or metabolism. The combination of tramadol with these drugs can cause serotonin toxicity with neuromuscular activity, tachycardia, fever, tachypnea and agitation (Indrawirawan and Mcalees 2014). Drugs include serotonin inhibitors (e.g., fluoxetine), monoamine oxidase inhibitors (i.e., selegiline) and tricyclic antidepressants (i.e., clomipramine) (Fitzgerald and Bronstein 2013).

In cats, doses of 4 mg/kg every six hours are recommended for oral administration based on a thermal threshold model (Pypendop et al. 2009), whereas 2–4 mg/kg every 12 hours has been used for osteoarthritis. Long-term administration of tramadol in cats has produced adverse effects when used for the treatment of osteoarthritis (Guedes et al. 2018). The injectable dose varies from 2 to 4 mg/kg IV, IM.

Oral analgesic prescription is still a challenge in veterinary medicine because there is no strong evidence for the use of tramadol, gabapentin or amantadine, especially when recommending compounded formulations. However, tramadol might have its place when administered in combination with NSAIDs and other analgesic therapies in acute and chronic pain control. In some countries, this may be the only available option for the veterinarian when NSAIDs are contraindicated.

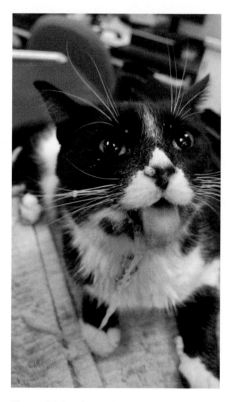

Figure 11.8 Cat salivating profusely after the oral administration of tramadol. Treatment compliance is the biggest challenge for the administration of tramadol orally in cats, since palatability is poor. *Source:* Courtesy of Dr. Paulo Steagall.

11.8.2 Partial μ-Opioid Agonist/κ-Antagonists

Buprenorphine is an agonist/antagonist. It has strong affinity for μ-receptors while having κ-antagonist properties (Cowan 2003). It is classed as a partial agonist, meaning that it does not induce the same degree of effect as a full agonist such as morphine. However, it is not clear if this "partial" effect applies to analgesia or only to some of the other effects of the drug (e.g., it is regarded as having a ceiling effect on respiratory depression). The onset is slow and the peak effect does not occur until about 45–60 minutes after intravenous administration. The strong affinity for μ-receptors means that it is hard to reverse its effects. The dissociation from the μ-receptors is also slow and the main advantage of buprenorphine is that it has a potential 8–12 hour duration of action, but in practice it rarely exceeds six hours. In cats, the elimination half-life exceeds six hours, but plasma concentrations of buprenorphine rarely correlate with analgesia (Taylor et al. 2001). The drug produces moderate sedation when used in the postoperative period. When given at 10 μg/kg in dogs 30 minutes before the end of anesthesia, it gave good analgesia at 15 minutes, but only half the dogs were pain-free at 45 minutes, and some still had some analgesia at four hours (Waterman and Kalthum 1992). Recent studies suggest that the subcutaneous administration of buprenorphine produces little effect at doses in the 10–20 μg/kg range, so it is essential that it be administered intramuscularly or intravenously (Steagall et al. 2014; Bortolami and Love 2015). The dose in the dog and cat is 10–40 μg/kg IM, IV.

There is an interest in using buprenorphine via buccal administration in cats for perioperative analgesia, because it appears to be tasteless and can be used in small volumes (Figure 11.10). However, the transmucosal uptake of the drug is limited and overall bioavailability has now been

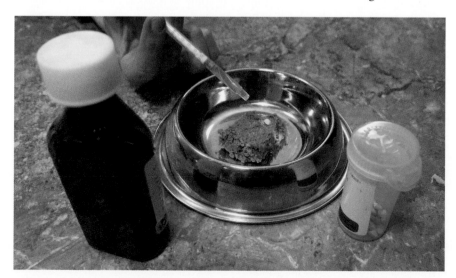

Figure 11.9 Several oral treatments (e.g., tramadol, gabapentin, amitriptyline, etc.) can be mixed with soft food for easy administration in cats. *Source:* Courtesy of Dr. Paulo Steagall.

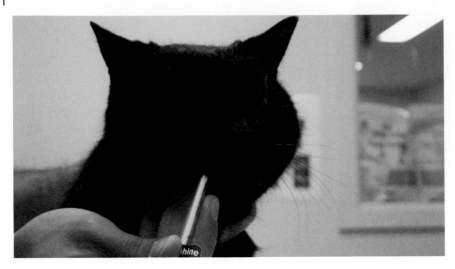

Figure 11.10 Oral transmucosal administration of buprenorphine in cat provides "hands-off" analgesia. The drug is tasteless and palatability is acceptable. There is some transmucosal uptake, and it should not be spilled or swallowed by the cat. *Source:* Courtesy of Dr. Paulo Steagall.

shown to be closer to 30% (Hedges et al. 2014a, b; Doodnaught et al. 2017). Buprenorphine is sometimes prescribed this way by veterinarians for postoperative pain relief after dental extractions, but cats with stomatitis had lower bioavailability and shorter absorption half-life than healthy cats following its buccal administration (Stathopoulou et al. 2017) and frequency and dose of administration should be adapted to the patient's needs. Other opioids such as morphine, methadone and hydromorphone have a similar bioavailability when the injectable solution is administered buccally (Pypendop et al. 2014). Small doses of buprenorphine are often mixed with local anesthetics for dental nerve blocks (see later).

One company has produced a high-concentration buprenorphine solution (1.8 mg/ml; Simbadol) that has a duration of action of 24 hours when administered at 0.24 mg/kg SC (Taylor et al. 2015; Doodnaught 2017). Because of its high concentration and high lipid solubility, this effectively forms a dermal depot that is slowly absorbed. The typical 0.3 mg/ml buprenorphine does not provide the same concentration gradient, so the absorption from a subcutaneous injection is so slow that it has a minimal effect. Simbadol provided similar analgesia in cats after dental procedures when administered once a day to the 0.3 mg/mL buprenorphine administered three times a day (Watanabe et al. 2020c). When Simbadol was administered at 0.24 mg/kg transmucosally it increased the thermal threshold for 8 hours but the pharmacokinetics of the administration of this concentrated buprenorphine have not been reported (Doodnaught et al. 2018).

11.8.3 Partial μ-Opioid Agonist/Partial κ-Agonists

Butorphanol is a partial agonist and its actions are slightly different than those of the other opioids. With increasing dosage, there is a ceiling effect on respiratory depression

such that further increases in dose do not increase respiratory depression. Its potential as an addictive drug is much less than that of the other opioids, and it is included as an antitussive in some human cough medicines. It causes mild sedation and appears to have a duration of activity of at least two hours or longer in some cases. Butorphanol has 7–10 times the receptor binding potency of morphine but does not seem to be as effective an analgesic in cases with severe pain. It does not cause histamine release when injected intravenously. Though early reports suggested a duration of analgesia in cats of at least six hours at a dose of 0.1 mg/kg IV in a model of visceral pain (Sawyer and Rech 1987), more recent studies suggest that it is a poor analgesic for clinical pain in cats (Warne et al. 2013, 2014). When given subcutaneously, it required 0.8 mg/kg to produce the same duration and consistency of analgesia (Sawyer and Rech 1987). In one study, butorphanol (0.5 mg/kg) failed to give complete analgesia in 2/12 dogs at 15 minutes postoperatively and wore off by 90 minutes in dogs given it after anesthesia, but had a longer duration if given during anesthesia (50% no analgesia at 90 minutes) (Waterman and Kalthum 1992). In various orthopedic studies in dogs, butorphanol (0.4 mg/kg) was inadequate in controlling pain; the duration of action was usually one hour or less, with questionable efficacy (Mathews et al. 1996; Pibarot et al. 1997). The duration of effect was up to two hours after laparotomy (Mathews et al. 1996). The dose is 0.1–0.4 mg/kg in dogs and 0.1–0.4 mg/kg IM, SC, IV in cats.

Nalbuphine is a partial κ-agonist and partial μ-agonist. It is more potent as an antagonist than any of the other commonly used mixed agonist/antagonist drugs. In trials as a postoperative analgesic in humans, it was as effective as pentazocine and meperidine. It does not produce much sedation and has a minimal effect on respiration. As with most of the opioids, it also has a minimal effect on the cardiovascular system (Sawyer et al. 1982). The dose in dogs and cats is 0.03–0.1 mg/kg IM, IV (intravenous injections may be slightly painful). In cats, doses from 0.75 to 3.0 mg/kg were equally effective for visceral analgesia and produced no behavioral side effects (Sawyer and Rech 1987). It is also used as a μ-opioid antagonist and has less sedative effect than butorphanol, while still leaving some analgesic action when compared with the pure antagonists.

11.8.4 Opioid Antagonists

Naloxone is the oldest of the pure opioid antagonists. These drugs bind to opioid receptors but have no effect, so they can be used to competitively displace the agonist. The most common use for the antagonists in the management of pain is to treat opioid-induced sedation, ventilatory depression, dysphoria and excitation. If a high dose of naloxone is used, it will antagonize the central effects of the opioid agonist, which may cause the animal to experience acute pain. Such an experience is intensely unpleasant for the patient and may precipitate immediate sympathetic stimulation, with serious consequences. In humans, this has led to pulmonary edema and even ventricular fibrillation, with several deaths attributed to the administration of naloxone. To this end, it is best to give the drug slowly and monitor the response of the patient. Doses for naloxone are 1–25 μg/kg. It is best to start at the low end of the range and titrate up to effect. As naloxone is supplied as a 400 or 1000 μg/ml (0.4 or 1 mg/ml) solution, it should be diluted down to a concentration that is easier to use. An effective method of reducing dysphoria, panting, sedation, or respiratory depression produced by an opioid overdose is to dilute 0.1–0.25 ml (0.4 mg/ml solution) in 10 ml normal saline and administer at 1 ml/minute to dogs, just to the point where the reversal of unwanted side effects has occurred. Using this technique, the analgesic effects of the opioid are not theoretically reversed. In dogs, naloxone is rapidly metabolized to naloxone glucuronide. It has a relatively short half-life in the brain and will only provide effective antagonism for about an hour, after which the animal may revert to the effects of the agonist (if it lasts longer) (Veng-Pedersen et al. 1995; Wilhelm et al. 1995). Since cats are deficient in glucuronyl transferase, it would be expected that naloxone might have a longer half-life in this species, but no direct comparison data are available.

11.8.5 Anti-Inflammatory Drugs

11.8.5.1 NSAIDs

NSAIDs are drugs that to some extent inhibit cyclooxygenase (COX) expression in cell membranes. There are two COX forms. COX-1 is commonly considered a constitutive form of the enzyme. It is responsible for regulation of normal homeostasis by controlling prostaglandin (PG) activity in the gastrointestinal tract, platelets and kidneys (Lomas and Grauer 2015). COX-2 is also expressed in a range of tissues and organs, and participates in normal homeostasis. However, it is primarily induced by tissue damage or injury and is commonly known as a pro-inflammatory enzyme. The release of COX-2 activates the production of various eicosanoids: inflammatory mediators that can amplify the inflammatory response and nociception (Luna et al. 2007; Kukanich et al. 2012). NSAIDs are metabolized mostly in the liver via glucuronidation in most species, making them potentially toxic to cats. Other pathways may be involved, depending on the NSAID and the species. For example, meloxicam is metabolized via oxidative pathways and has been successfully used for long-term administration in cats. NSAIDs are excreted predominantly via the biliary route (fecal) and urine.

Any NSAID can cause adverse effects, such as gastric irritation, protein-losing enteropathy, renal damage, or prolonged bleeding time by prevention of platelet aggregation. However, it is accepted that contemporary NSAIDs, which are more COX-2-specific, produce a lower prevalence of such effects when compared with older drugs (Luna et al. 2007; Monteiro-Steagall et al. 2013). Anorexia, diarrhea, vomiting and depression are common signs of NSAID toxicity but are normally observed with drug overdosing, concurrent steroid therapy, dosing errors, and when contraindications have not been respected. In such cases, treatment should be stopped immediately, and support therapy initiated. Contraindications include a history of gastrointestinal disease or NSAID intolerance, uncontrolled renal or hepatic disease, anemia, coagulopathies, hypovolemia or hypotension, concurrent corticosteroid administration, and close temporal administration of other NSAIDs. NSAID-induced acute renal injury in healthy cats after appropriate dosing/single injection is unlikely, but COX-2 is thought to play a role in preserving renal blood flow in the face of reduced perfusion. Many of the toxicity trials with current NSAIDs have demonstrated renal pathology in cats, and this has been the basis for the recommendation that these drugs only be used for a few days at most (robenacoxib, NADA 141-320 and meloxicam, NADA 141-219). However, new animal drug application; in cats with induced renal insufficiency (~85% reduction in renal tissue), neither aspirin nor meloxicam administered for seven days at standard doses caused any change in creatinine, glomerular filtration rate or urine protein creatinine ratio (Surdyk et al. 2013). Several studies have now shown that meloxicam and robenacoxib, at appropriate doses, can be administered to normal cats and those with chronic kidney disease (CKD) as long as urinary-tract infection, dental disease, hyperphosphatemia, and hypertension are controlled, and International Renal Interest Society (IRIS) stage I and II cats have normal appetite and drinking habits (Gowan et al. 2011, 2012; King et al. 2016). It is still important to monitor urea and creatinine concentrations during such therapy.

NSAIDs can cross the blood–brain barrier and produce central and peripheral analgesic, anti-inflammatory and antipyretic effects. Table 11.1 shows dosing recommendations for a variety of NSAIDs based on the WSAVA Global Pain Council guidelines. These drugs are widely available, and key players in the treatment of acute and chronic pain in small animal patients. There are major differences in labels, routes of administration, duration of treatment, and so forth among different NSAIDs and different countries. Veterinarians should be aware of the data in Table 11.1 and how they apply to their country of operation. The route of administration can impact pharmacokinetic variables, but the anti-inflammatory and analgesic effects (i.e., pharmacodynamics) are commonly equivalent. The majority of NSAIDs have good palatability and bioavailability after oral administration. This is one of their major advantages in terms of daily administration. On the other hand, some dental procedures may require long-term NSAID administration, and some of these drugs have been approved for daily administration "indefinitely" in dogs and with chronic pain. Additionally, some NSAIDs are approved for administration over several days in dogs and cats undergoing soft-tissue and orthopedic surgery. Thus, especially in cats, their use may be "off-label" for patients undergoing dental procedures or with chronic pain associated with dental conditions (Table 11.1). For example, full-mouth dental extractions for treatment of feline chronic gingivostomatitis commonly require at least five days of NSAID treatment. Long-term administration may be required for severe acute pain and to prevent persistent postsurgical pain. In cats, there is a particular concern around NSAID-induced toxicity, and the Association of American Feline Practitioners (AAFP) and International Society of Feline Medicine (ISFM) have published a review on this issue (Sparkes et al. 2010). Overall, the lowest effective dose should be administered when contraindications do not exist, and adverse effects should be monitored.

The timing of NSAID administration in the perioperative setting can be controversial. In general, healthy dogs and cats can tolerate preemptive administration, especially if fluid therapy is administered and blood pressure is monitored (Bostrom et al. 2002, 2006; Crandell et al. 2004; Frendin et al. 2006). However, NSAIDs are sometimes administered toward the end of the procedure and before extubation, to avoid any risk associated with intraoperative hypotension. There are no evidence-based studies that show benefit from pre- versus post-procedure administration, but it is known that patients benefit from the analgesic and anti-inflammatory effects that complement the use of other analgesics. The route of administration is also important. At the end of a procedure, the animal may be cold, and during recovery there is going to be some sympathetic activation, so dermal vasoconstriction is common during this period. This means that subcutaneous administration of the drug may be associated with significantly delayed peak effects (Lascelles et al. 1998). Intravenous administration is thus the best route to ensure the most immediate onset of the analgesic effect. As with most drugs, it is prudent to administer slowly over one to two minutes.

11.8.5.2 EP4 Receptor Antagonists

Grapiprant (2 mg/kg PO) is a US Food and Drug Administration (FDA)-approved EP4 prostaglandin receptor antagonist that has been licensed in different countries for management of pain and inflammation associated with osteoarthritis in dogs (Rausch-Derra et al. 2016b). The EP4 prostanoid receptor is usually activated by prostaglandin E2 during inflammatory states and is responsible for mediating pain, swelling and redness within the arachidonic acid cascade. It is the primary mediator of the PGE2-induced sensitization of sensory neurons. By blocking EP4 receptors, grapiprant should not impair the homeostatic activity of other prostaglandins, as observed with NSAIDs. The safety of grapiprant has been reported using different doses in research beagles over nine months. There were no drug-related effects on liver enzymes, blood urea nitrogen (BUN), creatinine values, or platelet function. However, some mild gastrointestinal effects may be observed, such as soft stool and sporadic vomiting (Rausch-Derra et al. 2015). Indeed, more dogs vomited with grapiprant (17%) when compared with a placebo group (6.25%) in a prospective, randomized, masked, placebo-controlled clinical study (Rausch-Derra et al. 2016a).

Many dogs that are treated with grapiprant for osteoarthritis may require dental treatment. It is not clear if it produces appropriate pain relief for dental extractions, for example. Though it makes sense to combine NSAIDs and grapiprant because of their different sites of action, to date the safety of such combinations has not been studied; until data are available, it would be prudent not to combine them. Despite its safety profile in healthy cats, grapiprant has not been licensed for use in this species (Rausch-Derra and Rhodes 2016).

Table 11.1 Nonsteroidal anti-inflammatory drugs (NSAIDs): canine and feline dosing recommendations. [a]

Drug	Indication	Species, dose,[b] route[c]	Frequency
Ketoprofen[d]	Surgical and chronic pain	**Dogs**	
		2.0 mg/kg, IV, SC, IM	Once postoperative
		1.0 mg/kg PO	Once per day for up to three additional days
		Cats	
		As for dogs	
Meloxicam[d]	Surgical pain/acute musculoskeletal	**Dogs**	
		0.2 mg/kg IV, SC	Once
		0.1 mg/kg PO	Once per day
		Cats	
		0.3 mg/kg IV, SC	One dose only; do not follow up with any additional dosing
		or	
		Up to 0.2 mg/kg SC	Once
		0.05 mg/kg PO	Once per day for up to four additional days
	Chronic pain	**Dogs**	
		0.2 mg/kg PO	Once on day 1
		0.1 mg/kg PO	Once per day to follow; use the lowest effective dose
		Cats	
		0.1 mg/kg PO	Once on day 1
		0.01–0.05 mg/kg PO	Once per day to follow; use the lowest effective dose
Cimicoxib[d]	Surgical pain	**Dogs**	
		2 mg/kg PO	Once daily for four to eight days
	Chronic pain	**Dogs**	
		2 mg/kg PO	Once daily; use lowest effective dose
Mavacoxib[d]	Chronic pain	**Dogs**	
		2 mg/kg PO	Dose on day 0, day 14, then once per month for up to five further months
Robenacoxib[d]	Surgical pain/acute musculoskeletal	**Dog**	
		2 mg/kg SC	Once followed by oral
		1 mg/kg PO	Once daily
		Cats	
		2 mg/kg SC	Once followed by oral
		1 mg/kg PO	Once daily for a total of six days or as licensed
	Chronic pain	**Dogs**	
		1 mg/kg PO	Once daily; use lowest effective dose
		Cats	
		1 mg/kg PO	Once per day to follow; use the lowest effective dose

(*Continued*)

Table 11.1 (Continued)

Drug	Indication	Species, dose,[b] route[c]	Frequency
Carprofen[d]	Surgical pain	**Dogs**	
		4 or 4.4 mg/kg SC, IV, PO	Once per day for up to four days
		2 or 2.2 mg/kg SC, IV, PO	Every 12 hours for up to four days
		Cats	
		2 to 4 mg/kg SC, IV	One dose only; do not follow up with any additional dosing
	Chronic pain	**Dogs**	
		4 or 4.4 mg/kg PO	Once daily; use lowest effective dose
		2 or 2.2 mg/kg PO	Once daily for up to three days
Firocoxib[d]	Surgical pain	**Dogs**	Once daily; use lowest effective dose
		5 mg/kg PO	
	Chronic pain	**Dogs**	Once daily for three to five days. Repeat once per **week**.
		5 mg/kg PO	
Tolfenamic acid	Acute and chronic pain	**Dogs**	
		4 mg/kg SC, IM, PO	
		Cats	
		As for dogs	
Flunixin meglumine	Pyrexia	**Dogs and Cats**	
		0.25 mg/kg SC	Once
		Dogs and Cats	
	Surgical and ophthalmological procedures	0.25–1.0 mg/kg SC	Every 12–24 hours for one or two treatments
Piroxicam	Inflammation of the lower urinary tract	**Dogs**	
		0.3 mg/kg, PO	Once daily for two treatments, then every two days
Paracetamol (acetaminophen)	Surgical/acute or chronic pain	**Dogs *Only***	
		10–15 mg/kg PO	Every 8–12 hours
		DO NOT USE IN CATS	
Aspirin	Surgical/acute or chronic pain	**Dogs**	
		10 mg/kg PO	Every 12 hours

[a] See text for details on the contraindications for use.
[b] Dose based on lean body weight.
[c] IV, intravenously; SC, subcutaneously; IM, intramuscularly; PO, *per os*.
[d] Indicates a veterinary-licensed version of this pharmaceutical exists in some countries. The label will provide the best information as to product use in a given country. Source: Modified from Mathews et al. (2014.)

11.8.5.3 Corticosteroids

Glucocorticosteroids are among the most misused classes of drugs in veterinary practice. There is little evidence-based medicine that supports their administration as analgesics in the clinical setting, particularly with regard to efficacy, optimal dosage and dosage interval, and physical and endocrine effects. However, these drugs are useful in the management of hypoadrenocorticism, allergic and autoimmune disorders, and specific inflammatory conditions. In cases involving a significant inflammatory component, the corticosteroids may help to reduce swelling and inflammation, which may reduce pain. But it is rare, in veterinary medicine, to use a corticosteroid alone for the management of this kind of case (Cray et al. 2018). Reported side effects include but are not restricted to behavioral changes, iatrogenic hyperadrenocorticism, polyphagia, diarrhea, hepatopathy, gastrointestinal perforation, polyuria, polydipsia, muscle atrophy, increased risk of infection, and poor wound healing, among other things (Aharon et al. 2017). The combination of glucocorticosteroids with NSAIDs is contraindicated due to the increased incidence of side effects (Boston et al. 2003).

11.8.5.4 Other Drugs with Analgesic and Potential Anti-Inflammatory Effects

Acetaminophen (Paracetamol) has analgesic and antypiretic effects but little if any anti-inflammatory activity (Table 11.1) (Chandrasekharan et al. 2002). Its mechanism of action seems to be related to the inhibition of a subtype of COX-1 enzymes in the central nervous system. It has been used for chronic pain in dogs as part of a multimodal approach with minimal gastrointestinal effects, and it has synergism with opioid analgesics. Acetaminophen toxicosis is usually associated with hepatotoxicity in dogs and methemoglobinemia in cats. This can be treated with intravenous fluids, N-acetylcysteine, ascorbic acid, and sodium bicarbonate. In dogs, clinical signs are generally seen with doses of 200 mg/kg, whereas cats are much more sensitive, exhibiting signs at doses of approximately 60 mg/kg. Early effects of acetaminophen toxicosis are progressive cyanosis, tachypnea, and dyspnea, depending on the degree of methemoglobinemia. In dogs, acetaminophen is conjugated with glucuronide and sulfate by transferase enzymes, which are deficient in the cat. For this reason, acetaminophen is contraindicated in cats.

Metamizole (Dypirone) is a weak NSAID with analgesic, antipyretic and spasmolytic properties (Table 11.1). Its mechanism of action seems to be related to the inhibition of a subtype of COX-1 enzyme in the central nervous system. This drug can decrease opioid consumption and its adverse effects. The administration of metamizole (25–35 mg/kg TID IV) has been shown to provide adequate postoperative analgesia after ovariohysterectomy in dogs (Imagawa et al. 2011). Since this is a phenolic compound, it should be used with caution in cats (Lebkowska-Wieruszewska et al. 2018).

11.8.6 Local Anesthetics

Blocking nociceptive input with a local anesthetic is the most effective method of pain management – all other treatments inhibit nociceptive input, but if the stimulus is strong enough it may overcome this inhibitory effect. A local anesthetic blocks conduction and therefore there is no central sensitization while it is preventing transmission. However, these drugs do not only block nociception but also remove all sensation, and therefore they can lead to dysesthesias and self-mutilation because of the altered sensation from the area. They will also block the motor component of nerves, but fortunately the main blocks carried out in dentistry only affect sensory nerves.

In the process of carrying out a block, it is imperative that the clinician uses appropriate doses and avoids intravascular injection. Syringes used by human dentists may have a ring on the end of the plunger so that the operator can aspirate without having to alter their hand position. This is more difficult with standard plastic syringes, but it can be done if the syringe is held correctly. With either method, it is essential to aspirate before injecting to ensure extravascular placement of the end of the needle (Aprea et al. 2011) (Figure 11.11). If the injection is started and there is a lot of resistance, the operator should stop and reposition the needle as this may indicate intraneural injection, which could lead to nerve damage.

11.8.6.1 Pharmacology

A detailed description of the pharmacology of the local anesthetics is beyond the scope of this chapter; the reader is referred to standard pharmacology texts. The four most commonly used local anesthetics in current dental practice are lidocaine, mepivacaine, ropivacaine and bupivacaine, all of which are classed as amides (Table 11.2). The drugs are listed here in order of onset and duration of action, but these are heavily influenced by proximity to the nerve and the concentration used, and are therefore very variable. If a drug is placed within the infraorbital canal, onset is rapid; even with bupivacaine, there is a good block by five minutes. However, onset may be significantly delayed if the drug is not deposited close to the nerve. In studies with infraorbital block in dogs, lidocaine (2%) lasted from 1 hour 20 minutes to 3 hours 40 minutes and bupivacaine (0.5%) from 2 hours 40 minutes to more than 13 hours (Pascoe, unpublished observations). The dog with the longest block with lidocaine had the shortest block with bupivacaine! A mixture of equal volumes of lidocaine and bupivacaine gave block durations that were intermediate, ranging from 3 hours 40 minutes to 5 hours 40 minutes. The duration of the block should exceed the surgical time, which may be beneficial during the early part of recovery. As the animal becomes less sedated, however, a prolonged block may be disadvantageous if it leads to dysesthesia and self-mutilation, though this seems to be rare in clinical practice. To date, no one has really examined the different concentrations of local anesthetic for dental blocks in dogs and cats, but given the size of the nerves and the failures we have seen with both inferior alveolar and infraorbital blocks, it is likely that the use of higher concentrations may be necessary to achieve the best effect. Hence, a smaller volume of 0.75% bupivacaine may be more effective than the same dose of 0.5% bupivacaine. Mixing local anesthetics such as bupivacaine and lidocaine will usually decrease the duration of action when compared with bupivacaine alone. Clinically, the onset is similar between the mixture and bupivacaine alone.

These drugs have a relatively narrow therapeutic margin, so the clinician should ensure that the total doses being used are less than those that might cause toxicity (Table 11.2).

11.8.6.2 Adjuncts

Veterinarians have combined more than one of the following adjuncts, based on the idea that they have different mechanisms of action, but there are no studies that define their additivity or synergism (Turner et al. 2018).

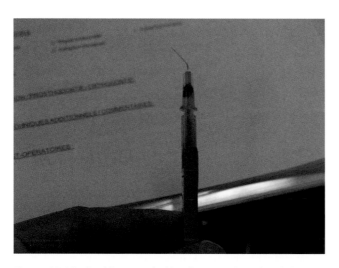

Figure 11.11 In this example, blood was aspirated and the injection of the local anesthetic solution for a maxillary nerve block was not performed. Given its high cardiotoxicity, intravenous administration of bupivacaine could be fatal in this case. *Source:* Courtesy of Dr. Paulo Steagall.

11.8.6.2.1 Catecholamines
For many years, vasoconstrictors have been added to local anesthetics to reduce vascular removal of the drug and limit systemic uptake. Epinephrine has been the most common additive and will prolong the action of lidocaine and mepivacaine. With the longer-acting drugs, the addition of epinephrine has little effect on the duration of action of a nerve block (Renck and Hassan 1992), but it has been added just to reduce the plasma concentrations of both ropivacaine and bupivacaine.

11.8.6.2.2 Alpha-2 Agonists
Dexmedetomidine may significantly increase the duration of action of a local anesthetic. The alpha-2 agonists cause vasoconstriction, but their effect is not reversed by alpha-2 antagonists, so the mechanism is neither vasoconstriction- nor alpha-2-mediated. Current hypotheses suggest that it is an inhibition of the hyperpolarization cation channels that are involved in the return to a resting membrane potential after a period of hyperpolarization (Brummett et al. 2011). In a study in children undergoing cleft palate repair, the addition of dexmedetomidine (1 µg/kg) to 0.25% bupivacaine for a palatine block increased the duration of postoperative analgesia by 50% (Obayah et al. 2010).

11.8.6.2.3 Opioids
Some opioids prolong the duration of local anesthetic blocks, but this is not an opioid effect, since there are no opioid receptors along the axonal part of a neuron. It has now been shown that many of these drugs block the same sodium channels affected by local anesthetics. Buprenorphine has the highest affinity (of the opioids tested) for sodium channel blockade, but fentanyl, sufentanil, methadone, meperidine, and tramadol all have IC_{50}s (inhibitory concentrations at which 50% of the sodium channels are blocked) that indicate a potency greater than or equal to that of lidocaine. In a human study, the addition of buprenorphine (7.5 µg/ml) to bupivacaine (0.5%) for intraoral nerve blocks increased the duration of postoperative analgesia from 8 to 28 hours (Modi

Table 11.2 Common local anesthetics used in veterinary anesthesia and pain management.

Local anesthetic[a]	Onset (min)	Common concentrations (%)	Duration of block (h)	Relative potency (lidocaine = 1)	Suggested maximum doses (mg/kg)
Lidocaine	5–15	1, 2	1–3	1	10
Mepivacaine	5–15	1, 2	1.5 – 2.5	1	4
Bupivacaine	5–20	0.25, 0.5, 0.75	4–10	4	2
Ropivacaine	10–20	0.5, 0.75	3–5	3	3
Levobupivacaine	10–20	0.5, 0.75	4–6	4	2

[a] Volumes of injection (0.25–1 ml) vary according to the size of the patient and their anatomy and body weight. Anesthetic blocks can be repeated according to the duration of the procedure, interest in postoperative analgesia, and the use of less than maximum recommended doses (see text).

et al. 2009). A study in dogs where the same concentrations of bupivacaine and buprenorphine were used for an infraorbital block showed evidence of an effect at 96 hours in 25% of the animals (Snyder et al. 2016), whereas none had analgesia at this time with bupivacaine alone.

11.8.6.2.4 *Dexamethasone*

Dexamethasone (4–8 mg added to local anesthetic) has been shown to increase the duration of block and of postoperative analgesia when it has been added to local anesthetics. It appears to be effective for both shorter- and longer-duration drugs (Huynh et al. 2015). The mechanism of action has not been defined, and several studies have shown no difference in postoperative analgesia with systemic versus locally applied dexamethasone (Marty et al. 2018).

11.8.6.3 Regional Techniques

The most common regional techniques are the infraorbital block and the inferior alveolar nerve block, though other blocks may also be important. The following descriptions are not comprehensive but give some idea of how they should be carried out.

11.8.6.3.1 *Inferior Alveolar Nerve Block*

The inferior alveolar nerve is blocked to remove sensation from the gingiva and teeth in the mandible. This nerve arises from the ventral branch of the mandibular nerve. It is typically blocked close to the point where it enters the mandibular foramen. The block is often not effective; in human dentistry, success can be as low as 25% (Aggarwal et al. 2017). Using an intraoral approach, the nerve can usually be palpated on the medial aspect of the mandible just rostral to the angular process. It is felt as a string-like structure that disappears as it enters the foramen. In large dogs, it is easy to place a finger on the nerve and advance the needle toward this site with the other hand. This becomes progressively more difficult with smaller patients because of the difficulty of getting both hands into the mouth. In such cases, the nerve may still be palpated, but the needle is advanced percutaneously from the ventral border of the mandible, in an attempt to slide it along the medial surface of the mandible so that the tip can be palpated close to the nerve with the other hand from inside the mouth. In dogs, there is often a concavity on the ventral border of the mandible (i.e., the vascular notch) where the bottom of this curve is close to the mandibular foramen, so this is a good landmark for needle placement (Figure 11.12). Some cats have a similar concavity, but it is much less common in this species. If the needle deviates more medially, there is the risk that the lingual nerve will be blocked. This nerve is sensory to the tongue and may make it more likely that the animal will injure the tongue as it is

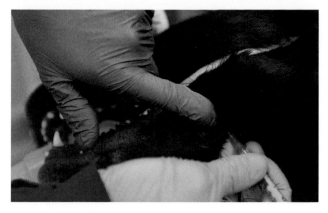

Figure 11.12 Inferior alveolar nerve block in a dog. *Source:* Dr. Ryota Watanabe, Université of Montréal.

recovering, even though motor function is intact (hypoglossal nerve). Since the dose needed for this block does not scale directly with body weight, a dose using metabolic size makes more sense. A suggested dose is $0.18\,ml/BW^{2/3}$, since the injection technique is less specific than when depositing the drug next to a nerve in a bony canal. The extraoral technique can be viewed at https://www.youtube.com/watch?v=2q8ndh5Bn6U.

11.8.6.4 Middle Mental Canal Injection

Injections into the middle mental canal are generally used to block the mandibular canine and incisor teeth (Krug and Losey 2011). The inferior alveolar nerve travels along this canal, so if the anesthetic were injected deeply into it, it might be possible to block all the mandibular teeth, but such an approach has not been validated. The middle mental canal exits ventral to the mesial root of the second premolar tooth and can be difficult to palpate because of the lower-lip frenulum that overlies this site. A needle should be advanced into the canal, advancing caudally, and injection made after ensuring that the needle is in the canal and not in a blood vessel by aspirating prior to injection. If there is any great resistance to injection, the needle should be repositioned to ensure that it is not going directly into the nerve or periosteum. In small dogs and cats, this foramen is very small, so few clinicians attempt this block in these patients. This technique can be viewed at https://www.youtube.com/watch?v=r9j06VVGvMw.

11.8.6.5 Infraorbital Block

The infraorbital nerve is a branch of the maxillary nerve that supplies the sensory innervation for the maxillary teeth and lateral gingiva. There are three groups of branches: the caudal, middle, and rostral superior alveolar nerves, which supply the caudal, middle and rostral maxillary teeth, respectively. The caudal superior alveolar nerves leave the infraorbital nerve before it enters the infraorbital canal, while the middle superior alveolar nerves branch off just after it does so. The rostral superior alveolar nerve branches off just before the nerve exits the canal and supplies the canine and incisor teeth. There is some evidence in the literature for a transmedian nerve supply for the maxillary canine teeth in cats, suggesting that a bilateral block may be necessary even when only one side is being operated on (Anderson and Pearl 1974; Pearl et al. 1977). The pterygopalatine nerve branches off from the maxillary nerve and gives rise to the accessory palatine and major palatine nerves, which supply the gingiva on the mesial side of the teeth. From this anatomy, it is expected that blocking of the canine and incisor teeth and the rostral premolars should result from an injection into the infraorbital canal but that blocking of the fourth premolar or molar teeth will require the local anesthetic to reach beyond the caudal end of the canal. Removal of sensation from the palate requires an even more caudal progression of the local anesthetic. In studies using needle injection into the canal and catheter injections beyond it, it has still been difficult to obtain consistent blocks for the maxillary teeth. Injection of local anesthetic into the caudal third of the infraorbital canal resulted in consistent blockade of stimuli from the canine tooth, about a 50% success rate for the fourth premolar, and minimal effect on the caudal molar tooth (Pascoe 2016) (Figure 11.13). Using a catheter to deposit local anesthetic beyond and at the caudal entrance to the canal resulted in more consistent blockade of the caudal teeth, but with minimal effect on the palatine nerve (Gross et al. 1997, 2000; Pascoe and Chohan 2017). The following technique is suggested as the most reliable: A catheter (e.g., a 22G 1.8″) is introduced into the canal through the gingival mucosa, advancing until the tip is roughly at a point on a line drawn vertically from the lateral canthus of the eye (Viscasillas et al. 2013). After depositing half the anesthetic at this location, the catheter is withdrawn to a point on a line drawn vertically from the medial canthus of the eye, and the rest of the drug is deposited here – this should be at the caudal end of the infraorbital canal (Viscasillas et al. 2013). In brachycephalic dogs and in cats the infraorbital canal is very short, so a 25- or 27-gauge needle may be easier to use for this block, and the local anesthetic can be deposited just caudal to the canal (Figure 11.14). Care should be taken not to advance the needle too far, to prevent penetration of the globe (Figure 11.15). All injections should be preceded by aspiration to ensure that the tip of the needle or catheter is not in a vessel. This applies even when there has been a negative aspiration for the distal injection and the needle or catheter has been withdrawn for a second injection. A suggested volume for this block is 0.11 ml/kg$^{0.67}$. The intraoral technique, without the introduction of a catheter, can be viewed at https://www.youtube.com/watch?v=H3L1LHBcM-g .

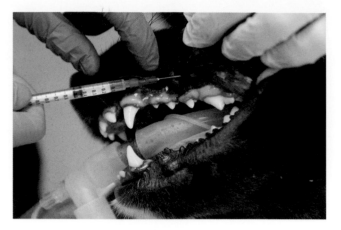

Figure 11.13 Infraorbital nerve block in a dog. (*Source:* Dr. Ryota Watanabe, University of Montréal).

11.8.6.6 Maxillary Nerve Block

Given the description of the preceding anatomy, some clinicians have chosen to use a maxillary approach to try to block the whole maxillary nerve. There are at least five approaches to this block described, but there are no comparative studies of the efficacy of each. The first three descriptions use the same anatomic landmarks but deposit the local anesthetic at different points along the maxillary nerve by varying the angle of the needle. The main landmark is the angle formed by the caudal border of the cranial ventral aspect of the zygomatic arch and the maxilla. If the needle is angled rostrally from this site toward the caudal end of the infraorbital canal, the drug is deposited in a similar location to that reached using the infraorbital approach with a long catheter. Care must be taken not to penetrate the globe by angling the needle too far dorsally (Perry et al. 2015; Loughran et al. 2016). The second method uses a more perpendicular needle direction to aim for the maxillary nerve before it branches into the pterygopalatine and infraorbital nerves. In both locations, the maxillary nerve lies on top of the medial pterygoid muscle, so if the needle is advanced until it touches bone, it should be withdrawn a few millimeters before injecting the drug. The pterygopalatine bone in this region is very thin and great care must be taken to avoid penetrating it and causing epistaxis. This more perpendicular approach also seems to increase the likelihood of penetrating the maxillary artery and causing a hematoma. The third approach is to angle the needle caudally and walk it off the cranial edge of the ramus of the mandible, aiming the needle toward the base of the skull and the foramen rotundum, where the maxillary nerve exits the skull. The fourth method is to use an intraoral approach, advancing the needle craniodorsally from behind the last molar tooth. Some authors have described using a needle bent to 45° for this method, to

Figure 11.14 Infraorbital nerve block in a cat. *Source:* Courtesy of Dr. Paulo Steagall.

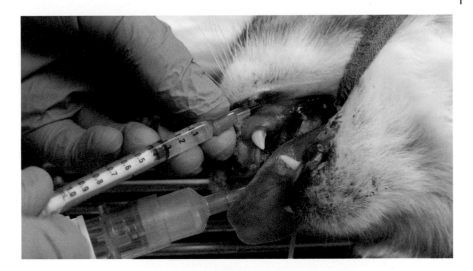

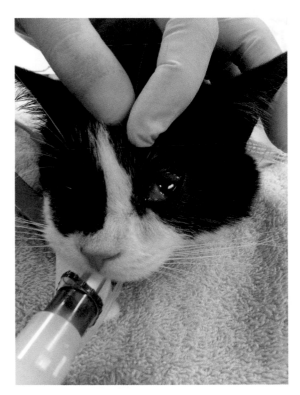

Figure 11.15 Bleeding observed after positioning the needle to perform an infraorbital nerve block in a cat. *Source:* Courtesy of Dr. Paulo Steagall.

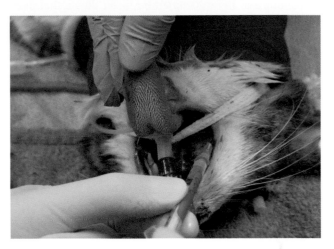

Figure 11.16 An intraoral approach for the maxillary nerve block in a cat. The needle is advanced in craniodorsally from behind the last molar tooth. Note that the needle is bent, to make the injection easier. *Source:* Courtesy of Dr. Paulo Steagall

deposit the drug in the right place in most cases, but in one animal it was deposited into the oral cavity, showing that care must be taken not to advance the needle too far (Langton and Walker 2017). The extraoral approach (the second method) can be viewed at https://www.youtube.com/watch?v=1AYNmsyzCv0 .

11.8.6.7 Palatine Block
This involves injecting local anesthetic into the palatine foramen to block the greater palatine nerve. The palatine foramen is not easy to find because of the density of the overlying tissue, and the nerve is accompanied by an artery, which increases the risk of hematoma/hemorrhage. Some authors have used this as an approach to the maxillary nerve, but there are much better and less risky ways to do this, as already described. This technique can be viewed at https://www.youtube.com/watch?v=-xsDqqGRrjI.

make the injection easier (Figure 11.16). This block requires very good spatial sense to get the needle to the right spot and not to go too shallow (ineffective block) or too deep (globe penetration) (Perry et al. 2015). The fifth method approaches the caudal end of the infraorbital canal from the orbital rim. The globe is gently displaced caudally and the needle is advanced from the middle of the ventral orbital rim through the skin and down toward the maxillary nerve. In a cadaver study, this technique appeared to

11.8.7 Systemic Lidocaine

Lidocaine has been studied extensively as an adjunct to general anesthesia and a way of providing some analgesia. Such studies have not been specifically applied to dental patients. Intravenous lidocaine at infusions up to 400 µg/kg/minute in dogs have shown a plateau effect on the minimum alveolar concentration (MAC) of inhalants, with a maximum reduction of 40–50% (Himes et al. 1977). In the clinical setting, it is unusual to exceed infusion of 200 µg/kg/minute, with an expectation that this will reduce MAC by ~30–40% (Steagall et al. 2006a). This high infusion rate should not be maintained for several hours due to the risk of lidocaine toxicity. Infusion rates of 120 µg/kg/minute after a bolus of 2 mg/kg have been well tolerated (Nunes De Moraes et al. 1998). While the results are similar in cats (Pypendop and Ilkiw 2005b), it has been shown that there is no cardiovascular benefit to the administration of lidocaine with inhalant anesthetics, so its use as an anesthetic adjunct in this species is not recommended (Pypendop and Ilkiw 2005a). Some studies have shown postoperative benefit to intravenous lidocaine administered intra- or postoperatively (Smith et al. 2004; Guimaraes Alves et al. 2014;Chiavaccini et al. 2017), despite the fact that no changes in antinociceptive threshold have been demonstrated in cats or dogs (Pypendop et al. 2006; Macdougall et al. 2009).

11.8.8 Ketamine

The primary excitatory neurotransmitter for nociception in the spinal cord is glutamate, which will activate the NMDA receptor if the incoming signal is persistent. This role of the NMDA receptor in central sensitization has led to renewed interest in NMDA receptor antagonists such as ketamine and amantadine (Pozzi et al. 2006). Ketamine may prevent central sensitization from occurring; doses associated with NMDA antagonism are lower than those required for induction of anesthesia.

Sub-anesthetic doses of ketamine have been used as an adjunctive analgesic in dogs and cats undergoing surgery (Slingsby and Waterman-Pearson 2000). Their administration reduces anesthetic requirements in both species (Pascoe et al. 2007). This could be an option during invasive oral surgery or in patients where central sensitization and severe pain are suspected. In dogs and cats, a loading dose (0.15–0.5 mg/kg) followed by a CRI (5–20 µg/kg/minute) is used. If anesthesia was induced with ketamine, the loading dose can be omitted. Such sub-anesthetic doses should be used cautiously in cats with renal insufficiency because of the requirement for renal excretion of both ketamine and its active metabolite, norketamine (dogs metabolize norketamine to dyhydronorketamine, which is an inactive form of the drug).

Ketamine had improved feeding behavior when administered as a CRI in dogs after mastectomy but did not provide an opioid-sparing effect (Sarrau et al. 2007). Pain scores after ketamine infusions were not significantly different than in a group receiving butorphanol, and the drug did not provide adequate analgesia in 37.5% of dogs undergoing ovariohysterectomy (Gutierrez-Blanco et al. 2015). When combined with opioids and other analgesic techniques, a CRI after a loading dose was associated with analgesia of longer duration in dogs undergoing limb amputation (Wagner et al. 2002) and with an anesthetic-sparing effect in dogs generally (Muir et al. 2003; Gutierrez-Blanco et al. 2013). This highlights that ketamine must be used as part of a multimodal analgesic approach and not as the sole method of pain relief after surgery. Its use is restricted to the hospital setting, since an intravenous infusion is required for long-term treatment.

11.8.9 Amantadine

Amantadine is only available as an oral formulation in most countries. The drug is administered with an NSAID for the treatment of chronic painful conditions that are refractory to NSAID administration alone. There is no indication for the use of amantadine as sole analgesic agent (Kukanich 2013). Scientific information on the use of amantadine as an analgesic in dogs and cats is almost non-existent (Madden et al. 2014). One study showed that physical activity was improved by the addition of amantadine in dogs with osteoarthritis-related pain refractory to an NSAID (Lascelles et al. 2008). Therefore, it is possible that the drug has potential as an adjuvant therapy for oral painful conditions.

Amantadine is well absorbed after oral administration (bioavailability ≈ 100%), with a peak plasma concentration one to four hours after administration. In both cats and dogs, it has a terminal elimination half-life of about six hours. Suggested doses range from 2 to 4 mg/kg every 12 hours, but more frequent administration would be suggested by the half-life. Treatment with NSAID and amantadine should be attempted for a minimum of three to four weeks for evaluation of its efficacy in chronic pain.

11.8.10 Gabapentin

Gabapentin is a structural analog of the inhibitory neurotransmitter GABA but it does not act at GABA receptors. Rather, it acts on voltage-gated calcium channels (Kukkar et al. 2013) to decrease neurotransmitter release. It has been used for neuropathic pain in different species. Based on meta-analysis and some systematic reviews, it has been recommended for perioperative pain control in humans (Mathiesen et al. 2007; Li et al. 2017). It can reduce the prevalence of opioid-induced adverse effects and chronic postsurgical pain and improve postoperative patient function. One study looked at the combination of gabapentin and buprenorphine in cats undergoing ovariohysterectomy and found that the analgesic effects were similar to those in cats receiving an NSAID and buprenorphine (Steagall et al. 2017).

Based on its high bioavailability and favorable pharmacokinetics in cats (Siao et al. 2010), there could be interest in using this drug in pain management of the dental patient. The WSAVA Global Pain Council suggests the administration of gabapentin in a multimodal protocol for the prevention of postsurgical pain. Doses are anecdotal in dogs and cats, but expert literature suggests 10–20 mg/kg every 12 hours for some number of days depending on the level of acute pain, and 5–10 mg/kg every 8–12 hours for a minimum of four weeks in chronic pain. Doses can be increased or decreased in individual animals according to their response. If the animal appears to be drowsy then the dose should be decreased, but it can be increased again if minimal effects are noted. At this time, there is no recommendation for the use of pregabalin – another gabapentinoid drug – in dogs or cats, especially given its high cost.

11.8.11 Mesenchymal Cells in Cats

These cells are commonly used for the treatment of immune-mediated and inflammatory disorders, since they can modulate the immune system response. Fresh, *autologous*, adipose-derived mesenchymal stem cells have been used safely and successfully in some cats for the treatment of feline chronic gingivostomatis complex (Arzi et al. 2016). In brief, nine cats received an intravenous injection with these cells experimentally. Immune cell subsets and serum protein and cytokine levels were evaluated up to six months after treatment. Five cats responded to treatment with remission, histological resolution, or clinical improvement with signs of systemic immunomodulation. A follow-up study showed that the use of fresh, *allogenic*, adipose-

derived mesenchymal cells in seven cats produced lower efficacy with a delayed response as compared with autologous cells (Arzi et al. 2017).

11.8.12 Maropitant

Maropitant (1 mg/kg) is a neurokinin-1 (NK-1) receptor antagonist used to treat and prevent emesis in dogs by blocking NK-1 receptors in the chemoreceptor trigger zone/emetic center in the central nervous system. Maropitant can reduce vomiting and discomfort in dogs and cats receiving opioids such as morphine (Lorenzutti et al. 2017) and hydromorphone and in cats receiving dexmedetomidine. However, injectable maropitant containing metacresol is associated with pain on injection; it appears that this can be lessened by using refrigerated (4 °C) drug (Narishetty et al. 2009). It is important to administer the maropitant about 60 minutes before the opioid/alpha-2 agonist in order to gain the most benefit from its effects (Hay Kraus 2014). Maropitant administered orally 2–20 hours before premedication was also effective at reducing, but not eliminating, vomiting and nausea in cats (Martin-Flores et al. 2016, 2017). However, nausca and ptyalism were not eliminated, and the use of maropitant had no effect on the incidence of intraoperative gastroesophageal reflux (Johnson 2014). Animals receiving maropitant tend to eat earlier and consume more food during the first 24 hours postoperation (Ramsey et al. 2014).

The NK-1 receptor and its ligand, substance P, have been isolated in spinal cord sensory afferents involved in nociceptive pathways. These sensory synaptic endings release substance P during noxious stimulation, and its vesicles are present in spinal cord-ascending projections to brain areas used for nociceptive processing. Studies in mice and rabbits have demonstrated that NK-1 receptor antagonists consistently induce analgesia in visceral noxious stimulation. Maropitant decreased inhalant anesthetic requirements after intravenous administration in dogs (Boscan et al. 2011). Many clinicians are adding maropitant to their anesthetic protocols in order to reduce nausea and vomiting, improve recovery and provide postoperative analgesia (Lotti et al. 2018; Corrêa et al. 2019).

References

Acs, G., Lodolini, G., Kaminsky, S., and Cisneros, G.J. (1992). Effect of nursing caries on body weight in a pediatric population. *Pediatr. Dent.* 14: 302–305.

Aggarwal, V., Singla, M., and Miglani, S. (2017). Comparative evaluation of anesthetic efficacy of 2% lidocaine, 4% articaine, and 0.5% bupivacaine on inferior alveolar nerve block in patients with symptomatic irreversible pulpitis: a prospective, randomized, double-blind clinical trial. *J. Oral Facial Pain Headache* 31: 124–128.

Aguiar, J., Chebroux, A., Martinez-Taboada, F., and Leece, E.A. (2015). Analgesic effects of maxillary and inferior alveolar nerve blocks in cats undergoing dental extractions. *J. Feline Med. Surg.* 17: 110–116.

Aharon, M.A., Prittie, J.E., and Buriko, K. (2017). A review of associated controversies surrounding glucocorticoid use in veterinary emergency and critical care. *J. Vet. Emerg. Crit. Care (San Antonio)* 27: 267–277.

Anderson, K.V. and Pearl, G.S. (1974). Transmedian innervation of canine tooth pulp in cats. *Exp. Neurol.* 44: 35–40.

Aprea, F., Vettorato, E., and Corletto, F. (2011). Severe cardiovascular depression in a cat following a mandibular nerve block with bupivacaine. *Vet. Anaesth. Analg.* 38: 614–618.

Arzi, B., Mills-Ko, E., Verstraete, F.J. et al. (2016). Therapeutic efficacy of fresh, autologous mesenchymal stem cells for severe refractory gingivostomatitis in cats. *Stem Cells Transl. Med.* 5: 75–86.

Arzi, B., Clark, K.C., Sundaram, A. et al. (2017). Therapeutic efficacy of fresh, allogeneic mesenchymal stem cells for severe refractory feline chronic gingivostomatitis. *Stem Cells Transl. Med.* 6: 1710–1722.

Bell, A., Helm, J., and Reid, J. (2014). Veterinarians' attitudes to chronic pain in dogs. *Vet. Rec.* 175: 428.

Benitez, M.E., Roush, J.K., Kukanich, B., and Mcmurphy, R. (2015). Pharmacokinetics of hydrocodone and tramadol administered for control of postoperative pain in dogs following tibial plateau leveling osteotomy. *Am. J. Vet. Res.* 76: 763–770.

Bortolami, E. and Love, E.J. (2015). Practical use of opioids in cats: a state-of-the-art, evidence-based review. *J. Feline Med. Surg.* 17: 283–311.

Boscan, P., Monnet, E., Mama, K. et al. (2011). Effect of maropitant, a neurokinin 1 receptor antagonist, on anesthetic requirements during noxious visceral stimulation of the ovary in dogs. *Am. J. Vet. Res.* 72: 1576–1579.

Boston, S.E., Moens, N.M., Kruth, S.A., and Southorn, E.P. (2003). Endoscopic evaluation of the gastroduodenal mucosa to determine the safety of short-term concurrent administration of meloxicam and dexamethasone in healthy dogs. *Am. J. Vet. Res.* 64: 1369–1375.

Bostrom, I.M., Nyman, G.C., Lord, P.E. et al. (2002). Effects of carprofen on renal function and results of serum biochemical and hematologic analyses in anesthetized dogs that had low blood pressure during anesthesia. *Am. J. Vet. Res.* 63: 712–721.

Bostrom, I.M., Nyman, G., Hoppe, A., and Lord, P. (2006). Effects of meloxicam on renal function in dogs with hypotension during anaesthesia. *Vet. Anaesth. Analg.* 33: 62–69.

Brodbelt, D.C., Taylor, P.M., and Stanway, G.W. (1997). A comparison of pre-operative morphine and buprenorphine for post operative analgesia for arthrotomy in the dog. *J. Vet. Anaesth.* 24: 42.

Brondani, J.T., Luna, S.P., and Padovani, C.R. (2011). Refinement and initial validation of a multidimensional composite scale for use in assessing acute postoperative pain in cats. *Am. J. Vet. Res.* 72: 174–183.

Brummett, C.M., Hong, E.K., Janda, A.M. et al. (2011). Perineural dexmedetomidine added to ropivacaine for sciatic nerve block in rats prolongs the duration of analgesia by blocking the hyperpolarization-activated cation current. *Anesthesiology* 115: 836–843.

Budsberg, S.C., Torres, B.T., Kleine, S.A. et al. (2018). Lack of effectiveness of tramadol hydrochloride for the treatment of pain and joint dysfunction in dogs with chronic osteoarthritis. *J. Am. Vet. Med. Assoc.* 252: 427–432.

Buset, S.L., Walter, C., Friedmann, A. et al. (2016). Are periodontal diseases really silent? A systematic review of their effect on quality of life. *J. Clin. Periodontol.* 43: 333–344.

Campbell, V.L., Drobatz, K.J., and Perkowski, S.Z. (2003). Postoperative hypoxemia and hypercarbia in healthy dogs undergoing routine ovariohysterectomy or castration and receiving butorphanol or hydromorphone for analgesia. *J. Am. Vet. Med. Assoc.* 222: 330–336.

Chandrasekharan, N.V., Dai, H., Roos, K.L. et al. (2002). COX-3, a cyclooxygenase-1 variant inhibited by acetaminophen and other analgesic/antipyretic drugs: cloning, structure, and expression. *Proc. Natl. Acad. Sci. U. S. A.* 99: 13926–13931.

Chiavaccini, L., Claude, A.K., and Meyer, R.E. (2017). Comparison of morphine, morphine–lidocaine, and morphine–lidocaine–ketamine infusions in dogs using an incision-induced pain model. *J. Am. Anim. Hosp. Assoc.* 53: 65–72.

Chung, G., Jung, S.J., and Oh, S.B. (2013). Cellular and molecular mechanisms of dental nociception. *J. Dent. Res.* 92: 948–955.

Corrêa, J. M. X., Soares, P. C. L., Niella, R. V. et al. (2019) Evaluation of the antinociceptive effect of maropitant, a neurokinin-1 receptor antagonist, in cats undergoing ovariohysterectomy. *Vet. Med. Int.* 2019: 9352528.

Cowan, A. (2003). Buprenorphine: new pharmacological aspects. *Int. J. Clin. Pract. Suppl.*: 3–8, disc. 23–24.

Crandell, D.E., Mathews, K.A., and Dyson, D.H. (2004). Effect of meloxicam and carprofen on renal function when administered to healthy dogs prior to anesthesia and painful stimulation. *Am. J. Vet. Res.* 65: 1384–1390.

Cray, M.T., Spector, D.I., and West, C.L. (2018). Acute masticatory muscle compartmental syndrome in a dog. *J. Am. Vet. Med. Assoc.* 253: 606–610.

De Vries, M. and Putter, G. (2015). Perioperative anaesthetic care of the cat undergoing dental and oral procedures: key considerations. *J. Feline Med. Surg.* 17: 23–36.

Dobromylskyj, P. (1993a). Assessment of methadone as an anaesthetic premedicant in cats. *J. Small Anim. Pract.* 34: 604–608.

Dobromylskyj, P. (1993b). The pharmacokinetics of methadone during the perioperative period. *J. Vet. Anaesth.* 20: 45.

Dohoo, S.E. and Dohoo, I.R. (1998). Attitudes and concerns of Canadian animal health technologists toward postoperative pain management in dogs and cats. *Can. Vet. J.* 39: 491–496.

Doodnaught, G. M., Monteiro, B. P., Benito, J., et al. (2017). Pharmacokinetic and pharmacodynamic modelling after subcutaneous, intravenous and buccal administration of a high-concentration formulation of buprenorphine in conscious cats. *PLoS One*, 12(4), e0176443.

Doodnaught, G. M., Monteiro, B. P., Edge, D. et al. (2018). Thermal antinociception after buccal administration of a high-concentration formulation of buprenorphine (Simbadol) at 0.24 mg kg-1 in conscious cats. *Vet. Anaesth. Analg.* 45: 714–716.

Dubin, A.E. and Patapoutian, A. (2010). Nociceptors: the sensors of the pain pathway. *J. Clin. Invest.* 120: 3760–3772.

Epstein, M., Rodan, I., Griffenhagen, G. et al. (2015). 2015 AAHA/AAFP pain management guidelines for dogs and cats. *J. Am. Anim. Hosp. Assoc.* 51: 67–84.

Evangelista, M.C., Watanabe, R., Leung, V.S.Y. et al. (2019). Facial expressions of pain in cats: the development and validation of a Feline Grimace Scale. *Sci. Rep.* 9: 19128.

Ferreira, M.C., Dias-Pereira, A.C., Branco-De-Almeida, L.S. et al. (2017). Impact of periodontal disease on quality of life: a systematic review. *J. Periodontal Res.* 52: 651–665.

Firth, A.M. and Haldane, S.L. (1999). Development of a scale to evaluate postoperative pain in dogs. *J. Am. Vet. Med. Assoc.* 214: 651–659.

Fitzgerald, K.T. and Bronstein, A.C. (2013). Selective serotonin reuptake inhibitor exposure. *Top. Companion Anim. Med.* 28: 13–17.

Frank, D. (2014). Recognizing behavioral signs of pain and disease: a guide for practitioners. *Vet. Clin. North Am. Small Anim. Pract.* 44: 507–524.

Frendin, J.H., Bostrom, I.M., Kampa, N. et al. (2006). Effects of carprofen on renal function during medetomidine–propofol–isoflurane anesthesia in dogs. *Am. J. Vet. Res.* 67: 1967–1973.

Gorman, A.L., Elliott, K.J., and Inturrisi, C.E. (1997). The d- and l-isomers of methadone bind to the non-competitive site on the N-methyl-D-aspartate (NMDA) receptor in rat forebrain and spinal cord. *Neurosci. Lett.* 223: 5–8.

Gowan, R.A., Lingard, A.E., Johnston, L. et al. (2011). Retrospective case-control study of the effects of long-term dosing with meloxicam on renal function in aged cats with degenerative joint disease. *J. Feline Med. Surg.* 13: 752–761.

Gowan, R.A., Baral, R.M., Lingard, A.E. et al. (2012). A retrospective analysis of the effects of meloxicam on the longevity of aged cats with and without overt chronic kidney disease. *J. Feline Med. Surg.* 14: 876–881.

Gross, M.E., Pope, E.R., O'brien, D. et al. (1997). Regional anesthesia of the infraorbital and inferior alveolar nerves during noninvasive tooth pulp stimulation in halothane-anesthetized dogs. *J. Am. Vet. Med. Assoc.* 211: 1403–1405.

Gross, M.E., Pope, E.R., Jarboe, J.M. et al. (2000). Regional anesthesia of the infraorbital and inferior alveolar nerves during noninvasive tooth pulp stimulation in halothane-anesthetized cats. *Am. J. Vet. Res.* 61: 1245–1247.

Guedes, A.G., Rude, E.P., and Rider, M.A. (2006). Evaluation of histamine release during constant rate infusion of morphine in dogs. *Vet. Anaesth. Analg.* 33: 28–35.

Guedes, A.G.P., Meadows, J.M., Pypendop, B.H., and Johnson, E.G. (2018). Evaluation of tramadol for treatment of osteoarthritis in geriatric cats. *J. Am. Vet. Med. Assoc.* 252: 565–571.

Guimaraes Alves, I.P., Montoro Nicacio, G., Diniz, M.S. et al. (2014). Analgesic comparison of systemic lidocaine, morphine or lidocaine plus morphine infusion in dogs undergoing fracture repair. *Acta Cir. Bras.* 29: 245–251.

Gutierrez-Blanco, E., Victoria-Mora, J.M., Ibancovichi-Camarillo, J.A. et al. (2013). Evaluation of the isoflurane-sparing effects of fentanyl, lidocaine, ketamine, dexmedetomidine, or the combination lidocaine–ketamine–dexmedetomidine during ovariohysterectomy in dogs. *Vet. Anaesth. Analg.* 40: 599–609.

Gutierrez-Blanco, E., Victoria-Mora, J.M., Ibancovichi-Camarillo, J.A. et al. (2015). Postoperative analgesic effects of either a constant rate infusion of fentanyl, lidocaine, ketamine, dexmedetomidine, or the combination lidocaine-ketamine-dexmedetomidine after ovariohysterectomy in dogs. *Vet. Anaesth. Analg.* 42: 309–318.

Harvey, C.E. (2005). Management of periodontal disease: understanding the options. *Vet. Clin. North Am. Small Anim. Pract.* 35 (4): 819–836, vi.

Hay Kraus, B.L. (2014). Effect of dosing interval on efficacy of maropitant for prevention of hydromorphone-induced vomiting and signs of nausea in dogs. *J. Am. Vet. Med. Assoc.* 245: 1015–1020.

Hedges, A.R., Pypendop, B.H., Shilo, Y. et al. (2014a). Impact of the blood sampling site on time-concentration drug profiles following intravenous or buccal drug administration. *J. Vet. Pharmacol. Ther.* 37: 145–150.

Hedges, A.R., Pypendop, B.H., Shilo-Benjamini, Y. et al. (2014b). Pharmacokinetics of buprenorphine following intravenous and buccal administration in cats, and effects on thermal threshold. *J. Vet. Pharmacol. Ther.* 37: 252–259.

Heyeraas, K.J., Kvinnsland, I., Byers, M.R., and Jacobsen, E.B. (1993). Nerve fibers immunoreactive to protein gene product 9.5, calcitonin gene-related peptide, substance P, and neuropeptide Y in the dental pulp, periodontal ligament, and gingiva in cats. *Acta Odontol. Scand.* 51: 207–221.

Himes, R.S., Difazio, C.A. Jr., and Burney, R.G. (1977). Effects of lidocaine on the anesthetic requirements for nitrous oxide and halothane. *Anesthesiology* 47: 437–440.

Hirvonen, T.J., Narhi, M.V., and Hakumaki, M.O. (1984). The excitability of dog pulp nerves in relation to the condition of dentine surface. *J. Endod.* 10: 294–298.

Hofmeister, E.H. and Egger, C.M. (2004). Transdermal fentanyl patches in small animals. *J. Am. Anim. Hosp. Assoc.* 40: 468–478.

Holmstrom, S.E., Bellows, J., Juriga, S. et al. (2013). 2013 AAHA dental care guidelines for dogs and cats. *J. Am. Anim. Hosp. Assoc.* 49: 75–82.

Huynh, T.M., Marret, E., and Bonnet, F. (2015). Combination of dexamethasone and local anaesthetic solution in peripheral nerve blocks: A meta-analysis of randomised controlled trials. *Eur. J. Anaesthesiol.* 32: 751–758.

IASP. (n.d.). Education. Available from https://www.iasp-pain.org/Education/ (accessed July 5, 2020).

Ikeda, H., Sunakawa, M., and Suda, H. (1995). Three groups of afferent pulpal feline nerve fibres show different electrophysiological response properties. *Arch. Oral Biol.* 40: 895–904.

Ikeda, H., Tokita, Y., and Suda, H. (1997). Capsaicin-sensitive A delta fibers in cat tooth pulp. *J. Dent. Res.* 76: 1341–1349.

Imagawa, V.H., Fantoni, D.T., Tatarunas, A.C. et al. (2011). The use of different doses of metamizol for post-operative analgesia in dogs. *Vet. Anaesth. Analg.* 38: 385–393.

Indrawirawan, Y. and Mcalees, T. (2014). Tramadol toxicity in a cat: case report and literature review of serotonin syndrome. *J. Feline Med. Surg.* 16: 572–578.

Johnson, R.A. (2014). Maropitant prevented vomiting but not gastroesophageal reflux in anesthetized dogs premedicated with acepromazine-hydromorphone. *Vet. Anaesth. Analg.* 41: 406–410.

Khanh, L.N., Ivey, S.L., Sokal-Gutierrez, K. et al. (2015). Early childhood caries, mouth pain, and nutritional threats in Vietnam. *Am. J. Public Health* 105: 2510–2517.

King, J.N., King, S., Budsberg, S.C. et al. (2016). Clinical safety of robenacoxib in feline osteoarthritis: results of a randomized, blinded, placebo-controlled clinical trial. *J. Feline Med. Surg.* 18: 632–642.

Kiyak, H.A., Beach, B.H., Worthington, P. et al. (1990). Psychological impact of osseointegrated dental implants. *Int. J. Oral Maxillofac. Implants* 5: 61–69.

Krug, W. and Losey, J. (2011). Area of desensitization following mental nerve blocks in dogs. *J. Vet. Dent.* 28: 146–150.

Kukanich, B. (2013). Outpatient oral analgesics in dogs and cats beyond nonsteroidal antiinflammatory drugs: an evidence-based approach. *Vet. Clin. North Am. Small Anim. Pract.* 43: 1109–1125.

Kukanich, B. and Papich, M.G. (2004). Pharmacokinetics of tramadol and the metabolite O-desmethyltramadol in dogs. *J. Vet. Pharmacol. Ther.* 27: 239–246.

Kukanich, B., Kukanich K., and Black, J. (2017) The effects of ketoconazole and cimetidine on the pharmacokinetics of oral tramadol in greyhound dogs. *J. Vet. Pharmcol. Ther.* 40: e54–e61.

Kukanich, B., Bidgood, T., and Knesl, O. (2012). Clinical pharmacology of nonsteroidal anti-inflammatory drugs in dogs. *Vet. Anaesth. Analg.* 39: 69–90.

Kukkar, A., Bali, A., Singh, N., and Jaggi, A.S. (2013). Implications and mechanism of action of gabapentin in neuropathic pain. *Arch. Pharm. Res.* 36: 237–251.

Langton, S.D. and Walker, J.J.A. (2017). A transorbital approach to the maxillary nerve block in dogs: a cadaver study. *Vet. Anaesth. Analg.* 44: 173–177.

Lascelles, B.D. and Robertson, S.A. (2004). Antinociceptive effects of hydromorphone, butorphanol, or the combination in cats. *J. Vet. Intern. Med.* 18: 190–195.

Lascelles, B.D., Cripps, P.J., Jones, A., and Waterman, A.E. (1997). Post-operative central hypersensitivity and pain: the pre-emptive value of pethidine for ovariohysterectomy. *Pain* 73: 461–471.

Lascelles, B.D., Cripps, P.J., Jones, A., and Waterman-Pearson, A.E. (1998). Efficacy and kinetics of carprofen, administered preoperatively or postoperatively, for the prevention of pain in dogs undergoing ovariohysterectomy. *Vet. Surg.* 27: 568–582.

Lascelles, B.D., Gaynor, J.S., Smith, E.S. et al. (2008). Amantadine in a multimodal analgesic regimen for alleviation of refractory osteoarthritis pain in dogs. *J. Vet. Intern. Med.* 22: 53–59.

Le Fur-Bonnabesse, A., Bodere, C., Helou, C. et al. (2017). Dental pain induced by an ambient thermal differential: pathophysiological hypothesis. *J. Pain Res.* 10: 2845–2851.

Lebkowska-Wieruszewska, B., Kim, T.W., Chea, B. et al. (2018). Pharmacokinetic profiles of the two major active metabolites of metamizole (dipyrone) in cats following three different routes of administration. *J. Vet. Pharmacol. Ther.* 41: 334–339.

Li, X.D., Han, C., and Yu, W.L. (2017). Is gabapentin effective and safe in open hysterectomy? A PRISMA compliant meta-analysis of randomized controlled trials. *J. Clin. Anesth.* 41: 76–83.

Lomas, A.L. and Grauer, G.F. (2015). The renal effects of NSAIDs in dogs. *J. Am. Anim. Hosp. Assoc.* 51: 197–203.

Lommer, M.J. (2013). Oral inflammation in small animals. *Vet. Clin. North Am. Small Anim. Pract.* 43: 555–571.

Lorenzutti, A.M., Martin-Flores, M., Litterio, N.J. et al. (2017). A comparison between maropitant and metoclopramide for the prevention of morphine-induced nausea and vomiting in dogs. *Can. Vet. J.* 58: 35–38.

Lotti, F., Boscan, P., Twedt, D. et al. (2018). Effect of oral maropitant and omeprazole on emesis, appetite and anesthesia recovery quality in dogs. *Vet. Anaesth. Analg.* 45: 885.e9.

Loughran, C.M., Raisis, A.L., Haitjema, G., and Chester, Z. (2016). Unilateral retrobulbar hematoma following maxillary nerve block in a dog. *J. Vet. Emerg. Crit. Care* 26: 815–818.

Lucas, A.N., Firth, A.M., Anderson, G.A. et al. (2001). Comparison of the effects of morphine administered by constant-rate intravenous infusion or intermittent intramuscular injection in dogs. *J. Am. Vet. Med. Assoc.* 218: 884–891.

Luna, S.P., Basilio, A.C., Steagall, P.V. et al. (2007). Evaluation of adverse effects of long-term oral administration of carprofen, etodolac, flunixin meglumine, ketoprofen, and meloxicam in dogs. *Am. J. Vet. Res.* 68: 258–264.

Lund, E.M., Armstrong, P.J., Kirk, C.A. et al. (1999). Health status and population characteristics of dogs and cats examined at private veterinary practices in the United States. *J. Am. Vet. Med. Assoc.* 214: 1336–1341.

Macdougall, L.M., Hethey, J.A., Livingston, A. et al. (2009). Antinociceptive, cardiopulmonary, and sedative effects of five intravenous infusion rates of lidocaine in conscious dogs. *Vet. Anaesth. Analg.* 36: 512–522.

Madden, M., Gurney, M., and Bright, S. (2014). Amantadine, an N-methyl-D-aspartate antagonist, for treatment of chronic neuropathic pain in a dog. *Vet. Anaesth. Analg.* 41: 440–441.

Magloire, H., Maurin, J.C., Couble, M.L. et al. (2010). Topical review. Dental pain and odontoblasts: facts and hypotheses. *J. Orofac. Pain* 24: 335–349.

Martin-Flores, M., Sakai, D.M., Mastrocco, A. et al. (2016). Evaluation of oral maropitant as an antiemetic in cats receiving morphine and dexmedetomidine. *J. Feline Med. Surg.* 18: 921–924.

Martin-Flores, M., Mastrocco, A., Lorenzutti, A.M. et al. (2017). Maropitant administered orally 2–2.5 h prior to morphine and dexmedetomidine reduces the incidence of emesis in cats. *J. Feline Med. Surg.* 19: 876–879.

Marty, P., Rontes, O., Chassery, C. et al. (2018). Perineural versus systemic dexamethasone in front-foot surgery under ankle block: a randomized double-blind study. *Reg. Anesth. Pain Med.* 43: 732–737.

Mathews, K.A., Paley, D.M., Foster, R.A. et al. (1996). A comparison of ketorolac with flunixin, butorphanol, and oxymorphone in controlling postoperative pain in dogs. *Can. Vet. J.* 37: 557–567.

Mathews, K., Kronen, P.W., Lascelles, D. et al. (2014). Guidelines for recognition, assessment and treatment of pain: WSAVA Global Pain Council members and co-authors of this document. *J. Small Anim. Pract.* 55: E10–E68.

Mathiesen, O., Moiniche, S., and Dahl, J.B. (2007). Gabapentin and postoperative pain: a qualitative and quantitative systematic review, with focus on procedure. *BMC Anesthesiol.* 7: 6.

Matthews, B. and Vongsavan, N. (1994). Interactions between neural and hydrodynamic mechanisms in dentine and pulp. *Arch. Oral Biol.* 39 (Suppl): 87S–95S.

Meintjes, R.A. (2012). An overview of the physiology of pain for the veterinarian. *Vet. J.* 193: 344–348.

Mengel, M.K., Stiefenhofer, A.E., Jyvasjarvi, E., and Kniffki, K.D. (1993). Pain sensation during cold stimulation of the teeth: differential reflection of A delta and C fibre activity? *Pain* 55: 159–169.

Modi, M., Rastogi, S., and Kumar, A. (2009). Buprenorphine with bupivacaine for intraoral nerve blocks to provide postoperative analgesia in outpatients after minor oral surgery. *J. Oral Maxillofac. Surg.* 67: 2571–2576.

Molony, V. (1997). Comments on Anand and Craig, PAIN, 67 (1996) 3–6. *Pain* 70: 293.

Molony, V. and Kent, J.E. (1997). Assessment of acute pain in farm animals using behavioral and physiological measurements. *J. Anim. Sci.* 75: 266–272.

Monteiro-Steagall, B.P., Steagall, P.V., and Lascelles, B.D. (2013). Systematic review of nonsteroidal anti-inflammatory drug-induced adverse effects in dogs. *J. Vet. Intern. Med.* 27: 1011–1019.

Muir, W.W., 3rd Wiese, A.J., and March, P.A. (2003). Effects of morphine, lidocaine, ketamine, and morphine–lidocaine–ketamine drug combination on minimum alveolar concentration in dogs anesthetized with isoflurane. *Am. J. Vet. Res.* 64: 1155–1160.

Narhi, M.V. and Hirvonen, T. (1987). The response of dog intradental nerves to hypertonic solutions of $CaCl_2$ and NaCl, and other stimuli, applied to exposed dentine. *Arch. Oral Biol.* 32: 781–786.

Narhi, M.V., Hirvonen, T.J., and Hakumaki, M.O. (1982). Activation of intradental nerves in the dog to some stimuli applied to the dentine. *Arch. Oral Biol.* 27: 1053–1058.

Narishetty, S.T., Galvan, B., Coscarelli, E. et al. (2009). Effect of refrigeration of the antiemetic Cerenia (maropitant) on pain on injection. *Vet. Ther.* 10: 93–102.

Ngassapa, D., Narhi, M., and Hirvonen, T. (1992). Effect of serotonin (5-HT) and calcitonin gene-related peptide (CGRP) on the function of intradental nerves in the dog. *Proc. Finn. Dent. Soc.* 88 (Suppl. 1): 143–148.

Niedfeldt, R.L. and Robertson, S.A. (2006). Postanesthetic hyperthermia in cats: a retrospective comparison between hydromorphone and buprenorphine. *Vet. Anaesth. Analg.* 33: 381–389.

Niemiec, B.A. (2008). Periodontal disease. *Top. Companion Anim. Med.* 23: 72–80.

Niemiec, B., Gawor, J., Nemec, A., Clarke, D., et al. (2020). World Small Animal Veterinary Association Global Dental Guidelines. *J. Small Anim. Pract.* 61: E36–161.

Nunes De Moraes, A., Dyson, D.H., O'Grady, M.R. et al. (1998). Plasma concentrations and cardiovascular influence of lidocaine infusions during isoflurane anesthesia in healthy dogs and dogs with subaortic stenosis. *Vet. Surg.* 27: 486 497.

Obayah, G.M., Refaie, A., Aboushanab, O. et al. (2010). Addition of dexmedetomidine to bupivacaine for greater palatine nerve block prolongs postoperative analgesia after cleft palate repair. *Eur. J. Anaesthesiol.* 27: 280–284.

Pascoe, P.J. (2016). The effects of lidocaine or a lidocaine-bupivacaine mixture administered into the infraorbital canal in dogs. *Am. J. Vet. Res.* 77: 682–687.

Pascoe, P. J. & Chohan, A. S. (2017). The effect of different volumes of injectate on the infraorbital block using lidocaine/bupivacaine in dogs. AVA Meeting, Prague.

Pascoe, P.J., Ilkiw, J.E., Craig, C., and Kollias-Baker, C. (2007). The effects of ketamine on the minimum alveolar concentration of isoflurane in cats. *Vet. Anaesth. Analg.* 34: 31–39.

Pearl, G.S., Anderson, K.V., and Rosing, H.S. (1977). Anatomic evidence revealing extensive transmedian innervation of feline canine teeth. *Exp. Neurol.* 54: 432–443.

Perez Jimenez, T.E., Mealey, K.L., Grubb, T.L. et al. (2016). Tramadol metabolism to O-desmethyl tramadol (M1) and N-desmethyl tramadol (M2) by dog liver microsomes: species comparison and identification of responsible canine cytochrome P-450s (CYPs). *Drug Metab. Dispos.* 44: 1963–1972.

Perry, R. and Tutt, C. (2015). Periodontal disease in cats: back to basics – with an eye on the future. *J. Feline Med. Surg.* 17: 45–65.

Perry, R., Moore, D., and Scurrell, E. (2015). Globe penetration in a cat following maxillary nerve block for dental surgery. *J. Feline Med. Surg.* 17: 66–72.

Pibarot, P., Dupuis, J., Grisneaux, E. et al. (1997). Comparison of ketoprofen, oxymorphone hydrochloride, and butorphanol in the treatment of postoperative pain in dogs. *J. Am. Vet. Med. Assoc.* 211: 438–444.

Popilskis, S., Kohn, D.F., Laurent, L., and Danilo, P. (1993). Efficacy of epidural morphine versus intravenous morphine for post-thoracotomy pain in dogs. *J. Vet. Anaesth.* 20: 21–25.

Posner, L.P., Gleed, R.D., Erb, H.N., and Ludders, J.W. (2007). Post-anesthetic hyperthermia in cats. *Vet. Anaesth. Analg.* 34: 40–47.

Pozzi, A., Muir, W.W., and Traverso, F. (2006). Prevention of central sensitization and pain by N-methyl-D-aspartate receptor antagonists. *J. Am. Vet. Med. Assoc.* 228: 53–60.

Pypendop, B.H. and Ilkiw, J.E. (2005a). Assessment of the hemodynamic effects of lidocaine administered IV in isoflurane-anesthetized cats. *Am. J. Vet. Res.* 66: 661–668.

Pypendop, B.H. and Ilkiw, J.E. (2005b). The effects of intravenous lidocaine administration on the minimum alveolar concentration of isoflurane in cats. *Anesth. Analg.* 100: 97–101.

Pypendop, B.H. and Ilkiw, J.E. (2008). Pharmacokinetics of tramadol, and its metabolite O-desmethyl-tramadol, in cats. *J. Vet. Pharmacol. Ther.* 31: 52–59.

Pypendop, B.H., Ilkiw, J.E., and Robertson, S.A. (2006). Effects of intravenous administration of lidocaine on the thermal threshold in cats. *Am. J. Vet. Res.* 67: 16–20.

Pypendop, B.H., Siao, K.T., and Ilkiw, J.E. (2009). Effects of tramadol hydrochloride on the thermal threshold in cats. *Am. J. Vet. Res.* 70: 1465–1470.

Pypendop, B.H., Ilkiw, J.E., and Shilo-Benjamini, Y. (2014). Bioavailability of morphine, methadone, hydromorphone, and oxymorphone following buccal administration in cats. *J. Vet. Pharmacol. Ther.* 37: 295–300.

Ramsey, D., Fleck, T., Berg, T. et al. (2014). Cerenia prevents perioperative nausea and vomiting and improves recovery in dogs undergoing routine surgery. *Int. J. Appl. Res. Vet. Med.* 12: 228–237.

Rausch-Derra, L.C. and Rhodes, L. (2016). Safety and toxicokinetic profiles associated with daily oral administration of grapiprant, a selective antagonist of the prostaglandin E2 EP4 receptor, to cats. *Am. J. Vet. Res.* 77: 688–692.

Rausch-Derra, L.C., Huebner, M., and Rhodes, L. (2015). Evaluation of the safety of long-term, daily oral administration of grapiprant, a novel drug for treatment of osteoarthritic pain and inflammation, in healthy dogs. *Am. J. Vet. Res.* 76: 853–859.

Rausch-Derra, L., Huebner, M., Wofford, J., and Rhodes, L. (2016a). A prospective, randomized, masked, placebo-controlled multisite clinical study of Grapiprant, an EP4 prostaglandin receptor antagonist (PRA), in dogs with osteoarthritis. *J. Vet. Intern. Med.* 30: 756–763.

Rausch-Derra, L.C., Rhodes, L., Freshwater, L., and Hawks, R. (2016b). Pharmacokinetic comparison of oral tablet and suspension formulations of grapiprant, a novel therapeutic for the pain and inflammation of osteoarthritis in dogs. *J. Vet. Pharmacol. Ther.* 39: 566–571.

Reddi, D. and Curran, N. (2014). Chronic pain after surgery: pathophysiology, risk factors and prevention. *Postgrad. Med. J.* 90: 222–227, quiz 226.

Reid, J., Nolan, A.M., Hughes, J.M.L. et al. (2007). Development of the short-form of the Glasgow composite measure pain scale (CMPS-SF) and derivation of an analgesic intervention score. *Anim. Welf.* 16 (S): 97–104.

Reid, J., Scott, E.M., Calvo, G., and Nolan, A.M. (2017). Definitive Glasgow acute pain scale for cats: validation and intervention level. *Vet. Rec.* 180: 449.

Reid, J., Nolan, A.M., and Scott, E.M. (2018). Measuring pain in dogs and cats using structured behavioural observation. *Vet. J.* 236: 72–79.

Renck, H. and Hassan, H.G. (1992). Epinephrine as an adjuvant to amino-amide local anesthetics does not prolong their duration of action in infraorbital nerve block in the rat. *Acta Anaesthesiol. Scand.* 36: 387–392.

Robertson, S.A., Hauptman, J.G., Nachreiner, R.F., and Richter, M.A. (2001). Effects of acetylpromazine or morphine on urine production in halothane-anesthetized dogs. *Am. J. Vet. Res.* 62: 1922–1927.

Robinson, E.P., Faggella, A.M., Henry, D.P., and Russell, W.L. (1988). Comparison of histamine release induced by morphine and oxymorphone administration in dogs. *Am. J. Vet. Res.* 49: 1699–1701.

Rolim, V.M., Pavarini, S.P., Campos, F.S. et al. (2017). Clinical, pathological, immunohistochemical and molecular characterization of feline chronic gingivostomatitis. *J. Feline Med. Surg.* 19: 403–409.

Rusbridge, C., Heath, S., Gunn-Moore, D.A. et al. (2010). Feline orofacial pain syndrome (FOPS): a retrospective study of 113 cases. *J. Feline Med. Surg.* 12: 498–508.

Sacerdote, P. and Levrini, L. (2012). Peripheral mechanisms of dental pain: the role of substance P. *Mediat. Inflamm.* 2012: 951920.

Sarrau, S., Jourdan, J., Dupuis-Soyris, F., and Verwaerde, P. (2007). Effects of postoperative ketamine infusion on pain control and feeding behaviour in bitches undergoing mastectomy. *J. Small Anim. Pract.* 48: 670–676.

Sawyer, D.C. and Rech, R.H. (1987). Analgesia and behavioral effects of butorphanol, nalbuphine, and pentazocine in the cat. *J. Am. Anim. Hosp. Assoc.* 23: 438–446.

Sawyer, D.C., Anderson, D.L., and Scott, J.B. (1982). Cardiovascular effects and clinical use of nalbuphine in the dog. *Proc. Assoc. Vet. Anaesth. G. B. Irel.* 10: 215–216.

Schutter, A.F., Tunsmeyer, J., and Kastner, S.B.R. (2017). Influence of tramadol on acute thermal and mechanical cutaneous nociception in dogs. *Vet. Anaesth. Analg.* 44: 309–316.

Sheiham, A. (2006). Dental caries affects body weight, growth and quality of life in pre-school children. *Br. Dent. J.* 201: 625–626.

Siao, K.T., Pypendop, B.H., and Ilkiw, J.E. (2010). Pharmacokinetics of gabapentin in cats. *Am. J. Vet. Res.* 71: 817–821.

Simon, B.T., Scallan, E.M., Carroll, G., and Steagall, P.V. (2017). The lack of analgesic use (oligoanalgesia) in small animal practice. *J. Small Anim. Pract.* 58: 543–554.

Slingsby, L. and Watermanpearson, A. (1998). Comparison of pethidine, buprenorphine and ketoprofen for postoperative analgesia after ovariohysterectomy in the cat. *Vet. Rec.* 143: 185–189.

Slingsby, L.S. and Waterman-Pearson, A.E. (2000). The post-operative analgesic effects of ketamine after canine ovariohysterectomy – a comparison between pre- or post-operative administration. *Res. Vet. Sci.* 69: 147–152.

Smith, L.J., Yu, J.K., Bjorling, D.E., and Waller, K. (2001). Effects of hydromorphone or oxymorphone, with or without acepromazine, on preanesthetic sedation, physiologic values, and histamine release in dogs. *J. Am. Vet. Med. Assoc.* 218: 1101–1105.

Smith, L.J., Bentley, E., Shih, A., and Miller, P.E. (2004). Systemic lidocaine infusion as an analgesic for intraocular surgery in dogs: a pilot study. *Vet. Anaesth. Analg.* 31: 53–63.

Snyder, C.J. and Snyder, L.B. (2013). Effect of mepivacaine in an infraorbital nerve block on minimum alveolar concentration of isoflurane in clinically normal anesthetized dogs undergoing a modified form of dental dolorimetry. *J. Am. Vet. Med. Assoc.* 242: 199–204.

Snyder, L.B., Snyder, C.J., and Hetzel, S. (2016). Effects of buprenorphine added to bupivacaine infraorbital nerve blocks on isoflurane minimum alveolar concentration using a model for acute dental/Oral surgical pain in dogs. *J. Vet. Dent.* 33: 90–96.

Sparkes, A.H., Heiene, R., Lascelles, B.D. et al. (2010). ISFM and AAFP consensus guidelines: long-term use of NSAIDs in cats. *J. Feline Med. Surg.* 12: 521–538.

Stathopoulou, T.R., Kouki, M., Pypendop, B.H. et al. (2017). Evaluation of analgesic effect and absorption of buprenorphine after buccal administration in cats with oral disease. *J. Feline Med. Surg* 20 (8): 704–710.

Steagall, P.V. and Monteiro, B.P. (2018). Acute pain in cats: recent advances in clinical assessment. *J. Feline Med. Surg.* 21 (1): 25–34.

Steagall, P.V., Teixeira Neto, F.J., Minto, B.W. et al. (2006a). Evaluation of the isoflurane-sparing effects of lidocaine and fentanyl during surgery in dogs. *J. Am. Vet. Med. Assoc.* 229: 522–527.

Steagall, P.V.M., Carnicelli, P., Taylor, P.M. et al. (2006b). Effects of subcutaneous methadone, morphine, buprenorphine or saline on thermal and pressure thresholds in cats. *J. Vet. Pharmacol. Ther.* 29: 531–537.

Steagall, P.V., Taylor, P.M., Brondani, J.T. et al. (2008). Antinociceptive effects of tramadol and acepromazine in cats. *J. Feline Med. Surg.* 10: 24–31.

Steagall, P.V., Monteiro-Steagall, B.P., and Taylor, P.M. (2014). A review of the studies using buprenorphine in cats. *J. Vet. Intern. Med.* 28: 762–770.

Steagall, P.V., Benito, J., Monteiro, B.P. et al. (2017). Analgesic effects of gabapentin and buprenorphine in cats undergoing ovariohysterectomy using two pain-scoring systems: a randomized clinical trial. *J. Feline Med. Surg.* 20 (8): 741–748.

Surdyk, K.K., Brown, C.A., and Brown, S.A. (2013). Evaluation of glomerular filtration rate in cats with reduced renal mass and administered meloxicam and acetylsalicylic acid. *Am. J. Vet. Res.* 74: 648–651.

Taylor, P.M. and Houlton, J.E.F. (1984). Post-operative analgesia in the dog: a comparison of morphine, buprenorphine and pentazocine. *J. Small Anim. Pract.* 25: 437–451.

Taylor, P.M., Robertson, S.A., Dixon, M.J. et al. (2001). Morphine, pethidine and buprenorphine disposition in the cat. *J. Vet. Pharmacol. Ther.* 24: 391–398.

Taylor, P.M., Luangdilok, C.H., and Sear, J.W. (2015). Pharmacokinetic and pharmacodynamic evaluation of high doses of buprenorphine delivered via high-concentration formulations in cats. *J. Feline Med. Surg.* 18: 290–302.

Turner, J.D., Dobson, S.W., Henshaw, D.S. et al. (2018). Single-injection adductor cCanal block with multiple adjuvants provides equivalent analgesia when compared with continuous adductor canal blockade for primary total knee arthroplasty: a double-blinded, randomized, controlled, equivalency trial. *J. Arthroplast.* 33: 3160–3166.e1.

Veng-Pedersen, P., Wilhelm, J.A., Zakszewski, T.B. et al. (1995). Duration of opioid antagonism by nalmefene and naloxone in the dog: an integrated pharmacokinetic/pharmacodynamic comparison. *J. Pharm. Sci.* 84: 1101–1106.

Viscasillas, J., Seymour, C.J., and Brodbelt, D.C. (2013). A cadaver study comparing two approaches for performing maxillary nerve block in dogs. *Vet. Anaesth. Analg.* 40: 212–219.

Vongsavan, N. and Matthews, B. (1992). Changes in pulpal blood flow and in fluid flow through dentine produced by autonomic and sensory nerve stimulation in the cat. *Proc. Finn. Dent. Soc.* 88 (Suppl. 1): 491–497.

Wagner, A.E., Walton, J.A., Hellyer, P.W. et al. (2002). Use of low doses of ketamine administered by constant rate infusion as an adjunct for postoperative analgesia in dogs. *J. Am. Vet. Med. Assoc.* 221: 72–75.

Warne, L.N., Beths, T., Holm, M., and Bauquier, S.H. (2013). Comparison of perioperative analgesic efficacy between methadone and butorphanol in cats. *J. Am. Vet. Med. Assoc.* 243: 844–850.

Warne, L.N., Beths, T., Holm, M. et al. (2014). Evaluation of the perioperative analgesic efficacy of buprenorphine, compared with butorphanol, in cats. *J. Am. Vet. Med. Assoc.* 245: 195–202.

Watanabe, R., Doodnaught, G., Proulx, C., et al. 2019. A multidisciplinary study of pain in cats undergoing dental extractions: a prospective, blinded, clinical trial. *PLoS One*, 14(3), e0213195.

Watanabe, R., Frank, D., and Steagall, P.V. (2020a). Pain behaviors before and after treatment of oral disease in cats using video assessment: a prospective, blinded, randomized clinical trial. *BMC Vet. Res.* 16 (1) 100.

Watanabe R, Doodnaught GM, Evangelista MC, Monteiro BP, Ruel HLM and Steagall PV (2020b). Inter-Rater Reliability of the Feline Grimace Scale in Cats Undergoing Dental Extractions. Front. Vet. Sci. 7:302.

Watanabe, R., Marcoux, J., Evangelista, M.C., et al. (2020c). The analgesic effects of buprenorphine (Vetergesic or Simbadol) in cats undergoing dental extractions: A randomized, blinded, clinical trial. *PLoS. One.* 15: e0230079.

Waterman, A.E. and Kalthum, W. (1992). Use of opioids in providing postoperative analgesia in the dog: A double-blind trial of pethidine, pentazocine, buprenorphine, and butorphanol. In: *Animal Pain*, 1e (eds. C.E. Short and A. Van Poznack), 466–476. New York: Churchill Livingstone.

Wilhelm, J.A., Veng-Pedersen, P., Zakszewski, T.B. et al. (1995). Duration of opioid antagonism by nalmefene and naloxone in the dog. A nonparametric pharmacodynamic comparison based on generalized cross-validated spline estimation. *Int. J. Clin. Pharmacol. Ther.* 33: 540–545.

Winer, J.N., Arzi, B., and Verstraete, F.J. (2016). Therapeutic Management of Feline Chronic Gingivostomatitis: A systematic review of the literature. *Front. Vet. Sci.* 3: 54.

Woodward, T.M. (2008). Pain management and regional anesthesia for the dental patient. *Top. Companion Anim. Med.* 23: 106–114.

Wu, W.N., Mckown, L.A., Gauthier, A.D. et al. (2001). Metabolism of the analgesic drug, tramadol hydrochloride, in rat and dog. *Xenobiotica* 31: 423–441.

Yang, S.E., Park, Y.G., Han, K. et al. (2016). Dental pain related to quality of life and mental health in south Korean adults. *Psychol. Health Med.* 21: 981–992.

12

Anesthesia of the Dental Patient
Victoria M. Lukasik

Southwest Veterinary Anesthesiology, Tucson, AZ, USA
University of Arizona College of Veterinary Medicine, Oro Valley, AZ, USA

12.1 Introduction

Patients must be comfortable and relaxed in order to provide comprehensive dental therapy (Figures 12.1 and 12.2). Though they may be sedated deeply enough to tolerate local anesthetic blocks and dental procedures, sedation leaves the airway and lungs unguarded. An unguarded airway predisposes to aspiration pneumonia, both from regurgitation and from the water and debris associated with the procedure. Placement of an endotracheal tube is the safest way to protect the lungs. With a tube in place, inhalant anesthesia becomes the best option for anesthetic maintenance in nearly every patient. Inhalant anesthesia has the advantage over heavy sedation because depth can be more precisely controlled. Further, post-anesthetic return of protective airway reflexes is usually rapid because inhalant drugs do not depend upon redistribution and hepatic metabolism – patients simply breathe to awaken.

The depth of anesthesia should be as light as possible while still providing unconsciousness, relaxation, analgesia, and amnesia. Physiology becomes less acceptable as anesthetic depth increases. Patient reserves are more heavily taxed and decompensation is more likely, especially in patients with pre-existing fragile physiology. Perioperative morbidity and mortality increase as depth of anesthesia increases (Petsiti et al. 2015). It is important to recognize that the duration of anesthesia also has a significant impact on morbidity and mortality (Johnston et al. 2002; Bidwell et al. 2007; Brodbelt et al. 2008). Though there are no strict guidelines as to the limit of anesthesia time, there is evidence that less than two hours is associated with significantly lower morbidity and mortality (Tevik 1983; Young and Taylor 1993). This supports breaking up procedures anticipated to take several hours into shorter anesthetic and surgical episodes. Staging is especially important in patients already compromised by fragile physiology and in geriatric patients.

12.2 Anesthesia Record Keeping

Each patient should have an anesthetic record that documents patient information, baseline physiologic and laboratory values, drug doses, administration routes, physiologic data during anesthesia, any anesthetic interventions, postoperative analgesia, recovery time, and recovery quality. There are many example forms and styles available in the public domain, but the use of a symbolic graphical trend record with physiologic data recorded every five minutes significantly reduces the number of major anesthetic interventions (Gurushanthaiah et al. 1995; Blike et al. 1999; Drews and Westenskow 2006). The graphical format allows physiologic trends to be identified significantly sooner compared to numeric tabular style records; this enables minor anesthetic adjustments to be instituted before major interventions become necessary.

12.3 Patient History and Physical Examination

Anesthetic planning begins with a thorough patient history and physical exam, which should include all body systems. Patients presented for dental therapy often have concurrent conditions that impact anesthetic planning and patient support. It is important to recognize and stabilize as many concurrent disease processes as possible prior to anesthesia. Chronic body pain, dehydration, muscle atrophy, and anorexia are all considerations for anesthetic

The Veterinary Dental Patient: A Multidisciplinary Approach, First Edition. Edited by Jerzy Gawor and Brook Niemiec.
© 2021 John Wiley & Sons Ltd. Published 2021 by John Wiley & Sons Ltd.
Companion website: www.wiley.com/go/gawor/veterinary-dental-patient

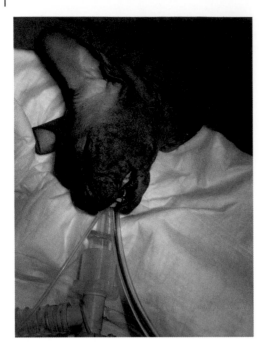

Figure 12.1 Patients prepared for dental procedures should be comfortable and relaxed when put under general anesthesia.

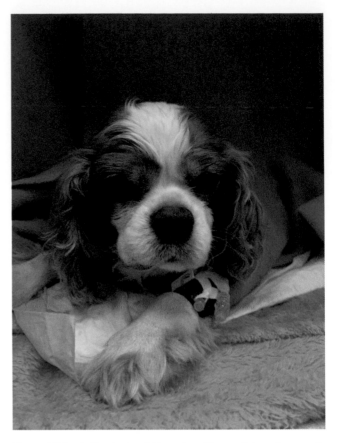

Figure 12.2 Patients should be calmed in a quiet environment, if possible when undergoing sedation.

planning. These conditions can impact patient management as much as diabetes mellitus, Cushing's disease, hyperthyroidism, and cardiac disease. All of these things impact drug and dose choices, fluid administration rates, and patient supportive measures. The physical examination also provides important baseline values for heart rate, respiratory rate, temperature, and blood pressure. Additional diagnostics (e.g., radiograph, echocardiogram [ECG]) may be dictated by patient history and physical examination. The only contraindication for general anesthesia is uncompensated cardiac failure. All other patients can be anesthetized successfully with appropriate planning, drug dosing, intraoperative support, and vigilant monitoring by an experienced practitioner.

12.4   Basic Laboratory Testing

Pre-anesthetic laboratory testing should include a complete blood count (CBC) with platelet count, serum chemistry, and urinalysis. Though the case for laboratory screening for all patients before general anesthesia is still debated, screening is highly recommended for patients that have concurrent disease (Alef et al. 2008; Bednarski et al. 2011). Occasionally, laboratory screening will reveal a clinically important unexpected abnormality, which indicates further work-up is necessary prior to anesthesia (Hargrove and Hofmeister 2015). Dental therapy should

then be postponed until advanced laboratory diagnostics are ordered and the cause of the abnormality is determined.

12.5   Anesthetic Management

12.5.1   Premedication

Once a patient has been fully evaluated, anesthetic planning can begin. There are many pre-anesthetic drugs and doses to choose from, with no single anesthetic protocol that will meet the needs of every patient. Balanced drug protocols include drugs from several different classes, each chosen for a specific purpose. This enables each drug to be administered at low to moderate doses, reducing unwanted side effects. Anesthesia induction, maintenance, and recovery are more likely to be smooth, quiet, and comfortable with balanced protocols. Patient factors influencing drug doses and choices include the physical status of the patient, body surface area, body fat, age, size, and temperament. Procedural considerations include anticipated procedure, analgesic requirements, possible complications, postoperative needs, expected duration of anesthesia, invasiveness, and dentist/anesthetist experience.

The goals of premedication include reducing anxiety and providing mild sedation. Other benefits are increased muscle relaxation, decreased drug side effects, suppression of vomiting and regurgitation, decreased doses of induction and maintenance drugs, and smoothing of induction and recovery. If a surgical procedure is anticipated, premedication should also include a preventive analgesic plan; this not only reduces short-term surgical pain, but also helps control long-term pain and any central sensitization that may develop during surgery (Vadivelu et al. 2014). Drugs combined in preventive analgesic protocols may be administered at any time in the perioperative period.

Administering pre-anesthetic combination injections intramuscularly into the semimembranosus muscles provides the most predictable onset and highest quality of sedation. In a study evaluating intramuscular injection sites, the semimembranosus site had a significantly higher sedation score compared to all others (Carter et al. 2013). Secondarily, the cervical injection site had a significantly higher sedation score compared to the lumbar and gluteal sites. The semimembranosus and cervical sites had significantly shorter sedation onset times compared to the gluteal and lumbar sites. Based on this evidence, it is recommended that premedication injections be administered intramuscularly into the semimembranosus muscles approximately 10–15 minutes prior to desired peak effects.

12.5.2 Selection of Drugs for Premedication

12.5.2.1 Suppression of Vomiting
Maropitant (Cerenia) is a neurokinin-1 (NK-1) receptor antagonist that blocks the pharmacologic action of substance P in the central nervous system. It has been shown to decrease vomiting precipitated by morphine and hydromorphone when administered subcutaneously 45 minutes prior to premedication (Hay Kraus 2013; Lorenzutti et al. 2016). There is also evidence that dogs receiving maropitant as part of their pre-anesthetic protocol resume normal eating behavior 16 hours sooner than those that do not receive it (Ramsey et al. 2014). Maropitant has thus become a routine addition to pre-anesthetic protocols.

12.5.2.2 Anticholergics
The routine addition of an anticholinergic to pre-anesthetic drug combinations has fallen out of favor. It is recommended that each patient be evaluated individually and anticholinergic addition be based upon individual patient needs. Administration in combination with an alpha-2 agonist is contraindicated (Alvaides et al. 2008). The myocardial hypoxemia precipitated by alpha-2 agonists predisposes the myocardium to greater hypoxemia, arrhythmia, and failure when faced with the extra burden of tachycardia.

The anticholinergics atropine and glycopyrrolate are used to treat pre-existing vagally induced bradyarrhythmia. They may also be used to prevent bradycardia precipitated by other drugs and to decrease salivary secretions. Anticholinergics should be avoided in patients with tachyarrhythmias. Anticholinergics decrease tear formation and dry the eye very shortly after administration (Doering et al. 2016). Decreased tear formation may last as long as 24 hours. It is recommended that artificial tears be applied to the eye at the time of anticholinergic administration and intermittently for 24 hours afterward. Atropine is a small molecule that crosses the blood–brain and placental barriers. Overdose may cause seizure. Glycopyrrolate is a large molecule that cannot cross the blood–brain barrier or placenta. It is less arrhythmogenic compared to atropine, and overdose will not cause seizure.

12.5.2.3 Mild to Moderate Tranquilizers
The benzodiazepines midazolam and diazepam are mild to moderate tranquilizers and are appropriate choices in compromised or geriatric patients. They have very little effect on cardiovascular function. Both drugs are reversible with flumazenil (Romazicon). Diazepam is supplied in a propylene glycol base and is not water-soluble. The propylene glycol base can make uptake from intramuscular or subcutaneous injection slow and unpredictable. Diazepam should be administered slowly intravenously because the propylene glycol carrier solution may cause hemolysis, thrombophlebitis, and cardiotoxicity. It is recommended that diazepam not be physically mixed with any other drugs or substances due to the risk of precipitate formation. Diazepam adsorbs to plastic within a few minutes of contact and should be drawn into plastic syringes immediately prior to administration. Midazolam is water-soluble and can be administered intramuscularly or subcutaneously with rapid and complete uptake. Midazolam does not adsorb to plastic and can be physically mixed with many other drugs and substances.

12.5.2.4 Sedative Analgesics
The addition of an opioid analgesic to premedication protocols will enhance sedation, allow a decrease in induction and maintenance drugs, and contribute to (but not replace) postoperative analgesia. Opioids commonly used in pre-anesthetic drug combinations include hydromorphone, oxymorphone, morphine, methadone, butorphanol, and buprenorphine. Fentanyl is more appropriately used at anesthesia induction due to its short duration of effect.

Hydromorphone, oxymorphone, methadone, fentanyl, and morphine are μ-receptor agonists and are good choices for patients that are expected to experience moderate to severe pain or that have chronic pain. All five drugs will provide excellent analgesia and have fair to good sedative properties. Full μ-agonist opioids may precipitate panting or pharmacologic (drug-induced) fever. Hydromorphone and oxymorphone have a slightly longer duration of effect compared to morphine. Morphine causes histamine release if given intravenously; therefore, intramuscular or very slow intravenous administration is preferred. Methadone also modulates the N-methyl D-aspartate (NMDA) receptor in addition to the μ-opioid receptor and may have an advantage in certain patients because of this (Doi et al. 2016). Depending upon the dose administered, full μ-opioid agonists can reduce the minimum anesthetic concentration (MAC) by up to 80%.

Butorphanol is classified as an agonist/antagonist, meaning that it will partially reverse some μ-opioid effects. It may reverse some of the analgesia provided by μ-opioid agonists, for example (Lascelles and Robertson 2004). Butorphanol has been shown to decrease isoflurane and sevoflurane MAC by 15–19% in both dogs and cats (Ko et al. 2000; Ilkiw et al. 2002; Yamashita et al. 2008). An opioid agonist/antagonist is more appropriately used in patients expected to experience mild pain.

Buprenorphine, a partial μ-agonist, has a dose-dependent analgesic duration and will provide mild analgesia. The onset of action is relatively slow, even with intravenous administration. It should be administered either intramuscularly or intravenously 30 minutes prior to the desired time of effect. It is not recommended to administer buprenorphine subcutaneously unless it is in a concentrated solution like Simbadol (Zoetis, Florham Park, NJ). At a dose of 0.05 mg/kg IV, buprenorphine was shown to decrease sevoflurane MAC by only 14% in cats (Ilkiw et al. 2002). It is appropriate choice for cats expected to experience mild to moderate pain.

12.5.2.5 Moderate to Heavy Sedatives

Patients requiring heavy sedation due to temperament are candidates to receive acepromazine or an alpha-2 adrenergic agonist in their premedication combination. These drugs are associated with a clinically important increase in unwanted side effects, even at lower doses, compared to the benzodiazepines and opioids. Caution should be exercised when using them, and doses should be minimized by the addition of other sedatives in balanced protocols. Both acepromazine and the alpha-2 agonist drugs (medetomidine, dexmedetomidine) block alpha receptors, which can precipitate additive unwanted drug effects. It is recommended to avoid using these two drugs together, or to exercise extreme caution (and use only low doses) if you do choose to combine them (Plumb 2008b).

Acepromazine is a phenothiazine tranquilizer with an onset of action between 30 and 60 minutes after subcutaneous or intramuscular injection. It has no analgesic properties and may cause profound vasodilation and hypotension. It can be overridden by catecholamines and cannot be relied upon as a sole restraining drug. Acepromazine predisposes patients to hypothermia, depresses ventilation, and can cause excessive vagal tone and bradycardia. It may decrease packed cell volume (PCV) by up to 50% within 30 minutes of administration due to vasodilation and interstitial fluid translocation. It should be used with caution in patients with cardiac dysfunction, decreased cardiac reserve, hepatic dysfunction, or general debilitation, as well as in pediatric and geriatric patients.

The alpha-2 agonists medetomidine, dexmedetomidine, detomidine, and xylazine have profound sedative effects and mild analgesic properties. Sedation will last considerably longer than analgesia. Alpha-2 agonist drugs are reversible with atipamezole (Antisedan). They can cause pulmonary hypertension, hyperglycemia, diuresis, and vomiting. Their sedative effects can be overridden by catecholamines. These drugs also interfere with thermoregulation. After administration, it may be difficult to raise peripheral veins due to altered hemodynamics and changes in vascular tone, both within the lungs and in the periphery. Patients given alpha-2 agonists may experience bradycardia and second-degree heart block. If bradycardia becomes severe enough to alter peripheral arterial blood pressure, it is recommended that an alpha-2 reversal drug be administered intramuscularly after anesthesia induction. The coadministration of anticholinergic drugs with alpha-2 agonists is contraindicated.

Alpha-2 agonists may precipitate muscle twitching, prolonged sedation, decreased arterial oxygenation, cyanosis, pulmonary edema, and decreased uptake of inhalant anesthetics (Keating et al. 2013). Their effects on peripheral arterial blood pressure are biphasic and include an initial period of hypertension lasting 20–40 minutes, followed by a longer period of hypotension, which can be profound. Pulmonary arterial vasoconstriction (pulmonary hypertension) occurs after dexmedetomidine administration and may be reflected as bradycardia, increased $PaCO_2$, and decreased PaO_2 (Zornow 1991; Kastner et al. 2005; Pypendop et al. 2011; Pascoe 2015). Alpha-2 agonists are contraindicated in patients with shock, hypotension, trauma, exercise intolerance, cardiac disease, increased afterload, respiratory disease or dysfunction, hepatic disease, renal disease, debilitation, or stress due to heat, cold, fatigue, or high altitude. Cardiopulmonary collapse may occur at two times the label dose of dexmedetomidine.

The proprietary combination of the dissociative tiletamine and benzodiazepine zolazepam (Telazol) can be used to premedicate dogs and cats. This drug combination may provide enough sedation to decrease the dose of subsequent anesthetics by 50% or more. Patients receiving this drug combination may experience vomiting, salivation, excess respiratory secretions, muscle twitching or rigidity, and pain at the injection site. They may vocalize and experience erratic or prolonged recoveries. Telazol provides very little analgesia and should not be used alone for procedures that precipitate anything beyond the mildest of pain.

Alfaxalone has also been administered intramuscularly in combination with other sedatives and analgesics to successfully sedate fractious patients. When combined in balanced premedication protocols, the intramuscular dose in dogs and cats is 1–5 mg/kg. Volume may be an issue when adding alfaxan to premedication combinations, and more than one injection site may be necessary (Tamura et al. 2015).

12.5.3 Creating Pre-Anesthetic Protocols

There are many potential pre-anesthetic combinations. In general, the combination of an opioid analgesic with a tranquilizer gives the most reliable and predictable results (Table 12.1).

Following administration of premedication drugs, it is important to allow sufficient time for peak drug effects to occur. If the injection is administered into the semimembranosus muscles, 10–15 minutes is sufficient. If it is administered subcutaneously or into the lumbar region, on the other hand, 20–90 minutes may be necessary for peak

effects and sedation quality is markedly reduced. After administering premedications, the patient should be placed in a quiet environment where they may be observed. An external heat source should be supplied or the ambient environmental temperature should be kept warm as thermoregulation and compensatory mechanisms begin to decrease. The patient should be placed on towels or other absorbent bedding to absorb urine or feces. Artificial tears should be applied if administering an anticholinergic, dexmedetomidine, telazol, or acepromazine.

12.5.4 Intravenous Catheter Placement and Fluid Support

All patients undergoing general anesthesia should have an intravenous catheter placed. The catheter should be a sufficient size to not impede administration of emergency drugs or fluids if they become necessary. The American Animal Hospital Association (AAHA) recently released new fluid guidelines for dogs and cats under general anesthesia (Table 12.2). Rates of administration have been reduced due to recognition that glomerular filtration rate (GFR) does not increase during general anesthesia and excess intravenous fluids translocate to become excess lung water (Davis et al. 2013).

12.5.5 Pre-Induction Support

Once peak drug effects from premedication have occurred and the intravenous catheter has been placed, the patient is ready to be moved to the procedure table, where induction of anesthesia will take place. External heat sources should

Table 12.1 Drugs used in pre-anesthetic combinations.[a]

Vomiting suppression	Anticholinergic (if indicated)	Tranquilizer	Opioid sedative	Opioid analgesic sedative	Opioid analgesic
Maropitant 1 mg/kg SQ	Atropine 0.01–0.04	Midazolam 0.1–0.4	Butorphanol 0.2–0.8	Hydromorphone 0.03–0.075	Buprenorphine 0.05–0.24
	Glycopyrrolate 0.01	Diazepam 0.1–0.4	Nalbuphine 0.2–0.4	Oxymorphone 0.03–0.075	
		Alfaxalone 1–2		Morphine 0.1–0.5	
		Acepromazine 0.03–0.05		Meperidine 2–5	
		Dexmedetomidine 0.001–0.005		Methadone 0.2–0.5	
		Medetomidine 0.002–0.01		Fentanyl 0.02–0.04 IV	

[a] Doses are mg/kg and are recommended to be administered intramuscularly into the semimembranous muscles unless otherwise indicated.

be available and pre-warmed. The table should be padded appropriately for patient comfort. At this time, physiologic values should be obtained and recorded. The application of all monitoring leads that the patient will allow should be done prior to anesthetic induction (ECG, Doppler ultrasound, indirect arterial blood pressure, SpO_2, etc.). Patients should be preoxygenated by facemask (without the rubber diaphragm) at 3 l/minute oxygen flow for 1–2 minutes prior to intravenous induction (Figure 12.3). In the event of apnea, this simple maneuver allows more time before oxygen desaturation occurs. Cardiac arrest in veterinary anesthesia is typically preceded by respiratory arrest, oxygen desaturation, and subsequent fatal ventricular arrhythmia due to myocardial hypoxemia (McMichael et al. 2012).

12.5.6 Anesthesia Induction

Induction of general anesthesia may be accomplished using injectable drugs or by the administration of inhalant anesthetic by facemask. In general, injectable inductions are preferred because they allow a more rapid loss of consciousness, less patient struggling, earlier control of the airway, and less danger of injury to the patient and staff. There are many drugs available for intravenous anesthetic induction. Popular ones include alfaxalone, propofol, a combination of diazepam or midazolam and ketamine, and etomidate. Balanced induction protocols are designed to reduce the dose of the individual induction drugs. Applied intravenously, they can be used with any premedication protocol and in compromised patients (Table 12.3).

Alfaxalone (Alfaxan) can be used for anesthetic induction in all patients, including fragile and geriatric ones. It is classified as a neuroactive steroid but is devoid

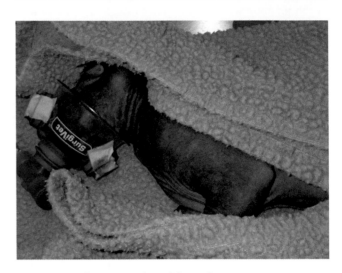

Figure 12.3 Preoxygenation of the patient.

Table 12.2 AAHA recommended intravenous fluid rates during general anesthesia.

Species	First hour	Second hour	Subsequent hours
Canine	5 ml/kg/hour	3.75 ml/kg/hour	2.8 ml/kg/hour
Feline	3 ml/kg/hour	2.25 ml/kg/hour	2 ml/kg/hour

Table 12.3 Anesthesia induction protocols for dogs and cats.

Flush the intravenous catheter and wait 15–30 seconds between drugs		
First injection	**Second injection**	**Third injection**
Alfaxalone 1–3 mg/kg		
Propofol 1–3 mg/kg		
Etomidate 1–2 mg/kg		
Midazolam 0.2 mg/kg	Ketamine 0.5–2 mg/kg	
Lidocaine 1 mg/kg	Propofol 0.5–2 mg/kg	
Lidocaine 1 mg/kg	Alfaxalone 0.5–2 mg/kg	
Midazolam 0.1 mg/kg	Alfaxalone 0.5–2 mg/kg	
Midazolam 0.1 mg/kg	Propofol 1–2 mg/kg	
Midazolam 0.2 mg/kg	Etomidate 1–2 mg/kg	
Ketamine 1 mg/kg	Alfaxalone 0.5–2 mg/kg	
Ketamine 1 mg/kg	Propofol 1–2 mg/kg	
Midazolam 0.1 mg/kg	Ketamine 1 mg/kg	Propofol 0.5–1 mg/kg
Lidocaine 1 mg/kg	Ketamine 1 mg/kg	Alfaxalone 0.5–1 mg/kg
Lidocaine 1 mg/kg	Midazolam 0.1 mg/kg	Alfaxalone 0.5–1 mg/kg

of endocrine activity. It exerts its mechanism of action by modulating neuronal cell-membrane chloride ion transport by binding to $GABA_A$ cell-surface receptors. It is administered slowly and steadily to effect over about 60 seconds. After appropriate pre-medication, induction doses are usually between 0.5 and 2 mg/kg IV. Anesthetic inductions using alfaxalone have similar qualities to propofol, providing relaxation and a smooth induction. Alfaxalone is cardiac-sparing compared to propofol, and apnea is less likely to occur. It can be administered as intermittent boluses, a low dose CRI (1 to 3 mg/kg/hr) to spare inhalant concentration, or for total intravenous anesthesia (TIVA) at 5 to 6 mg/kg/hr. This can be especially helpful if a particular patient cannot withstand the vasodilatory effects of the inhalant anesthetics. Like all anesthetics, Alfaxalone can depress cardiorespiratory function in a dose-dependent manner.

Propofol is a short-acting hypnotic that is unrelated to other general anesthetic drugs. Its onset of action is within seconds, and the duration of effect of a single bolus is two to five minutes. Induction is usually smooth, but muscle twitching can occur. Muscle twitching can be reduced if midazolam (or diazepam) is administered intravenously prior to propofol. Adverse effects include apnea (especially with rapid administration), hypotension, bradycardia or tachycardia, and an up to 50% decrease in cardiac output (Kurita et al. 2002). Repeated administration may cause Heinz body production in cats. Propofol should be used with caution in patients with decreased cardiac reserve. The addition of lidocaine 1 mg/kg IV, midazolam 0.1 mg/kg IV, or ketamine 1 mg/kg IV has been shown to decrease propofol induction dose by 25% (Griffenhagen 2013).

The combination of diazepam or midazolam and ketamine will induce anesthesia within 30–60 seconds. The duration of a single bolus is approximately two to five minutes. Intubation is slightly different because laryngeal reflexes are maintained. Patients may also exhibit salivation, apnea, and muscle stiffness, especially with a 1:1 volume: volume ratio of diazepam:ketamine. The author prefers a 2:1 volume ratio of midazolam:ketamine dosed at 0.5–1 ml/10 kg (midazolam 0.165–0.33 mg/kg and ketamine 1.65–3.3 mg/kg) to reduce muscle stiffness. Ketamine causes a central release of catecholamines, resulting in tachycardia, increased cardiac output, and increased blood pressure. In catecholamine-depleted patients, ketamine will act as a direct myocardial depressant and decrease cardiac output.

Etomidate (Amidate) is an imidazole derivative whose mechanism of action is not fully understood. It has little to no effect upon myocardial metabolism, cardiac output, peripheral circulation, or pulmonary circulation. It may depress ventilation slightly. Etomidate has been shown to decrease intraocular pressure. It is supplied in a propylene glycol base, and rapid intravenous injection may cause hemolysis. Its administration is associated with a six-hour reduction in plasma cortisol and aldosterone levels. This effect does not appear to have clinical significance after administration of a single induction dose.

Induction using inhalant anesthetics delivered by facemask is less desirable than intravenous induction. This is a relatively slow process that is stressful to the patient and staff. Even inductions with sevoflurane take several minutes, compared to 30–60 seconds with an injectable induction. Inhalant induction poses a greater potential for injury to patient and staff. The large amount of oxygen and liquid anesthetic used produces copious amounts of waste anesthetic gas, increasing staff health risks and significantly increasing cost. There is little documented hard evidence against mask inductions in dogs and cats. However, an equine mortality study definitely shows an increased risk of death (nearly threefold higher) (Johnston et al. 1995).

The concentration of inhalant necessary for intubation is much higher than that needed for surgical incision. This generally means that by the time a patient is deep enough to intubate, they will likely be very hypotensive and respiratory-depressed. Patients with pre-existing cardiovascular compromise or those that lack organ reserve due to illness are at great risk of decompensation and can experience catastrophic complications. The only patients that are appropriate candidates for inhalant induction are those in which intravenous access is impossible prior to induction. In these cases, an intravenous catheter should be placed as quickly as possible after patient relaxation. This may be before the patient is deep enough for endotracheal intubation.

Regardless of the induction method, the endotracheal tube is placed and the cuff inflated immediately following anesthetic induction. Caution must be exercised to avoid overinflation of the endotracheal tube cuff, because tracheal crush injury or tracheal rupture may occur (Mitchell et al. 2000) (Figure 12.4). One article recommended silicone-straight tubes for feline dentistry, postulating that these tubes might cause less tracheal mucosal injury when changing patient position frequently. The disadvantage of straight-silicone tubes is that they cannot be cut to a more appropriate length, increasing dead space, resistance to breathing, and the work of breathing. Very small patients or those with significant muscle wasting may become exhausted from the increased work of breathing. During placement, desensitization of the vocal cords and endotracheal-tube lubrication with lidocaine gel are indicated (Figure 12.5). Both count as part of the total dose of local anesthetic in cats (De Vries and Putter 2015).

The patient's respiratory rate, heart rate and rhythm, mucous membrane (MM) color, capillary refill time (CRT), arterial blood pressure, and other monitoring parameters should be checked immediately after induction and at intervals of no more than five minutes throughout anesthesia.

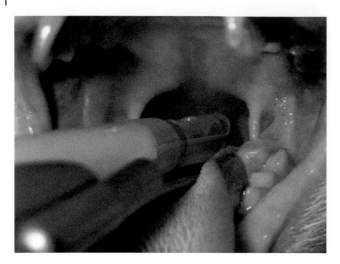

Figure 12.4   Straight silicone endotracheal tubes during intubation procedure.

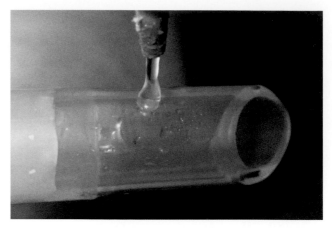

Figure 12.5   Lubrication of an endotracheal tube.

12.5.7   Inhalant Anesthetic Maintenance

To transition to inhalant more smoothly, it is recommended that the oxygen flow rate be continued at 3 l/minute for three minutes after the patient is connected to the anesthetic breathing circuit. This allows sufficient fresh gas flow and time to increase the inhalant concentration to a level that will maintain unconsciousness while the effects of the intravenous induction drug wane. For most patients, starting concentration for the inhalants should be similar to MAC, and increased or decreased based upon individual needs. Anesthetic depth should be determined every five minutes, and all physiologic variables should be documented each time. Small adjustments in inhalant concentration should be made based upon assessment of anesthetic depth.

Isoflurane and sevoflurane are currently the primary inhalant anesthetics in veterinary medicine. The MAC of sevoflurane is 2.4% in dogs and 2.6% in cats, while that of isoflurane is 1.3% in dogs and 1.6% in cats. By definition, half of patients are appropriately anesthetized at concentrations less than MAC, while the other half reach an appropriate depth of anesthesia by 1.3× MAC. MAC is a guide to initial vaporizer dial settings. The concentration an individual patient requires to maintain an appropriate depth of anesthesia is determined by monitoring changes in physical signs and physiologic variables. Physical signs that aid in determining anesthetic depth are the palpebral reflex, globe position, jaw tone, pinnal and withdrawal reflexes, and corneal reflexes. Physiologic monitoring of cardiovascular and respiratory parameters will also aid in determining the ideal vaporizer setting for each individual patient. Small vaporizer dial changes (0.1–0.25%)

should be made every time the patient is assessed (with physiologic data recorded at the same time) until the ideal depth of anesthesia is reached.

The concurrent use of opioids, sedatives, and tranquilizers will decrease MAC by as much as 60%. Physiologic conditions that decrease MAC are hypotension, hypothermia, PCV < 10%, $PaO_2 < 5.07$ kPa (38 mmHg), $PaCO_2 > 12.7$ kPa (95 mmHg), increasing age, and pregnancy. In patients with any of these indications, initial vaporizer dial settings should be slightly below MAC and adjusted as previously described.

MAC will be increased in patients that are experiencing painful surgical stimulus, have high catecholamine loads, have been administered ephedrine, are hyperthermic (up to 42 °C), or are neonatal. Vaporizer dial settings should be set slightly above MAC, and the inhalant concentration should be titrated appropriately.

MAC is not influenced by sex, duration of anesthesia, hypertension, PaO_2 between 5.07 and 66.7 kPa (38–500 mmHg), metabolic acidosis, metabolic alkalosis, hypocapnia, or hypercapnia up to 12.7 kPa (95 mmHg). MAC varies less than twofold between species and classes of animals. If an atypical species is presented for care, vaporizer dial settings will be similar to those used in dogs and cats.

Isoflurane and sevoflurane depress cardiovascular function to a similar degree. The primary unwanted side effect is hypotension due to vasodilation. Mild hypotension usually responds to decreasing depth of anesthesia and fluid administration. Profound hypotension may require administration of vasopressors or inotropes. Sevoflurane is superior to isoflurane in respiratory safety (Galloway et al. 2004). Adequate ventilation is better preserved as anesthetic depth increases under sevoflurane anesthesia.

12.5.8 MAC Sparing Techniques

Patients unable to compensate for the cardiorespiratory blunting effects of the inhalant anesthetics may benefit from application of a MAC sparing technique (Table 12.4). Local anesthetic blocks are commonly used in dental therapy to reduce the dose of inhalant anesthetics (see Chapter 11). If inhalant concentrations must be reduced for longer than a single injection will provide, a CRI may be considered as a sustainable method to reduce MAC (Table 12.5). A continuous infusion of anesthetic or analgesic drug has several advantages over intermittent boluses. It avoids "peak and valley" plasma drug concentrations and potentially slow onset of analgesia, and allows a continuous reduction in the vaporizer dial setting. It is important to administer intravenous loading doses of each drug before commencing a CRI. Loading doses ensure immediate therapeutic plasma drug concentrations. If loading doses are not administered prior to staring the CRI, it may take hours to achieve therapeutic blood levels.

12.5.9 Maropitant (Cerenia)

Maropitant has been shown to decrease sevoflurane MAC in dogs undergoing ovariohysterectomy by 24% after intravenous injection of 1 mg/kg followed by 0.03 mg/kg/hour CRI (Boscan et al. 2001). Sevoflurane MAC was further reduced (by 30% total) in dogs after 5 mg/kg IV followed by 0.15 mg/kg/hour CRI. In cats undergoing ovariohysterectomy, a dose of 1 mg/kg IV reduced sevoflurane MAC by 16%, while 5 mg/kg IV gave no further reduction (Niyom et al. 2013).

12.5.10 Midazolam CRI

Midazolam, a benzodiazepine, may be administered as a CRI to produce muscle relaxation or mild sedation. It has no intrinsic analgesic properties. It is usually administered in combination with fentanyl or any of the opioid CRIs listed in Table 12.5.

Table 12.4   Single injections of sedative or analgesic drugs used to decrease MAC.

Drug	Dog dose (mg/kg)	Cat dose (mg/kg)	Route
Fentanyl	0.002–0.005	0.002–0.005	IV
Hydromorphone	0.02–0.04	0.02–0.03	IV
Oxymorphone	0.02–0.04	0.02–0.03	IV
Dexmedetomidine	0.001–0.003	0.001–0.003	IV
Alfaxalone	0.5–2	0.5–2	IV
Propofol	0.5–1	0.5–1	IV

Table 12.5   Drugs used as CRIs during anesthesia to reduce MAC.

Drug	Loading dose (mg/kg IV)	Dogs (mg/kg/hour IV)	Cats (mg/kg/hour IV)
Fentanyl	0.002–0.005	0.001–0.01	0.001–0.005
Morphine	0.1–0.3	0.1–0.2	0.03–0.1
Hydromorphone	0.03–0.075	0.03–0.05	0.02–0.04
Oxymorphone	0.03–0.075	0.03–0.05	0.03–0.05
Methadone	0.1	0.1–0.3	0.1–0.3
Lidocaine	1 mg/kg	0.5–2	Not intra-op
Ketamine	0.25–0.5	0.12–1	0.12–0.1
Dexmedetomidine	0–0.001	0.00025–0.0005	0.00025–0.0005
Midazolam	0.2–0.4	0.2–0.4	0.2–0.4
Maropitant	1–5	0.03–0.15	Unknown at publication
Alfaxalone	0.5–2	1–6	1–3
Tramadol	1.5 mg/kg	2.6	Unknown at publication

12.5.11 Monitoring Patient Physiology

12.5.11.1 Noninvasive Arterial Blood Pressure

Arterial blood pressure is the measure of force per unit area exerted by the circulating blood on the blood vessel walls. Arterial blood pressure is included as one of the principal vital signs. Using the assumption that the arterial system is a static-elastic system, the only two physical determinants of arterial blood pressure are the blood volume within the arterial system and the compliance of the vessels. The physiologic factors affecting blood pressure are the cardiac output (heart rate × stroke volume) and peripheral resistance.

Noninvasive blood pressure (NIBP) is usually measured indirectly by either sphygmomanometry, utilizing a Doppler ultrasound, or oscillometric technique (Figure 12.6). Occulsion cuff width must be 40% limb circumference for accurate measurements. With either technique, the cuff should be placed snugly around the appendage, but not overly tight. If it is applied too tightly, the pressure readings will be lower than the actual pressure because the cuff will partially occlude the artery. If it is too loose, the pressure measurements will be falsely elevated because the cuff will need to be excessively inflated to occlude arterial blood flow. The degree of error is unknown and cannot be accurately estimated; however, awareness of potential measurement error does aid in clinical decision making.

Systolic blood pressure is primarily determined by stroke volume and arterial compliance. Systolic pressure, by definition, is the pressure in the arteries at the end of the rapid ejection phase of systole. During this phase, the blood volume forced into the arterial system exceeds that exiting into the arterioles. This corresponds to when maximal arterial blood volume and maximal arterial pressure are reached. Systolic hypotension is treated by increasing vascular tone or arterial blood volume.

Diastolic pressure is primarily determined by the systemic vascular resistance and heart rate. Peripheral runoff from the arterial system continues during diastole, even in the absence of ventricular ejection. This decreases the

arterial volume and pressure. Diastolic pressure is measured immediately preceding the next ventricular ejection, when arterial volume and pressure are the lowest. Normal disparity between systolic and diastolic pressures is between 4 and 5.33 kPa (30 and 40 mmHg). Diastolic hypotension is present when the disparity between systolic and diastolic blood pressure exceeds this range. Diastolic hypotension becomes important because it is the major contributing factor to hypotension of the mean arterial pressure (MAP). It is treated by increasing the heart rate, sometimes by as little as 10–20 bpm, or by increasing systemic vascular resistance.

MAP may provide the best estimate of adequate tissue perfusion, because it estimates an average driving perfusion

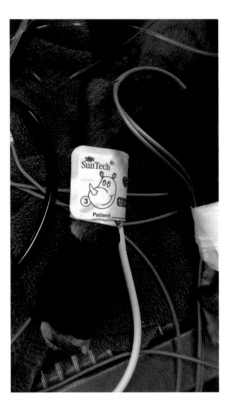

Figure 12.6   Noninvasive blood pressure measurement.

Table 12.6   Anesthetic management for obese patients.

Gastric management	Tranquilizer	Analgesic sedative	Induction	Analgesic	Reversal
Maropitant	Midazolam	Oxymorphone	Alfaxalone	Local block	Flumazenil
Metoclopramide	Diazepam	Buprenorphine	Midazolam Ketamine	NSAID	Naloxone
Proton Pump Inhibitor	Butrophanol	Hydromorphone	Propofol	Opioid	
		Morphine	Etomidate	Acetaminophen in dogs only	
		Fentanyl			

pressure. It is the pressure in the arteries averaged over time. MAP is a calculated value, generally represented by adding one-third the systolic/diastolic difference to the diastolic pressure. Complex algorithms exist in modern monitoring equipment that take heart rate into account when calculating it. Despite the influence of heart rate, MAP should be closer to the measured diastolic pressure. If the machine-generated numbers place diastolic pressure closer to systolic pressure, an error has occurred and the measurement should be retaken.

Normal values for arterial blood pressure in mammals are:

- Systolic: 14.7–18.66 kPa (110–140 mmHg)
- Diastolic: 8–13.33 kPa (60–100 mmHg)
- Mean: 10.66–16 kPa (80–120 mmHg)

12.5.11.2 Electrocardiogram

The electrocardiogram, commonly referred to as ECG or EKG, is a measurement of the electrical activity of the heart. The ECG rhythm strip is a valuable method for evaluating cardiac electrical rate and rhythm. It is the only means of specifically identifying arrhythmias. Changes in waveform morphology on ECG can imply derangements in oxygenation such as hypoxia/ischemia (ST changes) or electrolyte imbalances such as hyperkalemia (T, P wave morphology). Abnormal alterations in the ECG can indicate one or more of several heart-related conditions. Conditions that are not directly heart-related may also cause changes in the ECG, such as splenomegaly or gastric dilatation and volvulus. Arrhythmias are detrimental because they alter circulation, decrease tissue perfusion, and indicate decreased cardiac health.

An ECG represents only electrical activity of the heart. It provides no information about mechanical activity (quality of contraction), cardiac output, or blood pressure (perfusion). Electrical–mechanical dissociation, a form of cardiac arrest in whcih there is only electrical activity and no cardiac output, may demonstrate only subtle changes on ECG. A certain amount of expertise must be acquired to precisely interpret an ECG and distinguish artifacts from actual waveforms (Figure 12.7).

12.5.11.3 Monitoring Ventilation

The objective of monitoring ventilation is to ensure that the patient's breathing is adequately maintained. Though there are several basic methods of assessing the adequacy of ventilation, the single most useful indicator is $PaCO_2$ from blood gas analysis. When this is not available, measurement of CO_2 in the expired gas (capnography) provides a good estimate (Figure 12.8). Other methods of observation are helpful when no objective data related to the elimination of carbon dioxide are available.

A reservoir bag (of the correct volume for the patient) will give some indication regarding depth of ventilation (tidal volume). Usual tidal volumes in mammals are between 10 and 20 ml/kg. They can be estimated by observing how much volume leaves the reservoir bag during inspiration. This method is relatively inaccurate, but it can indicate severe hypoventilation if the bag is barely emptying. An appropriately sized reservoir bag empties by approximately one-fourth if the patient is moving its normal tidal volume of gas.

Capnography (end-expired CO_2 measurement [$ETCO_2$]) is very useful in most patients. The CO_2 in expired gas is measured by infrared spectrophotometry using either a

(a)

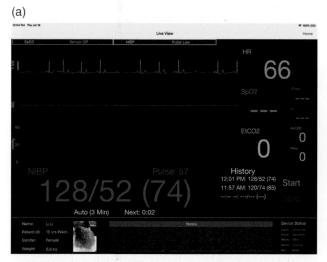

(b)

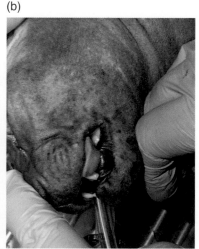

Figure 12.7 (a) ECG waveform on an anesthetic monitor displaying second-degree heart block. (*Source:* Victoria Lukasik.) (b) Esophagus probe Cardell introduced in a cat.

mainstream method or a sidestream sample of gas. For mainstream measurement, a spectrophotometer with a transparent window is inserted across the breathing circuit at the connection with the endotracheal tube. A continuous measurement is made of the CO_2 in the gas flowing through the circuit. During sidestream sampling, a fine tube is connected to a port in the breathing circuit located at the endotracheal tube adapter. A small sample of gas is continuously suctioned into a gas analyzer some distance from the patient and the CO_2 it contains is measured.

(a)　　　　　　　　　　　　　　　　　　(b)

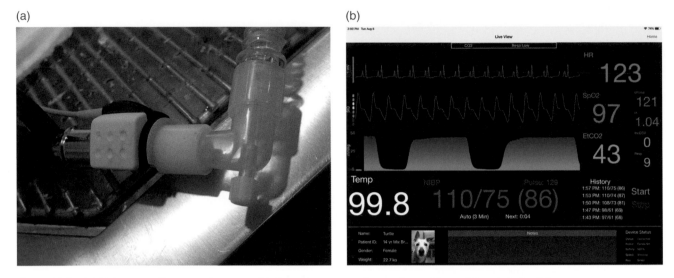

Figure 12.8　(a) Mainstream Capnography sensor. (b) Normal capnograph waveform.　(*Source:* Victoria Lukasik.)

(a)　　　　　　　　　　　　　　　　　　(b)

(c)

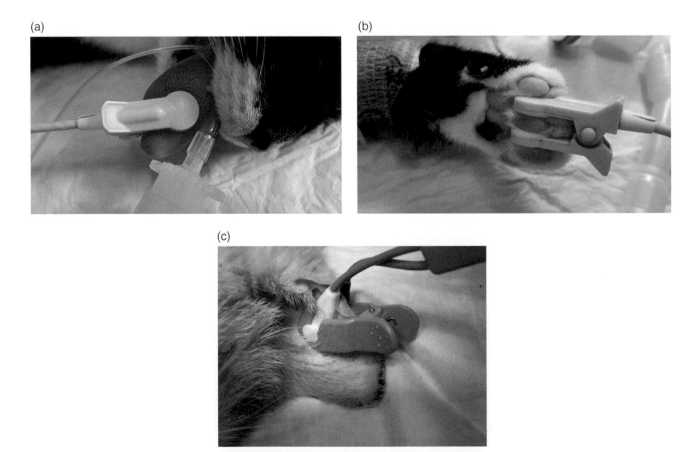

Figure 12.9　Pulsoximetry sensors on (a) tongue and (b) paws　(*Source:* Emilia Klim) and (c) pinna.

Ideally, the capnograph waveform should be displayed, as this gives much more information than numeric values alone (e.g., airway obstruction, rebreathing, leaks in the circuit, cardiac arrest). For more on capnograph waveforms and their interpretation, see www.capnography.com.

Capnography assumes that $ETCO_2$ is relatively close to arterial CO_2: about 0.66–1.33 kPa (5–10 mmHg) lower. Generally speaking, this is a safe assumption, but is not true in every case. Equipment should be calibrated periodically and occasionally correlated to an actual measurement of $PaCO_2$ (blood gas analysis). Sidestream measurement may provide imprecise values if the fine tubing becomes occluded by moisture or is kinked. There is some delay in measurement because of the distance the sample must travel, though this is not usually clinically important. The mainstream sampling unit is a bulky addition for small patients and may create traction on the endotracheal tube with certain patient positions. Both systems may report imprecise values from interference by halothane, though this is not necessarily true of the more modern inhalants (isoflurane, sevoflurane, desflurane).

When patients are awake, normal arterial CO_2 measured by blood gas analysis is 4.67–5.99 kPa (35–45 mmHg). Due to the respiratory depressant effects of the anesthetic drugs and increased airway resistance created by the endotracheal tube, acceptable $ETCO_2$ under anesthesia is between 5.99 and 7.99 kPa (35–60 mmHg). An arterial CO_2 greater than 7.99 kPa (60 mmHg) creates unacceptable acidemia that requires intervention. Unacceptable alkalemia is created by an arterial CO_2 less than 2.66 kPa (20 mmHg) and warrants intervention.

Hypoventilation is one of the most common anesthetic complications encountered in veterinary practice. Therapy for hypoventilation is very simple: assisted or controlled ventilation. Assisted ventilation is accomplished by squeezing the reservoir bag when the patient starts to inspire. Peak inspiratory pressures (PIPs) are usually between 0.98 and 2.94 (10 and 30 cm H_2O) in healthy patients; this may need to be increased to 5.88 kPa (60 cm H_2O) for patients with restrictive thoracic disease (pleural effusion, pneumothorax, thoracic mass, etc.). Disease of the lung tissue makes it very fragile, and positive-pressure ventilation may lead to pneumothorax even at very low PIP.

Controlled ventilation is accomplished by using a mechanical ventilator or continuously squeezing the reservoir bag until the patient is no longer attempting to ventilate on their own: the anesthetist has taken over the duty of moving gas into and out of the lungs. There are many types of mechanical ventilators, but the basic concepts are always the same: ensuring an adequate tidal volume (10–15 ml/kg), providing an appropriate number of breaths per minute (6–16), and avoiding barotrauma (most patients PIP < 2.95 kPa or 30 cm H_2O).

12.5.12 Pulse Oximetry

The pulse oximeter is actually a very poor way to assess ventilation until a patient is in hypoxemic crisis. The primary purpose of pulse oximetry is to determine the per cent oxygen saturation of hemoglobin (SpO_2). Acceptable SpO_2 values are between 90 and 100%. The pulse oximeter detects pulsatile flow in a capillary bed to determine SpO_2 and pulse rate (Figure 12.9). It does not give an indication of blood pressure. It often fails in situations of poor pulse quality, which may occur due to hypotension, hypothermia, poor local tissue perfusion, or vasoconstriction. The acquisition of a signal is also affected by pigmentation, debris, ambient light, lack of adequate patient contact, and motion.

The greatest value of pulse oximetry is during anesthetic recovery, where it ensures that patients transition to breathing room air appropriately. If a patient experiences oxygen desaturation during anesthetic recovery, oxygen should be supplemented until the patient can maintain hemoglobin oxygen saturation adequately on room air.

12.5.12.1 Hypothermia

Almost all patients that are sedated or anesthetized will lose body temperature. The exception is the Nordic dog breeds (Husky, Malamute, Samoyed, etc.), which may become hyperthermic under general anesthesia. The adverse effects of hypothermia include immune system depression, coagulopathy, myocardial depression, arrhythmia, decreased CO_2 production, alkalemia, hyperglycemia, hypovolemia due to cold diuresis, decreased hepatic metabolism, delayed drug elimination, and delayed anesthetic recovery. Confusion, stupor, and coma can also occur in hypothermic patients. MAC is decreased approximately 5% for each degree Celsius below normal body temperature.

Prevention of hypothermia is more desirable than trying to rewarm patients once they become cold. Effective rewarming cannot happen unless 60% of the body surface area is in contact with an external heat source. Desirable methods of preventing inadvertent hypothermia include controlling ambient temperature by keeping the operating room temperature at 24 °C (75 °F) or more, insulating patients using bubble wrap, plastic wrap, or warm blankets, warming skin prep and irrigation solutions, warming all intravenous fluids, humidifying and heating inspired gasses, applying circulating hot-water blankets at 40–41.5 °C (105–107 °F), forced-air heat-exchange blankets, or conductive heating blanket systems, and keeping patients dry or actively drying them postoperatively (Figure 12.10).

There are other methods for providing an external heat source, but they are not desirable due to the potential for thermal injury or electrocution. Radiant heaters or heat lamps ("French fry" lamps) cannot be easily regulated and

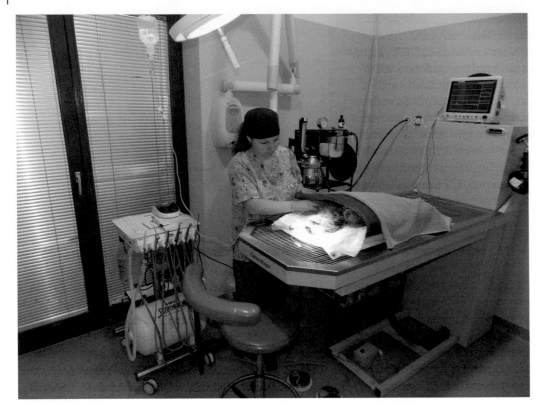

Figure 12.10   Temperature maintenance: forced hot-air blanket on top of a hot-water blanket.

can cause severe thermal injury to the skin. Electric heating pads and electric heating boards can develop hot spots or become wet and shock or electrocute the patient. Hot-water bottles can be used provided that they do not get above 41.5 °C (107 °F) and are removed when they become cool.

It is important to monitor a patient's temperature closely, because of the possibility of overshoot. Hyperthermia during surgery or rewarming can occur when the blood vessels in the periphery are vasodilated due to the anesthetic drugs. Heat is easily transferred to the core when peripheral vessels are vasodilated. The adverse effects of hyperthermia are numerous and can be detrimental to patient well-being.

12.5.13   Anesthetic Recovery

When discontinuing the inhalant anesthetic at the conclusion of a procedure, the oxygen flow rate should be increased to 3 l/minute for three minutes. This eliminates a significant amount of waste inhalant anesthesia from the machine and circuitry, decreasing staff exposure to anesthetic waste gas. The greatest risk of perianesthetic death is in the recovery phase. Monitoring should be continued, and an external heat source should be applied for several minutes into the recovery period (Figure 12.11). Mucus

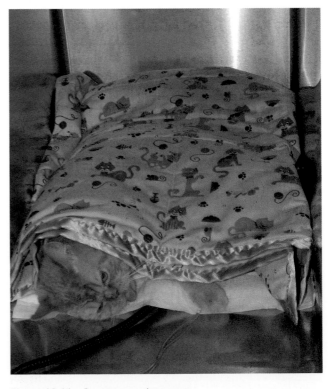

Figure 12.11   Recovery environment.

and other debris must be cleared from the pharynx prior to extubation. The patient should be extubated only when it has regained protective airway reflexes, not weak ineffective gagging. It should be post-oxygenated by face mask before and after extubation as needed. It is important to continue to monitor SpO_2 as patients transition to room air, approximately five minutes after discontinuing oxygen support. Occasionally, a patient will be oxygen-dependent for several minutes to a few hours post-anesthesia. Patients should be returned to their cages only after they have adequate muscle tone to breathe effectively and protect their airway properly. Postoperative analgesia is very important and is discussed in Chapter 11.

12.6 Special Patient Presentations

12.6.1 Geriatric Patients

In veterinary medicine, geriatric is usually defined as any animal exceeding 75–80% of its predicted lifespan. However, it is important to note that there may be little correlation between *chronologic age* and *physiologic age*, which necessitates careful individual patient assessment. Additionally, there may be coexisting diseases present that require additional consideration. The functional reserve of the cardiovascular system can be considerably reduced with age, and geriatric patients are less able to compensate for hypovolemia and vasodilation. The respiratory system undergoes mechanical changes leading to decreased compliance of the thorax, atrophy of the intercostal muscles and diaphragm, and decreased alveolar elasticity. This results in a linear decline in arterial oxygen tension with age. The ventilatory response to hypoxia and hypercarbia is also markedly blunted. These changes make the geriatric patient far more susceptible to hypoxia and hypercarbia in the perianesthetic period. There is some evidence that protective laryngeal and pharyngeal reflexes are reduced. Patients approaching life expectancy periodically awaken from anesthesia with nonspecific deficits in cognitive function. This "post-anesthetic fog" often resolves within a few hours, but it may last for two or three days or be permanent.

Anesthetic management of the geriatric patient should always be individualized. A full patient assessment should be performed, looking for evidence of age-associated changes, including mentation, as well as of concurrent disease. Scaling of drug doses based upon age alone is often appropriate in geriatric patients. Drug dosages should be scaled further when patients have moderate to severe coexisting disease(s). Appropriate scaling is based upon life expectancy, not a definitive number of years since birth. This is because life expectancies, even among dog breeds,

can vary by as much as 12–14 years. Doses are scaled approximately 10% at half life expectancy, 25% at three-quarters life expectancy, and 50% at life expectancy (Herminghaus et al. 2012). Some patients live well beyond life expectancy, and doses may be scaled even more in those circumstance. Drug dose is still influenced by temperament, species, procedure to be undertaken, and so on.

12.6.2 Obesity

The ventilatory system is greatly affected by the deposition of fat in and around the thoracic cavity. Obesity hypoventilation syndrome (OHS, Pickwickian syndrome) is a condition in which obese patients do not breathe well enough to properly oxygenate their blood or effectively remove carbon dioxide. It is caused by increased pressure on the diaphragm and thoracic organs due to excess adipose tissue. This compression leads to a reduced intrathoracic volume, compression of alveoli, and atelectasis. There is also a central nervous system component to OHS in which dysregulation of respiratory drive results in blunted responses to hypercapnea and hypoxemia. Additionally, the muscles of ventilation lack the ability to respond properly to hypoventilation. All of these factors lead to chronic hypoxemia and chronic respiratory acidemia, which is reflected as polycythemia and exercise intolerance.

The decrease in functional residual capacity (FRC) due to compressed alveoli impairs the obese patient's ability to tolerate apnea. Dorsal recumbency aggravates hypoxemia and hypercarbia. Increasing obesity leads to decreased pulmonary compliance and increased airway resistance, further impairing gas exchange through worsening ventilation/perfusion (V/Q) mismatch. Restrictive lung disease is frequently observed in obese patients. The rapid, shallow breathing seen in these patients increases the work of breathing.

Obese patients must have ventilatory support during anesthesia to avoid worsening of pulmonary function and further respiratory compromise in the post-anesthetic period. Ventilatory support should include pre-oxygenation for approximately three minutes, intermittent positive-pressure ventilation (IPPV) with positive end-expiratory pressure (PEEP), blood pressure monitoring to ensure that cardiac output does not suffer due to PEEP, and monitoring of arterial oxygenation (arterial blood gas or SpO_2) during the post-anesthetic period.

Obesity places an abnormal workload on the heart. Cardiomegaly and systemic hypertension reflect this increase in cardiac output. Pulmonary hypertension is common due to chronic hypoxemia and increased pulmonary blood volume.

Obese patients have an increased risk of aspiration pneumonia due to increased intra-abdominal (intragastric) pressure, increased gastric acidity, increased gastric fluid volume, and decreased gastric emptying. Pretreatment with Proton Pump Inhibitor, metoclopramide, and maropitant (Cerenia) is recommended (Marks, et al. 2018). It is especially important to avoid perianesthetic emesis in obese patients. This is not a reason to avoid opioid premedication, but it does necessitate obtunding the central vomiting effect of the opioids by administering an antiemetic (maropitant) prior to premedication.

Anesthetic drug protocols should be designed to provide minimal blunting of cardiac and respiratory function (Table 12.5). They should include appropriate analgesics, with preference given to techniques that are non-sedating, such as local anesthetic blocks, regional anesthesia, acetaminophen (in dogs only), and nonsteroidal anti-inflammatory drugs (NSAIDs). All induction drugs should be given slowly "to effect."

A cuffed endotracheal tube should be placed and the airway secured as quickly as possible. Injectable anesthetic inductions allow the most rapid securing of the airway. Extubation should be done after protective airway reflexes have been established, not after the first few ineffective gags. The head should be held up in recovery to reduce the chance of passive esophageal reflux reaching the pharynx. Sternal recumbency increases gastric pressure and decreases thoracic compliance. Recovery in a more oblique body position may be more suitable for obese patients.

Recovery should include post-oxygenation until the patient can once again maintain acceptable arterial oxygen saturation on room air. Baseline SpO$_2$ on room air should be obtained prior to the administration of any anesthetic drugs, to establish the individual patient's criteria for discontinuing oxygen support.

12.6.3 Cardiac Compromise

The only strict contraindication for general anesthesia is uncompensated cardiac disease. Patients who are fainting, have pulmonary edema, or are experiencing episodes of hypoxemia or runs of life-threatening arrhythmia do not tolerate the stress of general anesthesia and are at increased risk of death in the post-anesthetic period. An accurate cardiac diagnosis should be obtained prior to anesthesia in order to understand the hemodynamic and secondary effects of the cardiac disease. No single cardiac test can predict a patient's ability to withstand anesthesia. Elective procedures should be postponed until a patient's hemodynamics can be stabilized. Documentation of pre-existing cardiac arrhythmia is a consideration for choosing

anesthetic drugs and arrhythmias may need to be stabilized or treated before commencing anesthesia.

Patients with moderate to severe cardiac insufficiency are very sensitive to fluid administration, and intravenous fluids should be carefully titrated to avoid precipitating failure from volume overload. Intravenous fluid rates should be reduced to a minimal 1–3 ml/kg/hour for the first hour, and reduced an additional 25–50% in subsequent hours. Patients vary in how much fluid volume they can tolerate, but all those with cardiac insufficiency will be more sensitive to fluid overload. It is important to monitor systemic arterial blood pressure, heart rate and rhythm, and SpO$_2$ during anesthesia. It may also be helpful to auscult the lung sounds periodically during and after anesthesia.

All cardiac medications should be administered normally the day of surgery, and a small breakfast can be given six hours prior to the procedure if necessary. Some cardiac medications (angiotensin-converting enzyme [ACE] inhibitors, beta blockers) may predispose patients to hypotension. Administration of vasopressors or inotropes may be necessary to overcome these effects.

The anesthetics used should offset, rather than aggravate, any altered hemodynamics. The aim of the anesthetic protocol is to maintain or increase cardiac output and myocardial oxygenation. Multimodal anesthetic protocols that include benzodiazepines and opioid analgesics are more appropriate combinations in cardiac patients. Ketamine at low doses (0.5–1 mg/kg) may be well tolerated, but at higher doses it can increase heart rate beyond what patients can tolerate. This is especially true in cardiomyopathy patients. The alpha-2 agonists (e.g., dexmedetomidine) should not be used in cardiac patients, especially those with mitral valve insufficiency (Harvey and Ettinger 2007).

12.6.4 Diabetes Mellitus

Diabetic patients can pose some unique challenges in the perianesthetic period. Preoperative 12- or 24-hour blood glucose curves should be current and the insulin dose should be adjusted appropriately to maintain the patient as stable as possible. Preoperative fasting instructions should be designed to minimize disruption of the normal feeding routine. The author prefers patients to eat a full breakfast between 5:00 and 6:00 a.m., with the usual insulin dose administered immediately afterward. Arrival at the hospital is between 7:00 and 8:00 a.m. and the procedure should be scheduled after 11:00 a.m. to enable a six-hour fast.

Upon arrival, and 30 minutes later, the blood glucose should be checked and compared to the most recent curve. It should then be checked again every 30–60 minutes as necessary for patient management. The goal is to have the blood glucose between 150 and 250 mg/dl during the anesthetic procedure (Harvey and Schaer 2007). Patients outside of this range can have atypical drug effects. Commonly, the duration of effect is shortened or prolonged.

If the initial blood glucose is greater than 300 mg/dl and the second is higher, regular crystalline insulin (Humulin R) should be administered at a dose of 0.1–0.2 U/kg IM into the hamstring muscle. This may be repeated every 60 minutes as needed to reduce the blood glucose to between 150 and 250 mg/dl. The rate of blood glucose change should not exceed 75–100 mg/dl/hour. If it decreases rapidly, potassium may need to be supplemented intravenously. If it falls below 100 mg/dl, it may be treated with an intravenous dextrose solution as necessary (Plumb 2008a; Feldman and Nelson 2004a,b).

If the initial blood glucose is between 150 and 250 mg/dl and is stable in that range at subsequent checks, no intervention is necessary. If it is between 100 and 150 mg/dl and the second blood glucose is less than this, intravenous dextrose solutions should be administered to maintain it between 150 and 250 mg/dl.

Anesthesia induction should be by intravenous injection, and rapid airway control must occur. The anesthetic protocol should be nicely balanced and should include drugs that are short-acting or reversible. This type of protocol will also decrease the chance of delayed anesthetic recovery. The blood glucose should be checked every 30–60 minutes intraoperatively so that glycemic stability may be maintained. It should be checked again 30–60 minutes post-extubation. It may be checked more often if necessary, especially if recovery is slow. A regular feeding and insulin schedule should be resumed as quickly as possible post-procedure. In anorectic patients, particularly cats, the appetite can be stimulated by low doses of benzodiazepine (0.2 mg/kg IV q 24 hours) or mirtazepine (1–2 mg/kg PO q 48–72 hours).

12.6.5 Renal Disease

Renal blood flow is closely autoregulated in conscious, healthy patients, but anesthesia blunts or eliminates this ability. Maintenance of renal blood flow by maintaining normotension during anesthesia is thus vital to preserving renal function. Hypotension, even mild, can be devastating to a patient with renal failure. Preexisting hypovolemia will exaggerate it, and metabolic acidosis occurs frequently in renal patients. Renal excretion of drugs is usually impaired, causing delayed recoveries. PCV and total plasma protein (TPP) may be reduced and K^+ may be increased or decreased. Most geriatric patients have some degree of renal impairment, which may or may not be reflected by serum chemistry values.

Diuresis of moderately to severely azotemic patients prior to anesthesia may be beneficial. For diuresis, isotonic crystalloids are administered intravenously at 1.5–2 times maintenance fluid rates. Based upon the 2013 AAHA guidelines, maintenance rates in dogs are 2–6 ml/kg/hour IV and in cats 2–3 ml/kg/hour IV. Diuresis for 12–24 hours prior to anesthesia will decrease the severity of azotemia. Monitoring cardiac parameters and performing regular auscultation of the heart and lungs during diuresis is important.

There is no single anesthetic protocol that is recommended for renal disease. The most important aim of the protocol is to maintain or increase renal blood flow and oxygenation, and to maintain GFR and urine output. Choosing drugs that are less blunting to cardiac function such as benzodiazepines, opioids, and alfaxalone will help maintain circulatory integrity. The inhalant anesthetic drugs are powerful vasodilators, and incorporating MAC-reduction techniques into the anesthetic protocol may be necessary to maintain adequate blood pressure. There is some evidence that low-dose mannitol diuresis may be renal-protective if administered prior to renal ischemic events (Behnia et al. 1996; Fisher et al. 1998). Fluid administration into the postoperative period is dictated by individual patient needs.

12.6.6 Hepatic Dysfunction

It is important to recognize that elevated serum hepatic enzymes indicate only that hepatic cells are damaged and leaking enzyme, not that hepatic function is compromised. This section refers specifically to those patients with decreased liver function, not simply elevated serum hepatic enzymes. Prolonged clotting times, hypoglycemia, and hypoproteinemia are not uncommon and should be addressed prior to anesthesia. Dextrose supplementation or administration of fresh frozen plasma (FFP) may be necessary.

The duration of effect for drugs undergoing hepatic metabolism will be prolonged from delayed metabolism. Drug metabolism may be further decreased due to insufficient hepatic circulation from hypotension or hypovolemia. It is difficult to predict how long drug effects may persist; therefore, choosing drugs have a short duration of effect or are reversible creates the most desirable protocols. The inhalant anesthetics affect the liver primarily by changing circulatory patterns and precipitating hypotension and venous pooling. Maintaining cardiac output and systemic arterial blood pressure becomes a major priority. Administration of vasopressors or inotropes may be necessary to maintain adequate arterial blood pressure. If recovery is slow, administering reversal drugs is warranted, so long as appropriate analgesia remains.

References

Alef, M., von Praun, F., and Oechtering, G. (2008). Is routine pre-anaesthetic haematological and biochemical screening justified in dogs? *Vet. Anaesth. Analg.* 35 (2): 132–140.

Alvaides, R.K., Neto, F.J., Aguiar, A.J. et al. (2008). Sedative and cardiorespiratory effects of acepromazine or atropine given before dexmedetomidine in dogs. *Vet. Rec.* 162 (26): 852–856.

Bednarski, R., Grimm, K., Harvey, R. et al. (2011). AAHA anesthesia guidelines for dogs and cats. *J. Am. Anim. Hosp. Assoc.* 47 (6): 377–385.

Behnia, R., Koushanpour, E., and Brunner, E.A. (1996). Effects of hyperosmotic mannitol infusion on hemodynamics of dog kidney. *Anesth. Analg.* 82 (5): 902–908.

Bidwell, L.A., Bramlage, L.R., and Rood, W.A. (2007). Equine perioperative fatalities associated with general anaesthesia at a private practice – a retrospective case series. *Vet. Anaesth. Analg.* 34: 23–30.

Blike, G.T., Surgenor, S.D., and Whalen, K. (1999). A graphical object display improves anesthesiologists' performance on a simulated diagnostic task. *J. Clin. Monit. Comput.* 15 (1): 37–44.

Boscan, P., Monnet, E., Mama, K. et al. (2001). Effect of maropitant, a neurokinin 1 receptor antagonist, on anesthetic requirements during noxious visceral stimulation of the ovary in dogs. *Am. J. Vet. Res.* 72 (12): 1576–1579.

Brodbelt, D.C., Blissitt, K.J., Hammond, R.A. et al. (2008). The risk of death: the confidential enquiry into perioperative small animal fatalities. *Vet. Anaesth. Analg.* 35 (5): 365–373.

Carter, J.E., Lewis, C., and Beths, T. (2013). Onset and quality of sedation after intramuscular administration of dexmedetomidine and hydromorphone in various muscle groups in dogs. *J. Am. Vet. Med. Assoc.* 243 (11): 1569–1572.

Davis, H., Jensen, T., Johnson, A. et al. (2013). 2013 AAHA/ AAFP fluid therapy guidelines for dogs and cats. *J. Am. Anim. Hosp. Assoc.* 49 (3): 149–159.

De Vries, M. and Putter, G. (2015). Perioperative anesthetic care of the cat undergoing dental and oral procedures: key considerations. *J. Feline Med. Surg.* 17: 23–36.

Doering, C.J., Lukasik, V.M., and Merideth, R.E. (2016). Effects of intramuscular injection of glycopyrrolate on Schirmer tear test I results in dogs. *J. Am. Vet. Med. Assoc.* 248 (11): 1262–1266.

Doi, S., Mori, T., Uzawa, N. et al. (2016). Characterization of methadone as a β-arrestin-biased μ-opioid receptor agonist. *Mol. Pain* 12: 1744806916654146.

Drews, F.A. and Westenskow, D.R. (2006). The right picture is worth a thousand numbers: data displays in anesthesia. *Hum. Factors* 48 (1): 59–71.

Feldman, E.C. and Nelson, R.W. (2004a). Canine diabetes mellitus. In: *Canine and Feline Endocrinology and Reproduction* (eds. E. Feldman and R. Nelson), 486–538. St. Louis, MO: W.B. Saunders.

Feldman, E.C. and Nelson, R.W. (2004b). Feline diabetes mellitus. In: *Canine and Feline Endocrinology and Reproduction* (eds. E. Feldman and R. Nelson), 539–579. St. Louis, MO: W.B. Saunders.

Fisher, A.R., Jones, P., Barlow, P. et al. (1998). The influence of mannitol on renal function during and after open-heart surgery. *Perfusion* 13 (3): 181–186.

Galloway, D.S., Ko, J.C., and Reaugh, H.F. (2004). Anesthetic indices of sevoflurane and isoflurane in unpremedicated dogs. *J. Am. Vet. Med. Assoc.* 225 (5): 700–704.

Griffenhagen, G.M. (2013). A comparison of lidocaine, ketamine, and midazolam for co-induction of anesthesia with propofol in dogs. Abstracts presented at the American College of Veterinary Anesthesia and Analgesia Annual Meeting, 8th September, 2013, San Diego, CA, USA. *Vet. Anaesth. Analg.* 41: A1–A24.

Gurushanthaiah, K., Weinger, M., and Englund, C. (1995). Visual display format affects the ability of anesthesiologists to detect acute physiologic changes: a laboratory study employing a clinical display simulator. *Anesthesiology* 83 (6): 1184–1193.

Hargrove, K. and Hofmeister, E. (2015). Influence of pre-operative blood work and urinalysis on preanesthesia-related decision-making in healthy dogs undergoing elective orthopedic surgery. Abstracts presented at the American College of Veterinary Anesthesia and Analgesia Annual Meeting, 19th September, 2015, Washington DC, USA. *Vet. Anaesth. Analg.* 42: i–ii.

Harvey, R.C. and Ettinger, S.J. (2007). Cardivascular disease. In: *Lumb and Jones Veterinary Anesthesia and Analgesia*, 4e (eds. W.J. Tranquilli, J.C. Thurman and K.A. Grimm), 891–898. Ames, IA: Blackwell Publishing.

Harvey, R.C. and Schaer, M. (2007). Endocrine disease. In: *Lumb and Jones Veterinary Anesthesia and Analgesia*, 4e (eds. W.J. Tranquilli, J.C. Thurman and K.A. Grimm), 933–936. Ames, IA: Blackwell Publishing.

Hay Kraus, B.L. (2013). Efficacy of maropitant in preventing vomiting in dogs premedicated with hydromorphone. *Vet. Anaesth. Analg.* 40 (1): 28–34.

Herminghaus, A., Loser, S., and Wilhelm, W. (2012). Anesthesia for geriatric patients: Part 2: Anesthetics, patient age and anesthesia management. *Anaesthesist* 61 (4): 363–374.

Ilkiw, J.E., Pascoe, P.J., and Tripp, L.D. (2002). Effects of morphine, butorphanol, buprenorphine, and U50488H on the minimum alveolar concentration of isoflurane in cats. *Am. J. Vet. Res.* 63 (8): 1198–1202.

Johnston, G.M., Taylor, P.M., Homes, M.A. et al. (1995). Confidential enquiry of perioperative equine fatalities (CEPEF-1): preliminary results. *Equine Vet. J.* 27: 193–200.

Johnston, G.M., Eastment, J.K., Wood, J.L.N., and Taylor, P.M. (2002). The confidential enquiry into perioperative equine fatalities (CEPEF): mortality results of phases 1 and 2. *Vet. Anaesth. Analg.* 29 (4): 159.

Kastner, S.B., Kutter, A.P., Boller, J. et al. (2005). Cardiopulmonary effects of dexmedetomidine in sevoflurane-anesthetized sheep with and without nitric oxide inhalation. *Am. J. Vet. Res.* 66 (9): 1496–1502.

Keating, S.C., Valverde, A., Johnson, R.J., and McDonell, W.N. (2013). Cardiopulmonary effects of intravenous fentanyl infusion in dogs during isoflurane anesthesia and with concurrent acepromazine or dexmedetomidine administration during anesthetic recovery. *Am. J. Vet. Res.* 74 (5): 672–682.

Ko, J.C., Lange, D.N., Mandsager, R.E. et al. (2000). Effects of butorphanol and carprofen on the minimal alveolar concentration of isoflurane in dogs. *J. Am. Vet. Med. Assoc.* 217 (7): 1025–1028.

Kurita, T., Morita, K., Kazama, T. et al. (2002). Influence of cardiac output on plasma propofol concentrations during constant infusion in swine. *Anesthesiology* 96 (6): 1498–1503.

Lascelles, B.D. and Robertson, S.A. (2004). Antinociceptive effects of hydromorphone, butorphanol, or the combination in cats. *J. Vet. Intern. Med.* 18 (2): 190–195.

Lorenzutti, A.M., Martín-Flores, M., and Litterio, N.J. (2016). Evaluation of the antiemetic efficacy of maropitant in dogs medicated with morphine and acepromazine. *Vet. Anaesth. Analg.* 43 (2): 195–198.

Marks, SL., Kook, PH., Papich MG,. et al. (2018). ACVIM consensus statement: Support for rational administration of gastrointestinal protectants to dogs and cats. *J. Vet. Int. Med.* 32: 1823–1840.

McMichael, M., Herring, J., Fletcher, D.J. et al. (2012). RECOVER evidence and knowledge gap analysis on veterinary CPR. Part 2: Preparedness and prevention. *J. Vet. Emerg. Crit. Care* 22 (S1): S13–S25.

Mitchell, S.L., McCarthy, R., Rudloff, E. et al. (2000). Tracheal rupture associated with intubation in cats: 20 cases (1996–1998). *J. Am. Vet. Med. Assoc.* 216: 1592–1595.

Niyom, S., Boscan, P., Twedt, D.C. et al. (2013). Effect of maropitant, a neurokinin-1 receptor antagonist, on the minimum alveolar concentration of sevoflurane during stimulation of the ovarian ligament in cats. *Vet. Anaesth. Analg.* 40 (4): 425–431.

Pascoe, P.J. (2015). The cardiopulmonary effects of dexmedetomidine infusions in dogs during isoflurane anesthesia. *Vet. Anaesth. Analg.* 42 (4): 360–368.

Petsiti, A., Tassoudid, T., Vretzakis, G. et al. (2015). Depth of anesthesia as a risk factor for perioperative morbidity. *Anesthesiol. Res. Pract.* 2015: 829151.

Plumb, D.C. (2008a). Insulin. In: *Veterinary Drug Handbook* (ed. D. Plumb), 643–650. Stockholm, WI: Pharma Vet Publishing, Inc.

Plumb, D.C. (2008b). Dexmedetomidine. In: *Veterinary Drug Handbook* (ed. D. Plumb), 306–308. Stockholm, WI: Pharma Vet Publishing, Inc.

Pypendop, B.H., Barter, L.S., and Ilkiw, J.E. (2011). Hemodynamic effects of dexmedetomidine in isoflurane-anesthetized cats. *Vet. Anaesth. Analg.* 38 (6): 555–567.

Ramsey, D., Fleck, T., Berg, T. et al. (2014). Cerenia prevents perioperative nausea and vomiting and improves recovery in dogs undergoing routine surgery. *Vet. Med.* 12 (3): 228–237.

Tamura, J., Ishizuka, T., Fukui, S. et al. (2015). The pharmacological effects of the anesthetic alfaxalone after intramuscular administration to dogs. *J. Vet. Med. Sci.* 77 (3): 289–296.

Tevik, A. (1983). The role of anesthesia in surgical mortality of in horses. *Nord. Vet. Med.* 35: 175–179.

Vadivelu, N., Mitra, S., Schermer, E. et al. (2014). Preventive analgesia for postoperative pain control: a broader concept. *Local Reg. Anesth.* 7: 17–22.

Yamashita, K., Okano, Y., Yamashita, M. et al. (2008). Effects of carprofen and meloxicam with or without butorphanol on the minimum alveolar concentration of sevoflurane in dogs. *J. Vet. Med. Sci.* 70 (1): 29–35.

Young, S.S. and Taylor, P.M. (1993). Factors influencing the outcome of equine anesthesia: a review of 1314 cases. *Equine Vet. J.* 25: 147–151.

Zornow, M.H. (1991). Ventilatory, hemodynamic and sedative effects of the alpha 2 adrenergic agonist, dexmedetomidine. *Neuropharmacology* 30 (10): 1065–1071.

13

The Dental Patient and Its General Conditions

Cardiac Disease, Diabetes Mellitus, Pregnancy, History of Seizures, and Brachycephalic Syndrome

Eva Eberspächer-Schweda

Anaesthesiology and Perioperative Intensive Care, Department for Companion Animals and Horses, University of Veterinary Medicine Vienna, Vienna, Austria

13.1 Patients with Cardiac Disease

Patients with dental disease may suffer from comorbidities that need to be addressed before, during and after general anesthesia.

Before elective dental treatment, cardiac patients should be stabilized as much as possible. Treatment should be based on a thorough clinical examination and further diagnostic procedures such as electrocardiography, radiography, and cardiac ultrasound (Harvey and Ettinger 2007). Ideally, medical treatment should be initiated days or preferably weeks prior to dental surgery, in order to reach the following general goals in cardiac patients (Bednarski 1992):

- Maintain or improve cardiac contractility (positive inotropy)
- Reduce myocardial work (decrease afterload)
- Reduce (congestive) edema (diuresis)
- Reduce occurrence of arrhythmias

Most dental patients on cardiac medication should receive it as prescribed even on the day of surgery. Some medications may cause hypotension due to a decreased filling volume (angiotensin-converting enzyme [ACE] inhibitors) or Bradycardia (beta blockers), but these potential complications can be treated during anesthesia if necessary.

In general, a **balanced anesthesia** protocol is recommended, as in any other (compromised) patient (Clutton 2007). **Continuous monitoring** of the patient's vital parameters is mandatory and should include **electrocardiography** (heart rate and rhythm), **pulse oximetry** (arterial hemoglobin oxygen saturation), **capnography** (ventilation and circulation), **blood pressure measurement**, and core **body temperature** (Bednarski et al. 2011). Ideally, monitoring is placed before induction of anesthesia and lasts well into the recovery period in compromised

animals. The anesthetist's goal should be to "keep all parameters within normal limits," with the ultimate aim of maintaining oxygen delivery to the tissues. Ventilation and oxygenation can be supported with a modern anesthesia machine with mechanical ventilator. Physiological body temperatures can be maintained with active heating systems (i.e., forced warm air-blowing devices). **Stress** of the patient **should be avoided** as much as possible (i.e., by intramuscular administration of sedatives prior to induction of anesthesia in excited individuals), and continuous **oxygen supplementation** should be provided once they are sedated/anesthetized. **Intravenous access** and **endotracheal intubation** of the anesthetized patient are mandatory (Skarda et al. 1995a).

Doses for **emergency drugs** (at least atropine, epinephrine, and – depending on the cardiac disease – dopamine or dobutamine) should be calculated and the drugs should be readily available. Every precaution should be taken to save time during the procedure, in order to **keep anesthesia time as short as possible.**

In any case, during the pre-anesthetic evaluation, the owner should be made aware of the (increased) anesthetic risk and should sign a consent form. Dogs and cats should be fasted for six to eight hours prior to anesthesia, but should always have access to water.

In regard to the choice of anesthetics, there is often no true "right" or "correct" drug; in many cases, it may just be a matter of the dose (Eberspächer 2016). The challenge is that there is not one single type of cardiac disease but many different ones, with different stages of progression and severity. Therefore, the anesthetic plan should be individually tailored to each patient. It also helps to understand the basic physiology and anatomy of the heart, circulation, preload, and afterload, as well as the cardiovascular effects of the most important anesthetic drugs (Skarda et al. 1995b) (Table 13.1).

The Veterinary Dental Patient: A Multidisciplinary Approach, First Edition. Edited by Jerzy Gawor and Brook Niemiec.
© 2021 John Wiley & Sons Ltd. Published 2021 by John Wiley & Sons Ltd.
Companion website: www.wiley.com/go/gawor/veterinary-dental-patient

Table 13.1 Cardiovascular effects of important anesthetic drugs in physiologic doses.

Drug	Heart rate	Potential for arrhythmia	Inotropy	Cardiac output	Vascular resistance	Arterial blood pressure
Acepromazine	↔	↔	↔	↔	↓ to ↓↓	↓ to ↓↓
Midazolam/ Diazepam	↔	↔	↔	↔	↔	↔
Butorphanol	↔	↔	↔	↔	↔	↔
Buprenorphine	↔	↔	↔	↔	↔	↔
Methadone/ Morphine/ Fentanyl	awake ↔ anaesth ↓	↔ to ↑ (2nd degree AV-block)	↔	↔	↔	↔ with bradycardia ↓
Xylazine/ Medetomidine/ Dexmedetomidine	↓↓	↑	↔	↓ to ↓↓	↑ to ↑↑	First ↑ then ↔ to ↓ᵃ
Ketamine[b]	↑	↔	↑	↑	↑	↑
Propofol	↔	↔	↓	↓	↓	↓
Thiopental	↑	↑ (bigemini)	↓	↓	↓	↓
Alfaxalone	↑	↔	↓	↓	↓	↓
Etomidate	↔	↔	↔	↔	↔	↔
Isoflurane	↑	←	↓	↔ to ↓	↓ to ↓↓	↓
Sevoflurane	↔	↔		↔ to ↓	↓	↓

Source: Modified from Eberspächer (2016).
↔   no relevant influence.
↑   increase.
↑↑   pronounced increase.
↓   decrease.
↓↓   pronounced decrease.
awake   in an awake patient.
anaesth in an anesthetized patient.
ᵃ Represents the biphasic cardiovascular response of alpha-2 agonists.
ᵇ The indirect stimulating effect of ketamine on the cardiovascular system is diminished to non-existent during anesthesia.

As already mentioned, there are many cardiac diseases in dogs and cats, each requiring a different anesthetic approach (Pascoe 2005). The anesthetic management of the most commonly seen cardiac diseases in dental patients (dilated cardiomyopathy [DCM] and mitral valve insufficiency [MVI] in dogs and hypertrophic cardiomyopathy [HCM] in cats) is discussed next.

13.2 Dilated Cardiomyopathy in Dogs

13.2.1 Preoperative Considerations

The main concerns in patients with DCM are ventricular dilation and reduced contractility, resulting in **systolic dysfunction**, which is often compensated for by an increased preload. This increase in preload causes eccentric hypertrophy, leading to secondary MVI. When advanced, the disease will cause forward failure (lung edema) and backward failure (syncope).

Predisposed breeds include boxer, doberman, cocker spaniel, and giant breeds in general.

Pre- and peri-anesthetic management of dogs with DCM is largely similar to the management of patients with MVI (Steinbacher and Dörfelt 2012). Therefore, the two will be discussed together in the next section.

13.3 Mitral Valve Insufficiency in Dogs

13.3.1 Preoperative Considerations

MVI is the most common acquired heart disease in dogs and is characterized by progressive degeneration of the left atrioventricular valves. Due to mitral incompetence, the valves do not close properly during systole, which results in an abnormal leakage of blood backward from the left ventricle into the left atrium. This mitral regurgitation (MR) may lead to a reduction in cardiac output and lung edema, depending on the severity of the disease.

Predisposed breeds include cavalier King Charles spaniel, dachshund, and other small breeds such as toy poodles, Chihuahua, and Yorkshire terriers. Large-breed dogs are rarely affected, but they may suffer from MR secondary to dilated cardiomyopathy.

The required peri-anesthetic management intensity of dogs with DCM or MVI depends on the stage of the disease. However, the general plan should include (Fox et al. 1999):

- Improvement of myocardial contractility, avoidance of drugs with a negative inotropic effects.
- Reduction of peripheral vascular resistance, avoidance of drugs that cause vasoconstriction (medetomidine, xylazine) (Klide et al. 1975; Evans 1992).
- Maintenance of a physiological to high-physiological heart rate.
- Reduction of (lung) edema by diuresis, avoidance of fluid overload.
- Stabilization of cardiac rhythm, avoidance of arrhythmic drugs (thiopental).

13.3.2 Sedation

The aim of pre-anesthetic sedation should be a calm and relaxed animal, as well as reducing the oxygen requirement without compromising the cardiovascular system. In excited, stressed animals, intramuscular sedation is beneficial. The dose and choice of sedative drugs are based on availability and familiarity, the severity of the cardiac disease, and the patient's character. The following protocols and doses are examples. For further information or a more detailed discussion, please refer to veterinary anesthesia textbooks (e.g., Grimm et al. 2015).

In moderately excited but not overly compromised animals (Eberspächer et al. 2005):

Acepromazine 0.01–0.02 mg/kg PLUS butorphanol 0.2 mg/kg OR methadone 0.2 mg/kg OR morphine 0.2 mg/kg IM or IV.

In severely compromised, geriatric, and decompensated patients (Jones et al. 1979):

Morphine OR methadone OR butorphanol 0.2 mg/kg PLUS midazolam OR diazepam 0.2 mg/kg IM or IV; if necessary (i.e., low heart rate), atropine or glycopyrrolate can be administered.

In already compromised patients that may benefit from a more thorough sedation (i.e., because of aggression):

Ketamine OR alfaxalone 1–2 mg/kg PLUS midazolam OR diazepam 0.2 mg/kg PLUS/MINUS butorphanol 0.2 mg/kg in one syringe IM.

This sedation will never be as deep as when alpha-2 agonists (i.e., medetomidine or xylazine) are included in the protocol, but these drugs are contraindicated in DCM and MVI (Haskins et al. 1986; Pypendop and Verstegen 1998).

13.3.3 Induction of Anesthesia

During this phase, patients should be continuously monitored and oxygen should be administered at all times.

Intravenous induction is preferred over mask induction with inhalant anesthetics. Mask induction with volatile anesthetics like isoflurane and sevoflurane is considered more stressful (due to a period of excitement or struggle), takes longer, and gives the anesthetist poor control of the patient and (especially) the airway. In addition, it involves exposure of personnel to anesthetic vapors. Thus, it is generally not advised to "mask down" a patient. Arrhythmic drugs like thiopental should be avoided.

Appropriate intravenous induction drugs include **etomidate** 1–3 mg/kg slowly titrated IV, best combined with a benzodiazepine (midazolam OR diazepam 0.2 mg/kg) (Robertson 1992). Another option is **ketamine** 1–2 mg/kg IV after good sedation and potentially combined with a benzodiazepine and potentially **propofol** titrated to effect slowly IV (Ilkiw et al. 1992). **Alfaxalone** can also be used, but it can be expensive, especially in larger dogs (Fayyaz et al. 2009).

Patients should always be orotracheally intubated and continuously monitored, with proper hydration maintained by intravenous infusion of balanced electrolyte solutions. Vital parameters (i.e., blood pressure, heart rate, body temperature) should be kept within normal limits.

13.3.4 Maintenance Phase

Again, a balanced anesthesia technique should ideally be used. Often, a combination of an inhalant anesthetic (i.e., isoflurane, sevoflurane) (Rivenes et al. 2001) and opioids (i.e., fentanyl or methadone) or ketamine works very well in providing a stable maintenance phase of anesthesia (Klide 1976). To reduce doses and therefore side effects, local anesthetic techniques should be applied whenever possible.

13.3.5 Recovery and Postoperative Management

The degree of postoperative supervision and care depends on the patients' age the and severity of the cardiac disease as well as the invasiveness of the dental or oromaxillofacial surgery. Ideally, the vital parameters of the patient should be monitored and patient care should aim to maintain appropriate physiologic values. Oxygen saturation should be measured with a pulse oximeter, and supplemental oxygen should be provided, if necessary. Active warming should be started if patients are hypothermic after surgery. Volume status should be evaluated and the infusion rate adapted accordingly. Pain should be avoided by timely administration of the appropriate analgesic agents. In general, recovery should take place in a clean, calm, quiet, and warm environment (Skarda et al. 1996).

13.4 Hypertrophic Cardiomyopathy in Cats

13.4.1 Preoperative Considerations

Primary HCM in cats is an idiopathic or genetic disease of the myocardium characterized by concentric hypertrophy mainly of the left ventricle. Secondary HCM can be caused by diseases such as hyperthyroidism or systemic hypertension and must therefore be addressed as well. Underlying diseases must be treated before anesthetizing the patient, unless emergency treatment is necessary. Depending on the severity of the disease, myocardial ischemia and reduced myocardial relaxation will lead to a left-sided hypertrophy, diastolic dysfunction, and a dynamic outflow-tract obstruction (Poliac et al. 2006).

Predisposed breeds include Maine coon cats, Norwegian forest cats, Persian cats, ragdoll, Devon rex, and

American and British shorthair cats, but HCM can also affect European shorthair cats.

In contrast to most cardiac diseases in dogs, in which – based on history, clinical examination, and auscultation – a preliminary diagnosis can be made and confirmed with cardiac ultrasound, HCM in cats will often not cause any obvious symptoms (e.g., heart murmur). If there is a suspicion toward the disease, it is advisable to perform diagnostics such as a proBNP test or cardiac ultrasound.

The required peri-anesthetic management of cats with HCM depends on the stage of the disease. However, the general plan should include:

- Keeping myocardial contractility low, by not actively force the heart to work harder. Drugs that may increase contractility or cause tachycardia (e.g., ketamine, atropine) should be avoided.
- Decreasing stress! The cat should be handled gently in a calm and fear free environment and pre-anesthetic sedation should be used. Increased oxygen demand and increases in heart rate and blood pressure should be avoided (e.g., ketamine should be avoided).
- Maintenance of peripheral vascular resistance, avoidance of drugs that cause vasodilation (e.g., acepromazine).
- Maintenance of stroke volume.
- Maintenance of a physiological to low-physiological heart rate.
- Stabilization of the cardiac rhythm, avoidance of arrhythmic drugs (e.g., thiopental).
- Avoidance of (diastolic) hypotension; coronary perfusion depends on normotension.

13.4.2 Sedation

The aim of pre-anesthetic sedation should be stress reduction, maintenance of myocardial perfusion, and oxygenation, as well as normotension. Intramuscular sedation prior to catheter placement, gentle handling of the patient, and administration of oxygen will help fulfill these goals. The dose and choice of sedative drugs are based on availability and familiarity, the severity of the cardiac disease, and the patient's character. The following protocols and doses are again **examples**.

In severely compromised and decompensated patients:

Opioids (i.e., butorphanol OR methadone OR morphine 0.2–0.4 mg/kg) in combination with a benzodiazepine (midazolam OR diazepam 0.2 mg/kg) PLUS/MINUS alfaxalone 0.5–1 mg/kg in one syringe IM or one after the other IV.

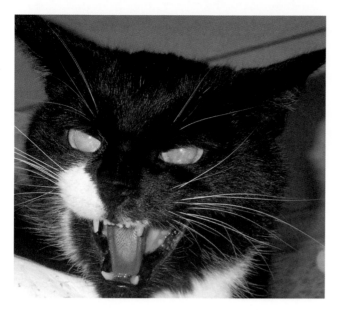

Figure 13.1 Aggressive cats should be sedated by intramuscular injection.

In compromised patients that may benefit from light sedation:

Butorphanol 0.2–0.4 mg/kg PLUS low-dose medetomidine 2–10 µg/kg in one syringe IM or one after the other in lower doses IV (Savola 1989).

In very aggressive cats that need to be sedated intramuscularly (Figure 13.1):

Alfaxalone 2–3 mg/kg PLUS medetomidine 2–10 µg/kg PLUS/MINUS butorphanol 0.2 mg/kg in one syringe IM.

In any case, immediately after sedation, an intravenous catheter should be placed (if not already done), oxygen should be provided, and monitoring devices should be attached.

13.4.3 Induction of Anesthesia

As already mentioned, during this phase compromised patients should be continuously monitored and oxygen should be administered at all times (preoxygenation). Intravenous induction is preferred over mask induction with inhalant anesthetics mostly due to stress. Arrhythmic drugs like thiopental should be avoided.

Intravenous induction drugs that may be used include:

Etomidate 1–3 mg/kg OR **alfaxalone** 1–3 mg/kg slowly titrated IV, both best combined with a benzodiazepine (midazolam OR diazepam 0.2 mg/kg) (Muir et al. 2009) OR **propofol** titrated slowly IV to effect after sedation to reduce side effects (Muzi et al. 1992).

Patients should always be orotracheally intubated and continuously monitored, fluid status should be main-

tained by intravenous infusion of balanced electrolyte solutions, and vital parameters (i.e., blood pressure, heart rate, body temperature) should be kept within normal limits.

13.4.4 Maintenance Phase

Again, a balanced anesthesia technique ideally should be used. Often, a combination of an inhalant anesthetic (i.e., isoflurane, sevoflurane) and opioids (i.e., fentanyl or methadone) works very well in providing a stable maintenance phase of anesthesia. To reduce doses, and therefore side effects, local/regional anesthesia should be applied whenever possible.

13.4.5 Recovery and Postoperative Management

The basic principles of cardiac disease management in dogs also apply in cats. In very aggressive cats, remember to take the intravenous catheter out while the patient is still slightly sedated to avoid unnecessary excitement in the postoperative phase.

13.5 Patients with Diabetes Mellitus

13.5.1 Preoperative Considerations

Diabetes mellitus (DM) results from a loss or dysfunction of the pancreatic beta-cells, often combined with a peripheral insulin resistance. It is a chronic disease leading to persistently high blood glucose concentrations. Typical clinical signs include polyuria/polydipsia, polyphagia, weight loss, and hind-limb weakness. Mobilization of fat can lead to hepatic lipidosis, which will lead in turn to hyperketonemia, ketonuria, and ketoacidosis if untreated. Hyperglycemia will lead to a dysfunction of the immune system, increased oxidative stress, and a pro-inflammatory status, among other symptoms.

A patient with DM should ideally be stabilized before anesthesia and surgery. The general treatment plan, beginning seven days prior to surgery at the latest, should include:

- Full blood panel, including chemistry (electrolytes, acid–base status, glucose, ketone bodies, liver enzymes, and kidney values).
- Urinalysis.
- Treatment of associated diseases (e.g., urinary tract infections, pancreatitis).
- Weight management and a special diet.
- Regular activity.
- Treatment with insulin.

Every change in the daily routine of the patient may have a significant influence on glucose status. General anesthesia will increase counter-regulatory hormones such as cortisol, catecholamines, and glucagon and may lead to an increase in insulin resistance. Therefore, it is crucial to stabilize patients prior to surgery. Anesthesia in an unstable, unregulated diabetic patient should be avoided unless the patient's life is in immediate danger.

During anesthesia, the general goal in these patients is to maintain euglycemia and avoid hypo- and hyperglycemic episodes. It is important to be prepared to treat both scenarios: have (very low doses of) insulin available to treat hyperglycemia and 2.5–5% glucose solutions available to treat hypoglycemia.

On the day of surgery, the patient will be fasted for six to eight hours. Therefore, only half of the usual insulin dose should be administered in the morning.

13.5.2 Anesthetic Management

Any protocol (balanced technique) can be used to sedate and anesthetize a stabilized patient with DM, but alpha-2 agonists (i.e., medetomidine, xylazine) significantly suppress insulin secretion and increase plasma glucose concentrations, and should therefore be avoided (Guedes and Rude 2013). Effective analgesic agents should be used systemically and locally to avoid stress, nociception, and pain, which would affect blood glucose concentrations.

13.5.3 Perioperative Management

Patient blood glucose concentrations should be checked regularly (every 30–60 minutes). In dogs, normal values range from 80 to 180 mg/dl; in cats, they range from 80 to 250 mg/dl. In both species, values up to 300 mg/dl are tolerable in stable DM patients.

- If blood glucose concentrations are below 80 mg/dl, infusion therapy with 2.5–5% glucose in balanced electrolyte solution should be started with about 3–5 ml/kg/hour. Recheck values after 10–60 minutes.
- If blood glucose concentrations are above 300 mg/dl, the patient should be treated with insulin (i.e., normal insulin 0.1–0.2 IE/kg IM or SC). Use insulin syringes for administration and repeat if necessary up to every hour, but not within four hours of when the next regular insulin dose will be administered.

Vital parameters also need to be monitored and kept within physiological range.

13.5.4 Recovery and Postoperative Management

During the postoperative phase, blood glucose concentrations should be monitored every two hours (in very stable patients, every four hours). If available, blood gases and acid–base status should be checked every 12 hours.

Patients should be offered food every two to four hours when awake.

13.6 Pregnant Patients

13.6.1 Preoperative Considerations

In pregnant cats and dogs, the physiology changes to accommodate the growing fetuses. This must be taken into account in anesthetic and perioperative management (Paddleford 1992).

Cardiovascular system: Cardiac output increases, mainly through an increase in heart rate. Therefore, bradycardia should be avoided. In dorsal recumbency, the uterus will (partially) occlude abdominal vessels and decrease venous return to the heart. This can lead to severe hypotension and even collapse if undetected.

Respiratory system: Minute ventilation and work of breathing increase due to increased abdominal pressure. Oxygen demand increases and respiratory depression without supplementation of oxygen quickly leads to hypoxemia.

Gastrointestinal system: There is an increased risk for reflux, regurgitation, and vomiting despite preoperative fasting. The use of antiemetic agents (i.e., metoclopramide and maropitant) and H2-receptor antagonists (i.e. ranitidine) is recommended. After induction, the airway should be secured quickly by intubation and inflation of the cuff to avoid aspiration.

Blood parameters: Plasma volume increases, so hematocrit and total protein will be reduced. This increases the free fraction of drugs, which in turn causes a more pronounced drug effect. Therefore, the dose of anesthetic drugs should be reduced, and if possible titrated to effect (Shnider 1978).

The indication for surgery in a pregnant animal must be carefully weighed against the life and health of the fetuses, since abortion is one of the most common complications. Regardless, the patient should be stabilized before anesthesia and surgery so as to start under best possible conditions. The general treatment plan should include (Holland 1991):

- Advance preparation to keep anesthesia as short as possible; only those dental procedures that are really necessary should be performed.

- Evaluation of blood parameters: at least hematocrit, total protein, glucose, creatinine, and electrolytes (if possible).
- Fetal perfusion and oxygenation depend on cardiac output and oxygenation of the mother. Hypotension and bradycardia should be avoided, and the cardiovascular system should be supported (by intravenous infusion).
- Use of local analgesia techniques to maintain the patient in a light plane of anesthesia.
- Constant oxygen administration and the use of manual or mechanical ventilation in case of hypoventilation.

13.6.2 Anesthetic Management

The anesthetic management and choice of drugs in pregnant patients will not necessarily be the same as would be used for a cesarean section. The management should focus on maintaining the patient's vital parameters within a physiological range to ensure adequate supply of oxygen and nutrients to the fetuses.

Drugs that negatively affect the cardiovascular system (i.e., alpha-2 agonists, acepromazine, thiopental) should be avoided (Gelissen et al. 1996). A balanced anesthesia technique based on opioids (i.e., butorphanol 0.1–0.4 mg/kg IM or IV), propofol (even as constant-rate infusion [CRI]), inhalant anesthetics, and a local analgesia technique will provide adequate anesthesia/analgesia (Ruiz et al. 2016). Remember that the minimum alveolar concentration (MAC) of inhalant anesthetics will be reduced in pregnant animals, so less inhalant is required to maintain anesthesia (Palahniuk et al. 1974).

13.6.3 Perioperative Management

Continuous monitoring, maintenance of vital parameters within a normal range, infusion of a balanced electrolyte solution, and constant administration of oxygen are mandatory in pregnant patients. The animal should be positioned comfortably in lateral recumbency (Kushnir and Epstein 2012). Dorsal recumbency should be avoided; if it is required, a reverse Trendelenburg position (head up and hind end down) may be beneficial.

13.6.4 Recovery and Postoperative Management

The patient should be monitored and supported until fully awake. A quiet, dry, warm, and stress-free environment is ideal for recovery. Adequate analgesia should be provided based on local analgesia and opioids, but nonsteroidal antiphlogistic agents should be avoided (Martinez et al. 1997). It is important to offer food and to send the patient home to a familiar environment as soon as possible.

13.7 Patients with a History of Seizures

13.7.1 Preoperative Considerations

Every dog and cat with a history of seizures should be neurologically examined and (when indicated) treated with anti-epileptic drugs (i.e., barbiturates, gabapentin) (Platt et al. 2006). Administration of these drugs should be continued on the day of surgery. Rarely will the induction of anesthesia trigger seizure-like activity. However, some general rules apply in the handling of these patients (Thomas 2000):

- Avoid stress of any kind and treat the patient gently. Opt for intramuscular sedation if intravenous catheter placement will be a struggle.
- Avoid drugs that may lower the seizure threshold, such as ketamine and potentially acepromazine (however, there is evidence that acepromazine actually inhibits seizure activity; Tobias et al. 2006).
- Administer oxygen at all times to avoid hypoxemia and hypoxia due to an increased oxygen demand caused by increased muscle activity.
- Calculate and prepare emergency drugs in case of a seizure event (e.g., midazolam or diazepam 0.2–0.5 mg/kg IV).

Obviously, an animal in immediate danger for seizure activity will most likely not undergo a dental procedure unless in a life-threatening situation

13.7.2 Sedation

Any protocol can be used so long as it is individually tailored to the patient's needs. As already mentioned, ketamine should be avoided, and the use of acepromazine is controversial. Ideally, drugs with muscle-relaxing properties should be used for sedation and anesthesia; midazolam or diazepam is part of the protocol. Opioids, alpha-2 agonists and other drugs can be combined to provide reliable sedation. In painful procedures, appropriate analgesia should be induced in a timely manner.

13.7.3 Induction of Anesthesia

Thiopental (if available) is considered a second-line anti-epileptic drug and may even have better anticonvulsive properties than propofol, which is considered third-line. Propofol may cause muscle twitching during induction if patients are not properly sedated, so it is recommended to reduce the dose by ensuring prior sedation, a quiet environment, and calm handling of the patient. If no benzodiazepine was used for premedication, it may be beneficial to add it to the induction agent.

13.7.4 Maintenance Phase

Again, a balanced anesthesia technique should ideally be used. Often, a combination of an inhalant anesthetic (i.e., isoflurane, sevoflurane) and opioids or local anesthesia techniques is used. Monitoring and perioperative support of the vital parameters should be self-evident.

13.7.5 Recovery and Postoperative Management

During the postoperative period, the patient should be on seizure-watch. Anticonvulsive emergency drugs (benzodiazepines, barbiturates, and potentially alpha-2 agonists) should be available in case of seizure activity. Recovery wards should be quiet, warm, and dry, and oxygen should be administered if necessary. If benzodiazepines were used in the course of anesthesia, they should not be antagonized in recovery (i.e., with flumazenil).

13.8 Brachycephalic Patients

13.8.1 Preoperative Considerations

The brachycephalic obstructive airway syndrome (BOAS) in dogs and cats is a consequence of misguided breeding standards for certain breeds. Brachycephalic breeds can be extremely "short-headed," which affects the shape of the muzzle and throat. This pathological condition can lead to breathing problems ranging from minor difficulties to severe respiratory distress.

If an animal is in respiratory distress, some general treatment options apply (Figure 13.2):

- Administration of oxygen via mask during induction of anesthesia.
- Rapid securing of the airways by endotracheal intubation.
- Active cooling in case of hyperthermia, often caused by the increased work of breathing.
- Possibly sedation, and in severe cases rapid sequence induction of anesthesia and intubation.

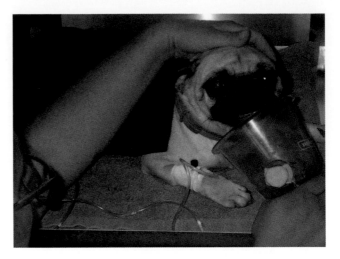

Figure 13.2   Patients with BOAS need special treatment and care.

Common comorbidities of brachycephalic breeds that need to be addressed include gastrointestinal problems (i.e., gastro-esophageal reflux caused by dyspnea). The administration of an antiemetic agent (i.e., metoclopramide or maropitant) and an H2-receptor antagonist to reduce gastric acid production (i.e. ranitidine) is recommended. If signs of pneumonia are detectable, the administration of antibiotics may be indicated.

13.8.2 Sedation

The main benefits of sedation are a reduction in stress (and therefore oxygen demand) and ease of handling. A combination of an opioid with low doses of acepromazine seems to work well for these patients. The use of butorphanol may decrease the coughing reflex in dogs. Small doses of an alpha-2 agonist intramuscularly in cardiovascularly healthy patients seem to be beneficial in facilitating intravenous catheter placement without struggle or stress (Downing and Gibson 2018).

13.8.3 Induction of Anesthesia

Before induction, the patient should always be preoxygenated. The route of oxygen supplementation is important, since a high percentage of oxygen should ideally reach the alveoli. With decreasing effectiveness, oxygen can be supplemented by flow-by with a mask or hose < well-fitted mask < oxygen cage < nasal tube < endotracheal tube. Flow rates are important: if they are too low (especially with narrow tubing), the effect is almost zero.

A rapid sequence induction with a fast-acting induction agent such as propofol potentially in combination with a benzodiazepine like midazolam or diazepam is ideal. The trachea in brachycephalic dogs is usually smaller in diameter than in mesaticephalic dogs (i.e., with a normal head form) of the same weight (Figure 13.3). Due to the short neck, the endotracheal tube can easily be placed too deep into the trachea and create a one-lung intubation. This can be prevented by measuring the length from the canine tooth to the thoracic inlet and memorizing the position marked on the endotracheal tube (in centimeters). If endotracheal intubation is not possible (e.g., due to mass, edema, or reduced opening of the jaw) but the airway needs to be secured, tracheotomy and placement of a (tracheostomy) tube is the treatment of choice. It may be advisable to clip and wash the ventral neck before surgery in brachycephalic breeds, in preparation for a potential tracheotomy.

13.8.4 Maintenance Phase

Beside regular monitoring, continuous evaluation of oxygenation is essential in these patients, especially during the induction and recovery phases. A pulse oximeter is very helpful, as it measures oxygen saturation in the arterial blood noninvasively and continuously. Any anesthetic protocol can be used as long as it is tailored to the individual patient's needs. Local analgesia techniques can be challenging due to the deformed skull anatomy. As in every dental patient, the oral cavity should be inspected after surgery and any debris, blood, or saliva/flushing solution cleaned out before moving on to recovery.

13.8.5 Recovery and Postoperative Management

A stress-free environment, oxygen, continuous supervision, and good airway management are extremely important in this phase. Brachycephalic patients tolerate intubation longer when sedated with opioids. An elevated head position facilitates the decongestion of the edema on the head. One person should supervise the recovery period, especially right after extubation, to ensure a patent airway with sufficient ventilation and oxygenation. Everything should be prepared for quick reintubation once extubated in case unexpected upper airway obstruction occurs (Figure 13.4).

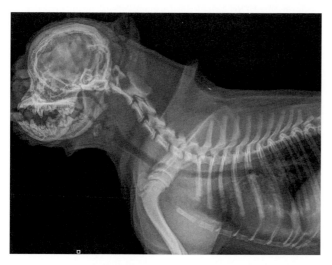

Figure 13.3 The trachea of brachycepalic dogs is smaller in diameter than those of other breeds of a comparable size.

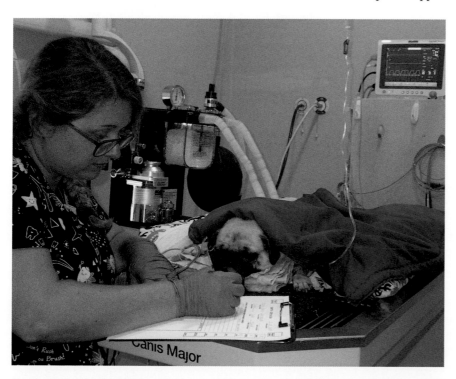

Figure 13.4 Brachycephalic patients must always be very carefully supervised immediately before and after extubation.

References

Bednarski, R.M. (1992). Anesthetic concerns for patients with cardiomyopathy. *Vet. Clin. North Am. Small Anim. Pract.* 22: 460–465.

Bednarski, R., Grimm, K., Harvey, R. et al. (2011). AAHA anesthesia guidelines for dogs and cats. *J. Am. Anim. Hosp. Assoc.* 47: 377–385.

Clutton, E. (2007). Cardiovascular disease. In: *BSAVA Manual of Canine and Feline Anaesthesia and Analgesia*, 2e (eds. C. Seymore and T. Duke-Nowakovski), 200–219. Gloucester: BSAVA.

Downing, F. and Gibson, S. (2018). Anaesthesia of brachycephalic dogs. *J. Small Anim. Pract.* 59: 725–733.

Eberspächer, E. (2016). *AnästhesieSkills*, 1e. Stuttgart: Schattauer.

Eberspächer, E., Baumgartner, C., Henke, J., and Erhardt, W. (2005). Invasive Blutdruckmessung nach intramuskulärer Verabreichung von Acepromazin als Narkoseprämedikation beim Hund. *Tierärztl Prax (K)* 33: 27–31.

Evans, A.T. (1992). Anesthesia for severe mitral and tricuspid regurgitation. *Vet. Clin. North Am. Small Anim. Pract.* 47: 631–635.

Fayyaz, S., Kerr, C.L., Dyson, D.H., and Mirakhur, K.K. (2009). Cardio-pulmonary effects of anesthetic induction with isoflurane, ketamine–diazepam or propofol–diazepam in the hypovolemic dog. *Vet. Anaesth. Analg.* 36: 110–123.

Fox, P.R., Sisson, D., and Moise, N.S. (1999). International small animal cardiac health council 1999: recommendations for diagnosis of heart disease and treatment of heart failure in small animals. In: *Textbook of Canine and Feline Cardiology*, 2e (eds. P.R. Fox, D. Sisson and N.S. Moise). Philadelphia, PA: W.B. Saunders.

Gelissen, H.P., Epema, A., Henning, R.H. et al. (1996). Inotropic effects of propofol, thiopental, midazolam, etomidate, and ketamine on isolated human atrial muscle. *Anesthesiology* 84: 397–403.

Guedes, A.G. and Rude, E.P. (2013). Effects of pre-operative administration of medetomidine on plasma insulin and glucose concentrations in healthy dogs and dogs with insulinoma. *Vet. Anaesth. Analg.* 40 (5): 472–481.

Grimm, K.A., Lamont, L.A., Tranquilli, W.J. et al. (eds.) (2015). *Veterinary Anesthesia and Analgesia: The Fifth Edition of Lumb and Jones*, 5e. Hoboken, NJ: Wiley-Blackwell.

Harvey, R.C. and Ettinger, S.J. (2007). Cardiovascular disease. In: *Lumb and Jones' Veterinary Anesthesia and Analgesia*, 4e (eds. W.J. Tranquilli, J.C. Thurmon and K.A. Grimm), 891–898. Ames, IA: Blackwell.

Haskins, S.C., Patz, J.D., and Farver, T.B. (1986). Xylazine and xylazine–ketamine in dogs. *Am. J. Vet. Res.* 47: 636–641.

Holland, M. (1991). Anesthesia for feline cesarean section. *Vet. Tech.* 12: 397–401.

Ilkiw, J.E., Pascoe, P.J., Haskins, S.C., and Patz, J.D. (1992). Cardiovascular and respiratory effects of propofol administration in hypovolemic dogs. *Am. J. Vet. Res.* 52: 2323–2327.

Jones, D.J., Stehling, L.C., and Zauder, H.L. (1979). Cardiovascular responses to diazepam and midazolam maleate in the dog. *Anesthesiology* 51: 430–434.

Klide, A.M. (1976). Cardiopulmonary effects of enflurane and isoflurane in the dog. *Am. J. Vet. Res.* 37: 127–131.

Klide, A.M., Calderwood, H.W., and Soma, L.R. (1975). Cardiopulmonary effects of xylazine in dogs. *Am. J. Vet. Res.* 36: 931–935.

Kushnir, Y. and Epstein, A. (2012). Anesthesia for the pregnant cat and dog. *Isr. J. Vet. Med.* 67: 19–23.

Martinez, E.A., Hartsfield, S.M., Melendez, L.P. et al. (1997). Cardiovascular effects of buprenorphine in anesthetized dogs. *Am. J. Vet. Res.* 58: 1280–1284.

Muir, W., Lerche, P., Wiese, A. et al. (2009). The cardiorespiratory and anesthetic effects of clinical and supraclinical doses of alfaxalone in cats. *Vet. Anaesth. Analg.* 36: 42–54.

Muzi, M., Berens, R.A., Kampine, J.P., and Ebert, T.J. (1992). Venodilation contributes to propofol-mediated hypotension in humans. *Anesth. Analg.* 74: 877–883.

Paddleford, R.R. (1992). Anesthesia for cesarean section in the dog. *Vet. Clin. North Am. Small Anim. Pract.* 22: 481–484.

Palahniuk, R.J., Shnider, S.M., Eger, E.I. III, and Lopez-Manzanara, P. (1974). Pregnancy decreases the requirements of inhaled anesthetic agents. *Anesthesiology* 41: 82–83.

Pascoe, P.J. (2005). Anaesthesia for patients with cardiovascular disease. Proceedings of the AVA spring meeting, Rimini, Italy.

Poliac, L.C., Barron, M.E., and Maron, B.J. (2006). Hypertrophic cardiomyopathy. *Anesthesiology* 104: 183–192.

Platt, S.R., Adams, V., Garosi, L.S. et al. (2006). Treatment with gabapentin of 11 dogs with refractory idiopathic epilepsy. *Vet. Rec.* 159: 881–884.

Pypendop, B. and Verstegen, J. (1998). Hemodynamic effects of medetomidine in the dog: a dose titration study. *Vet. Surg.* 27: 612–622.

Rivenes, S.M., Lewin, M.B., Stayer, S.A. et al. (2001). Cardiovascular effects of sevoflurane, isoflurane, halothane, and fentanyl–midazolam in children with congenital heart disease: an echocardiographic study of myocardial contractility and hemodynamics. *Anesthesiology* 94: 223–229.

Robertson, S. (1992). Advantages of etomidate use as an anesthetic agent. *Vet. Clin. North Am. Small Anim. Pract.* 22: 277–280.

Ruiz, C.C., Del Carro, A.P., Rosset, E. et al. (2016). Alfaxalone for total intravenous anaesthesia in bitches undergoing elective caesarean section and its effects on puppies: a randomized clinical trial. *Vet. Anaesth. Analg.* 43: 281–290.

Savola, J.M. (1989). Cardiovascular actions of medetomidine and their reversal by atipamezole. *Acta Vet. Scand. Suppl.* 85: 39–47.

Shnider, S.M. (1978). The physiology of pregnancy. In: *Annual Refresher Course Lectures* (ed. ASA), 1251–1258. Park Ridge, IL: American Society of Anesthesiologists.

Skarda, R.T., Bednarski, R.M., Muir, W.W. et al. (1995a). Sedation und Narkose bei Hund und Katze mit Herzkreislaufkrankheit 1. Teil: Narkoseplanung nach Risikobeurteilung, hämodynamische Wirkung der Pharmaka, Monitoring. *Schweiz. Arch. Tierheilkd.* 137: 312–321.

Skarda, R.T., Muir, W.W., Bednarski, R.M. et al. (1995b). Sedation und Narkose bei Hund und Katze mit Herzkreislaufkrankheit 2. Teil: Narkoseplanung an Hand der Pathophysiologie, Herzarrhythmien. *Schweiz. Arch. Tierheilkd.* 137: 543–551.

Skarda, R.T., Hubbel, J.A.E., Muir, W.W. et al. (1996). Sedation und Narkose bei Hund und Katze mit Herzkreislaufkrankheit 3. Teil: Ventilation, Überwachung der Atmung, postoperative Schmerzbehandlung. *Schweiz. Arch. Tierheilkd.* 138: 312–318.

Steinbacher, R. and Dörfelt, R. (2012). Übersichtsarbeit: Anästhesie bei Hunden und Katzen mit Herzerkrankung – ein unmögliches Unterfangen oder eine Herausforderung mit ueberschaubarem Risiko? *Wien. Tierärztl. Mschr.* 99: 27–43.

Thomas, W.B. (2000). Idiopathic epilepsy in dogs. *Vet. Clin. North Am. Small Anim. Pract.* 30: 183–206.

Tobias, K.M., Marioni-Henry, K., and Wagner, R. (2006). A retrospective study on the use of acepromazine maleate in dogs with seizures. *J. Am. Anim. Hosp. Assoc.* 42: 283–289.

14

Ophthalmic Considerations in the Veterinary Dental Patient
Jamie J. Schorling

American College of Veterinary Ophthalmologists, USA

14.1 Introduction

Ophthalmic considerations are an important component of complete care of the veterinary dental patient. Dental disease can cause ophthalmic abnormalities, and an understanding of these conditions can often provide guidance toward more accurate and successful diagnostics and treatment for the patient. Maxillofacial trauma can also cause significant ophthalmic damage, and careful ophthalmic and oral examinations are necessary in patients suspected of suffering trauma. Additionally, given the close proximity of the oral cavity to the eye and orbit, it is critical to protect these structures from trauma during dental procedures. There are also circumstances in which combined dental and periocular surgeries may be indicated, and the pros and cons of simultaneous procedures should be carefully considered. Ultimately, the veterinary dental patient benefits greatly when awareness of ophthalmic health is included in patient care.

14.2 Ophthalmic Manifestations of Dental Disease

Dental disease may cause a variety of ophthalmic disorders, including orbital, periorbital, conjunctival, nasolacrimal, neuro-ophthalmic, and uveal diseases (Ramsey et al. 1996). Knowledge of the anatomical relationship between the teeth and the orbit is vital for prompt and accurate recognition of ophthalmic manifestations of dental disease. Dogs and cats have an open bony orbit, meaning that it is incompletely surrounded by bone (Murphy and Pollock 1993). The orbital floor is soft tissue and includes the zygomatic salivary gland, medial pterygoid muscle, and orbital fat (Murphy and Pollock 1993)

(Figure 14.1). The area is richly supplied with blood vessels and nerves, including the maxillary artery, major and minor palatine areas, and maxillary branch of the trigeminal nerve (Murphy and Pollock 1993). Cranial nerves II, III, IV, ophthalmic branch of V, and VI, the extraocular muscles, and the vascular supply to the orbit and globe are housed within the periorbital cone (Murphy and Pollock 1993). Damage to any of these structures due to dental disease can result in ophthalmic abnormalities.

Clinical presentations of patients suffering from ophthalmic manifestations of dental disease range from chronic intermittent ocular discharge (Figure 14.2) to slow painless progressive exophthalmos, acute onset of unilateral painful periocular swelling with variable exophthalmos (Figure 14.3), blepharedema, conjunctival hyperemia and chemosis, nictitans protrusion, and mucopurulent ocular discharge (Figure 14.4) (Anthony et al. 2010). Pain on opening the mouth is common, due to impingement from the coronoid process of the mandible on the inflamed orbital soft tissues (Anthony et al. 2010). Uveitis is a less common manifestation of dental disease (Ramsey et al. 1996). Many of the acute-onset abnormalities warrant a diagnosis of orbital cellulitis or retrobulbar abscessation, with orbital neoplasia less likely as it tends to present with a more chronic painless progressive exophthalmos. Primary etiologic differentials for orbital cellulitis include dental disease, foreign body penetration (usually via the oral cavity), and hematogenous spread of bacteria to the highly vascular orbital space. In some cases, the etiology remains elusive. A patient presenting with ocular discharge, swelling, or exophthalmos should undergo a thorough ophthalmic examination, including Schirmer tear testing, fluorescein staining, tonometry, and gentle evaluation of the conjunctival fornices for a potential foreign body. Periocular inflammation can cause transient or

The Veterinary Dental Patient: A Multidisciplinary Approach, First Edition. Edited by Jerzy Gawor and Brook Niemiec.
© 2021 John Wiley & Sons Ltd. Published 2021 by John Wiley & Sons Ltd.
Companion website: www.wiley.com/go/gawor/veterinary-dental-patient

permanent keratoconjunctivitis sicca (KCS), monitoring of which permits early intervention to minimize potentially irreversible corneal damage. Exophthalmos, blepharedema, and chemosis can lead to impaired eyelid function and lagophthalmos, resulting in exposure keratitis and potential corneal ulceration (Figure 14.5). Intraocular pressure can be increased from impaired drainage due to orbital venous congestion (Anthony et al. 2010). Nasolacrimal disease should also be considered, as compression of the nasolacrimal duct due to dental disease can result in

ocular and nasal discharge (Ramsey and Fox 1997). When patients present with acute-onset, painful periocular swelling with no obvious primary ophthalmic disease, or if underlying dental disease is suspected, a complete oral examination with dental radiography or CBCT should be considered. Tooth root abscesses can cause retrobulbar abscesses or swelling with abscessation anterioventral to the globe (Figure 14.6). It is essential to maintain awareness that periodontal and endodontic disease and periapical abscessation of the caudal maxillary teeth may not be evident on routine oral examination, emphasizing the importance of dental radiographs (Ramsey et al. 1996).

In many cases of orbital cellulitis, empiric therapy is initiated prior to proceeding with general anesthesia for oral evaluation and imaging. Treatment of ophthalmic abnormalities often includes lubricants, with ointments preferred over solutions if there is any concern about corneal or conjunctival exposure and desiccation. Temporary tarsorrhaphies are warranted if exposure is severe, which is more common in brachycephalic patients. If the cornea is ulcerated, topical antimicrobials should be administered three to four times daily. It may also be appropriate to treat elevated intraocular pressure, if present, with antiglaucoma medications to prevent retinal and optic nerve damage until the orbital inflammation is controlled. It is just as important that the underlying orbital inflammation be addressed with broad-spectrum systemic antimicrobials and anti-inflammatories. Failure to address the systemic component of the illness can result in prolonged patient suffering, increased expense, and potentially unnecessary loss of vision, the globe, and teeth (Ramsey et al. 1996). When clinical signs do not improve, or if they recur after empiric medications are discontinued, further evaluation

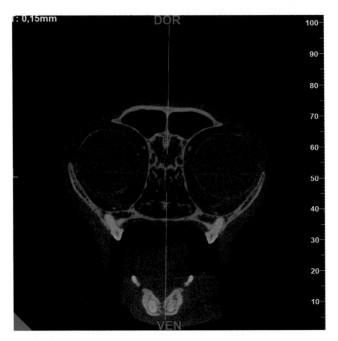

Figure 14.1 CT picture of the orbital area in a cat. Root apices are divided by a thin bony septum from the orbit.

(a)

(b)

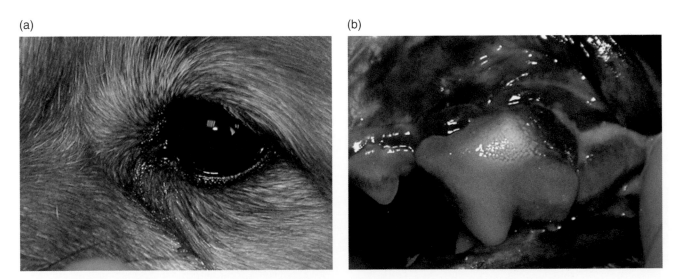

Figure 14.2 Nine-year-old dog with (a) chronic epiphora and conjunctivitis and (b) ipsilateral periodontal disease.

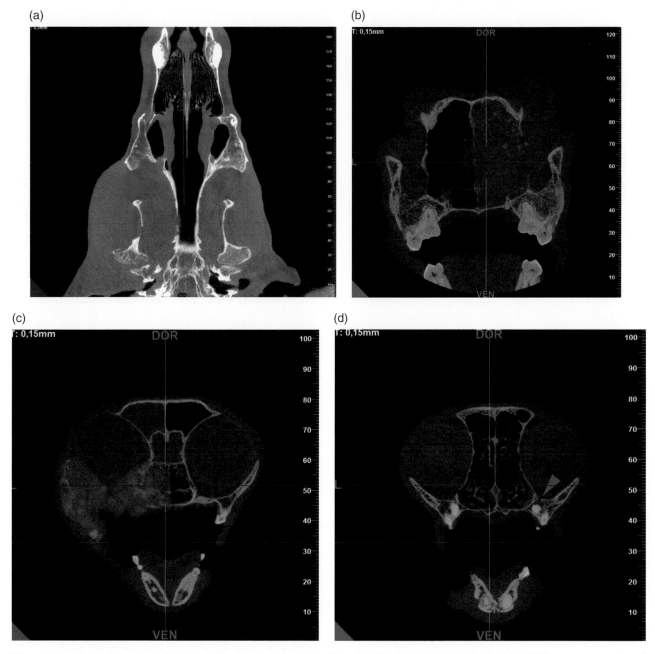

(a)

(b)

(c)

(d)

Figure 14.3 Exophthalmos can be associated with multiple oral pathologies: (a) left temporomandibular joint (TMJ) myxosarcoma in a dog; (b) adenocarcinboma of the right nasal cavity in a dog; (c) left side maxillary osteosarcoma in a cat; (d) odontogenic abscess in a cat (arrow).

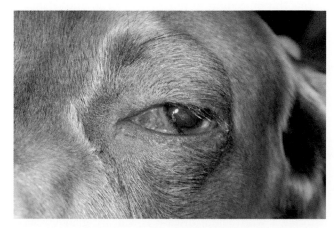

Figure 14.4 Two-year-old female spayed Weimaraner with acute left orbital cellulitis.

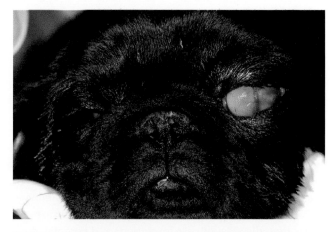

Figure 14.5 Young pug with severe left orbital cellulitis, exophthalmos, exposure keratitis, and corneal ulceration with abscessation.

(a)   (b)

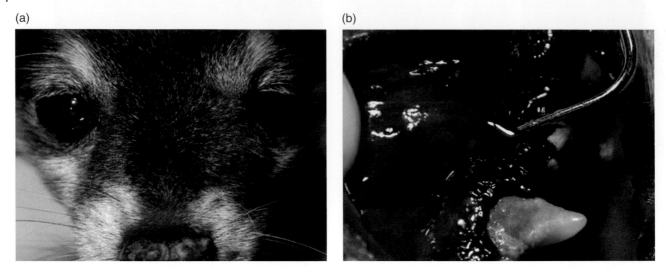

Figure 14.6   Aged terrier mix with (a) acute-onset painful fluctuant swelling anterioventral to the left globe due to (b) tooth root abscess.

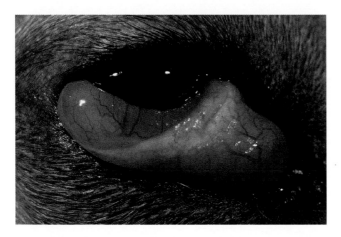

Figure 14.7   Three-year-old basset hound with marked ventral chemosis and nictitans protrusion associated with zygomatic sialadenitis.

for underlying oral disease, foreign body, or a systemic nidus of infection is warranted. Long-term ophthalmic sequelae to chronic orbital inflammation include chronic ocular discharge due to conjunctivitis, nasolacrimal obstruction (Figure 14.8), fistulous tract formation, KCS, persistent exophthalmos and exposure keratitis, development of enophthalmos, and impaired ocular motility due to atrophy and fibrosis of orbital muscles (Ramsey et al. 1996).

Drainage of retrobulbar abscesses via the transoral approach is somewhat controversial, as some individuals feel that drainage of an abscess, if present, is essential to successful therapy, while others feel that surgical drainage is usually low-yield (i.e., inflammation is more diffuse cellulitis than discrete abscess formation) and complications

can develop secondary to drainage attempts (Ramsey et al. 1996; Anthony et al. 2010; Shepard et al. 2011). Use of orbital ultrasound may provide guidance as to the value of surgical drainage. For instance, if a discrete hypoechoic abscess is present, surgical drainage may be more appropriate than with more hyperechoic inflammation.

To perform transmucosal drainage of an orbital abscess, the patient is placed under general anesthesia and intubated to protect the airway from any drainage. The eyes are lubricated with ointment or gel. The oral mucosa 0.5–1 cm caudal and medial to the dental arcade is prepared with povidone–iodine-soaked cotton swabs. A small incision is made caudomedially to the caudal maxillary second molar, with care taken to avoid penetration of the blade deeper than the mucosa so as not to cause laceration of regional arteries. A sterile blunt probe is inserted through the incision and pushed gently through the medial pterygoid muscle into the ventral caudal orbital space. If hemostatic forceps are used, they should not be opened and closed during this procedure, as this could inadvertently damage orbital vessels and nerves. If drainage occurs, it should be submitted for aerobic and anaerobic culture and sensitivity. Some authors recommend gently flushing the orbital space with saline or dilute 0.05% chlorhexidine gluconate solution, however this may exacerbate the degree of orbital swelling and exophthalmos and should be performed with caution. The surgical wound is left open to drain and heal by secondary intention, and postoperative medications pending results of culture and sensitivity are as stated in the previous paragraph (Ramsey et al. 1996; Anthony et al. 2010; Shepard et al. 2011).

A less frequent cause of conjunctivitis and exophthalmos associated with dental disease is salivary gland disease

(a)

(b)

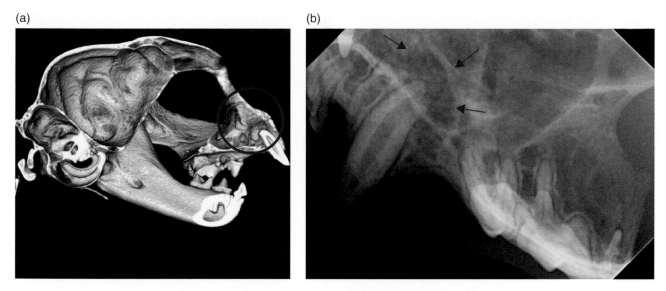

Figure 14.8 The nasolacrimal duct passes next to the apex of the left maxillary canine tooth, which causes an association of canine tooth pulp diseases (circled and arrowed) and epiphora: (a) CBCT and (b) radiograph.

(Ramsey et al. 1996). The zygomatic salivary gland resides in the ventral orbit just dorsal to the roots of the caudal maxillary teeth (Murphy and Pollock 1993). Zygomatic sialadenitis patients are often painful and febrile, with a ventral periocular swelling (Figure 14.7), variable exophthalmos or nictitans protrusion, and pain on opening the mouth (Cannon et al. 2011). Ultrasound-guided fine-needle aspiration yields a yellow tenacious salivary fluid with variable amounts of inflammatory cells. Aerobic and anaerobic cultures are indicated in affected patients (Cannon et al. 2011). Initial treatment includes broad-spectrum systemic antibiotics and anti-inflammatories, though advanced imaging and surgical exploration are often indicated (Cannon et al. 2011). Zygomatic salivary mucoceles (Figure 14.9) and retention cysts tend to cause acute onset of non-painful fluctuant periocular swelling with exophthalmos and nictitans elevation (Spiess and Pot 2013). A cystic structure in the ventral orbit is noted on ultrasound, and ultrasound-guided fine-needle aspiration yields yellow tenacious salivary fluid with minimal inflammation (Figure 14.6). Advanced imaging with CT or MRI is often necessary to delineate the lesion and allow for surgical excision by orbitotomy (Cannon et al. 2011; Spiess and Pot 2013).

Primary oral neoplasia that results in orbital involvement is another ophthalmic manifestation of dental disease. Though potential orbital tumors are primary and malignant, extension of neoplastic processes from surrounding structures has also been documented (Spiess and Pot 2013). If the primary oral neoplastic process is undetected, affected patients may present with a history of gradual non-painful progressive exophthalmos, though additional facial deformities, oculonasal discharge, and

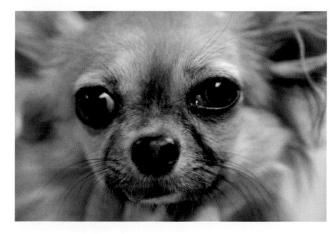

Figure 14.9 Two-year-old Chihuahua with a non-painful fluctuant swelling ventral to the left eye, mild nictitans protrusion, and subtle dorsal globe displacement. A zygomatic salivary mucocele was diagnosed.

other ipsilateral abnormalities are also frequently noted (Figure 14.10) (Spiess and Pot 2013). Advanced imaging and coordinated efforts by ophthalmologists, dentists, surgeons, and oncologists are often required to provide the best treatment options for these challenging cases, and the prognosis for long-term survival is normally guarded to poor, though there is increased survival time with early detection (Spiess and Pot 2013).

14.3 Maxillofacial Trauma

Maxillofacial trauma is not uncommon in veterinary patients, with vehicular trauma, other high-impact or blunt-force traumas, altercations with other animals, and falls from heights (high-rise syndrome) listed as the most common known etiologies (Soukup et al. 2013). Many of these patients also sustain ocular, periocular, and dentoalveolar trauma (Figure 14.11), as well as systemic injuries (Adamantos and Garosi 2011; Soukup et al. 2013). Full systemic assessment and emergency stabilization are of immediate importance. Thereafter, careful neuro-ophthalmic examination and thorough oral examination are essential to achieving complete patient care (Adamantos and Garosi 2011). Prompt intervention with regard to ophthalmic injuries may improve the prognosis for retention of the globe and vision, while in cases of severe proptosis or irreversible globe damage, enucleation will restore comfort for the patient as quickly as is possible. It should be expediently determined whether maxillofacial and dentoalveolar injuries require conservative supportive treatment or

surgical intervention to provide the best possible functional and cosmetic outcome long-term. Failure to properly address these issues can result in increased morbidity and even mortality due to chronic pain and decreased function (Figures 14.12 and 14.13).

14.4 Ophthalmic Care During Dental Surgery

Complete care of the veterinary dental patient necessitates attention to the eye during surgery. It is well documented that general anesthesia causes transient decreased tear production (Krupin et al. 1977; Vestre et al. 1979; Smith et al. 2003; Mouney et al. 2011; Peche et al. 2015). Lubrication of the eyes with ophthalmic ointment or gel

(a) (b)

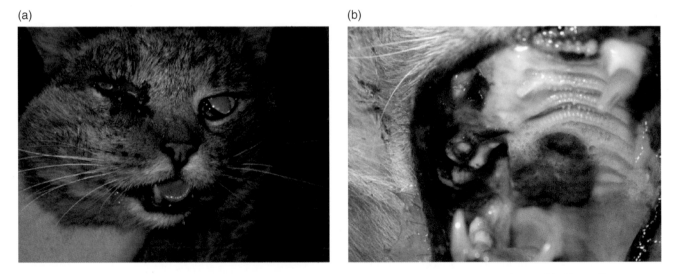

Figure 14.10 Twelve-year-old cat with (a) right side exophthalmos and periocular hemorrhage associated with (b) maxillary squamous cell carcinoma with sinus and orbital extension.

(a) (b)

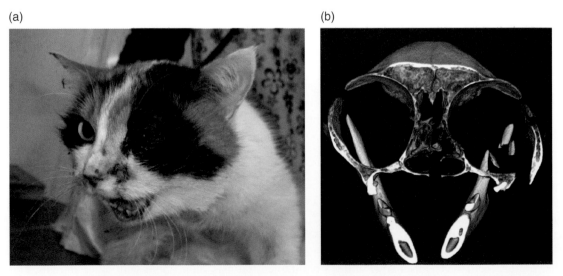

Figure 14.11 (a) High-rise syndrome in a cat, with hyphema OD, periocular hemorrhage OD, and a mandibular symphyseal separation. (b) CBCT imaging reveals extensive damage of orbitum coronoid process and zygomatic arch.

(Smith et al. 2003) is essential to protecting the ocular surface from desiccation and exposure to potential irritants. This is especially important when the oral cavity is irrigated with solutions that may be irritating to the ocular surface (e.g. CHX or sodium hypochlorite). Corneal exposure during general anesthesia and dentistry can result in corneal ulceration, infection, and the need for advanced corneal surgery to prevent potentially irreversible vision loss (Figure 14.14). During prolonged anesthesia, many surgeons recommend repeating ocular lubrication every 60 minutes (Figure 14.15).

Severe damage to the eye and orbital structures can occur during dental surgery due to inadvertent intraocular or orbital trauma from dental surgical instruments and nerve blocks (Guerreiro et al. 2014; Alessio and Krieger 2015; Perry et al. 2015; Troxel 2015). Brachycephalic dogs and cats (Figure 14.16) are at greater risk for such injuries, given the condensed anatomy in these patients (Ramsey et al. 1996; Guerreiro et al. 2014; Alessio and Krieger 2015; Perry et al. 2015; Troxel 2015). Preventative measures are essential, as inadvertent trauma typically leads to high morbidity, with loss of the eye, and even mortality, with potential patient death due to infection or brain trauma (Alessio and Krieger 2015; Perry et al. 2015; Troxel 2015). Key to the prevention of these disastrous events are awareness of the anatomical proximity of maxillary tooth roots and the orbit, accurate interpretation of dental radiographs, and proficiency with dental extraction techniques (Troxel 2015). However, should any type of

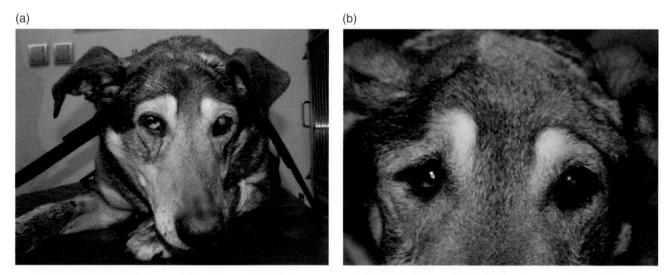

Figure 14.12 (a) Maxillofacial fractures due to vehicular trauma. (b) Severe temporalis muscle atrophy with enophthalmos and vision impairment at long-term follow-up.

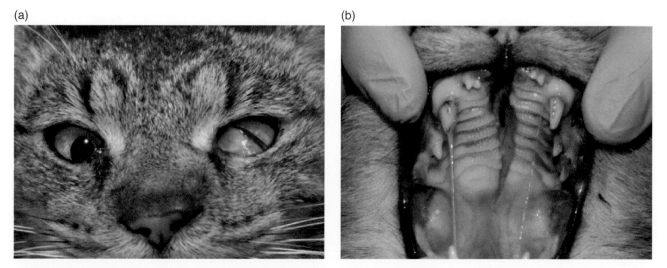

Figure 14.13 Cat with (a) Horner's syndrome secondary to (b) traumatic palatoschisis.

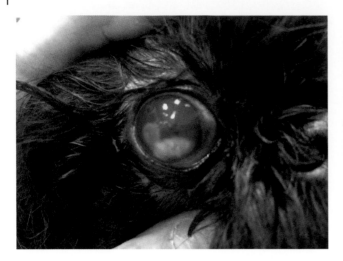

Figure 14.14 Eight-year-old female spayed shih-tzu with deep stromal corneal ulceration and hypopyon three days after dental extractions and cleaning. A conjunctival pedicle flap and aggressive medical management were required to prevent permanent vision loss.

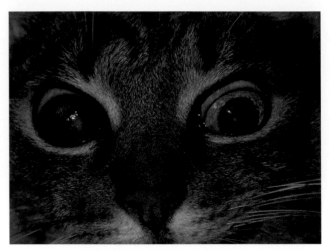

Figure 14.16 Panophthalmitis OD (right eye) in a cat after inadvertent globe penetration during dental extractions. Enucleation was required.

ocular or orbital trauma occur during dental surgery, prompt referral to or consultation with a veterinary ophthalmologist may improve the prognosis for globe retention in certain cases (Withrow 1979; Guerreiro et al. 2014).

14.5 Combined Oral and Ocular Surgery Considerations

In general, the veterinary dental surgeon should proceed with trepidation when considering combining dentistry with most other surgical procedures. Bacteremia and septicemia occur secondary to dental disease and surgery (Black et al. 1980; Nieves et al. 1997; English and Gilger 2007; Lobetti 2007; Westermeyer et al. 2013), while transitioning from dentistry to an ophthalmic or periocular procedure requires changing instrumentation, repositioning the patient, aseptic preparation, and prolonged anesthesia time. For these reasons, it is generally recommended to avoid simultaneous dental and ophthalmic procedures (Ramsey et al. 1996). However, when all aspects of ideal patient care are considered, there are likely a few periocular procedures that it may be reasonable to undertake in the veterinary dental patient: debulking small pedunculated eyelid masses in dogs is a relatively noninvasive procedure that may not require suturing and should heal quickly with minimal complications (Stades and Gelatt 2008), and minor entropion correction is also a low-risk procedure. But these are the only ophthalmic procedures that this author would consider in conjunction with dentistry. Larger eyelid mass excision that requires reconstruction carries greater risk of infection and dehiscence and should not be performed with dentistry (Stades and Gelatt 2008). Similarly, in cats, eyelid masses are

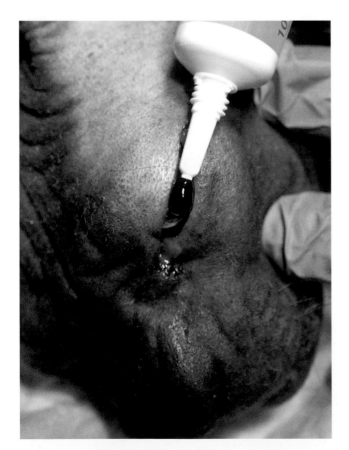

Figure 14.15 During dental procedures, it is necessary to repeat ocular lubrication every 60 minutes or even more often, depending on the ointment applied.

most often malignant and require more involved surgical resection (Stades and Gelatt 2008). Risk of infection and of complications increases with orbital surgeries, including nictitans repositioning and enucleation (Anthony et al. 2010; Shepard et al. 2011), so these surgeries should not be considered when dentistry is performed. Corneal, conjunctival, and intraocular surgeries should be absolutely avoided as the immunology of these tissues is unique (Stades and Gelatt 2008; Lee et al. 2014; De Andrade et al. 2015) and there is a risk of inflammation, infection, and significant damage to the eye and vision when complications arise.

14.6 Conclusion

There are several components of ophthalmology that are important for complete and proper care of the veterinary dental patient. The best possible patient care necessitates that the practitioner maintain an awareness of the close anatomical proximity of the oral cavity and orbital space, ocular manifestations of dental disease, and concerns and limitations of combined dental and ophthalmic procedures.

References

Adamantos, S. and Garosi, L. (2011). Head trauma in the cat: assessment and management of craniofacial injury. *J. Feline Med. Surg.* 13 (11): 806–814.

Alessio, T.L. and Krieger, E.M. (2015). Transient unilateral vision loss in a dog following inadvertent intravitreal injection of bupivicaine during a dental procedure. *J. Am. Vet. Med. Assoc.* 246 (9): 990–993.

Anthony, J.M., Sandmeyer, L.S., and Laycock, A.R. (2010). Nasolacrimal obstruction caused by root abscess of the upper canine tooth in a cat. *Vet. Ophthal.* 13 (2): 106–109.

Black, A.P., Crichlow, A.M., and Saunders, J.R. (1980). Bacteremia during ultrasonic teeth cleaning and extraction in the dog. *J. Am. Anim. Hosp. Assoc.* 16: 611–616.

Cannon, M.S., Paglia, D., Zwingenberger, A.L. et al. (2011). Clinical and diagnostic imaging findings in dogs with zygmoatic sialadenitis; 11 cases (1990–2009). *J. Am. Vet. Med. Assoc.* 239 (9): 1211–1218.

De Andrade, F.A., Fiorot, S.H., Benchimol, E.I. et al. (2015). The autoimmune diseases of the eyes. *Autoimmun. Rev.* 15 (3): 258–271.

English, R.E. and Gilger, B.C. (2007). Ocular immunology. In: *Veterinary Ophthalmology*, 5e, vol. 1 (ed. K.N. Gelatt), 273–299. Ames, IA: Wiley-Blackwell.

Guerreiro, C.E., Appelboam, H., and Lowe, R.C. (2014). Successful medical treatment for globe penetration following tooth extraction in a dog. *Vet. Ophthalmol.* 17 (2): 146–149.

Krupin, T., Cross, D.A., and Becker, B. (1977). Decreased basal tear production associated with general anesthesia. *Arch. Ophthalmol.* 95 (1): 107–108.

Lee, R.W., Nicholson, L.B., Sen, H.N. et al. (2014). Autoimmune and autoinflammatory mechanisms in uveitis. *Semin. Immunopathol.* 36 (5): 581–594.

Lobetti, R.G. (2007). Anaerobic bacterial pericardial effusion in a cat. *J. S. Afr. Vet. Assoc.* 78 (3): 175–177.

Mouney, M.C., Accola, P.J., Cremer, J. et al. (2011). Effects of acepromazine maleate or morphine on tear production before, during, and after sevoflurane anesthesia in dogs. *Am. J. Vet. Res.* 72 (11): 1427–1430.

Murphy, C.J. and Pollock, R.V.S. (1993). The eye. In: *Miller's Anatomy of the Dog*, 3e (ed. H.E. Evans), 1009–1057. Philadelphia, PA: Elsevier.

Nieves, M.A., Hartwig, P., Kinyon, J.M., and Riedesel, D.H. (1997). Bacterial isolates from plaque and from blood during and after routine dental procedures in dogs. *Vet. Surg.* 26 (1): 26–32.

Peche, N., Kostlin, R., Reese, S., and Pieper, K. (2015). Postanesthetic tear production and ocular irritation in cats. *Tieraztl Prax Aus K Kleintiere Heimtiere* 43 (2): 75–82.

Perry, R., Moore, D., and Scurrell, E. (2015). Globe penetration in a cat following maxillary nerve block for dental surgery. *J. Feline Med. Surg* 17 (1): 66–72.

Ramsey, D.T. and Fox, D.B. (1997). Surgery of the orbit. *Vet. Clin. North. Am. Small Anim. Pract* 27 (5): 1215–1264.

Ramsey, D.T., Marretta, S.M., Hamor, R.E. et al. (1996). Ophthalmic manifestations and complications of dental disease in dogs and cats. *J. Am. Anim. Hosp. Assoc.* 32: 215–224.

Shepard, M.K., Accola, P.J., Lopez, L.A. et al. (2011). Effect of duration and type of anesthesia on tear production in dogs. *Am. J. Vet. Res.* 72 (5): 608–612.

Smith, M.M., Smith, E.M., La Croix, N., and Mould, J. (2003). Orbital penetration associated with tooth extraction. *J. Vet. Dent.* 20 (1): 8–17.

Soukup, J.W., Mulherin, B.L., and Snyder, C.J. (2013). Prevalence and nature of dentoalveolar injuries among patients with maxillofacial fractures. *J. Small Anim. Pract.* 54 (1): 9–14.

Spiess, B.M. and Pot, S.A. (2013). Diseases and surgery or the canine orbit. In: *Veterinary Ophthalmology*, 5e (eds. K.N. Gelatt, B.C. Gilger and T.J. Kern), 793–831. Ames, IA: Wiley-Blackwell.

Stades, F.C. and Gelatt, K.N. (2008). Diseases and surgery of the canine eyelid. In: *Essentials of Veterinary*

Ophthalmology, 2e (ed. K.N. Gelatt), 74–77. Ames, IA: Wiley-Blackwell.

Troxel, M. (2015). Iatrogenic traumatic brain injury during tooth extraction. *J. Am. Anim. Hosp. Assoc.* 51 (2): 114–118.

Vestre, W.A., Brightman, A.H. 2nd, Helper, L.C., and Lowery, J.C. (1979). Decreased tear production associated with general anesthesia in the dog. *J. Am. Vet. Med. Assoc.* 174 (9): 1006–1007.

Westermeyer, H.D., Ward, D.A., Whittemore, J.C., and Lyons, J.A. (2013). Actinoyces endogenous endophthalmitis in a cat following multiple dental extractions. *Vet. Ophthalmol* 16 (6): 459–463.

Withrow, S.J. (1979). Dental extraction as a probable cause of septicemia in the dog. *J. Am. Anim. Hosp. Assoc.* 15: 345–346.

15

Oral Health in the Context of Other Planned Surgeries
Daniel Koch

Daniel Koch Small Animal Surgery Referrals, Diessenhofen, Switzerland

15.1   Introduction

Though there is agreement among most veterinarians that oral treatment may affect other parts of the body, no proof of this concept can be found in the literature. There are only sparse comments on the management of timely coordinated interventions. Grove (1985) mentions that a premedication with antibiotics is wise if another surgery in addition to that in the mouth is performed. If periodontal treatment has been provided on the same day, postoperative antibiotic therapy should be given for three days. This concept may be a good rule of thumb and work for healthy patients. Other veterinarians and dental specialists, however, choose a more prudent approach and never combine oral with other surgeries. However, this in turn raises the question whether repeated anesthesia is the better choice for an older animal.

In the past, in young healthy animals, interceptive orthodontics (e.g., persistent or supernumerary deciduous teeth extraction) was recommended alongside neutering. While there is a risk involved in extracting retained teeth at the same time as a sterile procedure, due to the potential for infection at the sterile site, performing both procedures under the same anesthetic might be preferable to administering a separate anesthetic later. Further, clients may neglect to return their pet for extraction at a later date.

Spaying/neutering at the age of six to eight months provides a great opportunity to perform a thorough oral, clinical, and radiographic examination under general anesthesia (Fulton et al. 2014) (Figure 15.1).

One would think that the human literature would provide meaningful answers and offer distinct guidelines. Oral healthcare in animals, however, is significantly different from that in humans. Specialists make most interventions in human beings. There is no question of treating oral conditions in humans while performing other surgeries elsewhere in the body. Risk factors in human surgeries differ considerably from those in animals, and include socioeconomic and behavioral factors. The oral periodontal status in animals is typically significantly worse than in humans because oral cleansing is not routinely performed. On the other hand, the simple fact that in veterinary medicine, the patient and practitioner are of different species significantly reduces the transmission possibilities between the two and lowers the risk of nosocomial infections.

Together, these differences have led to numerous manuscripts dealing with basic information on pathophysiological pathways and precautionary guidelines for prosthetic implants and patients with heart diseases. No single recommendation regarding interventions in the oral cavity and other planned surgeries is to be found.

This chapter summarizes the pertinent information for the veterinarian and provides a working protocol. The author is fully aware that the recommendations lack a fundamental research basis in either veterinary or general surgery. Therefore, the reader is urged to take the information provided and use their clinical judgment to adapt it on a case-by-case basis.

15.2   Pathways Linking Oral Disease to Remote Locations

There are three mechanisms that link oral infections to secondary systemic effects: (i) transient bacteremia; (ii) metastatic injury from microbial toxins; and (iii) immunological injury induced by microorganisms. Most bacteria are anaerobic and, Gram-negative rods (Davis et al. 2013). The close vicinity of the microflora to the bloodstream facilitates bacteremia and systemic spread of products and immunocomplexes (Li et al. 2000).

The Veterinary Dental Patient: A Multidisciplinary Approach, First Edition. Edited by Jerzy Gawor and Brook Niemiec.
© 2021 John Wiley & Sons Ltd. Published 2021 by John Wiley & Sons Ltd.
Companion website: www.wiley.com/go/gawor/veterinary-dental-patient

(a)
(b)

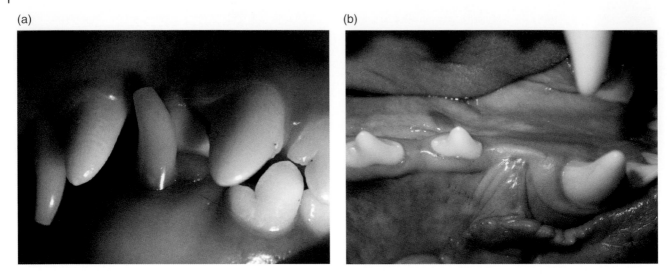

Figure 15.1 Spaying at age six to eight months can be a convenient opportunity for oral diagnostics and possibly for interventions like (a) interceptive orthodontics or (b) operculectomy or extraction of impacted teeth.

15.2.1 Bacteremia

Bacteremia following dental procedures has been well documented in human literature. Bacteremia is observed in 100% of patients after dental extraction, in 70% after dental scaling, in 55% after molar surgery, in 20% after endodontic treatment, and in 55% after bilateral tonsillectomy (Heimdahl et al. 1990). There is even detectable bacteremia before the start of treatment in 9% of children, and simple measures like brushing the teeth increases its prevalence (Roberts et al. 1997).

The estimated rate of dental problems in dogs and cats is 80% (Harvey and Emily 1993), or 90% according to some more recent studies (Fernandes et al. 2012; Queck et al. 2018). Therefore, it is more than reasonable to assume that animals will have similar or even higher risks than humans for developing bacteremia during dental procedures. In an attempt to quantify the timing and quality of bacteremia, Nieves et al. (1997) took blood samples and cultivated them before, during, and after dental scaling in dogs with different types of gingivitis (Table 15.1). Bacteremia was seen in all dogs treated, with no differences in amount or duration between different stages of periodontal disease. It was typically noted at between 10 and 20 minutes after the start of dental scaling and lasted between 50 and 70 minutes in all groups. This study clearly showed that visual inspection of the oral cavity cannot adequately assess the likelihood of a dog or cat developing bacteremia during a simple dental procedure. Furthermore, Gram-negative, Gram-positive, and anaerobic bacteria can be found in the blood of all dogs undergoing dental scaling, regardless of the severity of oral pathology.

Table 15.1 Bacterial genera cultured from both blood and plaque in different classes of gingivitis.

Bacterial genera	Class 1	Class 2	Class 3
Gram-negative			
Pasteurella	*	*	*
Pasteurella/actinomyces	*	*	*
Pseudomonas	*	*	
Atypical pseudomonas	*	*	*
Gram-positive			
Actinomyces	*		*
Corynebacterium	*	*	*
Alpha-hemolytic streptococcus	*	*	*
Gamma streptococcus		*	*
Anaerobic			
Bacteroides	*	*	*
Porphyromonas			*
Prevotella	*		*
Fusobacterium			*
Lactobacillus			*
Propionibacterium			*

Source: After Nieves et al. (1997).
Class 1, mild gingivitis; class 2, moderate gingivitis; class 3, severe gingivitis and periodontitis. n = 20 dogs.
* denotes genera common to blood and plaque.

Rates of bacteremia after dental procedures do vary significantly with the type of intervention, however. Pertinent data can be obtained from human research (Watters et al. 2013). The riskiest procedures are dental extractions and periodontal treatment, including gingivectomy and scaling, with an average incidence of about

65% for developing a bacteremia (Figure 15.2). Even probing in patients with periodontal disease results in bacteremia in about 30% of cases. Orthodontic and most of endodontic treatments are less at risk, mainly because the indications are not infection. In summary, the veterinarian must realize that even a brief, minor scaling in a dog with mild gingivitis results in the same bacteremia as is seen in general dental treatment in a dog with severe periodontitis – and that dental extractions carry a significant risk for severe short-term bacteremia.

Nevertheless, daily activities such as mastication and tooth brushing in humans result in more bacteremia than does a professional cleaning (Guntheroth 1984; Glass et al. 1989; Hartzell et al. 2005) (Table 15.2).

15.2.2 Entotoxins

Some oral bacteria – mainly the Gram-negative ones – have the ability to produce endotoxins, which are composed of lipopolysaccharides (LPSs). These are released from the

(a)

(b)

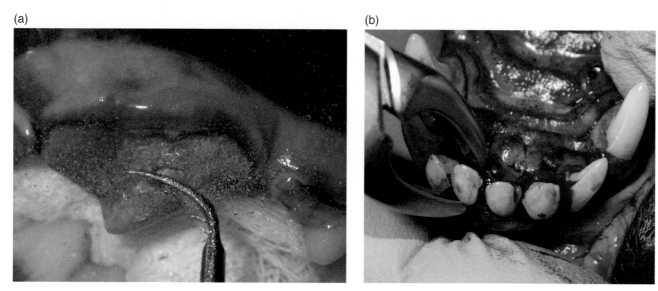

Figure 15.2   Teeth descaling (a) and dental extractions (b) are both associated with bacteremia.

Table 15.2   Incidence of bacteria by procedure group in human dentistry.

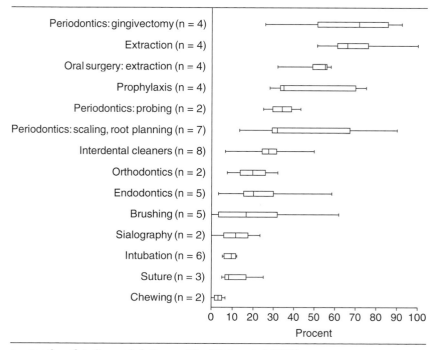

n = number of studies pooled. *Source:* After Watters et al. (2013).

cell wall during cell death and division. The polysaccharide portion varies considerably and is not responsible for the toxic effect, whereas the lipid-A portion remains constant between bacterial species and initiates the pathological alterations. During the course of periodontal disease, the portion of Gram-negative bacteria increases, and so too does that of LPSs, which are released into the gingival crevicular fluid and enter the gingival epithelium. There, they stimulate cells to release cytokines associated with inflammation (interleukin 1, interleukin 6, prostaglandin E_2, tumor necrosis factor alpha) and induce a B-cell response (plasma cells, antibody response). Together with the bacteria, LPSs, cytokines, and other inflammatory mediators can enter into the circulation and cause systemic effects (DeBowes 1998; Rawlinson et al. 2011; Nemec et al. 2013).

15.2.3 Immunological Injury

The third link from oral infection to systemic disease is provided by metastatic immunological injury. Soluble antigens may enter the bloodstream, react with specific antibodies, and form a macromolecular complex. These immunocomplexes can give rise to a variety of acute and chronic inflammatory reactions at the site of deposition, such as polyarthritis, uveitis, nerve paralysis, and neutrophil dysfunction (Thoden van Velzen et al. 1984).

15.2.4 Impact on Other Organs

While it is proven that bacteria and endotoxins enter the general circulation in large amounts mainly during scaling and extractions and in smaller amounts on a daily basis, the question must be raised: "Do they create any harm in the body?" Human research focuses mainly on the risks that come along with existing periodontal disease. Proven relations are reported on atheroma and thrombus formation, leading to atherosclerosis and myocardial infarction (Hamilton et al. 2017). People with preexisting heart disease are at risk for endocarditis when their teeth are scaled or extracted. Old and immunocompromised patients develop bacterial pneumonia by means of direct aspiration of bacteria or hematogenous spread during dental procedures. Low birth weight is strongly correlated to the periodontal status of the mother. Diabetes mellitus is a risk factor for periodontal disease, and simultaneously periodontal infection induces a chronic state of insulin resistance (Li et al. 2000).

Similar research was conducted in dogs by DeBowes et al. (1996), who compared a periodontal disease score to histopathological changes in several organs at necropsy. They found an association between the periodontal tissue and hepatic parenchymal inflammation, fibrotic myocytes,

and low-grade insulted kidney, whereas lung, spleen, tonsils, and submandibular lymph nodes showed no correlation. Pavlica et al. (2008) even demonstrated that periodontal disease burden is linked to the gross and histopathology scores in liver, kidney, and atrioventricular valves. These studies imply that plaque bacteria resulting in periodontitis contribute to the development of chronic systemic tissue alterations in most parts of the body, in cats and dogs as well as in humans.

In the liver, oral bacterial invasion has been shown to increase parenchymal inflammation and portal fibrosis (DeBowes et al. 1996). Pavlica et al. (2008) showed a significant relationship between periodontal disease burden and inflammation in the hepatic parenchyma. Furthermore, generalized bacteremias (some of which are plausibly oral in origin) have been shown to cause cholestasis in dogs (Taboada and Meyer 1989; Center 1990).

Periodontal disease has been proposed as a risk factor for the development of chronic kidney disease in dogs and cats (O'Neill et al. 2013; Finch et al. 2016). A large retrospective study showed increased risk in cats of both chronic kidney disease and cystitis incidence with increasing periodontal scores (Trevejo et al. 2018). These changes are proposed to be due to chronic inflammation and secondary scarring of the organ, resulting in decreased function over time (DeBowes et al. 1996; Pavlica et al. 2008).

Ultimately, the relationship between oral health and orthopedic implants must be cleared. Steel implants have a three times lower resistance to infection than titanium ones (Arens et al. 1996), which is explained by their different biocompatibility characteristics: soft tissue adheres firmly to titanium implant surfaces, while around steel implants, a fibrous capsule enclosing a dead space filled with liquid forms, in which bacteria can spread and multiply and are less accessible to defense mechanisms and antibiotics. In the presence of a bacteremia after oral intervention, however, the tissue around such implants was not infected by these bacteria in an otherwise healthy patient (Waldman et al. 1997; LaPorte et al. 1999). Prophylactic antibiotic use has no effect on the occurrence of implant infections. Therefore, the recommendation is to perform a preoperative exam and test for concurrent general diseases, and to evaluate whether risks factors other than oral disease might contribute to infection of an orthopedic or prosthetic implant.

In conclusion, chronic periodontal disease leads to tissue alterations, which may predispose to specific organ failures or make an organ susceptible for infection during stress, trauma, or surgery. All dental procedures – but mainly scaling and probing in the presence of a gingivitis, as well as extractions – lead to short-term bacteremia, but healthy tissue and orthopedic implants are not affected by it.

Unfortunately, no studies can be found that evaluate probable deleterious effects of dental interventions conducted at the same time as surgeries on other parts of the body. In human medicine, such a study concept finds no clinical analog. In veterinary medicine, however, it can be assumed that many veterinarians have performed dental scaling before or after spaying or other soft-tissue surgery without being aware that the risk for an infection was dramatically increased. Because objective data are lacking, the following recommendations are based on current knowledge and must be evaluated by future research projects.

15.3 Guidelines for the Veterinarian

15.3.1 Classification Systems

15.3.1.1 Dental Procedures
Class A, intervention in minor infected tissue:

- no preexisting systemic effects expected
- causes mild transient bacteremia
- examples: orthodontic and endodontic procedures

Class B, intervention in major infected tissue:

- mainly preexisting infections and inflammations
- causes transient bacteremia
- examples: scaling, gingivectomy, extractions, periodontal interventions

15.3.1.2 Other Planned Surgeries (Established Classification)
Class I, clean surgeries:

- uninfected, no inflammation
- respiratory, gastrointestinal, and urogenital tract not entered
- closed primarily
- examples: explorative laparotomy, splenectomy, mastectomy, many orthopedic surgeries, closed-fracture stabilization

Class II, clean–contaminated surgeries:

- respiratory, gastrointestinal, and urogenital tract entered and controlled
- no unusual contamination
- examples: liver and gastrointestinal surgery, cystotomy, ovariohysterectomy

Class III, contaminated surgeries:

- open, fresh, accidental wounds
- major break in sterile technique, gross spillage from gastrointestinal tract
- acute nonpurulent inflammation
- examples: rectal surgery, penetrating wounds, traumatic abrasions

Class IV, dirty surgeries:

- old traumatic wounds, devitalized tissue
- existing infection or perforation
- bacteria present before procedure
- examples: old abscessation on skin or internal organs, bowel perforation

15.3.2 Considerations

When the veterinarian must decide if procedures may be combined or staged, a rough estimation of tissue healing and bacteremia time is mandatory. Class A dental procedures may result in short-term bacteremia, whereas class B will lead to a longer bacteremia duration. In a similar way, class I–IV surgeries result in bacteremia lasting minutes to hours. Infection of distant organs can be prevented by perioperative antibiotics.

The healing ability of the oral cavity is very good and is rarely affected by other surgeries. Most tissues in the other parts of the body, however, should remain sterile and are at greater risk for complications as a result of infection form a dental procedure (e.g., intestines, joints).

During the healing period of these specific organs (Table 15.3), the injured tissue may be susceptible to infection, because the vascularization and host-defense mechanisms are not yet established. Bacteria from the oral cavity may cause infection and challenge the expected normal outcome. It is therefore not recommended to burden the body with extra microbials from the oral cavity (Figure 15.3).

Different conclusions may be drawn when a dog or cat is old or has a specific risk for anesthesia. The veterinarian must then weigh the risks of a second anesthesia against the risk of infection in a distant organ. In an emergency situation, however, they must open the thorax or abdomen or approach a bone even when dental treatments have recently been performed.

15.3.3 Recommendations

For a complete list of recommendations, see Table 15.3.

Table 15.3 Expected healing times for different tissues.

Skin, subcutis, small intestines	7 days
Joint capsule, large intestines	14 days
Muscle, fascia, ligaments	7 weeks
Bone, tendon	12–15 weeks
Neurotissue	Weeks to years

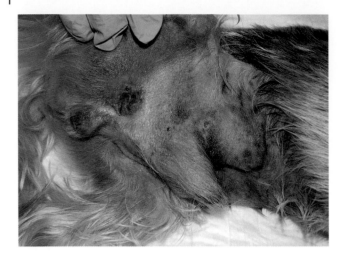

Figure 15.3 This patient, a 9-year-old Yorkshire terrier underwent castration and under the same anaesthesia teeth descaling was performed. 2 days after was presented with severe signs of sepsis and the surgical wounds were dehiscent and infected.

Table 15.4 Recommendations when dental (class A or B) and other surgeries (class I, II, III, or IV) are planned.

	Dental procedure Class A (endodontics, orthodontics)	Dental procedure Class B (periodontal, extractions)
Other planned surgery Class I, clean	Combination: no Order: dental at least one day before Antibiotics: only perioperative Exceptions: no	Combination: no Order: dental at least seven days before or after Antibiotics: 10 days, depending on periodontal status Exceptions: no
Other planned surgery Class II, clean–contaminated	Combination: no Order: dental at least one day before Antibiotics: no preventive or prolonged needed Exceptions: anesthesia risk	Combination: no Order: dental at least seven days before or after Antibiotics: 10 days, depending on periodontal status Exceptions: no
Other planned surgery Class III, contaminated	Combination: yes Order: dental first Antibiotics: peri- and postoperative Exceptions:	Combination: no Order: dental at least three days after Antibiotics: peri- and postoperative Exceptions: anesthesia risk
Other planned surgery Class IV, dirty	Combination: yes Order: dental first Antibiotics: at least 10 days, depending on other surgery tissue status Exceptions:	Combination: yes Order: dental after Antibiotics: at least 10 days, depending on other surgery tissue status Exceptions:

Source: After Hosgood (2003).

References

Arens, S., Schlegel, U., Printzen, G. et al. (1996). Influence of materials for fixation implants on local infection. An experimental study of steel versus titanium DCP in rabbits. *J. Bone Joint Surg. Br.* 78: 647–651.

Center, S.A. (1990). Hepatobilliary infections. In: *Infectious Diseases of the Dog and Cat* (ed. C.E. Green), 146–156. Philadelphia, PA: W.B. Saunders.

Davis, I.J., Wallis, C., Deusch, O. et al. (2013). A cross-sectional survey of bacterial species in plaque from client owned dogs with healthy gingiva, gingivitis or mild periodontitis. *PLoS One* 8 (12): e83158.

DeBowes, L.J. (1998). The effects of dental disease on systemic disease. *Vet. Clin. North Am. Small Anim. Pract.* 28: 1057–1062.

DeBowes, L.J., Mosier, D., Logan, E. et al. (1996). Association of periodontal disease and histologic lesions in multiple organs from 45 dogs. *J. Vet. Dent.* 13: 57–60.

Fernandes, N.A., Batista Borges, A.P., Carlo Reis, E.C. et al. (2012). Prevalence of periodontal disease in dogs and owners' level of awareness – a prospective clinical trial. *Rev. Ceres Viçosa* 59 (4): 446–451.

Finch, N.C., Syme, H.M., and Elliott, J. (2016). Risk factors for development of chronic kidney disease in cats. *J. Vet. Intern. Med.* 30 (2): 602–610.

Fulton, A.J., Fiani, N., and Verstraete, F.J.M. (2014). Canine Pediatric Dentistry. *Vet. Clin. Small Anim.* 44: 303–324.

Glass, R.T., Martin, M.E., and Peter, L.J. (1989). Transmission of disease in dogs by toothbrushing. *Quintessence Int.* 20 (11): 819–824.

Grove, T.K. (1985). Periodontal disease. In: *Veterinary Dentistry* (ed. C.E. Harvey), 59–78. Philadelphia, PA: W.B. Saunders.

Guntheroth, W.G. (1984). How important are dental procedures as a cause of infective endocarditis. *Am. J. Cardiol.* 54 (7): 797–801.

Hamilton, J.A., Hasturk, H., Kantarci, A., Serhan, C.N., and Van Dyke, T. (2017). Atherosclerosis, Periodontal Disease, and Treatment with Resolvins. *Curr Atheroscler Rep.* Nov 6;19 (12): 57. doi: 10.1007/s11883-017-0696-4. PMID: 29110146.

Hartzell, J.D., Torred, K.P., and Wortmann, G. (2005). Incidence of bacteremia after routine tooth brushing. *Am. J. Med. Sci.* 329: 178–180.

Harvey, C.E. and Emily, P.P. (eds.) (1993). *Veterinary Dentistry*. Philadelphia, PA: W.B. Saunders.

Heimdahl, A., Hall, G., Hedberg, M. et al. (1990). Detection and quantitation by lysis-filtration of bacteremia after different oral surgical procedures. *J. Clin. Microbiol.* 28: 2205–2209.

Hosgood, G. (2003). Wound repair and specific tissue reponse to injury. In: *Textbook of Small Animal Surgery* (ed. D. Slatter), 66–86. Philadelphia, PA: W.B. Saunders.

LaPorte, D.M., Waldman, B.J., Mont, M.A., and Hungerford, D.S. (1999). Infections associated with dental procedures in total hip arthroplasty. *J. Bone Joint Surg. Br.* 81: 56–59.

Li, X., Kolltveit, K.M., Tronstad, L., and Olsen, I. (2000). Systemic diseases caused by oral infection. *Clin. Microbiol. Rev.* 13: 547–558.

Nemec, A., Verstraete, F.J., Jerin, A. et al. (2013). Periodontal disease, periodontal treatment and systemic nitric oxide in dogs. *Res. Vet. Sci.* 94 (3): 542–544.

Nieves, M.A., Hartwig, P., Kinyon, J.M., and Riedesel, D.H. (1997). Bacterial isolates from plaque and from blood during and after routine dental procedures in dogs. *Vet. Surg.* 26: 26.

O'Neill, D.G., Elliott, J., Church, D.B. et al. (2013). Chronic kidney disease in dogs in UK veterinary practices: prevalence, risk factors, and survival. *J. Vet. Intern. Med.* 27 (4): 814–821.

Pavlica, Z., Petelin, M., Juntes, P. et al. (2008). Periodontal disease burden and pathological changes in organs of dogs. *J. Vet. Dent.* 25: 97–105.

Queck, K.E., Chapman, A., Herzog, L.J. et al. (2018). Oral-fluid thiol-detection test identifies underlying active periodontal disease not detected by the visual awake examination. *J. Am. Anim. Hosp. Assoc.* 54 (3): 132–137.

Rawlinson, J.E., Goldstein, R.E., Reiter, A.M. et al. (2011). Association of periodontal disease with systemic health indices in dogs and the systemic response to treatment of periodontal disease. *J. Am. Vet. Med. Assoc.* 238 (5): 601–609.

Roberts, G.J., Holzel, H.S., Sury, M.R. et al. (1997). Dental bacteremia in children. *Pediatr. Cardiol.* 18: 24–27.

Taboada, J. and Meyer, D.J. (1989). Cholestasis in associated with extrahepatic bacterial infection in five dogs. *J. Vet. Intern. Med.* 3: 216–220.

Thoden van Velzen, S.K., Abraham-Inpijn, L., and Moorer, W.R. (1984). Plaque and systemic disease: a reappraisal of the focal infection concept. *J. Clin. Periodontol.* 11: 209–220.

Trevejo, R.T., Lefebvre, S.L., Yang, M. et al. (2018). Survival analysis to evaluate associations between periodontal disease and the risk of development of chronic azotemic kidney disease in cats evaluated at primary care veterinary hospitals. *J. Am. Vet. Med. Assoc.* 252 (6): 710–720.

Waldman, B.J., Mont, M.A., and Hungerford, D.S. (1997). Total knee arthroplasty infections associated with dental procedures. *Clin. Orthop. Relat. Res.*: 164–172.

Watters, W. 3rd, Rethman, M.P., Hanson, N.B. et al. (2013). Prevention of orthopaedic implant infection in patients undergoing dental procedures. *J. Am. Acad. Orthop. Surg.* 21: 180–189.

16

Systemic Diseases Influencing Oral Health and Conditions

Jerzy Gawor

Veterinary Clinic Arka, Kraków, Poland

16.1 Introduction

The oral cavity is not an isolated area and many systemic conditions will influence the condition of the oral structures. In carnivores, it is not only the beginning of the alimentary tract also it serves as a sensory apparatus, is an important part of thermoregulation, plays a role in behavioral communication, and is critical for self-defense. It also provides grooming support in cats. Due to the possibility of the veterinarian being bitten, it is often not thoroughly inspected, which results in many missed pathologies.

Once an oral lesion is noticed, veterinarians and owners can mistakenly classify the pathology as only a local problem, often associated with the teeth. Attention to the patient as a whole is important to avoid this "tunnel vision" creating a misdiagnosis where an oral lesion is only a part of a wider clinical syndrome. Thus, it is important to take into account the varied possible causes of an oral lesion, collect a complete history, and perform a thorough general physical examination.

The conditions presented in this chapter include selected systemic diseases that, in their clinical appearance, affect the oral health or its functionality. More information can be found in Chapters 10 and 18.

16.2 Genetic and Developmental Disorders

Cleft lip or palate, hydrocephalus, and deformations of the palate, nose, pharynx, lip, or tongue are not only associated with malfunction of the oral cavity but can lead to severe consequences or even death. Evaluation for these conditions should be part of every first "well puppy or kitten"

examination and of all visits during the first six months of life (Figure 16.1).

Cleft palates result from incorrect development of either the primary or the secondary palate. The primary palate forms from fusion of the nasal prominences, while secondary palate formation relies on fusion of maxillary processes (Kelly and Bardach 2012). A thorough examination of the entire maxillofacial area, preferably with 3D imaging (CT scan), is indicated in animals affected by cleft palate to rule out other abnormalities (Nemec et al. 2015) (Figure 16.2).

Congenital hydrocephalus can lead to significant malformations of the head and subsequent changes of the relations of the jaw length, and thus create a malocclusion (Figure 16.3). It can also be associated with other congenital conditions such as cleft palate.

All of these problems negatively influence suckling and intake of nutrients, and therefore the affected patient typically does not develop correctly and may differ from the rest of the litter. Some conditions are lethal (i.e., microglossia or aglossia) (Figure 16.4), but others, despite causing significant difficulties in function and quality of life (QOL), do not always result in death. Corrective surgery is possible in many cases and can improve QOL and functionality of the mouth.

Siamese twins in cats and dogs are rare and most do not survive long (Mazzullo et al. 2009). Fused heads or dicephalic individuals are prone to serious anatomic disorders of the entire body and are often associated with cleft lips and palates, which makes their survival very limited.

Masticatory muscle myositis (MMM), craniomandibular osteopathy (CMO), and temporomandibular joint (TMJ) dysplasia all affect the functionality of the masticatory apparatus and the comfort of the patient. A commercial laboratory test is available to detect patients with CMO (or

The Veterinary Dental Patient: A Multidisciplinary Approach, First Edition. Edited by Jerzy Gawor and Brook Niemiec.
© 2021 John Wiley & Sons Ltd. Published 2021 by John Wiley & Sons Ltd.
Companion website: www.wiley.com/go/gawor/veterinary-dental-patient

those that carry the genetic predisposition), which is worth performing in predisposed breeds. Diagnosing MMM requires a laboratory test for antibodies and is only effective in the acute period. Muscle biopsy has supportive

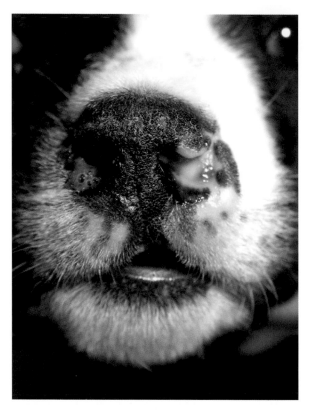

Figure 16.1 Oral and maxillofacial assessment in young individuals should be focused on the presence of developmental defects and their signalments. Nasal discharge in a puppy can be associated with cleft palate.

value, but the final diagnosis is based on laboratory results (Barone and Reiter 2011). The diagnosis of TMJ dysplasia requires advanced radiographic techniques, including the use of 3D imaging.

Von Willebrand's disease is another genetic syndrome that can be diagnosed using a commercial test (Meyers and Hoeppe 2014). In predisposed breeds (e.g., Doberman pinschers), this test should be performed as a qualification for any surgery, but particularly for oral surgery (e.g., tooth extractions) due to the rich vascularity of the oral cavity. It is covered in more detail in Chapter 10.

MMM mainly affects large-breed dogs, but it can affect any breed. The immune system of the patient recognizes the 2M protein as foreign and produces antibodies against the 2M fibers, thus initiating an inflammatory process. Affected muscles include the temporal, masseter, and lateral pterygoid muscles, while the digastrics contain 2A fibers and are free of disease. Diagnosis is based on laboratory testing, which identifies the specific antibodies of the disease. If steroids are used prior to blood collection, this can cause a false negative result. Biopsy can add information and help to rule out other pathologies, but it is more invasive. One other advantage of histopathology is that the results are generally available faster than antibody titers. Treatment consists of anti-inflammatory drugs in high-dose (Fink et al. 2013; Gracis et al. 2018).

CMO is a non-neoplastic, proliferative bony disease of the dog, affecting primarily the mandible, tympanic bullae, and occasionally other bones of the head. Most reported cases occur in Scottish terriers, West Highland white terriers, and cairn terriers. Biopsy and histopathological evaluation are essential for making decisions in CMO, but

(a)

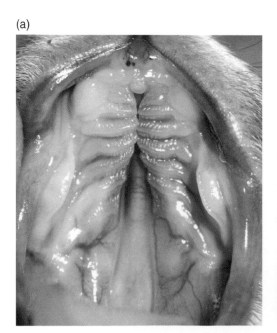

(b)

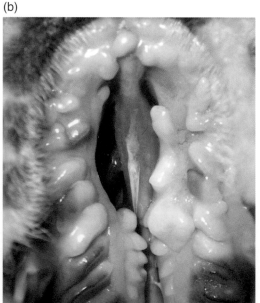

Figure 16.2 Cleft palate in (a) kitten and (b) puppy.

(a)

(b)

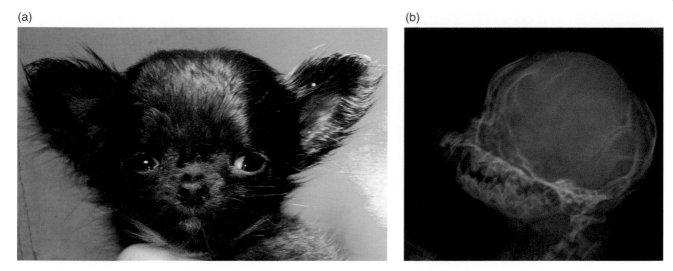

Figure 16.3   Hydrocephalus associated with malocclusion: (a) clinical picture; (b) radiograph.

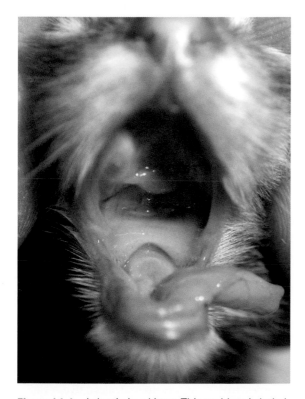

Figure 16.4   Aglossia in a kitten. This problem is lethal.

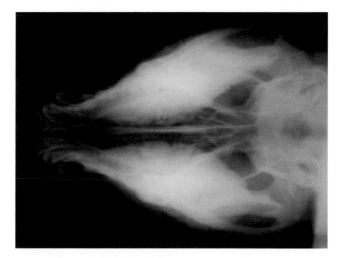

Figure 16.5   Radiographic appearance of CMO in a dog on extraoral dorsoventral view of the head.

radiographic appearance is very typical for this condition (Figure 16.5) and currently a commercial laboratory test is also available. Early diagnosis, particularly before joint involvement, increases the likelihood of a speedy recovery. Anti-inflammatory therapy is considered the basis of treatment (Gawor 2004) (Figure 16.6).

Ankyloglossia is a genetic disorder to which the Anatolian shepherd is predisposed. The lingual frenulum is abnormally short and thickened, which limits tongue function by attaching it to the floor of the mouth, compromising panting and drinking. This condition is relatively easy to cure, through a procedure called a frenotomy (Figure 16.7).

Enamel hypoplasia is analogous to a form of autosomal recessive amelogenesis imperfecta (ARAI) in humans has been recently characterized in Samoyed (Pedersen et al. 2017), as well as in standard Poodle (Mannerfelt and Lindgren 2009) and Italian Greyhounds (Gandolfi et al. 2013).

TMJ dysplasia is a very uncommon presentation (Lantz 2012). In fact, in one study of 41 dogs with TMJ disorders, only seven showed features of dysplasia (Arzi et al. 2013). It can be asymptomatic, and an incidental finding during cranial imaging or occlusion assessment (Figure 16.8). Major features include a flattened

(a)

(b)

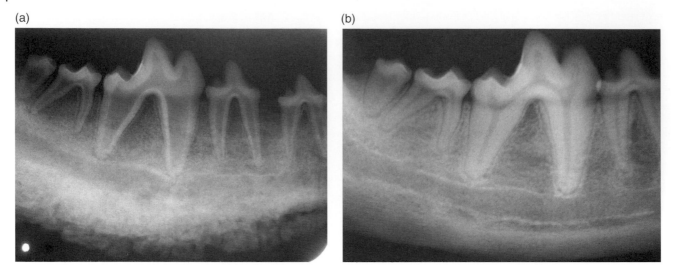

Figure 16.6 Treatment of CMO can be successful and the condition of the bone can recover to normal. (a) Right mandible in an eight-month-old Doberman (a). The same mandible, 1.5 years after recovery.

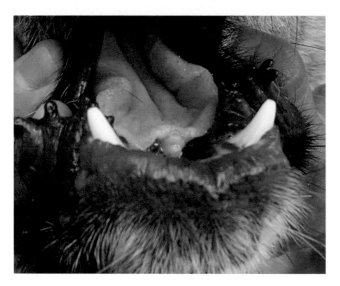

Figure 16.7 Ankyloglossia affects drinking and panting, limiting life comfort (Source: Courtesy of Dr. Efe Onur).

mandibular fossa and its articular eminence, thickening and shortening of the retroarticular process, and abnormal angulation and surface of the mandibular condyle, all of which often make the articular space wider than normal. Two forms of TMJ dysplasia exist: the luxating form, with flattened articular space and lack of retroarticular process, and the chondrodystrophic form, with curved fossa and condyle. The former results in jaw locking or luxation, while the latter is asymptomatic (Schwarz 2011).Treatment is based on clinical signs and the severity of disease.

16.3   Systemic Diseases

16.3.1   Infectious Disease

Diseases that are caused by viruses and are associated with oral lesions in cats include feline calicivirus (FCV), feline immunodeficiency virus (FIV), feline leukemia virus (FeLV), and feline herpesvirus-1. FCV has been mentioned in the etiopathogenesis of chronic gingivostomatitis syndrome, but the lesions that are typically described are lingual ulcerations (Hurley and Sykes 2003) (Figure 16.9). A report from a survey of 226 cats showed that those infected solely with FIV appeared to have not only a greater prevalence of oral cavity infections, but a more severe disease. However, FIV- or FeLV-infected cats that were coinfected with FCV had the highest prevalence and most severe form of oral cavity infections/lesions (Tenorio et al. 1991) (Figure 16.10). Recent studies show that the severity of lesions in cats suffering from caudal stomatitis is not related to FCV load (Druet and Hennet 2017).

Feline herpesvirus-1 can create oral ulcerative lesions, which can resemble other conditions such as eosinophilic granuloma and therefore require accurate diagnosis prior to empiric treatment with immunosuppressive drugs (Lommer 2013).

In dogs, viral papillomatosis is an infectious and contagious condition mostly seen in puppies who have contracted the disease from other dogs. It can also be recognized in immune-compromised individuals (Figure 16.11). Normally, it is self-limiting, but in severe cases surgical treatment or immune therapy may be indicated (Lange and Favrot 2011).

(a) (b)

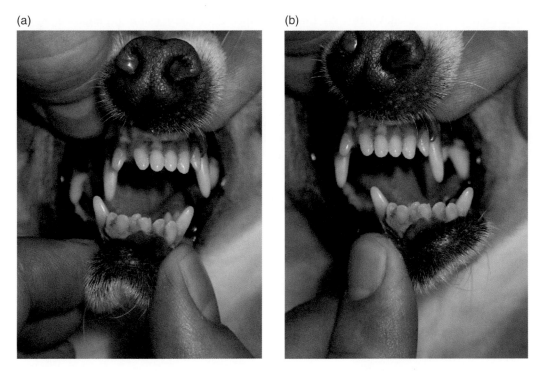

Figure 16.8 Clinical signalments of TMJ dysplasia can be diagnosed during occlusal assessment: an unequal and asymmetric lateral movement of the jaws (a) to the right and (b) to the left.

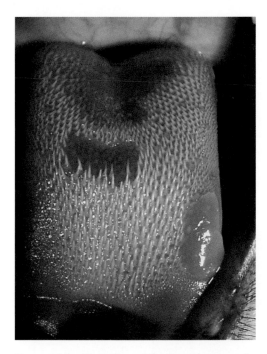

Figure 16.9 Ulceration of the lingual mucosa, frequently associated with FCV infection.

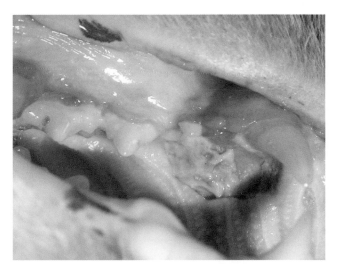

Figure 16.10 Oral lesions in a cat suffering from a mixed infection of FIV and FCV.

Oral manifestations accompanying canine venereal transmissible tumor are rare but have been reported (Ganguly et al. 2016).

Canine distemper can, due to fever and epitheliotropism of the virus, affect enamel development and quality in dogs. Likewise, infectious hepatitis, or any other disease that creates hyperthermia, can cause damage to or death of ameloblasts and affect amelogenesis. This damage will result in enamel hypocalcification/hypoplasia (EH). However, it is important to note that these infectious etiologies are often fatal and thus are a rare cause of this condition. Further, the enamel produced during the infection is the only area that is damaged, creating a horizontal line of disease, rather than the whole tooth being affected. When the whole tooth *is* involved, this indicates a genetic condition known as amelogenesis imperfecta (Boy et al. 2016) (Figure 16.12).

Any infectious conditions that cause regurgitation or vomiting can also negatively affect the enamel because of frequent contact of the teeth with acidic material from the stomach. It is important to note that enamel formation for deciduous dentition starts at approximately the 30th day of gestation, while development of the permanent teeth enamel occurs gradually and terminates prior to permanent teeth eruption (at three to six months of life).

In general, infectious diseases that cause loss of appetite or indigestion can be associated with certain nutritional deficits and thus affect the development of oral structures.

Chlamydia spp., *Clostridium tetani*, *Leptospira canicola*, and *Fusobacterium* are microorganisms that cause infections which may affect the function of the oropharynx. Chlamydia is mentioned here mostly because it involves adjacent anatomic compartments (e.g., eyes, nasal cavity) (Figure 16.13). Easy-to-perform commercial tests are now available that aid in immediate determination of the particular causative factor, allowing treatment to focus on the diagnosis rather than being empiric.

Though mycotic infections of the oral cavity are uncommon, Candida species can appear as opportunistic agents in stomatitis (Jadhav and Pal 2006). Additionally, mycotic infections may occur in immunocompromised patients. Aspergillus infection mostly

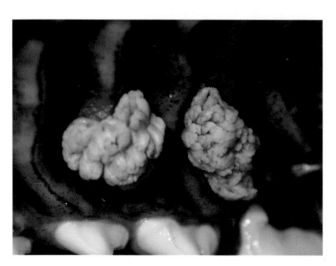

Figure 16.11   Oral papillomatosis in a puppy.

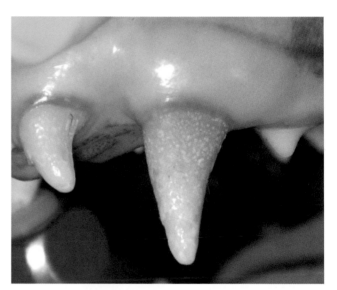

Figure 16.12   Generalized amelogenesis imperfecta in Akita Inu.

(a)   (b)

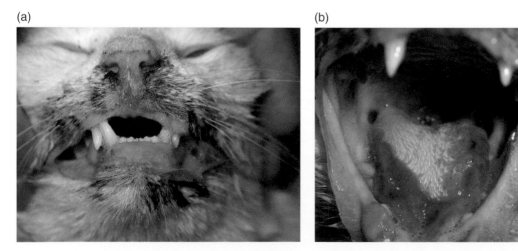

Figure 16.13   Chlamydia infection in cats causes (a) drooling nasal discharge and often (b) loss of appetite due to oral mucosa ulcerations.

(a)

(b)

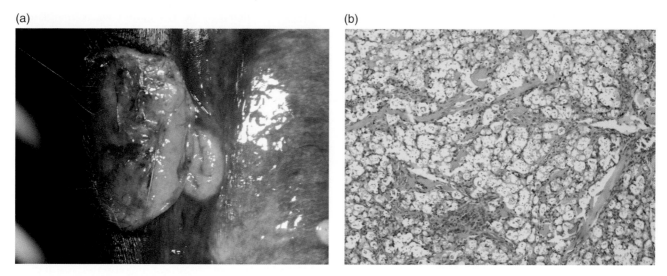

Figure 16.14 *Cryptococcus* infection: (a) oral lesion; (b) microscopic slide illustrating infected tissue.

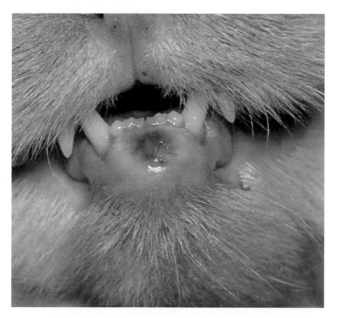

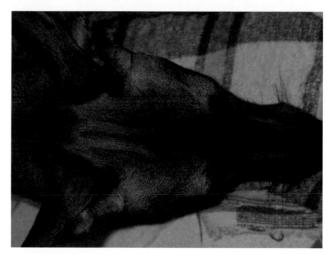

Figure 16.16 Seizures and muscle tension are part of the clinical picture of tetanus in dogs.

Figure 16.15 Biopsy of a lower-lip lesion, revealed the typical histopathologic appearance of actinomycosis.

affects the nasal cavity and sinus, but it may penetrate the nasopalatine ducts and cause oral lesions (Harvey 1993). Blastomycosis (Salinardi et al. 2003) and cryptococcus (Santin et al. 2013) are reported as causative factors of oral or oropharyngeal lesions (Figure 16.14). Actinomyces in rabbits should be considered when a differential diagnosis for facial abscesses is considered (Tyrrell et al. 2002). However, in this author's experience, labial nodular lesions in some cats are also associated with Actinomyces infection (Figure 16.15).

Tetanus is rare in dogs and cats compared with many other domestic species and humans, because of a relative inability of the toxin to penetrate and bind to nervous tissue in these species (Greene 2006). It has been described in cats without any oral signs (Tomek et al. 2004), but in dogs (which are less resistant to tetanus than cats) the clinical picture may include contracted facial musculature, erect ears, and raised lips, in addition to seizures, opisthotonus, and vocalization (Sprott 2008) (Figure 16.16).

In canine leischmaniosis, oral manifestations are rare, though they have been reported ((Viegas et al. 2012)) (Figure 16.17). In areas where this vector-borne disease is common (mostly Mediterranean countries), differential diagnosis of oral lesions should include leischmania. However, there are now reports of canine leischmania from countries where the vectors (sandfly gen. Phlebotomus) are not present.

16.3.2 Immune-Related Disorders

Erythema multiforme (EM), eosinophilic granuloma complex (EGC), pemphigus vulgaris, mucous membrane pemphigoid, epidermolysis bullosa aquisita, and systemic lupus erythematosus are on the list of immune-related inflammatory diseases causing oral lesions and other clinical signs. Pemphigus foliaceus and bullous pemphigoid do not usually present with oral lesions (Lommer 2013).

Lesions caused by these diseases are in general inflammatory, with appearance of erosions, vesicles, pustules, ulcers, and areas of sloughing, but mostly have a mixed character (Figure 16.18). Despite the proposed categorization of oral mucosal diseases into ulcerative, vesicobullous, and proliferative (Lommer 2013), it is impossible to see any of these signalments as pathognomic for a specific disease,

so definitive diagnosis by laboratory test is mandatory before a treatment plan can be designed (Figure 16.19).

In this group should also be included problems exclusively related to the oral cavity and surroundings that severely affect the animal, including feline chronic gingivitis stomatitis (caudal stomatitis), plaque-associated stomatitis in dogs (chronic ulcerative paradental stomatitis (CUPS), and feline juvenile gingivitis. In puppies, juvenile facial dermatitis may cause difficulty in eating due to pain (Figure 16.20).

EGC is a group of conditions that share a common etiology and some histopathological features. While these lesions have been reported in dogs (especially Siberian huskies, Malamutes, and cavalier King Charles spaniels), they are much more common in cats. The disease process is similar in both species. The true etiology of these conditions is unknown, but local accumulation of eosinophils (and their release of inflammatory agents) is thought to initiate the inflammation and necrosis seen in most such lesions. The presence of eosinophils suggests that they result from an immune-mediated or hypersensitivity reaction. This reaction may occur due to a local (food) or systemic (flea allergy or atopy) allergy, though these lesions have been seen in cases where allergic and infectious disease have been essentially ruled out. Additional causes may include a response to irritation, such as chronic grooming, or a traumatic malocclusion (Niemiec 2010). Finally, there appears to be a genetic predisposition to this condition in Norwegian forest cats (see more in Chapter 24).

16.3.3 Metabolic Diseases

Severe clotting disorders can be associated with bone marrow issues or thrombocytopenia, as well as von Willebrand's disease and toxic problems (poisoning by some rodenticides).

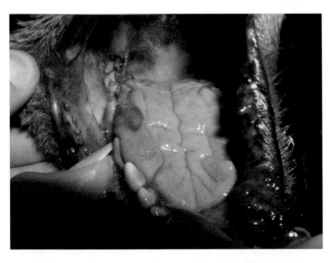

Figure 16.17 Oral lesions caused by *Leischmania* spp. (*Source:* Courtesy of Prof. Alexander Koutinas).

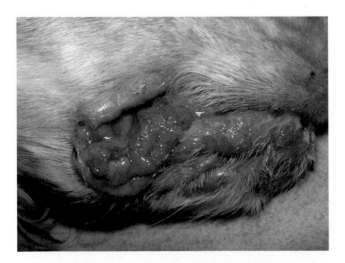

Figure 16.18 Pemphigus foliaceus lesion present on the lips of a cocker spaniel.

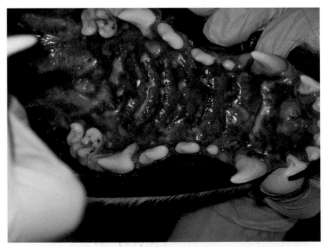

Figure 16.19 Pemphigoid oral lesion (*Source:* Courtesy of Dr. Leonard Gugala).

This may cause spontaneous gingival bleeding, particularly when the animal has an active process disrupting the integrity of the soft oral tissues (e.g., teeth eruption, periodontal disease, oral mucosa ulcerations) (Figure 16.21).

Osteopenia juvenalis very often is caused by malnutrition, particularly in rescued stray cats fed an unbalanced diet (e.g., exclusively raw meat). It creates an abnormal phosphorus/calcium ratio in the serum, with hyperphosphatemia and hypocalcemia. This situation can lead to significant hypomineralization of long and flat bones (the latter in the head), pathologic fractures, and compromised strength of alveolar bone. Treatment is based on provision of a balanced diet and pharmacologic action with supplementation of calcium and decreasing phosphorus based on monitoring of serum levels (Figure 16.22).

Hyperparathyroidism can be associated with renal failure or parathyroid tumor, and results in rapid decalcification of the jaws, causing abnormal loss of rigidity of bones or "rubber jaw" (Figures 16.23 and 16.24).

Diabetes mellitus weakens the immune system and increases the risk of infection. Thus, the patient can be more prone to periodontal disease (Delamaire et al. 1997). Observations of the relationship between the prevalence of diabetes in periodontally affected patients and faster development of periodontal diseases in diabetic individuals

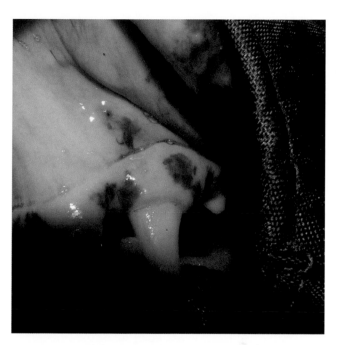

Figure 16.21 Punch test in a Doberman pinscher to observe mucosal bleeding time (MBT), and blood clotting efficiency. The only reliable test for von Willebrand's disease is a genetic one.

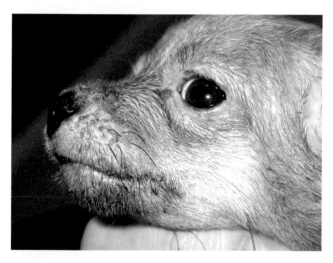

Figure 16.20 Juvenile facial dermatitis in a puppy.

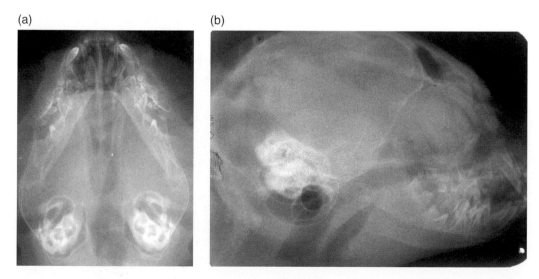

Figure 16.22 Osteopenia juvenalis in a kitten with malnutrition: (a) lack of readable nasal structures; (b) thinned maxillofacial bones.

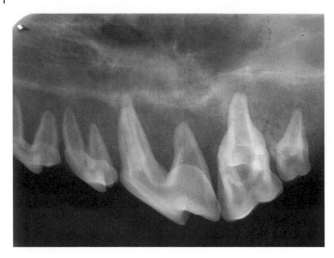

Figure 16.23 Hyperparathyroidismus associated with renal insufficiency causing "rubber jaw" syndrome in a puppy.

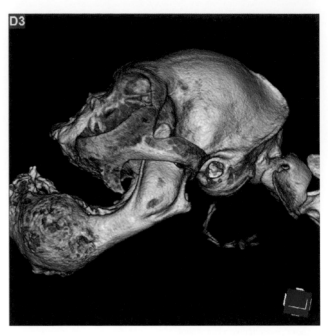

Figure 16.25 Hyperostosis of the rostral mandible, mimicking acromegaly.

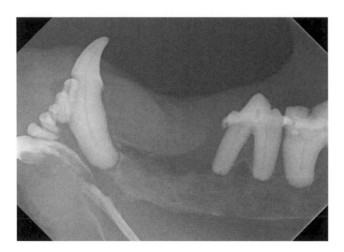

Figure 16.24 Hyperparathyroidismus associated with a geriatric parathyroid tumor causing similar signalments to rubber jaw in an old cat.

come directly from human medicine. The same resources show improved diabetic control in patients without periodontal disease, as active periodontal disease increases insulin resistance in humans. Intervention studies have demonstrated that the treatment of periodontal disease improves the glycemic control of diabetes mellitus patients (Bascones-Martínez et al. 2014).

In some cats, the reported clinical features of acromegaly related to the head and face include prognathia inferior and the enlargement of jaws, tongue, and forehead. Thus, acromegaly must be taken into account when a differential diagnosis for oral and maxillofacial problems related to growth of the rostral part of the mandible is considered. Hyperostosis, osteomyelitis or neoplasia may cause similar signalments (Figure 16.25). Most but not all cats with acromegaly also have diabetes mellitus (Federico Fracassi et al. 2016).

Children with thyroid disorders (both hypo- and hyperthyroid) have high caries prevalence and poor periodontal health. Additionally, other oral abnormalities such as macroglossia, problems with eruption, and malocclusion are more frequent in this group than in healthy children (Venkatesh Babu and Patel 2016).

Congenital feline hypothyroidism was described in a 10-month-old kitten. The kitten appeared to have disproportionate dwarfism, with the clinical signs of incompletely erupted permanent dentition covered by thickened gingival tissue, short stature, a broad, flattened face, and short neck. After Thyroxine supplementation, the kitten appeared like a normal healthy cat at 22 months of age (Jacobson and Rochette 2018).

Systemic diseases require stabilization and control to efficiently manage periodontal disease and associated oral dysfunctions.

The oral mucosa can change color in some systemic conditions: pale in anemia, cyanotic in hypoxia, yellow in jaundice, and intense red in hyperemia, fever, and some toxic conditions (warfarin poisoning). Any abnormal colors of oral structures should be investigated (Harvey 1993). Azotemia associated with renal failure can cause ulcerations in the oral cavity, typically on the lateral part of the tongue or on the cheek mucosa (Figure 16.26), which are commonly called uremic ulcers or uremic stomatitis (Gracis et al. 2018).

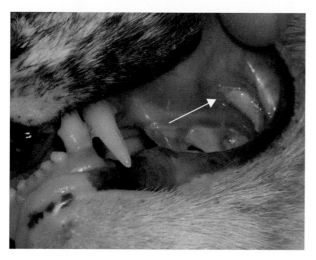

Figure 16.26 Uremic ulcerations and mucositis in a cat with chronic renal insufficiency (arrow).

16.3.4 Toxic Conditions

The toxic influence of some medicines can result in intrinsic staining of the dentition, tooth discoloration, or proliferation of the gingiva. Poisons, chemical burns, and snake and insect bites that affect the animal through the oral cavity can cause lesions in the oral mucosa (Figure 16.27). Adverse effects of drugs may also be present in the oral cavity (Guillaumin, 2020).

16.3.5 Traumatic Conditions

Neuropraxia (Robins and Robins 1976) is a disorder of the peripheral nervous system in which there is a temporary loss of motor and sensory function due to blockage of nerve conduction, lasting an average of six to eight weeks before full recovery. It often occurs after overuse of the jaws, for example due to carrying heavy branches or tires.

Seizures accompanying epilepsy or other neurological disorders may cause tongue injury (Figure 16.28). Similar injuries can happen after prolonged desensitization of the tongue following an incorrectly performed mandibular nerve block.

Idiopathic problems like vitiligo, myositis atrophicans, and proliferative stomatitis involve the face or oral cavity. Despite the fact that etiology remains unknown, some empiric efforts at treatment have been performed, with various effects (Figure 16.29).

(a)

(b)

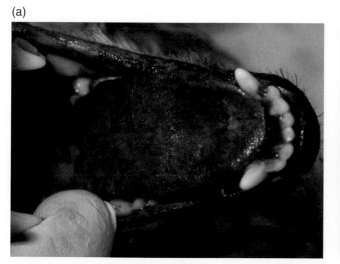
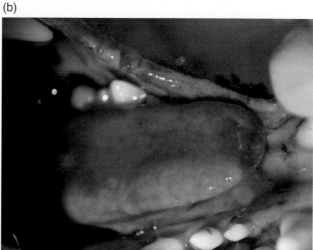

Figure 16.27 Chemical burn of the oral mucosa caused by caustic soda: (a) immediately after burn; (b) after two weeks of treatment.

(a)

(b)

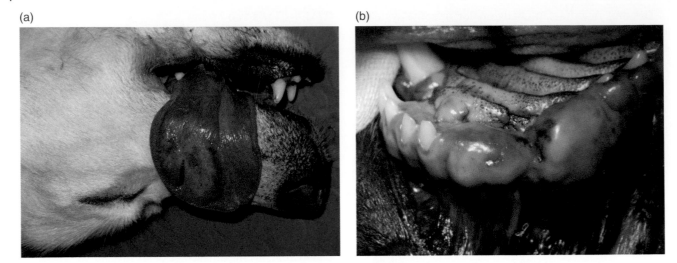

Figure 16.28 (a) Lingual mucosa damage and (b) multiple teeth fractures in a dog (b) with frequent seizures.

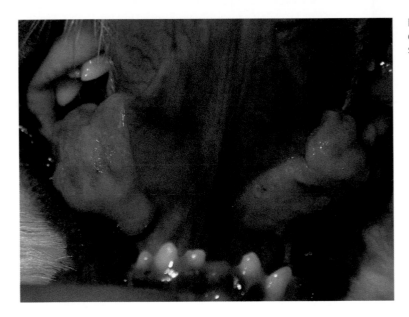

Figure 16.29 Mucosal proliferation in a Japanese chin of unknown origin treated successfully by surgical excision.

References

Arzi, B., Cissell, D.D., Verstraete, F.J. et al. (2013). Computed tomographic findings in dogs and cats with temporomandibular joint disorders: 58 cases (2006–2011). *J. Am. Vet. Med. Assoc.* 242 (1): 69–75.

Barone, G. and Reiter, A.M. (2011). *Masticatory Myositis in Clinical Veterinary Advisor*, 2e (ed. E. Cote), 704–705. St. Louis, MO: Mosby.

Bascones-Martínez, A., González-Febles, J., and Sanz-Esporrín, J. (2014). Diabetes and periodontal disease. Review of the literature. *J. Am. J. Dent.* 27 (2): 63–67.

Boy, S., Crossley, D., and Steenkamp, G. (2016). Developmental structural tooth defects in dogs – experience from veterinary dental referral practice and review of the literature. *Front. Vet. Sci.* 3: 9.

Delamaire, M., Maugendre, D., Moreno, M. et al. (1997). Impaired leucocyte functions in diabetic patients. *Diabet. Med.* 14 (1): 29–34.

Druet, I. and Hennet, P. (2017). Relationship between feline calicivirus load, oral lesions, and outcome in Feline chronic gingivostomatitis (caudal stomatitis): retrospective study in 104 cats. *Front. Vet. Sci.* 4: 209.

Fink, L., Lewis, J., and Reiter, A. (2013). Biopsy of the temporal and masseter muscles in dog. *J. Vet. Dent.* 30 (4): 276–280.

Fracassi, F., Salsi, M., Sammartano, F. et al. (2016). Acromegaly in a non-diabetic cat. *J. Feline Med. Surg. Open Rep.* 2 (1).

Gandolfi, B., Liu, H., Griffioen, L., and Pedersen, N.C. (2013). Simple recessive mutation in ENAM is associated with amelogenesis imperfecta in Italian Greyhounds. *Anim. Genet.* 44 (5): 569–578.

Ganguly, B., Das, U., and Das, A.K. (2016). Canine transmissible venereal tumour: a review. *Vet. Comp. Oncol.* 14 (1): 1–12.

Gawor, J. (2004). Report of four cases of craniomandibular osteopathy. *Eur. J. Comp. An. Pract.* 14: 209–213.

Gracis, M., Reiter, A.M., and Ordeix, L. (2018). Management of selected non-periodontal inflammatory, infectious and reactive conditions. In: *BSAVA Manual of Canine and Feline Dentistry and Oral Surgery* (eds. M. Gracis and A.M. Reiter), 190–192. Quedgeley: BSAVA.

Greene, C.E. (2006). Tetanus. In: *Infectious Diseases of the Dog and Cat*, vol. 3 (ed. C.E. Greene), 395–402. St. Louis, MO: Saunders-Elsevier.

Guillaumin J. (n.d.) Image gallery: adverse drug reactions. Available from https://www.cliniciansbrief.com/article/image-gallery-adverse-drug-reactions (accessed July 5, 2020).

Harvey, C.E. (1993). Oral lesions of soft tissue and bone: differential diagnosis. In: *Small Animal Dentistry*, 42–49. St. Louis, MO: Mosby.

Hurley, K.F. and Sykes, E.S. (2003). Update on feline calicivirus: new trends. *Vet. Clin. North Am. Small Anim. Prac.* 33 (4): 759–772.

Jacobson, T. and Rochette, J. (2018). Congenital feline hypothyroidism with partially erupted adult dentition in a 10-month-old male neutered domestic shorthair cat: a case report. *J. Vet. Dent.* 35 (3): 178–186.

Jadhav, V.J. and Pal, M. (2006). Canine mycotic stomatitis due to Candida albicans. *Rev. Iberoam Micol.* 23 (4): 233–234.

Kelly, M.K. and Bardach, J. (2012). Biologic basis of cleft palate and palatal surgery. In: *Oral and Maxillofacial Surgery in Dogs and Cats* (ed. F.J.M. Verstraete), 343–350. Philadelphia, PA: Elsevier.

Lange, C.E. and Favrot, C. (2011). Canine papillomaviruses. *Vet. Clin. North Am. Small Anim. Pract.* 41 (6): 1183–1195.

Lantz, G.C. (2012). Temporomandibular joint dysplasia. In: *Oral and Maxillofacial Surgery in Dogs and Cats* (eds. F.J.M. Verstraete and M.J. Lommer), 531–538. Edinburgh: W.B. Saunders.

Lommer, M.J. (2013). Oral inflammation in small animals. *Vet. Clin. Small Anim.* 43: 555–571.

Mannerfelt, T. and Lindgren, I. (2009). Enamel defects in standard poodle dogs in Sweden. *J. Vet. Dent.* 26 (4): 213–215.

Mazzullo, G., Macri, F., Rapisarda, G., and Marino, F. (2009). Deradelphous cephalothoracopagus in kittens. *Anat. Histol. Embryol.* 38 (5): 327–329.

Meyers E, Hoepp N (2014). Canine Von Willebrand disease for veterinary technicians. *NAVTA J.* Available from https://www.vetmedteam.com/class.aspx?ci=600 (accessed July 5, 2020).

Nemec, A., Daniaux, L., Johnson, E. et al. (2015). Craniomaxillofacial abnormalities in dogs with congenital palatal defects: computed tomographic findings. *Vet. Surg.* 44 (4): 417–422.

Niemiec, B.A. (2010). Pathologies of the oral mucosa. In: *A Color Handbook Small Animal Dental Oral and Maxillofacial diseases* (ed. B.A. Niemiec), 186–188. London: Manson.

Pedersen, N.C., Shope, B., and Liu, H. (2017). An autosomal recessive mutation in SCL24A4 causing enamel hypoplasia in Samoyed and its relationship to breed-wide genetic diversity. *Canine Genet. Epidemiol.* 4: 11.

Robins, G.M. and Robins, G.M. (1976). Dropped jaw – mandibular neurapraxia in the dog. *J. Small Anim. Pract.* 17: 753–758.

Salinardi, B., Marretta, S.M., McCullough, S.M. et al. (2003). Pharyngeal–laryngeal blastomycosis in dog. *J. Vet. Dent.* 20 (3): 146–147.

Santin, R., Mattei, A.S., Waller, S.B. et al. (2013). Clinical and mycological analysis of dog's oral cavity. *Braz. J. Microbiol.* 44 (1): 139–143.

Schwarz, T. (2011). Temporomandibular joint and masticatory apparatus. In: *Veterinary Comnputed Tomography* (eds. T. Schwarz and J. Saudners), 125–136. Hoboken, NJ: Wiley-Blackwell.

Sprott, K.R. (2008). Generalized tetanus in a Labrador retriever. *Can. Vet. J.* 49 (12): 1221–1223.

Tenorio, A.P., Franti, C.E., Madewell, B.R., and Pedersen, N.C. (1991). Chronic oral infections of cats and their relationship to persistent oral carriage of feline calici-, immunodeficiency, or leukemia viruses. *Vet. Immunol. Immunopathol.* 29 (1–2): 1–14.

Tomek, A.L., Kathmann, I., Faissler, D. et al. (2004). Tetanus in cats: 3 case descriptions. *Schweiz Arch. Tierheilkd.* 146 (6): 295–302.

Tyrrell, K.L., Citron, D.M., Jenkins, J.R., and Goldstein, E.J. (2002). Periodontal bacteria in rabbit mandibular and maxillary abscesses. *J. Clin. Microbiol.* 40 (3): 1044–1047.

Venkatesh Babu, N.S. and Patel, P.B. (2016). Oral health status of children suffering from thyroid disorders. *J. Indian Soc. Pedod. Prev. Dent.* 34 (2): 139–144.

Viegas, C., Requicha, J., Albuquerque, C. et al. (2012). Tongue nodules in canine leishmaniosis – a case report. *Parasit. Vectors* 5: 120.

17

Common Situations of Malpractice and Mistakes, and How Best to Avoid Them

Jerzy Gawor[1] and Brook Niemiec[2]

[1] *Veterinary Clinic Arka, Kraków, Poland*
[2] *Veterinary Dental Specialties and Oral Surgery, San Diego, CA, USA*

17.1 Introduction

Veterinary medicine, like most aspects of contemporary society, is becoming more litigious. Veterinary dentistry provides many opportunities for malpractice and mistakes. This is commonly due to lack of training and proper equipment rather than true neglect. However, the prudent practitioner will take all possible steps to avoid poor technique and malpractice. This chapter will outline the most common causes of malpractice in veterinary dentistry and how best to avoid them. These include: anesthesia, oral examination, therapy/surgery, and client communication. The best way to avoid these problems is through proper training and equipment.

There is a difference between error and true malpractice. Errors may occur for many reasons, but when proper protocols are not followed or a practitioner attempts procedures in which they are not proficient (without the client's informed consent), this is a clear case of malpractice. It is important to note that specialists are subject to more scrutiny than general practitioners, and therefore a higher level of care is expected.

17.2 Anesthesia

It is well established that anesthesia is required for proper oral examination, as well as all dental therapies. Dental procedures are often lengthy, which increases the chances of adverse outcomes. Furthermore, many dental patients are geriatric or small in stature, which may likewise increase the complication rate. Therefore, well-performed anesthesia is critical in veterinary dentistry.

The first step in qualifying a patient for a dental procedure is a proper and complete physical exam. The most important part of this is auscultation of the heart and lungs. Make sure to listen to the heart and feel pulses for some time to help find infrequent arrhythmias. A proper exam will go a long way to ensuring fitness for anesthesia. Any physical finding (heart murmur, arrhythmia, pallor of mucous membranes, abdominal masses, etc.) should be fully worked up, ideally by an appropriate specialist, prior to anesthesia.

Even an outwardly normal animal may still have comorbidities that will complicate anesthesia. Therefore, preoperative testing is now a very common recommendation in veterinary medicine. The recommendations for various species, breeds, and ages are listed in Chapter 12 and appendix A.

The anesthesia procedure starts before the pet arrives and does not end until after it has returned home. Providing proper pre- and postoperative instructions is very important to patient safety (see later). Once in the clinic, keep the patient as stress-free as possible and strive to maintain normal body temperature.

Always use current and acceptable anesthetic protocols and monitor the patient continually throughout the procedure. Remember the adage, "if it's not written down, it didn't happen." Make sure to follow the standards in the practice act or regulations for your particular region. In the state of Nevada, for example, *something* must be recorded every five minutes during anesthesia. Multimodal monitoring is always recommended, which should always include blood pressure. Also, remember to monitor temperature, as hypothermia greatly increases the risk of anesthesia overdose and other complications.

Always monitor the patient in recovery, ideally until standing. It has been reported that more pets die in recovery

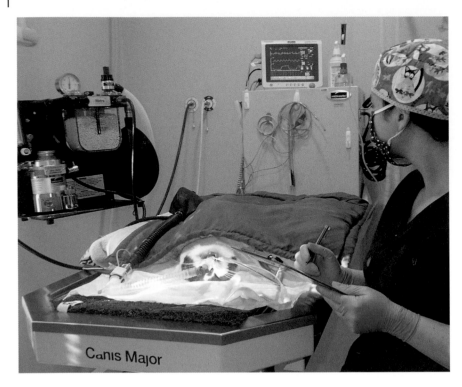

Figure 17.1   Monitoring until completely awake is crucial for safety.

than during anesthesia itself (Figure 17.1). Only release anesthetized pets following complete recovery (once they are able to walk) (Brodbelt 2009).

17.3   Oral Exam and Diagnostics

As discussed in Chapter 20, a complete oral exam is a required part of every dental procedure. A visual examination of the pharyngeal area should be made during intubation. Following anesthetic induction, a visual examination of the entire oral cavity can be performed. This examination *must* include periodontal probing around every tooth. In addition, tactile exam for pulp exposure and tooth resorption is strongly mandated. One common area of missed pathology is on the lingual/palatal aspect of the teeth. This is an area that is very difficult to evaluate visually (especially in small dogs), so a tactile exam with a periodontal probe and explorer is strongly recommended (Figure 17.2).

The oral exam findings *must* be recorded on a dental chart (Figure 17.3). This should be of adequate size to allow for recording of all pathology and therapy. At least half a page is recommended, although a full page is ideal. Some practices use two charts: one for diagnosis and one for

treatment. Note that a Veterinary Medical Board (VMB) in the United States recently reprimanded a veterinarian who wrote down their findings in detail in the medical record, but did not have a dental chart.

Dental radiographs are quickly becoming the standard of care; if they are not yet in your area, they will be soon. There is a significant amount of infectious/painful oral pathology that will be left untreated without the benefit of dental radiology. In addition, many of the complications of oral surgery listed in the next section can be avoided with properly exposed and interpreted dental radiographs. The lack of radiographs as well as using nondiagnostic images are quite common and are as much malpractice as is misinterpretation. Numerous studies support the value of full-mouth radiographs in all patients. (Verstraete et al. 1998) Further, in many cases (e.g., neoplasia, trauma), 3D imaging has been shown to be superior to standard and intraoral dental radiographs, and should be recommend if available in your practice area (Figure 17.4).

Transillumination may be a more sensitive technique for the diagnosis of non-vital teeth (Figure 17.5). Dental radiographic changes take time to occur, but transillumination will often reveal them. However, recent studies reveal this test is accurate in only 76% of tested teeth (Proulx et al. 2019).

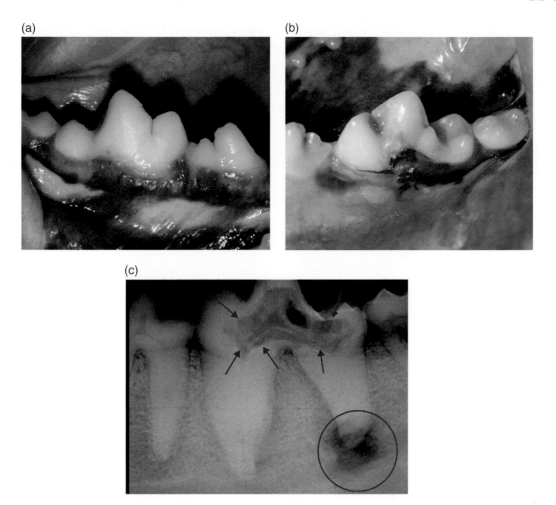

(a)

(b)

(c)

Figure 17.2 (a) A mandibular right first molar (409) which is clinically unremarkable from the buccal side. (b) Inflammatory lesion from the lingual aspect. (c) Radiograph showing resorption (arrows) and periapical lesion (circle).

Figure 17.3 Dental charting is a mandatory part of oral examination. It should preferably be done in a four-handed manner (veterinarian plus assistant). Additionally, radiographs should be available.

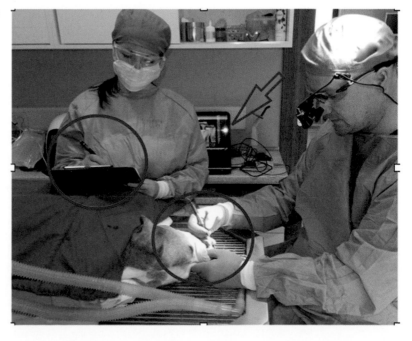

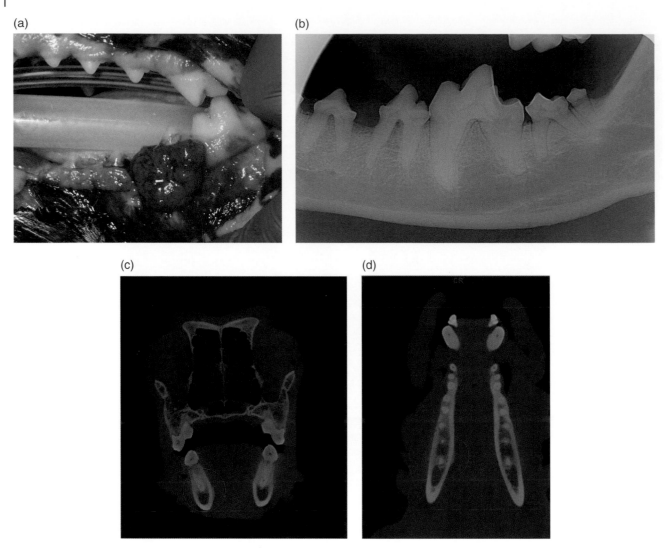

Figure 17.4 Mandibular tumor (melanoma malignum) in (a) clinical, (b) radiographic, and (c,d) CBCT assessment. Subtle bone reaction is visible in CBCT scans (circle).

Histopathology of all suspect growths is strongly recommended to avoid missed pathology. Malignancies will look very benign in the early stages, and treatment at this stage has the best prognosis.

17.4 Improper Therapy and Iatrogenic Damage

There are numerous reasons why dental procedures might fail, so care must be taken to ensure success. On occasion, iatrogenic problems (jaw fracture, eye damage) will result in an emergency visit to a specialist as obvious issues that must be corrected immediately. These are the complications that are most likely to result in a malpractice suit. Other times (such as in surgical dehiscence), a mistake is found later and may be fixed by the veterinarian. Most often, however, iatrogenic failures (e.g., retained roots,

improper cleanings) go unnoticed, allowing a false sense of security. It is important to note that these pets still suffer in silence.

Improper/incomplete scaling is a *very* common occurrence in veterinary dentistry. It is actually typical for referral dentists to find uncleaned periodontal pockets and other pathology on examination of patients who just recently received a cleaning. Further, residual calculus is often found on the lingual/palatal aspect of teeth following cleaning at a general practitioner's (especially in small-breed dogs) (Figure 17.6). This may result in continued pain and infection for the patient. While it would almost never result in a lawsuit, it is not best medicine and should be avoided. Hands-on training will greatly help in avoiding such a situation, as well as speeding up the process. However, the best way to avoid such issues is to perform the oral exam *after* cleaning. In this way, it provides a final check of cleaning quality. If a clinic has a policy of performing

(a)

(b)

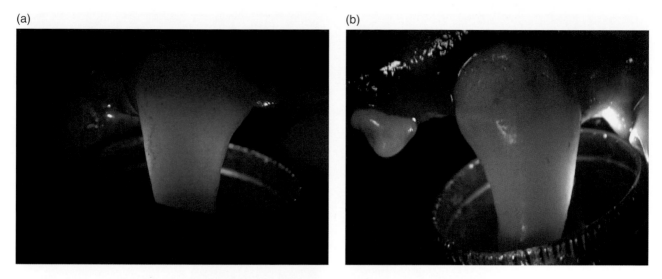

Figure 17.5 Transillumination of (a) the vital tooth is different than that of (b) the nonvital tooth.

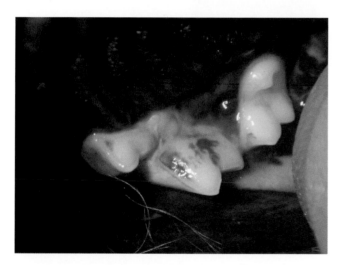

Figure 17.6 Calculus on the palatal aspect of the teeth is often missed during routine prophylaxis.

the exam preoperatively, a quick post-cleaning check by the responsible veterinarian is recommended. Other means of avoiding residual plaque/calculus include drying the teeth with air and using a plaque-disclosing solution. Only by proper and complete cleanings will periodontal disease be effectively treated.

Retained tooth roots are also very common. In fact, a recent study found that 82.4% of canine patients and 92.8% of feline had retained roots from "extracted" carnassial teeth (Moore and Niemiec 2014) (Figure 17.7). Furthermore, over 50% of the patients in the study had radiographic changes consistent with infection over 50% of the time. Note that these patients had *no clinical signs* of infection, but many clients reported improved attitudes following extraction of the roots (Figure 17.7).

While retained roots most commonly fester without any outward evidence of disease, they are still a source of pain and infection for the patient. Occasionally, they will result in a draining abscess, requiring immediate therapy. In these cases, the clinic is generally found liable and at risk of a malpractice suit. It is important to note, however, that even "quiet" retained roots are unacceptable and below the standard of care.

Using proper surgical technique (preoperative dental radiographs, small sharp elevators, gentle patient elevation) will help avoid root fracture. However, by far the best way to avoid this scenario is to *always* expose a postoperative radiograph. This author has found numerous retained roots on teeth that he has deemed to be completely extracted. If a boarded dentist can be wrong, so can a general practitioner. Additionally, in some cases, facial abscesses may have a different cause from the tooth. This author had a case with an abscess created by a foxtail (grass awn foreign body) that was in the correct position for a maxillary carnassial abscess. The tooth was also fractured with periapical lucencies. Therefore, the presumption was a tooth root abscess. The tooth was extracted completely, but no postoperative radiograph was exposed. When the swelling returned two weeks later, the client was upset and brought the pet in for radiographs and suspected tooth root extraction. No roots were found, and subsequently the foreign body was discovered by a surgeon. If a postoperative radiograph had been exposed, it would not only have sped the process of healing, but also have saved the client and veterinarian unnecessary angst and expense (Figure 17.8).

If retained roots are found on the postoperative dental radiograph, surgical removal is recommended. Do not delve after these roots blind, as they can be pushed into the

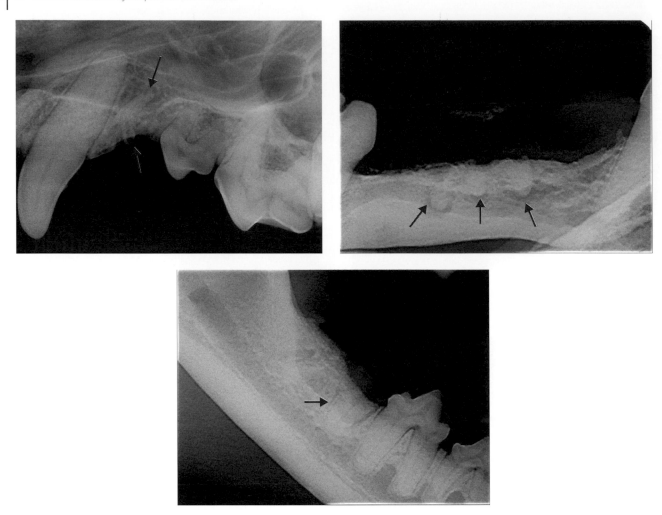

Figure 17.7 Retained root tips and roots that require action after poorly performed extractions.

(a)   (b)

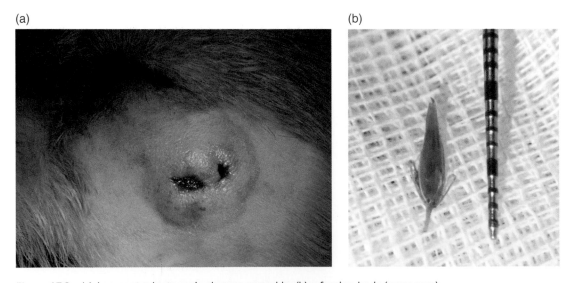

Figure 17.8 (a) Apparent odontogenic abscess caused by (b) a foreign body (grass awn).

mandibular canal or nasal cavity (see later). If roots are found on routine dental radiographs, it is currently recommended to surgically remove them regardless of a lack of clinical signs of infection. The exception is where the roots are significantly resorbed/ankylosed and without radiographic evidence of infection (Figure 17.9).

Oronasal fistulas typically result from maxillary canine extractions, but can occur following extraction of any maxillary tooth. There is minimal bone between the maxillary tooth roots and the nasal cavity, and it can be destroyed by periodontal or endodontic disease or damaged during extraction. The best way to avoid this complication is to ensure that there is no tension on the incision line prior to closure. This is accomplished by creating a sufficiently

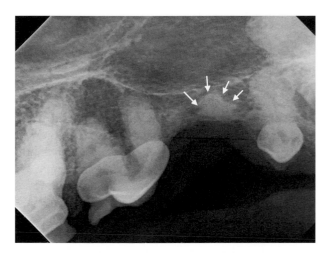

Figure 17.9 Incidental discovery of a retained root of the right maxillary second premolar (106) (arrows) left for monitoring due to limited anesthesia time.

large flap and fenestrating the periosteum (see Chapter 21). If the flap stays in place without sutures, tension is released (Figure 17.10). If it fails and an oronasal fistula occurs, referral rather than an additional closure attempt is recommended, as each surgery creates additional scar tissue, which makes closure increasingly difficult.

Pathologic mandibular fractures are an increasing problem in veterinary dentistry. They are most common in the mandibular canines of all small-animal patients, as well as the mandibular first molar of small- and toy-breed dogs. The main cause is excessive force on the mandible when extracting teeth as well as minimal bone around the first molar tooth. By using small sharp elevators and patience, this complication can usually be avoided.

The main reason for the increase in incidence of such fractures is the increased popularity of small- and toy-breed dogs. These breeds have proportionally larger roots in comparison to their mandibles than do large-breed dogs, especially in the case of the mandibular first molar (Figure 17.11).

Chronic alveolar bone loss from periodontal disease weakens the bone in the affected area and can lead to mandibular fractures during extraction attempts. In addition, dentoalveolar ankylosis can make extractions more challenging and therefore increase the risk of iatrogenic fracture. Preoperative dental radiographs will elucidate these conditions and greatly decrease the chances of this complication occurring. The possibility of iatrogenic fracture should be discussed with all clients before a mandibular tooth extraction, especially if dental radiology reveals an area of increased susceptibility. In these cases, referral to a qualified veterinary dentist is strongly recommended. If the client declines this, note it in the medical record.

(a)

(b)

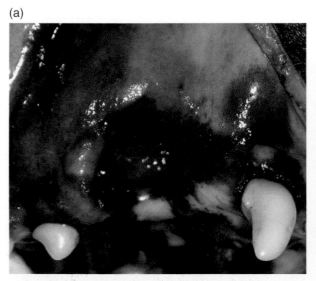 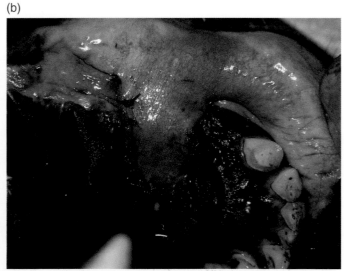

Figure 17.10 (a) Oronasal fistula. (b) After repair.

If the mandible does fracture, immediate referral is recommended. Fixing a fractured mandible (especially one with advanced periodontal disease) is very challenging, and attempts by a general practitioner are often unsuccessful and increase trauma to the patient. A (tape) muzzle is generally recommended for stabilization prior to definitive therapy.

Damage of the structures and tissue adjacent to a surgical area or linked to a procedure requires repair and follow-up, and a detailed explanation must be offered to the pet owner. Some such damage may be delayed, such as cortical blindness or periapical tissue irritation caused by chemical debridement of the root canal, or soft-tissue inflammation or defects due to stabilizations or appliances.

Some complications can also appear due to lack of understanding by the owner about planned postoperative care and the necessary intervention if a problem occurs. Therefore, all instructions must be given in writing at the time of discharge and signed by the owner, and a signed copy must be attached to the medical record. Hard dental tissues require at least preservation of the exposed dentin or pulp by appropriate techniques, along with adequate follow-up. Soft-tissue lacerations and other defects require at least local treatment and topical cleansing gel application (Figure 17.12).

Forcing of roots into the mandibular or nasal cavity is generally caused by attempts to remove retained roots "blind." Proper elevation is achieved *only* when the instrument is within the periodontal ligament space. When the space is not visualized, it often results in apical pressure being placed directly on the whole root. Since the apices of the roots are very close to (or even within) the mandibular canal/nasal cavity, it is easy to push them in (Figure 17.13).

When a root breaks, don't panic. This is a very common problem. The way to retrieve a retained root is to make a surgical flap and remove buccal cortical bone to a level where you can identify the root and the periodontal ligament space. Once this has been done, proceed with extraction as normal. Always make sure not to put too much apical pressure on the root, and instead to utilize a gentle twisting elevation. If it continues to crumble, continue removing bone until the root is removed.

If a root does go into the nasal cavity or mandibular canal, *do not* attempt to retrieve it. There are large blood vessels and important nerves in these areas and significant hemorrhage is common (see later). Even with suction and magnification, extraction is challenging for veterinary dentists. Inform the client of the problem and refer the pet to a qualified dentist for extraction.

Iatrogenic orbital or brain damage typically occurs during extraction of the maxillary molar teeth in small-breed dogs. There is minimal space between the roots of these teeth and the orbit, and this, coupled with a weakened

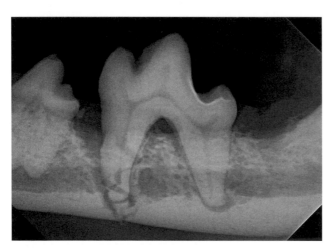

Figure 17.11 Iatrogenic left mandibular fracture caused during an extraction attempt of 309. Note that this tooth should been sectioned.

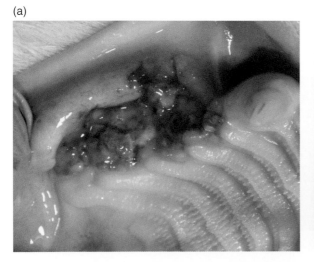
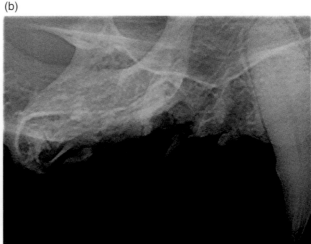

Figure 17.12 (a) Poor extraction technique in this cat and lack of suturing caused wound dehisence and infection. (b) radiograph.

(a)

(b)

(c)

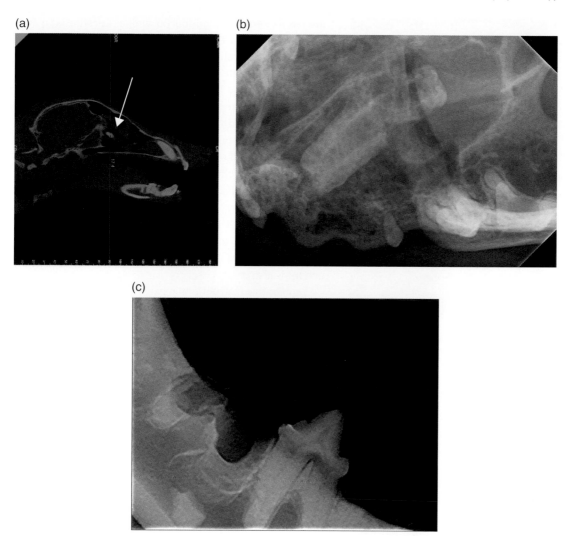

Figure 17.13 Root pushed into nose, diagnosed after several months of nasal discharge (a) CBCT scan of the dog (b) radiograph of the left maxilla in a cat. (c) Intraoperative complication of a root intruded into mandibular canal.

bone, can allow the elevator to enter/damage the eye. In general, this results in loss of the eye. In addition, the elevator may penetrate the brain, resulting in death of the patient. To avoid these disastrous issues, do not place excessive apical pressure on roots of the caudal maxillary teeth. Keeping a finger within a few millimeters of the instrument tip will avoid the instrument traveling very far in case of slippage (Figure 17.14). In case of orbital penetration, *immediate* referral to an ophthalmologist is necessary if there is to be any hope of saving the eye (see Chapter 14) (Perry et al. 2015).

The oral cavity has a tremendous vascular supply. The three main vessels are the infraorbital, palatine, and mandibular. Not only are there numerous large vessels in this area, but the tissues are very well perfused. In addition, the nasal cavity has a significant diffuse vascular supply. Therefore, oral and maxillofacial surgery will typically result in at least some hemorrhage. However, if one of the major vessels is transected or the nasal cavity entered, **excessive hemorrhage** can ensue.

The best way to avoid this complication is to have a firm knowledge of oral anatomy. This will help avoid cutting the vessels inadvertently. If this occurs, or if transection is part of the planned surgery, the best way to control the hemorrhage is to ligate the vessel. This should always be performed in cases of large vessel transection. If at all possible, identify and clamp the vessel prior to cutting it. If not, be prepared to clamp it as soon as it is cut, and follow with ligation. Significant bleeding should be expected from extractions of maxillary canine teeth with oronasal fistulas, as the vascular rich nasal tissues will also be inflamed. Another extraction that can result in significant hemorrhage is the mandibular fist molar of small-breed dogs, where the roots often lie in (or sometimes even through) the mandibular canal. This puts the mandibular artery at risk for cutting with the elevator or bur during the extraction. Occasionally, however, a root will be adhered to the vessel, which can cause tearing of the vessel during even simple extraction.

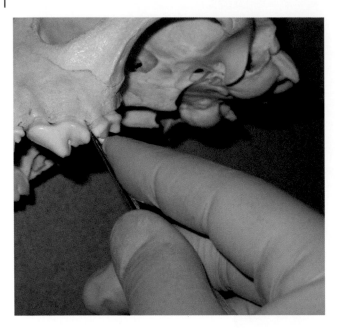

Figure 17.14 Keeping an index finger close to the working tip of the elevator prevents excessive penetration in case of instrument slippage from the extraction site.

In cases where the vessel retracts and cannot be found or where there is severe, diffuse bleeding, the first step is to apply pressure. Application of a collagen sponge or a hemostatic agent could also be performed. This author finds that collagen sponges are very effective in nasal or alveolar bleeding (i.e., with oronasal fistulas or mandibular first molar extractions). If the hemorrhage is severe and life-threatening, ligation of the carotid artery may be attempted as a last resort.

Finally, when extracting a tooth via an open (surgical) approach, be careful not to damage the surrounding teeth. This is most common when performing extractions on the mandibular first molar in small-breed dogs. If these teeth are damaged, it is considered malpractice and the issue must be treated appropriately (restoration or extraction). Furthermore, appropriate gentle soft-tissue handling techniques must be employed or the tissue may become nonvital, necessitating a significant surgery.

17.5 Client Communication

Proper communication can go a long way to avoiding client displeasure and complaints. It is imperative to completely discuss all dental procedures (as well as anesthesia) before performing them. Thus, as complete an oral exam as the patient will allow should be performed in order to allow for the most complete discussion possible. Such discussion should include the possibility of extractions and any other therapies found necessary. The client should also be forewarned that additional pathology is often found on exam, and to be prepared for a phone call to approve additional therapy. All of this will go a long way toward avoiding a disgruntled client.

A thorough dialog regarding the risks and benefits of any planned procedures will help alleviate client concerns and avoid future complaints. The discussion should include the option of referral to a specialist if necessary and feasible. Covering the risks of anesthesia tailored to the particular patient is also critical.

Preoperative instructions regarding work-up and fasting are critical. Ideally, these should be presented in both verbal and written forms. The client should sign and be given a copy of these instructions to avoid any danger of miscommunication. This will also serve as evidence of proper instruction in the medical record. On the day of surgery, the client should be queried to ensure that the instructions have been followed, and should fill out and sign an anesthesia release form. This should include space to again declare that fasting instructions were followed and to list any medications the patient is currently taking.

The anesthetized exam and radiographs will often uncover pathology that was not seen on conscious oral exam. The client should be contacted to obtain permission for any additional therapy, and a cost estimate should be given for the revised treatment plan. Texting or emailing clinical pictures or dental radiographs can aid in client understanding. If the client cannot be reached, performing additional therapy (especially extractions) is not recommended. Remember, you can extract a tooth any time, but you can never put it back in.

The client should receive written and verbal postoperative instructions.

Contacting the client the day after surgery is an excellent way of quickly resolving any issues that may have resulted from the dental procedure or anesthesia. This will also give them the opportunity to ask any questions and may alert them that a behavior is concerning. This communication should again be documented in the medical record.

References and Further Reading

Brodbelt D. Perioperative mortality in small animal anaesthesia. Vet J. 2009 Nov;182(2):152-61. doi: 10.1016/j.tvjl.2008.06.011. Epub 2008 Jul 26. PMID: 18658000.

Eisner E. Standard of Care in North American Animal Dental Service. in Clinical Veterinary Dentistry. Vet Clin Small Anim 43 2013, 447–469.

Moore, JI; Niemiec, B. (2014). Evaluation of extraction sites for evidence of retained tooth roots and periapical pathology. *J. Am. Anim. Hosp. Assoc.* 50(2): 77–82.

Perry R, Moore D, Scurrell E. Globe penetration in a cat following maxillary nerve block for dental surgery. J Feline Med Surg. 2015 Jan;17(1):66–72. doi: 10.1177/1098612X14560101. PMID: 25527494.

Proulx, C., Dumais, Y., Beauchamp, G., and Steagall, P. (2019). Reliability of electric pulp test or tooth transillumination to assess pulpal health in permanent canine teeth. Proceedings of the Veterinary Dental Forum, Orlando, FL, September 26–29.

Verstraete FJ, Kass PH, Terpak CH. Diagnostic value of full-mouth radiography in dogs. Am J Vet Res. 1998 Jun;59(6):686–91.

Verstraete FJ, Kass PH, Terpak CH. Diagnostic value of full-mouth radiography in cats. Am J Vet Res. 1998 Jun;59(6):692–5.

18

Dentistry Through Life

Pediatric and Geriatric Dentistry

Jerzy Gawor[1] and Brook Niemiec[2]

[1]*Veterinary Clinic Arka, Kraków, Poland*
[2]*Veterinary Dental Specialties and Oral Surgery, San Diego, CA, USA*

18.1 Pediatric Dentistry

Pediatric dentistry covers the period between birth and seven months of age, when the adult teeth are fully erupted. There are numerous problems that can occur during this time. Some are similar to conditions seen in the adult dentition, but others are only seen in juvenile patients.

Deciduous dental formulae are as follows (Table 18.1):

- **Canine:** Three incisors, one canine, and three premolars in each quadrant for a total of 28 teeth.
- **Feline:** Three incisors and one canine in each quadrant, plus three maxillary premolars per side and two mandibular premolars per side for a total of 26 teeth.

There are no deciduous molars in either species; however, the deciduous mandibular and maxillary third premolars function as – and look like – molar teeth.

Teeth eruption is a natural process typical for diphyodent animals (having two generations of teeth: deciduous and permanent). It is caused by progressive growth of the roots, and occurs at specific times for each tooth and species (Table 18.2). The deciduous teeth starts eruption at about 3 weeks of age in dogs and 2 weeks in cats. During the third month of life, shedding of the deciduous dentition associated with eruption of permanent successors occurs. The eruptive process involves a balance between the osteoclastic and odontoclastic activity above the tooth and the osteoblastic activity below it (Stapleton and Clarke 1999). The time of permanent teeth eruption is between three and seven months.

Teeth eruption consists of three stages:

- **Preeruptive stage:** Development of the crown and formation of the tooth.
- **Prefunctional eruptive stage:** Begins with onset of root development.
- **Functional post eruptive stage:** Begins when the tooth moves into occlusion (Mendoza et al. 2001).

The central role in the eruption process is played by the dental follicle (Taney and Smith 2006).

18.1.1 Problems of the Teeth

The most common problem seen in pediatric dentistry is **persistent deciduous dentition**. This is most frequently encountered in toy and small-breed dogs, but it can occur in any breed, as well as in cats. The teeth most often retained are the canines, followed by the incisors and then the premolars. This is a serious condition, since it causes both orthodontic and periodontal problems (Niemiec 2010) (Figure 18.1).

The main reason for a deciduous tooth to be persistent is an incorrect eruption path or ectopic position of the permanent tooth, but persistence can also occur due to a mechanical blockage of the eruptive path (Hobson 2005; Niemiec 2010; Carle and Shope 2014), as well as a thickened gingiva, dentigeroust cyst, enamel/dentin hypoplasia, ameloblastoma, or odontoma (Hoffman 2008).

When the permanent tooth erupts along its natural path, it places pressure on the apex of the deciduous tooth, resulting in root-end resorption in the latter.

Delayed eruption or impaction can occur due to a variety of reasons. The most common is the presence of an overlying structure that interferes with normal eruption (Shipp and Fahrenkrug 1992). Another could be abnormal and asynchronic growth of maxilla and mandible (Gracis

The Veterinary Dental Patient: A Multidisciplinary Approach, First Edition. Edited by Jerzy Gawor and Brook Niemiec.
© 2021 John Wiley & Sons Ltd. Published 2021 by John Wiley & Sons Ltd.
Companion website: www.wiley.com/go/gawor/veterinary-dental-patient

Table 18.1 Dental formulae for cats and dogs. I (incisors); C (canines); P (premolars); M (molars).

Dog	Deciduous dentition	2 x	I	3	C	1	P	3	M	0	= 28
				3		1		3		0	
	Permanent dentition	2 x	I	3	C	1	P	4	M	2	= 42
				3		1		4		3	
Cat	Deciduous dentition	2 x	I	3	C	1	P	3	M	0	= 26
				3		1		2		0	
	Permanent dentition	2 x	I	3	C	1	P	3	M	1	= 30
				3		1		2		1	

Table 18.2 Estimated timing of eruption of different teeth in different species.

	Deciduous dentition		Permanent dentition	
	Dog	Cat	Dog	Cat
Incisors	3–4	2–3	3–5	3–4
Canines	3–5	3–4	4–6	4–5
Premolars	4–5	3–6	4–6	4–6
Molars	N/A		5–7	4–5
End of eruption	5		5–7	
	Weeks		Months	

et al. 2000). Also, teeth crowding or supernumerary teeth can cause problems with permanent teeth eruption.

During assessment of dentition and occlusion in young animals, attention should be paid to whether the eruption process is progressing properly and is completed at the appropriate age. The clinical examination must be complemented by radiography in all situations of delayed eruption, persistent deciduous teeth, impaction or retention of the teeth, or missing teeth.

Juvenile gingivitis in both dogs and cats can also be associated with eruption problems and persistent deciduous dentition, as it normally appears at the time of permanent teeth eruption (Perry and Tutt 2015) (Figure 18.2). Orthodontically, the adult tooth will erupt in an unnatural position, which can cause tooth, gingival, or palatine trauma. The sooner such a tooth is removed, the better the chances of self-correction. The classic belief was that retention of the deciduous tooth caused the adult tooth to erupt in an unnatural position, but current knowledge suggests that it is the other way round: the adult tooth erupting in the wrong place causes the deciduous to be retained (Niemiec 2010).

The periodontal ramifications occur due to the fact that the gingival and periodontal apparatus is attached to the persistent deciduous in that area and therefore does not form a normal attachment to the erupting permanent tooth (Hobson 2005) (Figure 18.3). This results in a weakened periodontal attachment and susceptibility to future periodontal disease. This is even more concerning given that the patients who tend to retain teeth (toy and small breeds) be predisposed to periodontal disease.

The adult tooth does not need to be completely erupted for these problems to occur; In fact, the problems begin as soon as the permanent tooth begins to erupt. Therefore, the tooth should be extracted as early as possible to lessen the untoward effects. Do not wait until six months of age to perform the extraction alongside neutering.

In human dentistry, a tooth is considered retained when its enamel touches the permanent successor (Figure 18.4). This allows for prompt therapy: there is no point in delaying extraction once the enamels of the two teeth are in contact. Human dentists also call this pseudopolyodontia.

Malocclusions in deciduous teeth are fairly common (Niemiec 2010). In some cases (especially mild mesioclusion of the mandibular canines), the patient may be genetically programmed for a normal bite and only temporarily maloccluded (Niemiec 2010). This is due to the fact that the maxilla and mandible grow at varying rates (Hennet and Harvey 1992). However, the deciduous dentition may interfere with jaw movement and subsequent correction. This situation is called an **adverse dental interlock** (Gawor 2013) (Figure 18.5). The interlock may be removed via extraction of the deciduous teeth that are creating it, through a procedure known as **interceptive orthodontics**. If this is done promptly in a patient that is genetically programmed to have a normal bite, self-correction may occur (Hale 2005). Classically, it was recommended that teeth be extracted from the jaw on which movement was desired. However, this author recommends extracting any tooth that may cause a problem. Interceptive orthodontics

(a)

(b)

(c)

(d)

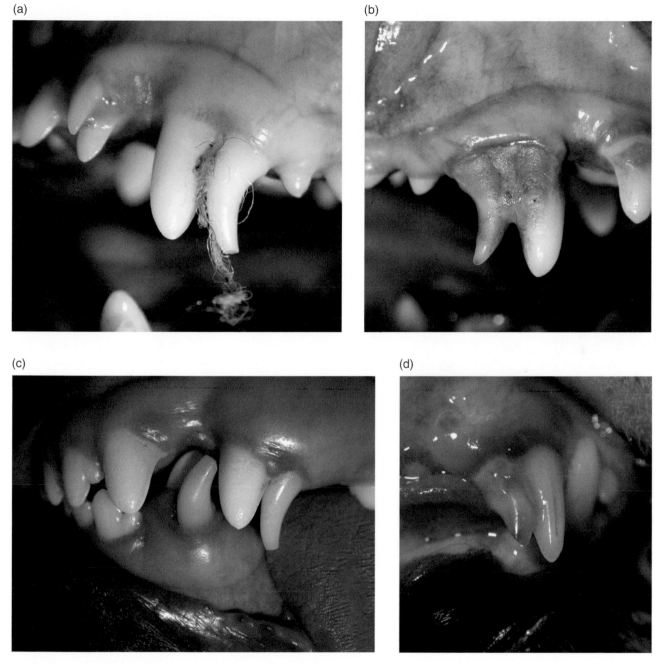

Figure 18.1   Persistent deciduous dentition causes numerous problems, including (a) entrapment of foreign objects, (b) faster deposition of dental calculus, (c) malocclusion, and (d) gingivitis.

should be performed as soon as possible (six to eight weeks) for maximum effect (Wiggs and Lobprise 1997).

In class II (overshot) and IV (wry) malocclusions, the patient often suffers from palatine trauma secondary to the tooth malalignment (Niemiec 2010) (Figure 18.6). This hurts like a thorn in the paw. Extraction will alleviate this discomfort, as well as possibly allowing movement of the jaw.

Malocclusions in the adult dentition can be treated in various ways. These include extraction, coronal amputation and vital pulp therapy, and orthodontic appliances (Niemiec 2013). Early recognition and proper therapy are essential to successful outcomes.

Deciduous teeth are weaker than adult teeth and therefore have an increased susceptibility to **fracture** (Hale 2005). Combined with the fact that the pulp chamber is very large,

(a)

(b)

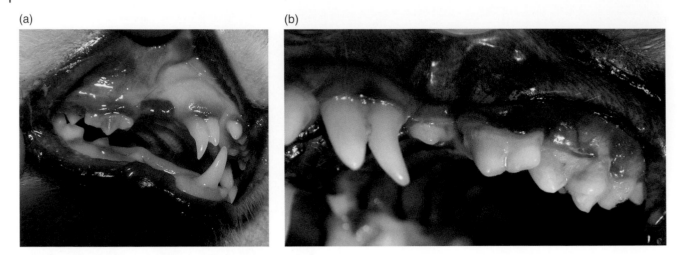

Figure 18.2   Juvenile gingivitis in (a) cats and (b) dogs can be associated with persistent deciduous dentition.

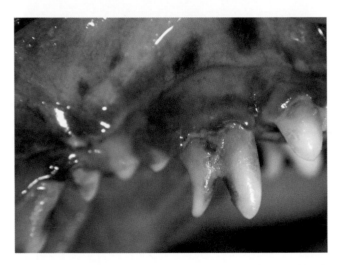

Figure 18.3   The gingival sulcus cannot be correctly developed in the presence of persistent deciduous teeth leading to faster development of periodontal diseases.

this makes pulp (nerve) exposure a fairly common occurrence. This is a very painful experience for the patient, though they may not demonstrate it outwardly (Golden et al. 1982). In addition, deciduous teeth can quickly become infected in the same manner as a permanent tooth. All deciduous teeth which are fractured with direct pulp exposure need to be extracted; ignoring them is *not* an option (Ulbricht et al. 2003). Do not wait until neutering as they will be painful and infected on a daily basis (Figure 18.7).

In addition to the previously mentioned arguments for immediate extraction of fractured deciduous teeth, one more is important: infection of their pulp, and subsequent pulp necrosis and abscess, can affect the permanent tooth developing near the periapical area (Figure 18.8).

Unerupted teeth can occur for a variety of reasons. Generally, they are due to a failure of passive eruption. There is no practical therapy for this condition. On occasion, however, there may be bony or soft-tissue interference

(Shipp and Fahrenkrug 1992). If this is suspected, an **operculectomy** (surgical removal of the barrier to eruption) should be performed as soon as possible (Stapleton and Clarke 1999). This *must* be performed prior to root-end closure (at approximately one year of age) in order for the tooth to naturally erupt. If this fails to bring about resolution of the problem, the cause is likely failure of passive eruption. The most common teeth to be impacted or embedded are the mandibular first premolars in brachycephalic dogs (Niemiec 2010).

The biggest issue with unerupted teeth is that they may lead to the formation of **dentigerous cysts** (Figure 18.9). Such cysts have been reported to occur in 29% of impacted teeth in dogs (Babbitt et al. 2016). They are created by fluid leaking from ameloblasts (which would normally be exfoliated during eruption). (MacGee et al 2012) They can become quite large and disfiguring, necessitating major surgical correction. In addition, they can result in pathologic fracture (Niemiec 2017). For this reason, all "missing" teeth should be radiographed at an early age.

The radiographic appearance of such cystic structures is classically a radiolucent structure surrounding the crown of an impacted tooth (Gawor et al. 2017a) (Figure 18.10). If a cyst is found, treatment should be performed right away. The treatment of choice is currently surgical extraction of the offending tooth and thorough debridement of the cystic lining (Anderson and Harvey 1993; Neville et al. 2002; Taney and Smith 2006). To rule out early malignancy, it is always reasonable to submit the removed tissue samples for histopathologic evaluation.

Enamel hypoplasia/hypocalcification results from a malformation of the enamel occurring prior to tooth eruption (Wiggs and Lobprise 1997). Once the tooth erupts into the mouth, the weakened enamel flakes off, exposing the underlying dentin (Niemiec 2014a). The dentinal exposure causes significant discomfort for the patient as the dentinal tubules produce significant pain

(a) 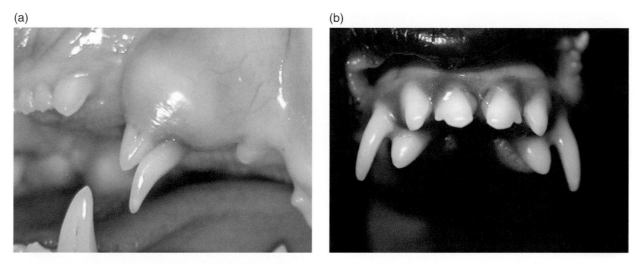 (b)

Figure 18.4 (a) By definition, persistent deciduous teeth are those whose enamels are touching one another. (b) However this situation does not always occur.

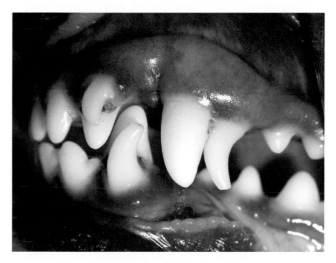

Figure 18.5 Adverse dental interlock caused by persistent deciduous dentition.

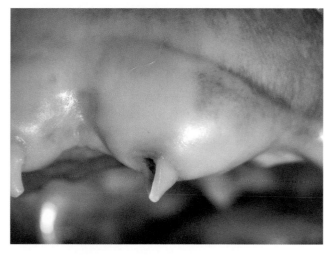

Figure 18.7 A fractured deciduous tooth always requires action.

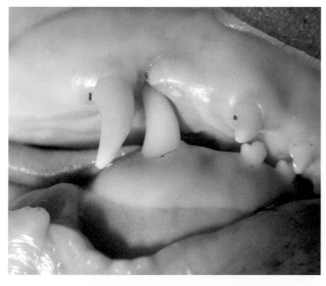

Figure 18.6 Class II malocclusion is very often traumatic, regardless of whether it occurs in the deciduous or permanent dentition.

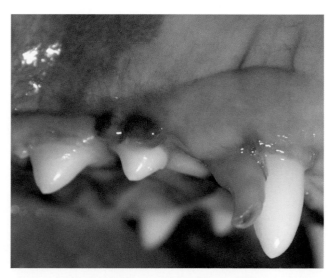

Figure 18.8 Complications of neglected tooth fracture: periapical lesion in a nonvital fractured infected deciduous tooth.

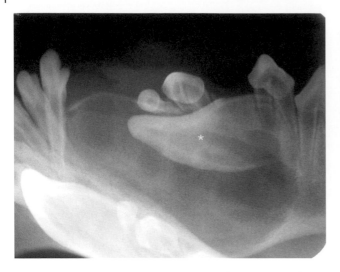

Figure 18.9 Dentigerous cyst associated with an impacted canine tooth (Asterisk) in a young dog.

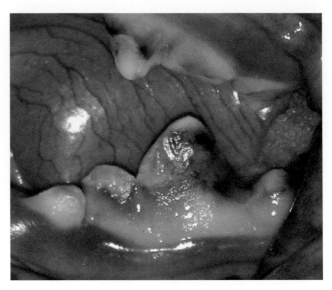

Figure 18.11 Enamel hypoplasia present on multiple teeth.

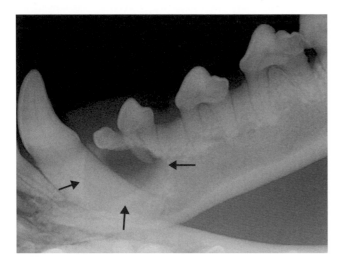

Figure 18.10 Radiographic appearance of a dentigerous cyst associated with an impacted first mandibular premolar tooth.

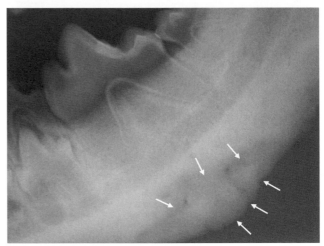

Figure 18.12 Periostitis ossificans visible in a young dog mandible as a "double cortex" (arrows).

(Startup 2014). In addition, the exposed tubules can act as a conduit for bacterial infection of the pulp (or root canal system), which may initiate endodontic disease. The dentinal surface is much rougher than enamel, and its exposure increases plaque and calculus deposition, which in turn increases periodontal inflammation. Finally, the dentin will become stained (Figure 18.11). For all of these reasons, prompt and definitive therapy of such teeth is critical to the health of the patient. The best treatment is restorative: ideally a composite restoration, though in smaller teeth or in cases of financial limitations, bonded sealants can be performed (Niemiec 2014a). A properly placed restoration will alleviate all of the deleterious effects associated with this condition. Finally, in severe cases where increased strength is necessary to

avoid a fracture, a cast-metal crown could be performed (Niemiec 2014b). Congenital enamel defects may also be associated with genetic factors (see Chapter 10).

Periostitis ossificans in large-breed puppies result from an inflamed or infected dental follicle, developing from an unerupted tooth (typically the mandibular first molar) or secondary to pericoronitis. The presented cases were seen in males aged three to five months with unilateral mandibular swelling. This condition generally resolves with no treatment (Blazejewski et al. 2010) (Figure 18.12).

Other anatomic anomalies include gemination, fusion, concrescence of the teeth, presence of supernumerary teeth, supernumerary roots, dilaceration of crowns or roots, invagination of teeth, and enamel pearls. Intrinsic tooth discoloration may be caused by systemic and local factors. Though changes caused by systemic tetracycline administration do not require treatment, other staining may be associated with internal resorption or pulp disease.

All of the preceding conditions must be evaluated radiographically in order to design a good treatment plan and to determine a prognosis (Gawor et al. 2017b) (Figure 18.13).

18.1.2 Problems of the Oral Soft Tissues

Cleft palates are a fairly uncommon occurrence. They can be fairly mild to major and may involve the hard and/or the soft palate. The length of the cleft is not the major prognostic factor, but the width: the wider the cleft, the more guarded the prognosis. Clefts can generally be corrected surgically, but this can be quite challenging due to the lack of pliability of the palate (Niemiec 2010). Many flap techniques have been devised for the correction of these defects (Marretta 2012). These are very challenging procedures with a less than excellent prognosis, and thus referral to a qualified veterinary dentist is strongly recommended. If the practitioner attempts repair (either by choice or due to circumstances), they are encouraged to study and practice these techniques first. The major point to consider in these cases is the need to create closure without tension. In addition, every effort must be made to successfully cure the problem on the first attempt, as subsequent surgeries will be more difficult due to scar tissue formation. It is important to note that in dogs with congenital palatal defects, other craniomaxillofacial abnormalities may occur. This is why advanced imaging, including CT, is recommended for all dogs with such defects, in order to better assess associated craniofacial defects and better plan surgical repair (Nemec et al. 2014).

Oral papillomatosis is the most common proliferative condition in puppies. It appears as whitish cauliflower growths on the gingiva and oral mucosa. It is viral-induced and generally self-limiting (Harvey and McKeever 1998). However, it can become infected and can mimic more aggressive tumors (Niemiec 2010). Therefore, excisional biopsy may be recommended to ensure the diagnosis, especially in questionable cases.

Eruptive gingivitis is inflammation of the gingiva during and just after tooth eruption. It is self-limiting in most cases, but home care (brushing or chlorhexidine rinses) is recommended to decrease the inflammation. Juvenile gingivitis in cats can progress into juvenile periodontitis if untreated. If the condition does not resolve in a short period of time, additional diagnostics and therapy are recommended, as this could actually represent juvenile periodontitis.

Juvenile periodontitis is an emerging problem in felines (Niemiec 2012a). The etiology is currently unknown, but in humans there is a period of increased susceptibility to gingivitis during the pubertal period (puberty gingivitis) (Neville et al. 2002; Niemiec 2010). Furthermore, a genetic predisposition has been reported in Siamese, Somali, and Maine Coon cats (Wiggs and Lobprise 1997). Onset is usually during the eruptive period of the permanent dentition, and bleeding during mastication and on oral exam may occur (Niemiec 2010). Many cases are associated with proliferation of the free gingival margin and creation of pseudopockets (Figure 18.14). These patients are not typically painful, but halitosis as well as bilateral mandibular lymphadenopathy is common. If left untreated, juvenile periodontitis typically proceeds quickly to periodontal disease (Niemiec 2010). This in turn results in significant early bone loss, periodontal pocket formation, and furcation exposure (Wiggs and Lobprise 1997), which is most significant around the

(a)

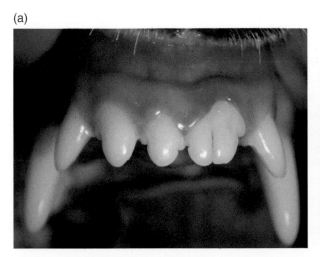

(b)

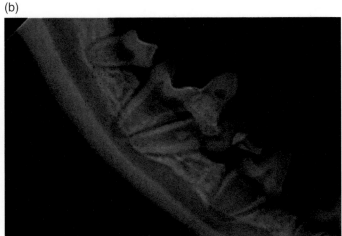

Figure 18.13   (a) Fused incisor teeth in a six-month-old whippet. (b) Invagination of a tooth (409) in a Chihuahua. Note missing 311 and convergence of the roots in all teeth.

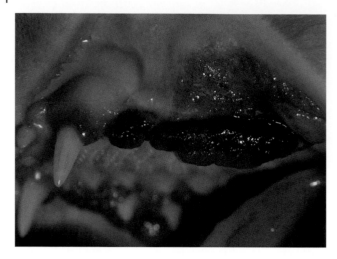

Figure 18.14 Proliferative juvenile gingivitis in a Maine Coon cat.

mandibular first molars. This condition is commonly mistaken for caudal stomatitis. The distinguishing clinical sign is the lack of caudal inflammation in cases of periodontitis. The therapeutic goal is the same as in all cases of periodontitis: plaque control (Niemiec 2012a). However, due to the level of inflammation, this must be much stricter than in classic chronic periodontitis. Early (nine months of age) and frequent (q six to nine months) dental prophylaxis and strict home care are critical to decreasing inflammation (Niemiec 2010). Ideally, home care should consist of daily brushing, which is the gold standard of plaque control. Other home-care alternatives include chlorhexidine rinses (Maxi/Guard, Addison Labs) and plaque-control diets (t/d Canine and Feline, Hills Pet Nutrition, Topeka, KS) and treats. In cases where gingival hyperplasia is present, early gingivectomy is recommended to remove psuedopockets, decrease inflammation, and facilitate plaque control (both professional and home-care) (Niemiec 2012a). Finally, extraction of any significantly diseased teeth is warranted, to decrease the degree of inflammation (Niemiec 2010). Susceptibility appears to subside at approximately two years of age (Wiggs and Lobprise 1997). If this does not occur, effective management is often exceedingly difficult (Niemiec 2010).

Other conditions seen in juvenile patients (e.g., infantile calvarial hyperostosis [ICH], craniomandibular osteopathy [CMO], cleft lip, microglossia, and malocclusion) are discussed in Chapters 10 and 18.

18.2 Geriatric Dentistry

The lifespan of small-animal patients is getting increasing, mostly due to advances in medicine as well as the continuous efforts of veterinarians to prevent and treat dis-

eases. In addition, since pets are now part of the family, clients are investing more in proper care.

With age, oral health generally worsens, so older patients suffer from a higher degree of pain and infection. For this reason, senior-care programs for veterinary patients should very strongly highlight oral care, and regular oral examinations must become part of any prophylactic regime (Metzger 2005).

Periodontal disease has been associated with numerous local and systemic conditions that negatively affect the quality of life (QOL), and possibly the lifespan, of animal patients (Niemiec 2012b,c). These consequences, along with the general trend toward ownership of smaller-breed dogs and the increasing lifespan of all breeds, make treatment of periodontal disease in senior pets critical.

The potential systemic consequences of periodontal disease are numerous, and while there is no direct cause and effect, the staggering number of references is significant. One of the organs most affected is the heart. The highest hazard ratios are for endocarditis (6.36) and hypertrophic cardiomyopathy (3.96) for dogs with a prior diagnosis of stage 3 periodontal disease (Glickman et al. 2009). Further, the kidney and liver are responsible for filtration of the blood and thus will also be negatively affected by periodontal infection (Taboada and Meyer 1989; Debowes et al. 1996; Pavlica et al. 2008; Finch et al. 2016). Human studies have additionally linked periodontal disease to strokes and pulmonary infections, as well as an increased risk of malignancies (Hayes et al. 1998; Hujoel et al. 2003). There are also numerous reports of increased risk of diabetes mellitus in patients with periodontal disease (Nishimura et al. 2005; Nagata 2009).

There is increasing evidence for a benefit of periodontal care on systemic disease, with improvements noted in heart, liver, and kidney function and diabetic control (Stewart et al. 2001; Tomofuji et al. 2009; Graziani et al. 2010). Thus, patients with comorbidities that do not severely affect anesthetic risk should receive a recommendation for dental care (Niemiec 2012c).

Speaking of anesthesia, there are numerous myths and misconceptions related to dental care in older patients, the most prominent of which is that age itself a significant risk factor. In fact, age has minimal effect on anesthetic risk. Such risk is always a concern, but it must be weighed against the potential benefits to the patient of management of their oral pain and infection. Most owners accept anesthetic risk when it is significantly exceeded by the potential benefits to their pet, and the improvement in their QOL. Fatal complications (death from anesthesia) are reported at 0.17% in dogs and 0.24% in cats (Brodbelt et al. 2008). Furthermore, most of these cases are associated with the use of xylazine or a lack of heart-rate monitoring (Dyson et al. 1998). Since xylazine is

(a)

(b)

(c)

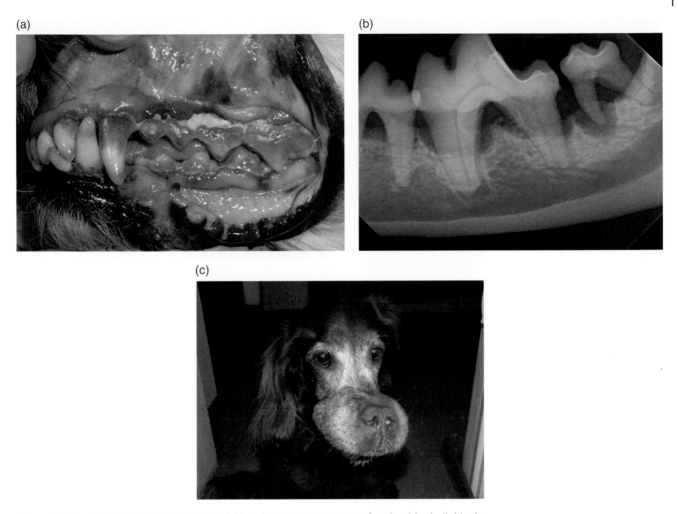

Figure 18.15   (a,b) Periodontal disease and (c) oral tumors occur more often in older individuals.

currently recognized as substandard care and the level of monitoring is vastly improved, both factors are less of a problem today. The safety of anesthesia and the composition of the anesthetic protocol are thoroughly covered in Chapter 12.

Due to the generalized lack of quality dental care in veterinary patients and the common occurrence of significant dental diseases, extraction of most or all of a patient's teeth is not an uncommon occurrence. A common question among pet owners is, "How can my dog or cat survive (eat) without teeth?" The veterinary dental community fully agrees with the opinion of Hale (2003) that "The dog is far better off having no teeth than having bad teeth . . . preserving bad teeth in the face of a poor or questionable prognosis serves no positive purpose." This comes from the fact that dogs, as well as cats, have less and less need to express their territorial instinct and defend their area, and the hunting and killing of prey animals is becoming even less common.

Periodontal disease affects the vast majority of dogs and cats (Lund et al. 1999), and age is a predilecting factor for this disease (Gawor et al. 2006) (Figure 18.15). Teeth resorption

(Fig. 18.16) and increased risk of oral tumors (Figure 18.15c.) are related to age (Peralta et al. 2010). Therefore, in old patients, radiographic and clinical evaluation must be focused on these problems. Due to a reported association between the presence of oral tumors and teeth resorption after the discovery of signs of resorption, examination must look for any suggestion of proliferation (Nemec et al. 2012) (Figure 18.17).

Worn teeth due to attrition or abrasion may likewise be more frequently diagnosed in older animals. Attrition from malocclusions generally reaches an equilibrium by about 18 months of age, but abrasion from ball chewing or pruritus (self-chewing) will worsen with age (Figure 18.18). Tooth resorption is more common in older cats (up to 75% at age over nine years) (Lommer and Verstraete 2001), and extrusion (movement of a tooth beyond its normal occlusal plane) is more common in older patients (Lewis et al. 2008) (Figure 18.19).

Aging of orodental structures is an ongoing process that must be taken into account when planning oral surgery in

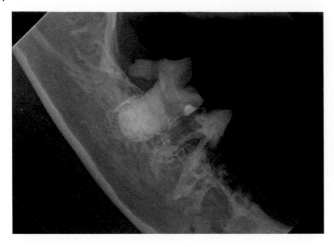

Figure 18.16 Ankylosis and teeth resorption are more frequent in geriatric patients.

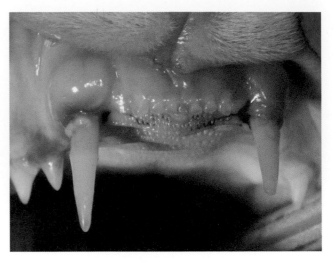

Figure 18.19 Right maxillary canine tooth (104) extrusion in a cat can be associated with tooth resorption.

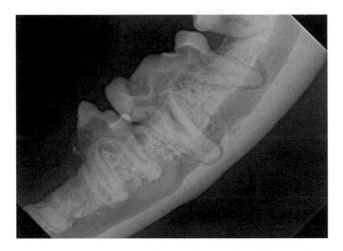

Figure 18.17 Tooth resorption may be associated with oral tumors. In this dog, the contralateral mandible was affected by squamous-cell carcinoma (SCC).

older pets. Thinning and decreased keratinization of the gingival epithelium, a decresing number of fibroblasts, and decreased synthesis of collagen makes recovery potentials lower than in younger individuals. Periodontal ligaments have a more irregular structure and fewer fibroblasts, so their number and elasticity may decrease. This can compromise their major function, which is absorbing the forces applied during mastication (Needleman 2006). In young animals, the periodontal ligament space is relatively wide and thick, but with age and thickening of the cementum and alveolar bone, it becomes narrower. This results in extractions being more difficult in older patients, unless there is advanced periodontal disease (Figures 18.20 and 18.21).

Standards for procedures, equipment, instrumentation, and materials remain the same no matter the patient's age. Older patients deserve the same level of care as younger

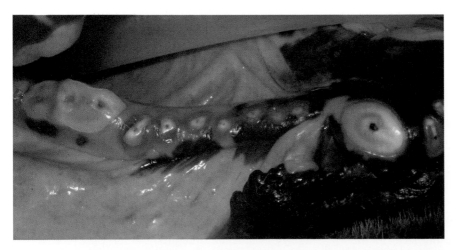

Figure 18.18 Bad habits like chewing on hard objects cause generalized teeth abrasion with time often with pulp chamber exposure.

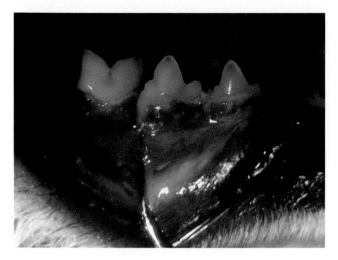

Figure 18.20 Transparent and brittle enamel can be one of the signs of teeth aging.

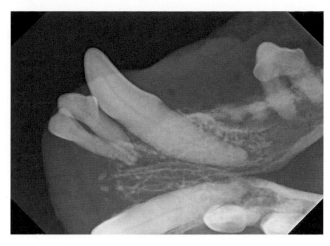

Figure 18.21 Alveolar bone atrophy is often diagnosed in older toy-breed dogs.

ones: if a root canal treatment is the superior choice, it should be offered. However, the anesthesia time required and the need for reexamination under general anesthesia may make extraction a more logical choice in these pets, rather than an advanced procedure.

As a final note, several factors make companion dogs a powerful animal model for understanding age-related diseases in humans, including their comparatively accelerated rate of aging, their high prevalence of oral diseases, and their cohabitation of the human environment.

References

Anderson, J.G. and Harvey, C.E. (1993). Odontogenic cysts. *J Vet. Dent.* 4: 5–9.

Babbitt, S.G., Krakowski Volker, M., and Luskin, I.R. (2016). Incidence of radiographic cystic lesions associated with Unerupted teeth in dogs. *J. Vet. Dent.* 33 (4): 226–233.

Blazejewski, S.W., Lewis, J.R., Gracis, M. et al. (2010). Mandibular periostitis ossificans in immature large breed dogs: 5 cases (1999–2006). *J. Vet. Dent.* 27 (3): 148–159.

Brodbelt, DC. et. al. (2008). The risk of death: the confidential enquiry into perioperative small animal fatalities. *Vet. Anaesth. Anal.* 35 (5): 365–373.

Carle, D. and Shope, B. (2014). Soft tissue tooth impaction in a dog. *J. Vet. Dent.* 31 (2): 96–105.

Debowes, L.J., Mosier, D., Logan, E. et al. (1996). Association of periodontal disease and histologic lesions in multiple organs from 45 dogs. *J. Vet. Dent.* 13 (2): 57–60.

Dyson, D.H., Maxie, M.G., and Schnurr, D. (1998). Morbidity and mortality associated with anesthetic management in small animal veterinary practice in Ontario. *J. Am. Anim. Hosp. Assoc.* 34: 325–335.

Finch, N.C., Syme, H.M., and Elliott, J. (2016). Risk factors for development of chronic kidney disease in cats. *J. Vet. Intern. Med.* 30 (2): 602–610.

Gawor, J. (2013). Genetics and heredity in veterinary orthodontics. In: *Veterinary Orthodontics*, vol. 20 (ed. B.A. Niemiec), 8–12. Tustin, CA: Practical Veterinary Publishing.

Gawor, J. (2017a). Dental radiograph interpretation, Part G: Proliferative lesions. In: *Practical Veterinary Dental Radiology* (eds. B.A. Niemiec, J. Gawor and V. Jekl), 193–219. Boca Raton, FL: CRC Press.

Gawor, J. (2017b). Dental radiograph interpretation, Part E: Hard tissue diseases. In: *Practical Veterinary Dental Radiology* (eds. B.A. Niemiec, J. Gawor and V. Jekl), 156–172. Boca Raton, FL: CRC Press.

Gawor, J., Reiter, A., Jodkowska, K. et al. (2006). Influence of diet on oral heath in cats and dogs. *J. Nutr.* 136 (7 Suppl): 2021S–2023S.

Glickman, L.T., Glickman, N.W., Moore, G.E. et al. (2009). Evaluation of the risk of endocarditis and other cardiovascular events on the basis of the severity of periodontal disease in dogs. *J. Am. Vet. Med. Assoc.* 234 (4): 486–494.

Golden, A.L., Stoller, N.S., and Harvey, C.E. (1982). A survey of oral and dental diseases in dogs anesthetized at a veterinary hospital. *J. Am. Anim. Hosp. Assoc.* 18: 891–899.

Gracis, M., Keith, D., and Vite, C.H. (2000). Dental and craniofacial findings in 8 miniature schnauzer dogs affected by myotonia congenita. *J. Vet. Dent.* 17 (3): 119–127.

Graziani, F., Cei, S., La Ferla, F. et al. (2010). Effects of non-surgical periodontal therapy on the glomerular filtration rate of the kidney: an exploratory trial. *J. Clin. Periodontol.* 37 (7): 638–643.

Hale, F.A. (2003). The owner–animal–environment triad in the treatment of canine periodontal disease. *J. Vet. Dent.* 20 (2): 118–122.

Hale, F.A. (2005). Juvenile veterinary dentistry. *Vet. Clin. North Am. Small Anim. Pract.* 35: 789–817.

Harvey, R.G. and McKeever, P.J. (1998). Nodular dermatoses. In: *A Colour Handbook of Skin Diseases of the Dog and Cat*, 57–80. London: Manson.

Hayes, C., Sparrow, D., Cohen, M. et al. (1998). The association between alveolar bone loss and pulmonary function: the VA dental longitudinal study. *Ann. Periodontol.* 3 (1): 257–261.

Hennet, P.R. and Harvey, C.E. (1992). Craniofacial development and growth in the dog. *J. Vet. Dent.* 9 (2): 11–18.

Hobson, P. (2005). Extraction of retained primary canine teeth in the dog. *J. Vet. Dent.* 22 (2): 132–137.

Hoffman, S. (2008). Abnormal tooth eruption in a cat. *J. Vet. Dent.* 25 (2): 118–122.

Hujoel, P.P., Drangsholt, M., Spiekerman, C., and Weiss, N.S. (2003). An exploration of the periodontitis-cancer association. *Ann. Epidemiol.* 13: 312–316.

Lewis, J., Eked, A., Shofer, F. et al. (2008). Significant association between tooth extrusion and tooth resorption in domestic cats. *J. Vet. Dent.* 25 (2): 86–95.

Lommer, M.J. and Verstraete, F.J.M. (2001). Radiographic patterns of periodontitis in cats: 147 cases (1998–1999). *J. Am. Vet. Med. Assoc.* 218: 230–234.

Lund, E.M., Armstrong, P.J. et al. (1999). Health status and population characteristics of dogs and cats examined at private veterinary practices in the United States. *J. Am. Vet. Med. Assoc.* 214: 1336–1341.

MacGee, S; Pinson, D; Shaiken, L. (2012). Bilateral dentigerous cysts in a dog. *J. Vet. Dent.* 29 (4): 242–249.

Marretta, S.M. (2012). Cleft palate repair techniques. In: *Oral and Maxillofacial Surgery in Dogs and Cats*, 1e (eds. F.J. Verstraete and M.J. Lommer), 351–362. Edinburgh: W.B. Saunders.

Mendoza, K.A., Marretta, S.M., Behr, M.J., and Klippert, L.S. (2001). Facial swelling associated with impaction of the deciduous and permanent maxillary fourth premolars in a dog with patent ductus arteriosus. *J. Vet. Dent.* 18 (2): 69–74.

Metzger, F.L. (2005). Senior and geriatric care programs for veterinarians. *Vet. Clin. Small Anim.* 35: 743–753.

Nagata, T. (2009). Relationhip between diabetes and periodontal disease. *Clin. Calc.* 19 (9): 1291–1298.

Needleman, I. (2006). Aging and the periodontium. In: *Carranza's Clinical Periodontology* (eds. F.A. Carranza,

M.G. Newman, H.H. Takei and P.R. Klokkevold), 93–98. St. Louis, MO: Elsevier.

Nemec, A., Arzi, B., Murphy, B. et al. (2012). Prevalence and types of tooth resorption in dogs with oral tumors. *Am. J. Vet. Res.* 73 (7): 1057–1066.

Nemec, A., Danbiaux, L., Johnson, E. et al. (2014). Craniomaxillofacial abnormalities in dogs with congenital palatal defects: computed tomographic findings. *Vet. Surg.* 9999: 1–6.

Neville, B.W., Damm, D.D., Allen, C.M., and Bouquot, J.E. (2002). Periodontal diseases. In: *Oral and Maxillofacial Pathology*, 2e (eds. J.P. Sapp, L. Eversole and G. Wysocki), 137–162. Philadelphia, PA: W.B. Saunders.

Niemiec, B.A. (2010). Pathology in the pediatric patient. In: *Small Animal Dental, Oral and Maxillofacial Disease, a Color Handbook* (ed. B.A. Niemiec), 189–126. London: Manson.

Niemiec, B.A. (2012a). Unusual forms of periodontal disease. In: *Veterinary Periodontology* (ed. B.A. Niemeic), 101–103. Ames, IA: Wiley-Blackwell.

Niemiec, B.A. (2012b). Local and regional consequences of periodontal disease. In: *Veterinary Periodontology* (ed. B.A. Niemiec), 69–80. Ames, IA: Wiley-Blackwell.

Niemiec, B.A. (2012c). Systemic manifestations of periodontal disease. In: *Veterinary Periodontology* (ed. B.A. Niemiec), 81–90. Ames, IA: Wiley-Blackwell.

Niemiec, B.A. (2013). *Veterinary Orthodontics*. Tustin CA: Practical Veterianry Publishing.

Niemiec, B.A. (2014a). Restoration of enamel hypocalcification. In: *Veterinary Restorative Dentistry for the General Practitioner* (ed. B.A. Niemiec), 56–64. San Diego, CA: Practical Veterinary Publishing.

Niemiec, B.A. (2014b). Indications for restoration. In: *Veterinary Restorative Dentistry for the General Practitioner* (ed. B.A. Niemiec), 36–47. San Diego, CA: Practical Veterinary Publishing.

Niemiec, B.A. (2017). The indications for and importance of dental radiographs. In: *Practical Veterianry Dental Radiology* (eds. B.A. Niemiec, J. Gawor and V. Jekel), 5–30. Boca Raton, FL: CRC Press.

Nishimura, F., Soga, Y., Iwamoto, Y. et al. (2005). Periodontal disease as part of the insulin resistance syndrome in diabetic patients. *J. Int. Acad. Periodontol.* 7 (1): 16–20.

Pavlica, Z., Petelin, M., Juntes, P. et al. (2008). Periodontal disease burden and pathological changes in the organs of dogs. *J. Vet. Dent.* 25 (2): 97–108.

Peralta, S., Verstraete, F.J.M., and Kass, P.H. (2010). Radiographic evaluation of the types of tooth resorption in dogs. *Am. J. Vet. Res.* 71 (7): 784–793.

Perry, R. and Tutt, C. (2015). Periodontal disease in cats back to basis with an eye on the future. *J. Feline Med. Surg.* 17: 45–65.

Shipp, A.D. and Fahrenkrug, P. (1992). *Practitioner's Guide to Veterinary Dentistry*. Beverly Hills, CA: Dr. Shipps Laboratories.

Stapleton, B.L. and Clarke, L.L. (1999). Mandibular canine tooth impaction in a young dog. Treatment and subsequent eruption: a case report. *J. Vet. Dent.* 16 (3): 105–108.

Startup, S. (2014). Tooth defense and response. In: *Veterinary Restorative Dentistry for the General Practitioner* (ed. B.A. Niemiec), 16–35. San Diego, CA: Practical Veterinary Publishing.

Stewart, J.E., Wager, K.A., Friedlander, A.H., and Zadeh, H.H. (2001). The effect of periodontal treatment on glycemic control in patients with type 2 diabetes mellitus. *J. Clin. Periodontol.* 28: 306–310.

Taboada, J. and Meyer, D.J. (1989). Cholestasis in associated with extrahepatic bacterial infection in five dogs. *J. Vet. Intern. Med.* 3: 216–220.

Taney, K.G. and Smith, M.M. (2006). Surgical extraction of impacted teeth in a dog. *J. Vet. Dent.* 23 (3): 168–177.

Tomofuji, T., Ekuni, D., Sanbe, T. et al. (2009). Effects of improvement in periodontal inflammation by tooth brushing on serum lipopolysaccharide concentration and liver injury in rats. *Acta Odontol. Scand.* 67: 200–205.

Ulbricht, R.D., Marretta, S.M., and Klippert, L.S. (2003). Surgical extraction of a fractured, nonvital deciduous tooth in a tiger. *J. Vet. Dent.* 20 (4): 209–212.

Wiggs, R.B. and Lobprise, H.B. (1997). Domestic feline oral and dental disease. In: *Veterinary Dentistry: Principles and Practice* (eds. R.B. Wiggs and H.B. Lobprise), 482–517. Philadelphia, PA: Lippincott-Raven.

Part III

Dentistry in Daily Practice

What Every Veterinarian Should Know

19

Management of the Dental Patient

Jerzy Gawor[1] and Brook Niemiec[2]

[1]*Veterinary Clinic Arka, Kraków, Poland*
[2]*Veterinary Dental Specialties and Oral Surgery, San Diego, CA, USA*

19.1   Identifying Problems

There are three major routes to identifying a possible oral/dental problem:

1) **Routine oral examination** during the annual physical or when presented for another condition. The oral cavity assessment in a conscious patient can provide sufficient information to proceed with additional examination and testing (typically under general anesthesia), and as such is a critical part of any clinical examination. Regular oral rechecks are part of the oral prophylactic program (see Chapter 5). The veterinary dental patient is in general a lifelong patient. Simple scoring systems based on interviews and short clinical assessment provide the **oral health index (**OHI**)** (see Chapters 4 and 5), based on which the veterinarian can categorize patients into one of three groups: prophylactic recommendations; significant change or surgery required; and immediate surgery mandatory.
2) **Owner's initiative**, as a result of bad breath, blood in the saliva, drooling, deformation of the head, or difficulty eating. This is why education of the public is so important, and waiting-room posters, smartphone applications, and public campaigns focusing on these signs are essential to pet health (Figure 19.1). A sufficiently educated owner may even perform their own assessment at home and, using the available scoring systems, decide whether their pet is a candidate for dental consult or prophylaxis.
3) **Incidental finding during anesthesia.** This is a very common situation, especially in patients that are difficult to examine or do not show any clinical signs (Figure 19.3). It is important for all members of the veterinary team to evaluate the oral cavity when an animal is sedated or anesthetized, regardless of the reason why anesthesia was performed.

19.2   First Consultation or Discussion with the pet owner

This includes qualification for surgery and anesthesia, dental history, and preliminary estimates of time and cost. During the first consultation, the following subjects should be discussed: safety of anesthesia, professional dental cleaning, reasons for surgery, and the suspected category of the health problem (e.g., trauma, pulp diseases, malocclusion, periodontal diseases, extractions, oral tumor, developmental disorder).

Specialists and general practitioners often have different perspectives, communication styles, and expectations during the first consultation:

1) Specialist perspectives. The owner is already aware that an oral problem exists, so the dental specialist will inform them mostly about possible actions and scenarios, as well as the necessity of anesthesia. Clients normally expect that a specialist will share their thoughts about the preliminary diagnosis. Quite often, they will ask, "What would you do if it was your pet?" At this point, the specialist should not promote a particular treatment option, but should present all available modalities and decide with the owner which best to pursue, based on the patient's condition. Depending on their skill level, they might draw a picture for the owner, showing the origin of the problem, the mechanisms of pathology, and the treatment goals (Figure 19.3).

The Veterinary Dental Patient: A Multidisciplinary Approach, First Edition. Edited by Jerzy Gawor and Brook Niemiec.
© 2021 John Wiley & Sons Ltd. Published 2021 by John Wiley & Sons Ltd.
Companion website: www.wiley.com/go/gawor/veterinary-dental-patient

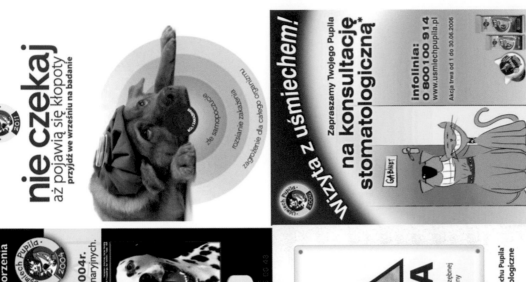

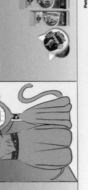
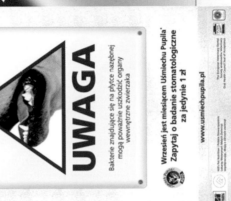
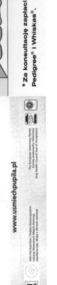
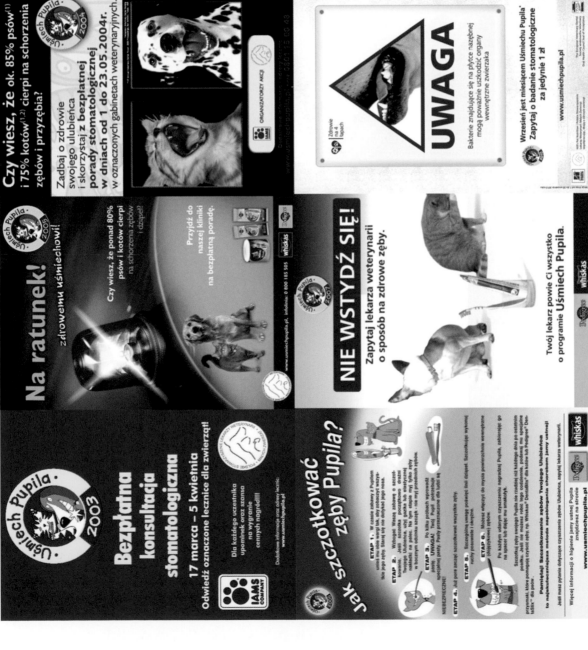

Figure 19.1   PetSmile Campaign posters.

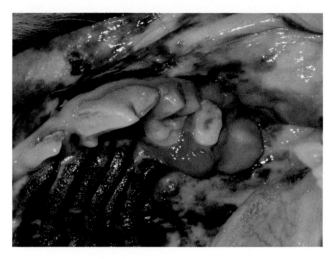

Figure 19.2 Incidental finding of oral growth in a patient undergoing nondental surgery.

2) GP perspectives. General practitioners struggle with a general lack of oral health awareness in the public. Relatively few patients (<10%) come to veterinarians with a dental complaint. Therefore, in many cases, the first-contact veterinarian faces two important challenges when presented with oral disease. The first is to convince the owner that the identified problem has clinical importance and requires treatment. The second is to avoid the temptation to help the patient without a diagnosis, by providing relief of pain or infection with an empiric treatment. Even if the patient is eventually referred, such an action quite often postpones the moment of surgery, because antibiotics and anti-inflammatory drugs can temporally improve the situation and give a false feeling that the problem has been solved.

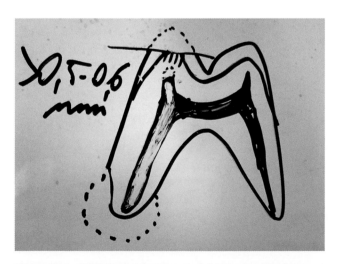

Figure 19.3 Whiteboard drawing explaining a problem to a pet owner.

19.3 Additional Consultations: Internal Medicine, Cardiologist, Neurologist, Anesthesiologist

These should always be a part of any anesthesia assessment in patients with comorbidities, regardless of who is going to operate (general practitioner or specialist). Minimizing anesthesia risk and estimating the maximum amount of time for which the patient can be anesthetized can be accomplished using a multidisciplinary approach. Otherwise, such consultations are not required routinely, but if there is any doubt – or on request of the pet owner – they should be carried out.

19.4 Day of Surgery

1) It is common for clients to decline some part of recommended care. "Against medical advice" (AMA) is the term used in healthcare institutions when a patient leaves a hospital against the advice of their doctor. There is widespread ethical and legal consensus that competent patients (or their authorized surrogates) are entitled to decline recommended treatment (Levy et al. 2012). An example AMA form is shown in Figure 19.4.
2) Sedation is commonly used to introduce the patient into general anesthesia, reducing patient stress and allowing the owners to participate in the process. This is a convenient moment to introduce the nurse who is going to take care of the patient. Many owners will want to spend this time with their pet, and in most cases the pet will benefit from such contact, allowing for easier catheterization and induction into general anesthesia. Sedation should ideally be performed in a quiet room with low lighting. If there is no such room available, the patient should be taken into the back office or another private area.
3) Anesthesia safety should be discussed at the time of first consultation, and a consent form highlighting the level of risk involved should be signed by the client (see Figure 19.5). All medical aspects of anesthesia are described in Chapter 12.
4) COHAT consists of two episodes: diagnostic and prophylactic. The owner is presented with the final (or at least, preliminary) diagnosis, while a qualified nurse carries out the cleaning and prepares the oral cavity for further procedures. COHAT in unhealthy patients or those with limitations on their anesthesia time can be simplified: radiography is carried out prior to teeth cleaning, only teeth that will remain in the oral cavity

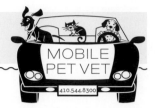

Less stress for you and your pet

MOBILE
PET VET
410.544.8300

Against Medical Advice Release

Date: _____/_____/_____

Against Medical Advice Release

> **Patient:**
> **Species:**
> **Breed:**
> **Gender:**
> **DOB:**   **Age:**
>
> **Client:**

Please initial the appropriate statement below:

Please initial the appropriate statement below:

_____ I, the undersigned, do fully understand that I am taking my pet, _____, out of the care of Mobile Pet Vet against the advice of the medical staff. Because of my decision to remove my pet from the doctors care, I have been informed that there may be further complications in her condition. These conditions may include, but are not limited to, further deterioration of her condition and/or death.

_____ I, the undersigned, do fully understand that I have elected services for my pet, _____, that do not represent the optimal care as advised by Mobile Pet Vet. The ramification of such a decision on my part may include further deterioration of her condition and/or her death.

_____   _____
Authorized Signature   Date

Figure 19.4   Example "against medical advice" (AMA) release form.

are descaled, discussion with the owner is kept brief or done prior to sedation, and the owner is given only a rough treatment plan. If there is no time pressure and the status of the patient allows for a thorough discussion, however, the priorities and staging of the procedure should be presented to the owner, and different scenarios should be discussed. Some actions must be agreed with the owner, such as any resective surgeries, extractions, or other irreversible procedures. Though it takes time, it is necessary to reach an agreement to avoid confusion and problems at discharge.

Some procedures (e.g., resective surgery, any long-term anesthesia) require hospitalization and owner agreement. It is best to inform the owner that the decision regarding discharge will be made two to three hours postoperatively.

5) Procedures that are planned and agreed by the owner are performed in order according to a list of priorities. For example, endodontic treatment of a vital tooth should be done first, to give sufficient time for possible bleeding control and to allow for staging of the procedure. Endodontic treatment can be done prior to

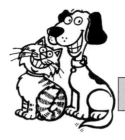

HALE VETERINARY CLINIC
DENTAL AND ORAL SURGERY FOR PETS
ESTIMATE AND CONSENT FORM

Problem(s):_____

_____

_____

Planned Treatment:_____

_____

_____

_____

• My veterinarian has referred me to Hale Veterinary Clinic specifically regarding a dental or oral problem with my pet. Hale Veterinary Clinic will be unable to provide treatment for conditions other than those related to this referral.

• The fees related to the above treatment plan are outlined on the other side of this document. I understand that this is an estimate only and is based on a pre-anesthetic examination. New information which comes to light during the more detailed oral examination and radiographs taken following induction of general anesthesia may make the estimate invalid.

• Reasonable attempts will be made to work within this estimate or to obtain authorization for procedures not outlined above. If contact is not possible, I understand that other procedures may be carried out at the discretion of the doctor and that I will be responsible for charges related to these treatments. I agree to pay all fees related to the treatment of the named animal at discharge. Payment may be made by Visa®, MasterCard®, debit card, cash or a combination.

• I understand that the practice of veterinary dentistry is not an exact science and that guarantees as to outcome are not possible. Treatment options and procedures have been explained to my satisfaction and I give my informed consent to Fraser Hale to carry out these treatments.

• I understand that the ultimate success of the proposed treatment may depend on adequate home-care and follow-up and acknowledge my responsibility in this regard. This is particularly so with the management of periodontal disease.

• I understand that any anesthetic poses some risk to the patient and that precautions will be taken to minimize such risks. In the unlikely event of an anesthetic complication, I authorize Hale Veterinary Clinic to carry out such procedures and treatments as are deemed appropriate.

• I give Hale Veterinary Clinic permission to photograph my pet for the purpose of documenting the treatment and I understand that the photographs may be used for educational purposes. Confidentiality is assured.

• I have read and understand "Who Does What at Hale Veterinary Clinic".

• When it is time for my pet's follow-up appointment with Hale Veterinary Clinic, I wish to be (a) contacted by Hale Veterinary Clinic or (b) contacted by my regular veterinarian (circle one).

OWNER/AGENT:_____ **DATE:**_____ **PHONE:**_____

Figure 19.5   Example estimate and consent form.

extractions to avoid contamination of the surgical site. The presence of an oral mass that may require major surgery leads to the prioritization of biopsy over other surgeries. Any surgical procedures should be performed after onset of the local nerve block and before the end of its duration. Finally, general health status should determine the maximum anesthesia time. Thus, in compro-mised patients, the duration of a procedure is an important selective criterion, and the focus of the operating team should be on the fastest possible completion of anesthesia. All perioperative and postoperative aspects of patient's care are discussed in chapters 11, 12, 13. An anesthesia record form should be filled out (see Figure 19.6)

Anesthesia Record

Date _____

Surgical_____Animal ID# _____ Owner# _____
Procedure:
_____

Pre-anesthetic: _____

Induction_____

Intubation Time: _____ Extubation Time: _____

Fluids Given: _____

Surgery Start: _____

Surgery End: _____

Surgeons: _____

Personel assistants: Signature
_____

Time	Isoflurane conc Sevoflurane conc	Other anesthetics Nerve blocks	Add. drugs	Heart rate	Blood pressure	% O$_2$ Saturation	Temp	Resp rate
Recovery:								

Figure 19.6   Example anesthesia record.

6) Prior to discharge, the patient is carefully inspected in terms of status, consciousness, and vital parameters. The catheter is removed and the skin is cleaned. Good estimates for discharge are the time needed to recover and the time to completely recover.

7) A pharmacologic plan of the postoperative treatment should be prepared in writing as part of the discharge documentation and verbally explained to the client. All medicines should be prepared in labeled envelopes or packages, with the dose, frequency, and duration clearly marked.

8) The most important thing to provide at discharge are clear instructions for the immediate postoperative period, in both verbal and written form. The owner is typically under a significant level of stress, and will be more focused on their pet than on whoever is discharging them. The instructions must include the recommended drug doses and time of administration, dietary recommendations, and when the next visit is scheduled. At the end of the discharge form, there should be a note to contact the clinic in case of any concerns. This author avoids making home-care recommendations at the time of discharge, if possible, and advises setting up the next visit for within 10–14 days. During this period, the only dental treatment should consist of pain management, infection prevention, and the use of topical products to enhance healing.

19.5 Follow-Up

1) This author offers the first post-surgery recheck for free (in fact, for the legal reasons, the price is included in the cost of the surgery) to motivate client compliance. The application of a barrier sealant (e.g., Oravet, BI) will retard the accumulation of plaque, so tooth brushing and passive home care are not yet required. However, the owner should be made aware that this is only temporary.

2) The lifelong prophylactic program should be tailored to each patient. Different frequencies of visit are required for periodontal disease, orthodontic patients, oncologic patients, and working dogs. Aside from oncologic patients, the most common recheck program is based on the color code described in point 4 (below).

3) Distant follow-up (with or without anesthesia) will depend on the procedure outcome and prognosis. Radiographic changes (e.g., periapical lucency) require a minimum of six months to evaluate, but periodontal pockets heal quicker and can be assessed six to eight weeks after the procedure.

4) The following color code is easy to implement and depends on the oral condition of the patient as subjectively defined by the veterinarian: green indicates annual dental rechecks are requried, orange indicates rechecks every six months, and red indicates rechecks every three months. In addition, every time the owner identifies any suspicious lesions, an immediate visit is recommended. Other diagnostic tests such as disclosing solutions, UV lights, ora-strips, and the OHI will improve the diagnostic value of these rechecks.

19.6 What Every Vet Should Know About Dental Problems

Human dentistry is a separate profession from human medicine, with a strong community, growing industry, and very active scientific field. The veterinary dental field is slowly improving but is still underdeveloped. The list of dental skills that every small-animal veterinarian should possess is described in the Joint European Veterinary Dental Society (EVDS)/European Veterinary Dental College (EVDC) Statement on Clinical Competencies in Small Companion Animal Dentistry and Oral Surgery (EVDS/EVDC 2014) (see Chapter 3).

It can be somewhat confusing when we look at veterinary education and realize how much attention is paid to, say, diabetes, which affects 1 dog in 170, when compared to periodontal disease, which affects 90% of dogs at one year of age. It must be possible to teach them in more sensible proportions.

19.6.1 Key Points

1) Oral health must be a part of the common program of healthcare individually tailored to each patient.

2) The simple diagnostic tools available to pet owners cannot provide accurate diagnosis but aid in developing public awareness about oral problems.

3) Oral pain perception is not always associated with an expression of discomfort. Despite intense pain, many patients eat, drink, and behave almost normally.

References and Further Reading

Bellows J, Berg ML, Dennis S, Harvey R, Lobprise HB, Snyder CJ, Stone AES, Van de Wetering AG. 2019 AAHA Dental Care Guidelines for Dogs and Cats. J Am Anim Hosp Assoc. 2019 Mar/Apr;55(2):49–69. doi: 10.5326/JAAHA-MS-6933. PMID: 30776257.

EVDS and EVDC (2014) Competencies in Dentistry and Oral Surgery for Small Companion Animals. Available from https://www.evds.org/images/pdf/Competencies.pdf (accessed July 5, 2020).

Levy, F., Mareiniss, D.P., and Iacovelli, C. (2012). The importance of a proper AGAINST-MEDICAL-Advice (AMA) discharge: how signing out AMA may create significant liability protection for providers. *J. Emerg. Med.* 43 (3): 516–520.

Niemiec B, Gawor J, Nemec A, Clarke D, McLeod K, Tutt C, Gioso M, Steagall PV, Chandler M, Morgenegg G, Jouppi R. World Small Animal Veterinary Association Global Dental Guidelines. J Small Anim Pract. 2020 Jul;61(7):E36-E161. doi: 10.1111/jsap.13132. Erratum in: J Small Anim Pract. 2020 Dec;61(12):786. PMID: 32715504.

20

Professional Dental Cleaning

Brook Niemiec

Veterinary Dental Specialties and Oral Surgery, San Diego, CA, USA

20.1   Introduction

The first step in any periodontal therapy (other than instituting home care in immature pets [under a year of age]) is a Professional Dental Cleaning. This procedure may also be called a complete oral health assessment and treatment (COHAT) or oral assessment, treatment, and prevention (Oral ATP) (Bellows 2010). These newer names are designed to convey the fact that a proper dental cleaning in veterinary medicine is rarely just a cleaning, as other treatments are typically required.

Regardless of the name, the goal of this procedure is clean and smooth teeth. However, a critical part of any dental procedure is evaluation of the periodontal tissues, as well as the entire oral cavity. This step is as important as the cleaning, but it is often poorly performed or completely omitted. Any professional periodontal therapy for veterinary patients must be performed under general anesthesia (see Chapter 11), with a well-cuffed endotracheal tube (Holmstrom et al. 2002a; Niemiec 2003; Bellows 2004a; Colmery 2005). Only when the patient is properly anesthetized can a safe and effective cleaning and oral evaluation be performed (Huffman 2010). In addition, anesthesia provides a much more pleasant experience for the dental patient.

General anesthesia should be multimodal and balanced. The endotracheal tube must be properly inflated (not over-inflated) to avoid aspiration of procedural water, oral contaminants, or regurgitation, any of which could cause aspiration pneumonia. Finally, since these can be lengthy procedures, it is critical that the patient be provided heat support and be well monitored (Colmery 2005) (see Chapter 12).

Proper periodontal/dental/oral therapy takes time and patience. A minimum of one hour should be allotted for *all*

dental cases, and often much more. Professional periodontal therapies must be performed with quality (not quantity) in mind.

20.2   Procedure

A complete dental prophylaxis should include all of the steps listed in this section. Note that there are almost as many recipes for a dental cleaning as there are veterinary dentists, but the basic procedure is essentially the same. The sequence presented below is this author's personal recommendation. The reader is encouraged to research the procedure in other texts and develop a protocol of their own (see Wiggs and Lobprise 1997a; Holmstrom et al. 2002a; Niemiec 2003; Bellows 2004b).

20.2.1   Step 1: Presurgical Exam and Consultation

A complete oral and physical exam is a critical but often only cursorily performed (or completely neglected) step. The physical exam, in combination with preoperative testing, screens for general health issues that compromise anesthetic safety (e.g., cardiopulmonary disease, anemia, hepatopathy) (Joubert 2007; Huffman 2010). The conscious oral examination should identify any obvious oral pathologies (fractured, intrinsically stained, or mobile teeth; masses; large tooth-resorptive [TR] lesions) as well as provide a *preliminary* assessment of periodontal health. All disease processes identified can then be discussed along with the available treatment options. It is recommended to utilize visual educational materials during discussions with clients (Figure 20.1), including by making

The Veterinary Dental Patient: A Multidisciplinary Approach, First Edition. Edited by Jerzy Gawor and Brook Niemiec.
© 2021 John Wiley & Sons Ltd. Published 2021 by John Wiley & Sons Ltd.
Companion website: www.wiley.com/go/gawor/veterinary-dental-patient

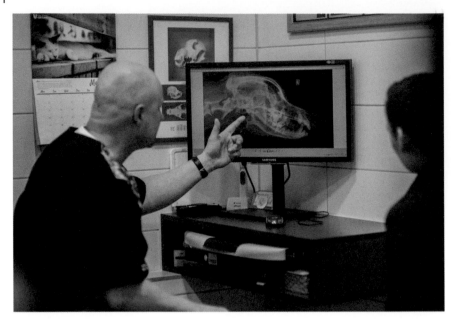

Figure 20.1 Use of visual educational materials during conversation with a pet owner.

use of a "smile" book or computer slideshow of common cases. This face-to-face discussion will improve client understanding of the disease processes, and should thus increase compliance with recommended therapy.

Based on the oral examination findings, the practitioner can create a somewhat accurate estimate of both procedure time and financial costs. The client should be informed that a complete oral examination is *not* possible on a conscious patient, and thus that the preoperative estimate is only preliminary. In addition, the number of dental procedures should be determined based on the anticipated time *for each case*, as procedures vary widely in the time they require; for example, two stage IV dental procedures can take longer than five stage I and II ones. This small investment of time prior to the procedure will improve the experience for everyone involved (veterinarian, technician, receptionist, client, and patient) (Holmstrom et al. 1998a; Niemiec 2003; Bellows 2004b; Huffman 2010).

20.2.1.1 Staff and Patient Protection

Numerous studies have shown that mechanical scalers create highly contaminated aerosols containing bacteria, fungi, and viruses (Pederson et al. 2002; Harrel 2004; Szymańska 2007). These infectious organisms come not only from the patient's mouth, but also from the water lines of the mechanized handpieces (Shearer 1996; Meiller et al. 1999; Wirthlin et al. 2003).

Furthermore, low levels of aersolization occur even during hand scaling and oral examination (Huntley and

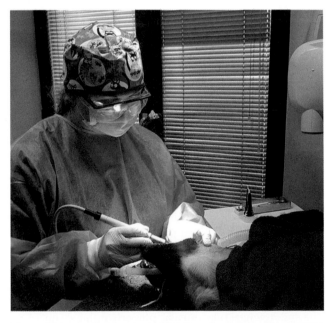

Figure 20.2 A veterinary technician (nurse) properly attired in PPE.

Campbell 1998). Such pathogenic aerosols have been linked to numerous deleterious effects on veterinary staff. Therefore, staff members performing dental procedures should be instructed to wear personal protective equipment (mask, goggles, and gloves) at all times (Harrel et al. 1998; Holmstrom et al. 1998b; Bellows 2004a,b; Pattison and Pattison 2006) (Figure 20.2). Dental procedures must *not* be performed in "sterile" environments such as surgical suites. Furthermore, they should not be performed near any sick or compromised patients, nor any "clean" procedures (blood draws and catheterizations) (Bellows 2004c). Ideally, procedures should be confined to their own designated room, preferably with a high-efficiency particulate air filter (HEPA) on the ventilation ducts, as airborne aerosols have been shown to affect entire offices (Legnani et al. 1994; Osorio et al. 1995; Leggat and Kedjarune 2001; Al Maghlouth et al. 2007). Finally, it is important to remember that aerosols will contaminate clothing (Huntley and Campbell 1998), so it is recommended that disposable gowns be worn in the dental operatory (Holmstrom et al. 1998b).

20.2.2 Step 2: Chlorhexidine Lavage

The oral cavity is a "dirty" area and dental procedures are at least mildly invasive, which often results in transient bacteremia (Lafaurie et al. 2007). This will be worsened with increasing periodontitis (Daly et al. 2001; Forner et al. 2006). As previously stated, scaling (especially mechanical) causes bacterial aersolization. While the incidence of pneumonia is related to the duration of intubation, it can occur with even short surgical procedures, so the number of oral pathogens should be minimized whenever intubation is planned (Okuda et al. 2003).

Rinsing the oral cavity with a 0.12% solution of chlohexidine gluconate will decrease the bacterial load (Fine et al. 1993; Niemiec 2003; Bellows 2004b; Harrel and Molinari 2004; Day et al. 2006; Jahn 2006a). One minute of contact time has been recommended as an effective minimum, as this has been shown to decrease the degree of bacteremia following extractions (Tomas et al. 2007) and would be expected to be beneficial in cases of periodontal therapy as well. The effectiveness of this technique is demonstrated by a study showing that open-heart surgery patients had better survival rates when their mouths were rinsed with chlorhexidine (CHX) gluconate prior to surgery (Limeback 1998). Not only does the reduction of oral bacteria benefit the patient, it also lowers the number of aerosolized bacteria and thus reduces staff contamination (Fine et al. 1992; Jahn 2006a).

20.2.3 Step 3: Supragingival Cleaning

Large calculus accumulations can be quickly removed with calculus (or extraction) forceps (Wiggs and Lobprise 1997a; Bellows 2004b) (Figure 20.3). However, this must be done very carefully to avoid tooth and gingival damage (Holmstrom et al. 1998c). Since mechanical scalers are very effective in removing large deposits (Pattison and Pattison 2006), this author does not often use forceps.

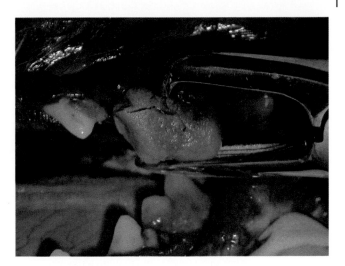

Figure 20.3 Manual descaling forceps in action.

This step can be performed via mechanical or hand scaling, but is best with a combination of the two (Pattison and Pattison 2006).

20.2.3.1 Mechanical Scaling

Mechanical scalers come in sonic and ultrasonic types, with the ultrasonic more common in veterinary dentistry. There are two main subtypes of ultrasonic scalers: magnetostrictive and piezoelectric (Wiggs and Lobprise 1997b). Both are electrically driven, vibrating at approximately 25000–45000 Hz (Wiggs and Lobprise 1997b; Bellows 2004a; Pattison and Pattison 2006). **Magnetostrictive units** have an elliptical pattern of vibration, which means all sides of the instrument are useful (Bellows 2004a). **Piezoelectric units** were previously thought to have a linear pattern of vibration, so that only the sides (and not the front or back) were effective at plaque removal (Bellows 2004a; Jahn 2006a). However, a recent study has shown that piezoelectrics also have an elliptical motion, and thus are effective on all surfaces (Lea et al. 2009). An additional advantage of piezoelectrics is that they produce significantly less heat than magnetostrictives and are less damaging to the enamel, which means they may be the safer choice (Holmstrom et al. 1998c).

Both types of ultrasonic scalers are very efficient and provide the additional benefit of creating an antibacterial effect in the coolant spray (cavitation) (Bellows 2004a; Jahn 2006a; Arabaci et al. 2007; Felver et al. 2009) (Figure 20.4).

In contrast, sonic scalers run on compressed air and vibrate at only 2000–6500 Hz (Holmstrom et al. 1998c; Bellows 2004a; Jahn 2006a; Pattison and Pattison 2006). Most reports indicate that this slower speed results in a longer scaling time compared to ultrasonics (Loose and

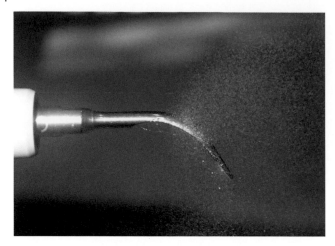

Figure 20.4 Cooling spray (cavitation) from an ultrasonic scaler, associated with a bactericidal effect.

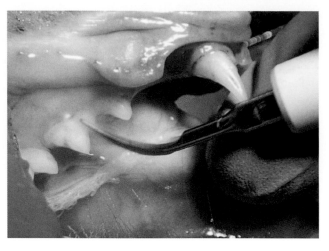

Figure 20.5 Use of the terminal 1–3 mm of a mechanical scaler tip is recommended.

Kiger 1987). However, some indicate an equal time (Lie and Leknes 1985), and at least one suggests that sonic scalers may actually be faster (Clinical Research Associates, Provo, UT). At slower speeds, sonic scalers generate minimal heat, making them a safer alternative to ultrasonics (Holmstrom et al. 2002b). Sonic scalers also have an elliptical pattern of vibration, so all sides of the instrument are useful (Jahn 2006a). It was classically believed that they did not offer the antibacterial effects of the ultrasonics, but this is being challenged (Hermann et al. 1995; Derdilopoulou et al. 2007). They run on a higher amplitude (10× or more as compared to ultrasonics), which may be more damaging to the root surface (Jacobson et al. 1994; Bellows 2004a).

When using mechanical scalers, it is important to select the correct power level setting for the instrument. Ultrasonic tips have a recommended vibrational speed

(Hz) range, and this should be determined and set prior to initiating scaling. The power should be set low and adjusted upward to the *minimum* required (Pattison and Pattison 2006). Note that there may be a different setting for the same instrument/tip when it is utilized subgingivally. The area of maximum vibration for all ultrasonic scalers is 1–3 mm from the tip (Holmstrom et al. 1998c; Debowes 2010) (Figure 20.5). Piezoelectric scalers *only* function in these last 3 mm, but magnetostrictive scalers are useful (though not nearly as effective) over a much larger area (Bellows 2004a). Do not use the very tip of the instrument as it is not effective and can damage or roughen the tooth surface (Bellows 2004a; Pattison and Pattison 2006). Adequate coolant *must* be delivered through the working end of the scaler. A fine but significant spray should be seen when the unit is activated (Pattison and Pattison 2006) (Figure 20.6). If inadequate

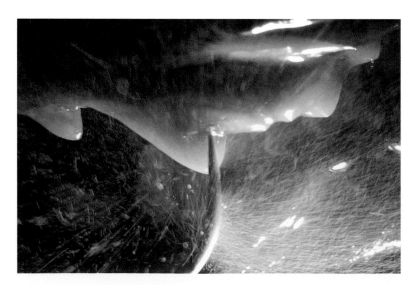

Figure 20.6 The cooling spray prevents thermal injury to vital tissue by the hot working tip of a scaler.

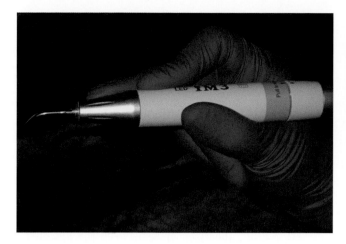

Figure 20.7 Correct grasp of a mechanical scaler handpiece.

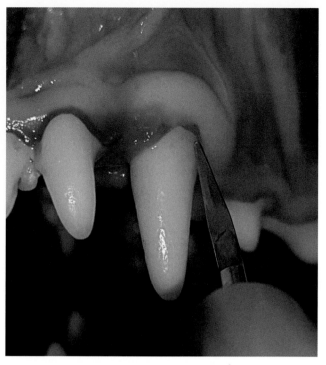

Figure 20.8 The working tip must be placed almost parallel to the tooth surface while descaling.

or excessive coolant is released, adjust the water flow to an appropriate level. Utilizing a mechanical scaler without sufficient coolant can cause numerous deleterious effects, including tooth death (Nicoll and Peters 1998; Holmstrom et al. 2002a). It is important to note that standard periodontal tips must *not* be introduced under the gingival margin as the coolant will not reach the working area of the instrument (Wiggs and Lobprise 1997b; Jahn 2006a), resulting in overheating and possible tooth damage. Specific low-powered periodontal tips are available for subgingival use.

The instrument should be *gently* grasped with the fingertips (Holmstrom et al. 1998a; Pattison and Pattison 2006) (Figure 20.7). Avoid using a palm grip as this reduces tactile sensitivity, increases operator fatigue, and can lead to too much downward pressure being placed on the tooth (see later). Next, place the *side* of the instrument in contact with the tooth surface with a very light (feather) touch (Wiggs and Lobprise 1997a; Holmstrom et al. 2002a; Pattison and Pattison 2006; Debowes 2010). Additional downward pressure will *not* improve the instrument's efficiency. In fact, applying excessive pressure on the tooth surface dampens the vibration, making it *less* effective (Trenter et al. 2003), and damages the instrument and the tooth (Brine et al. 2000; Holmstrom et al. 2002a). Keep the tip parallel to the tooth and run across the *entire* tooth surface using numerous overlapping strokes in different directions (Holmstrom et al. 1998c; Pattison and Pattison 2006) (Figure 20.8). Keep the instrument in motion at all times to avoid tooth damage (Pattison and Pattison 2006).

It has long been recommended that the amount of time an ultrasonic scaler is used on a single tooth be limited to no more than 15 seconds (Wiggs and Lobprise 1997a;

Holmstrom et al. 1998c; Pattison and Pattison 2006), with some authors recommending only 5–7 seconds (Debowes 2010). However, an exhaustive literature search can find no primary research that indicates a length of time that actually causes pulp damage, *providing that the instrument has adequate water cooling* (Nicoll and Peters 1998; Vérez-Fraguela et al. 2000). Though the classic recommendations may therefore be somewhat arbitrary, if the calculus in not removed from a tooth in 15 seconds, it may be best to move to another and return to the "tough" tooth later. Inefficient cleaning likely indicates either that the equipment is not working properly or that operator technique is faulty. Often, slow cleaning is caused by worn-out tips, as the loss of the terminal 1 mm of the tip reduces the efficiency of an ultrasonic scaler by 25%, and loss of 2 mm by 50% (Bellows 2004d) (Figure 20.9). Check the equipment thoroughly, and make sure that the side of the terminal 1–3 mm is in contact with the tooth. If calculus appears "tough," consider rotating the instrument slightly to ensure the proper orientation. A tiny adjustment may lead to a dramatic improvement in cleaning efficiency.

As soon as the instrument loses contact with the tooth, the scaler becomes ineffective. Keep it in constant motion, running *slowly* over the tooth surface to cover each square millimeter (Holmstrom et al. 1998c; Pattison and Pattison 2006; Niemiec 2008). Plaque and incipient calculus are

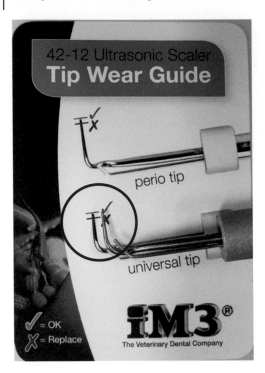

Figure 20.9 The quality of the working tip must be checked on a frequent basis.

difficult to visualize. Therefore, assume that the entire tooth is "dirty" and clean it completely (Figure 20.10).

Mechanical scalers are very efficient in plaque and calculus removal. This can decrease operator fatigue (versus hand scaling), which may decrease the incidence of repetitive motion injuries (e.g., carpal tunnel) (Holmstrom et al. 2002c; Jahn 2006a). They can, however, be more damaging to the tooth surface (Fichtel et al. 2008; Niemiec 2008) and may not completely clean the teeth. Therefore, it is recommended that a combination of hand and ultrasonic scaling be performed (Pattison and Pattison 2006; Niemiec 2008).

Rotosonic scaling, while popular in the past, is no longer recommended (Bellows 2004a). Rotosonic scalers produce a significantly rougher surface compared to hand and ultrasonic/sonic power scalers (Brine et al. 2000) and are *by far* the most damaging mechanical scaling instruments (Wiggs and Lobprise 1997b; Holmstrom et al. 1998c).

20.2.3.2 Hand Scaling

Supragingival hand scaling is best performed with a scaler. The blade of the scaler is triangular in shape, with two sharp cutting edges and a sharp back and tip (Wiggs and Lobprise 1997b; Bellows 2004a; Pattison and Pattison 2006; Niemiec 2008). It is typically positioned at 90° to the shaft (universal scaler) (Pattison and Pattison 2006). However, area-specific scalers with different

terminal angles are also available, which may improve cleaning ability (Holmstrom et al. 1998c; Pattison and Pattison 2006). Scalers are designed for *supragingival* use only, as the shape of the instrument and the sharp back and tip can easily damage the gingiva (Wiggs and Lobprise 1997b; Pattison and Pattison 2006; Niemiec 2008) (Figure 20.11). The sharp tip is very useful in cleaning tight interproximal spaces and developmental grooves (Bellows 2004a).

Periodontal hand instruments (scalers and curettes) are typically held with a modified pen grasp (Holmstrom et al. 2002a; Pattison and Pattison 2006; Niemiec 2008) (Figure 20.12). The instrument is gently held at the end of the textured or rubberized area, between the *tips* of the thumb and index finger. The middle finger is placed near the terminal end of the shaft and used to feel for vibrations, which signal residual calculus or diseased/rough tooth/root surfaces. Finally, the ring and pinkie fingers are rested on a stable surface, generally the target tooth or nearby teeth. Other grips such as the extended or open grasp and long reach can be necessary in certain situations (Holmstrom et al. 1998c).

All hand instruments *must* be used with a gentle touch (Pattison and Pattison 2006; Niemiec 2008). The instrument should be positioned so that the terminal shank is parallel to the tooth surface (if using a universal scaler, the handle will also be parallel) and the blade is placed at the gingival margin (Figure 20.13). Hand scalers should always be used in a pull-stroke fashion, away from the gingiva, to avoid inadvertent laceration (Holmstrom et al. 1998c; Niemiec 2008). The scaler's cutting surface should be drawn against the tooth numerous times in overlapping strokes until the tooth feels smooth (Pattison and Pattison 2006).

20.2.4 Step 4: Subgingival Plaque and Calculus Scaling

This is *the most important step* in dental cleaning, as supragingival plaque control is insufficient to treat periodontal disease (Holmstrom et al. 1998c; Westfelt et al. 1998; Niemiec 2008). Unfortunately, it is also the most difficult, for several reasons (Pattison and Pattison 2006):

- Subgingival calculus is harder than supragingival and tends to be locked into tooth-surface irregularities (Zander 1953; Canis et al. 1979).
- Visualization of subgingival deposits is difficult, and may be limited by bleeding from the inflamed tissues. This means a good tactile sense is required.
- The gingival sulcus (or periodontal pocket) limits the movement of the instrument (Pattison and Pattison 2006).

(a)

(b)

(c)

(d)

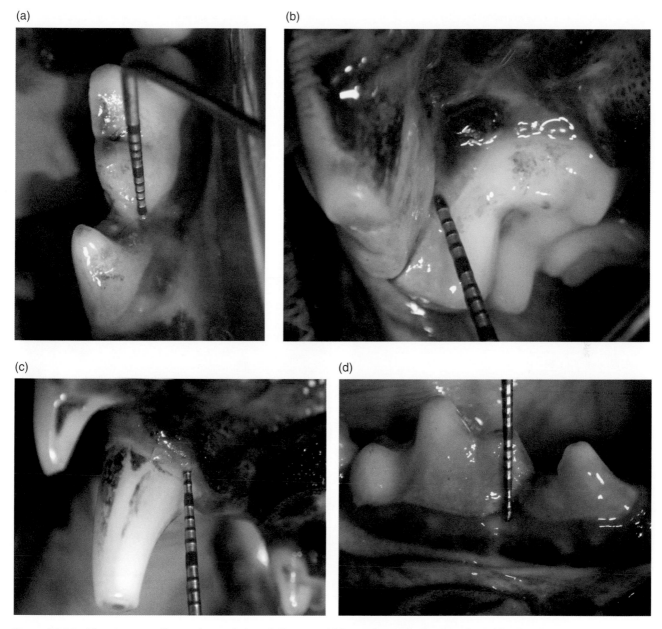

Figure 20.10 The places predisposed to periodontal diseases which require particular attention while cleaning: (a) lingual aspect of the fourth mandibular premolar and first molar; (b) palatal aspect of the maxillary fourth premolar; (c) palatal aspect of the maxillary canine tooth; and (d) buccal aspect of the mandibular fourth premolar and mandibular molar.

Figure 20.11 A manual scaler can only be applied supragingivally.

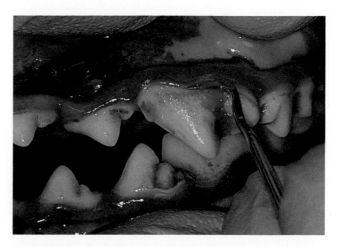

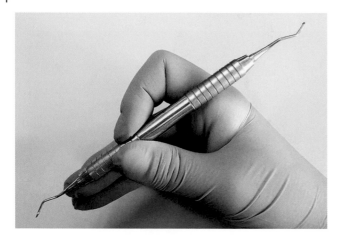

Figure 20.12   Modified pen grasp of a curette Source: Emilia Klim.

(a)   (b)

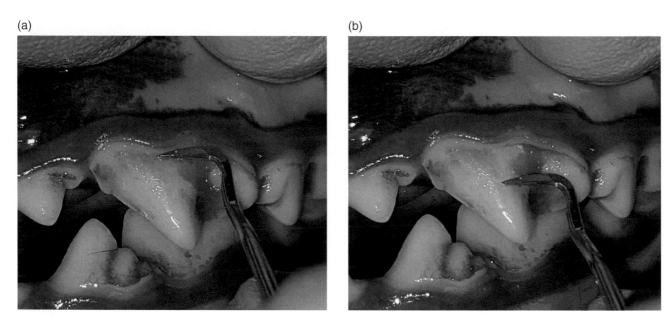

Figure 20.13   Position of a scaler's blade (a) at the gingival margin and (b) after an effective strike.

Due to these limitations, the incidence of residual calculus increases with increasing pocket depth (Caffesse et al. 1986).

Subgingival scaling was classically performed by hand with a curette, but advances in sonic and ultrasonic tips now allow their use under the gingival margin (Wiggs and Lobprise 1997b; Pattison and Pattison 2006). Numerous studies have shown that sonic and ultrasonic scaling are equal in effectiveness to traditional hand scaling (Thornton and Garnick 1982; Copulos et al. 1993; Beuchat et al. 2001; Obeid et al. 2004) and may even be superior for cleaning class II and III furcations (Leon and Vogel 1987). Therefore, it is recommended that a combination of ultrasonic and hand scaling be used for best results (Pattison and Pattison 2006).

A curette has two cutting edges, with a blunted toe and bottom (Wiggs and Lobprise 1997b; Pattison and Pattison 2006; Niemiec 2008). With proper, gentle use, the blunted bottom will not cut through the delicate periodontal attachment (Pattison and Pattison 2006). There are two types of curette in common use: universal and Gracey (Figure 20.14). Universal curettes usually have a 90° angle and are designed to be used throughout the mouth. Gracey curettes are designed with different angles to provide superior cleaning on different surfaces of the teeth in different areas of the mouth (i.e., area-specific cleaning).

Curettes are labeled by number; the lower the number (i.e., 1–2), the smaller the terminal angle of the shank, and the further forward in the mouth the instrument is designed to be used (Pattison and Pattison 2006; Niemiec 2008).

Figure 20.14 (a) Universal curette. (b) Gracey curette.

(a)　　　　　　　　　(b)

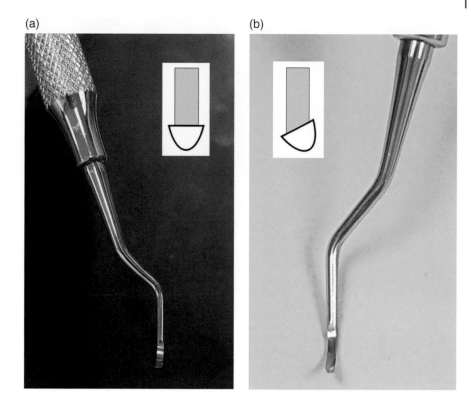

However, these numbers correspond to human dentition, so the veterinary practitioner needs to make selections carefully.

Manual subgingival scaling is a very technically demanding procedure, and therefore it is recommended that anyone performing this technique attends a hands-on continuing education program to hone their skills (Holmstrom et al. 2002b). It involves the following steps (Wiggs and Lobprise 1997a; Holmstrom et al. 1998a; Pattison and Pattison 2006; Niemiec 2008):

- Place the blade of the instrument on the tooth surface just coronal to the gingival margin, with the lower shank parallel to the surface (Figure 20.15).
- Rotate the curette so that the flat "face" of the blade is against the tooth surface (Figure 20.16). This decreases the profile of the instrument during insertion, and allows the blade to slide over the calculus.
- Insert the curette *gently* up to the base of the sulcus or periodontal pocket (Figure 20.17).
- Once the bottom of the pocket is reached, rotate the instrument so that the terminal portion (or shank) is parallel to the tooth. This will create a 90° angle between the working edge and the tooth, which is the correct "working angle" for cleaning. Once properly positioned, apply *slight* pressure down on to the tooth surface. Finally, remove the instrument from the pocket with a firm/short stroke (Figure 20.18).

This technique is then repeated with numerous overlapping strokes in different directions until the tooth/root feels smooth (Niemiec 2008).

20.2.4.1 Mechanical Scaling

Traditional ultrasonic scalers should not be used subgingivally, in order to avoid damage to the gingiva, periodontal tissues, and pulp (Jahn 2006a). Such damage may occur due to excessive power settings and because the large tips cannot properly access the tight subgingival area. However, the biggest danger is thermal, as the water coolant cannot effectively reach the tip of the instrument. Sonic and ultrasonic scalers with specialized periodontal tips have therefore been developed for subgingival use (Pattison and Pattison 2006) (Figure 20.19). These instruments are much easier to use and may thus provide a superior cleaning in the hands of novices, though this has not been confirmed by clinical study (Kocher et al. 1997a,b). Additionally, ultrasonic scaling may result in decreased levels of bacteria and endotoxins on the root surface (Drisko 1998), due to the fact that the ultrasonic waves produce cavitational activity, acoustic turbulence, and acoustic microstreaming, resulting in bacterial disruption (Walsley et al. 1988; Bellows 2004b; Jahn 2006a; Arabaci et al. 2007). These activities may improve plaque removal and root-surface cleanliness (Walsley et al. 1988; Khambay and Walmsley 1999).

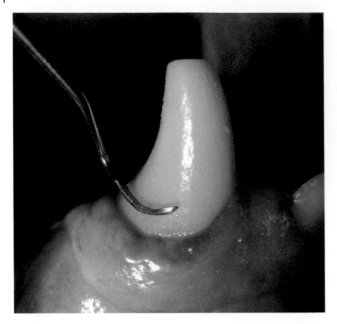

Figure 20.15 Manual subgingival scaling step one: The blade of the instrument is placed on the tooth surface just coronal to the gingival margin, with the lower shank parallel to the tooth surface.

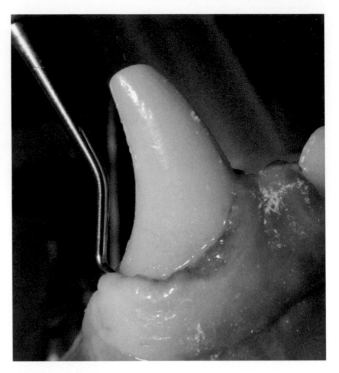

Figure 20.17 Manual subgingival scaling step three: The curette is inserted *gently* to the base of the sulcus or periodontal pocket.

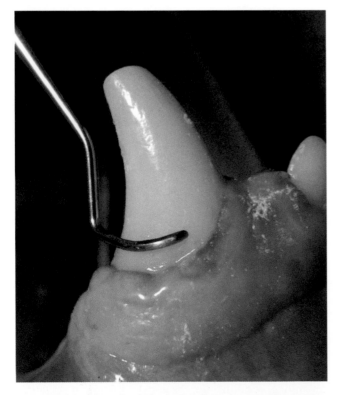

Figure 20.16 Manual subgingival scaling step two: The curette is rotated so that the flat "face" of the blade is against the tooth surface.

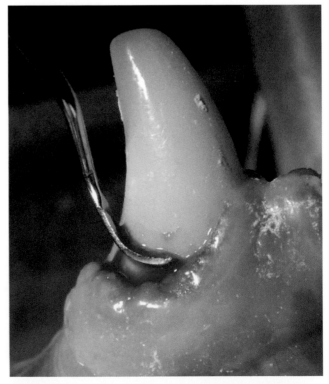

Figure 20.18 Manual subgingival scaling step four: Once the bottom of the pocket is reached, the instrument is rotated so that the terminal portion (or shank) is parallel to the tooth. Then, *slight* pressure is applied down on to the tooth surface. Finally, the instrument is removed from the pocket with a firm/short stroke.

Figure 20.19 Mechanical subgingival scalers.

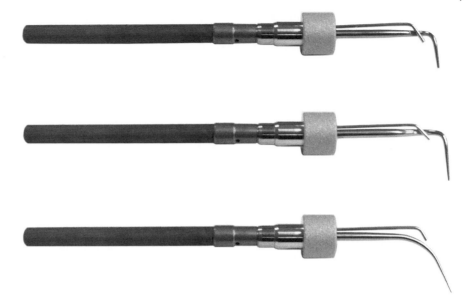

Figure 20.20 Mechanical smoothing of the root surface: (a) removal of the calculus covering the root; (b) roughly cleaned of the calculus root surface; (c) smoothing the root surface with the use of a curette.

(a)   (b)   (c)

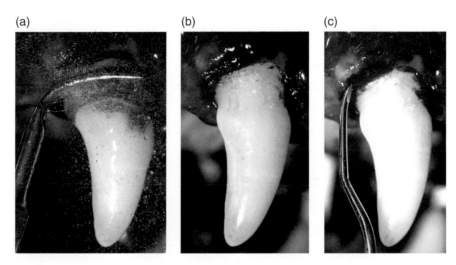

Mechanical scalers are used subgingivally as already described for supragingival mechanical scaling, but more care must be taken not to damage the delicate root surface. Again, this technique is performed with a *gentle* touch using numerous overlapping strokes until the root feels smooth (Pattison and Pattison 2006) (Figure 20.20).

20.2.5 Step 5: Residual Plaque and Calculus Identification

After scaling, it is recommended to check the teeth with an explorer for any rough areas that indicate residual calculus or small areas of dental pathology (such as TRs) (Holmstrom et al. 2002a; Pattison and Pattison 2006) (Figure 20.21). Residual plaque and calculus may also be identified by utilizing a plaque-disclosing solution (Reveal, Covetrus) or by drying the tooth surfaces (residual calculus will appear chalky) (Wiggs and Lobprise 1997c; Holmstrom et al. 2002a; Bellows 2004b).

20.2.6 Step 6: Polishing

All dental scaling results in microabrasion and roughening of the tooth surface (Wiggs and Lobprise 1997a; Bellows 2004b), leading to increased plaque adherence (Silness 1980; Holmstrom et al. 1998c; Berglundh et al. 2007). Polishing smooths the surface of the teeth, thereby retarding plaque attachment (Bellows 2004b). In human dentistry, the polishing step is controversial, due to the cumulative loss of enamel throughout life and the fact that proper scaling leaves a very smooth surface (Pattison and Pattison 2006). However, veterinary dental cleanings are often performed by less experienced operators who may leave the tooth surface rough, leading to increased plaque attachment. For this reason, combined with the fact that veterinary patients receive far fewer cleanings in their lifetime than humans, polishing continues to be recommended in veterinary patients (Wiggs and Lobprise 1997a; Niemiec 2003; Fichtel et al. 2008; Debowes 2010).

Practices may use a commercially available polish or make their own. This author recommends a slurry of flour of pumice and CHX solution mixed in a dappen dish. This not only is less messy than standard prophy paste, it also contains an antimicrobial.

The polishing procedure is typically performed with a rubber prophy cup on a slow-speed handpiece with a 90° angle (prophy angle) (Pattison and Pattison 2006; Fichtel et al. 2008; Niemiec 2010). The handpiece should be run at a slow speed, no greater than 3000 rpm (Wiggs and Lobprise 1997a; Niemiec 2008). Faster rotation does not improve the speed or quality of the procedure, and may result in overheating of the tooth. An adequate amount of polish should be used at all times, as running the prophy cup without paste is not only inefficient, but can overheat the tooth (Pattison and Pattison 2006). Therefore, coating the teeth with paste prior to polishing is recommended

(Figure 20.22), and the prophy cup should then be supplemented as needed. This also saves time, as the technician will not need to return to the polishing supply as often.

As with scaling, every square millimeter of tooth surface should be polished. *Slight* pressure should be placed downward on the tooth in order to flare the edges of the prophy cup to polish the subgingival areas (Figure 20.23). A tooth may be polished for a *maximum* of five seconds at a time, to avoid overheating (Wiggs and Lobprise 1997a; Holmstrom et al. 1998c; Bellows 2010). It can then be further polished after a short break (during which other teeth may be polished).

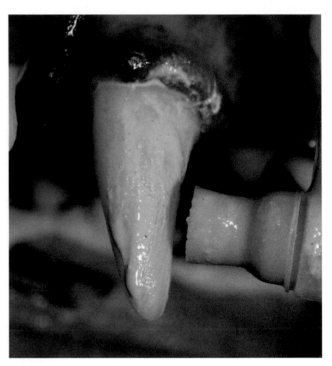

Figure 20.22 Coating the tooth surface prior to polishing.

Figure 20.23 Polishing the crown starts from the gingival margin.

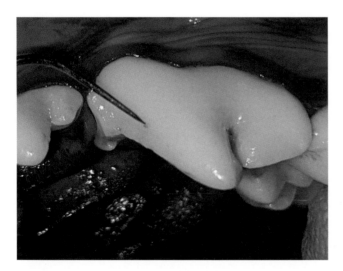

Figure 20.21 Checking the descaled crown surface with an explorer.

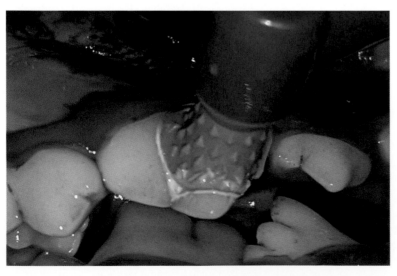

20.2.7 Step 7: Sulcal Lavage

During cleaning and polishing, debris such as calculus and prophy paste accumulates in the periodontal space (Wiggs and Lobprise 1997a; Niemiec 2008). In some cases, there are visible deposits, but in *all* cases there is microscopic debris. The presence of these substances allows for continued infection and inflammation, and therefore a gentle lavage of the sulcus is strongly recommended (Wiggs and Lobprise 1997a; Holmstrom et al. 2002a; Niemiec 2008). Sulcal lavage is performed with a small (22–25)-gauge blunt-ended cannula, which is placed gently into the sulcus. The solution is then injected while slowly moving along the arcade (Figure 20.24).

Sterile saline can be used as a lavage solution, but most dentists favor a 0.12% chlohexidine rinse (Wiggs and Lobprise 1997a; Bellows 2004b; Jahn 2006b). The use of CHX was discouraged by some veterinary dentists due to

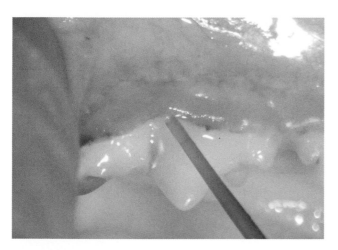

Figure 20.24 Gingival sulcus lavage with the use of a blunt-ended cannula.

its cytotoxic effects on periodontal ligament cells *in vitro* (Chang et al. 2001), but recent studies have proven that it does not delay wound healing and may even speed recovery and decrease pain (Tatnall et al. 1990; Quirynen et al. 2000; Jahn 2006b). There is even evidence that postoperative CHX may actually improve healing and alveolar bone height (Brägger et al. 1994).

20.2.8 Step 8: Fluoride Therapy (Optional)

This is a controversial step, with some dentists recommending that it be performed in all cases, and some recommending that it never be done (Holmstrom et al. 2002a; Bellows 2004b). The positive aspects of fluoride include (Wiggs and Lobprise 1997a; Holmstrom et al. 2002a; Bellows 2004b, 2010; Spackman and Bauer 2006):

- Antiplaque and antibacterial activities.
- Hardening of the tooth structure.
- Decreasing of tooth sensitivity.

Minimizing tooth sensitivity is most important in patients with gingival recession and secondary root exposure. Cementum is removed during root planning, which may expose underlying dentin (Klokkevold et al. 2006); this leads to sensitivity of the teeth, which is worst in the cervical area (Fischer et al. 1991; Klokkevold et al. 2006). Human literature reports that approximately 50% of patients experience sensitivity following subgingival scaling and root planing (Von Troil et al. 2002). The application of fluoride should help decrease this condition (Bellows 2004b; Klokkevold et al. 2006).

The fluoride preparation should be placed on the teeth and allowed to sit for the manufacture's recommended contact time (3 minutes for foam and 10 minutes for gel) (Figure 20.25). It can then be removed either by wiping or by blowing it off with compressed air (Bellows 2004b).

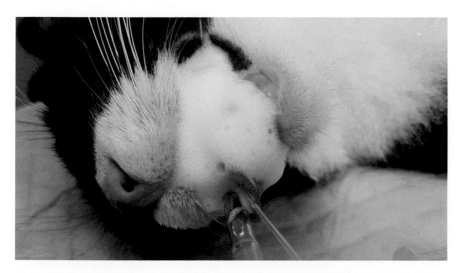

Figure 20.25 Application of fluoride foam in a cat following professional teeth cleaning. *Source:* Emilia Klim.

Fluoride should not be rinsed away with water as this decreases its efficacy (Bellows 2004b; Klokkevold et al. 2006).

20.2.9   Step 9: Periodontal Probing, Oral Evaluation, and Dental Charting

This is a *critically* important part of a professional dental cleaning, but is unfortunately often poorly performed or even completely omitted (Holmstrom et al. 2002a; Bellows 2004b). The *entire* oral cavity must be systematically evaluated using both visual and tactile senses.

Careful visual examination should be performed alongside periodontal evaluation. Possible findings include (but are not limited to): fractured, mobile, or intrinsically stained teeth; tooth defects (e.g., caries or tooth resorption); and oral masses. This author recommends that the patient be placed in dorsal recumbency for the oral exam, as it improves visualization (Huffman 2010).

The periodontal evaluation should begin with a determination of the plaque, calculus, and gingivitis indices. These key pieces of information are frequently noted prior to dental cleaning. Next, the periodontal status should be measured. The only accurate method for detecting and measuring periodontal pockets is through the use of a periodontal probe, as pockets are not always diagnosed by radiographs and are often not seen on visual exam (Carranza and Takei 2006; Tetradis et al. 2006; Niemiec 2010).

The periodontal evaluation should be initiated at the first incisor of one of the quadrants and then continued distally, one tooth at a time. This decreases the chance of a tooth being skipped. Periodontal probing is performed by gently inserting the probe into the pocket until it stops and then slowly "walking" it around the tooth (Bellows 2004b; Carranza and Takei 2006; Niemiec 2008) (Figure 20.26). Depth measurements should be taken at six spots around *every* tooth (Holmstrom et al. 2002a; Bellows 2004a; Carranza and Takei 2006; Niemiec 2008) (Figure 20.27). The normal sulcal depth in dogs is 0–3 mm, while that in cats is 0–0.5 mm (Wiggs and Lobprise 1997c; Bellows 2004b; Debowes 2010; Niemiec 2010). This author considers normal sulcal depth in toy-breed dogs to be ≤2 mm (Figure 20.28).

Probing is focused on oral soft tissues, including the gingival sulcus area, furcation area, diastemata, and gingiva. After soft-tissue assessment, the next step is to evaluate the dentition using a dental explorer and mirror. Quite often, the explorer will be combined with a periodontal probe, so most of the oral examination can be performed with just one instrument. The explorer should be inserted in all developmental grooves, areas of roughness, and defects, while the dental mirror should be used to view the lingual

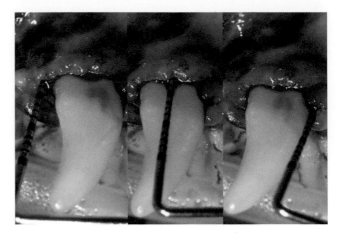

Figure 20.26   Probing the gingival sulcus of the right maxillary canine tooth in a dog from the buccal side. This is the most important part of the periodontal clinical assessment.

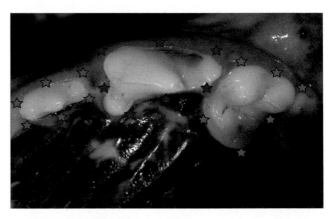

Figure 20.27   The minimum six places around the tooth that should be probed (stars).

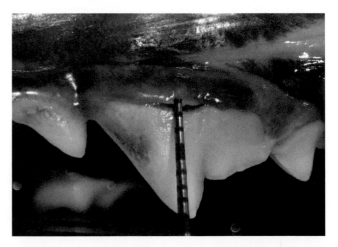

Figure 20.28   Normal probing depth in toy-breed dogs (≤2 mm).

and palatal sides of the crowns; the same instrument is also used to reflect light in order to illuminate caudal parts of the mouth.

(a)

(b)

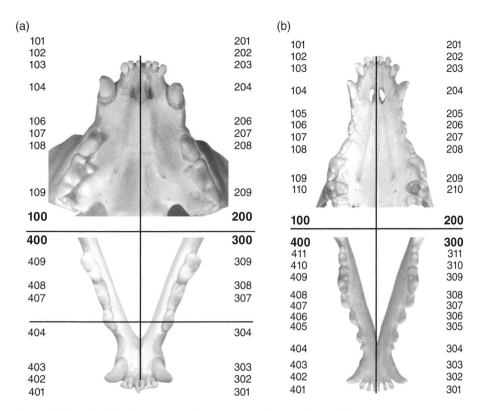

Figure 20.29 The Triadan system of dental nomenclature: (a) cat; (b) dog.

All abnormal findings must be recorded on a dental chart. Dental charting is easier and more efficient if performed four-handed (Bellows 2004c; Huffman 2010): this is where one person evaluates the mouth and calls out all pathological findings to another, who records it on the chart. Using the modified Triadan system will greatly increase the efficiency of this step.

The modified Triadan system (Floyd 1991) uses numbers to identify the teeth (Niemiec 2008; Huffman 2010). First, each quadrant is numbered, starting with the maxillary right quadrant as the 100 series and progressing clockwise so that the maxillary left is 200, the mandibular left is 300, and the mandibular right is 400 (Figure 20.29). Next, starting at the rostral midline, the teeth are counted distally starting with the first incisor, which is tooth 01. The canines are always number 04 and the first molars are 09. For example, the maxillary left fourth premolar is tooth 208. This has been extrapolated from the fact that the complete dentition of the ancestral carnivore has been determined to consist of four quadrants containing three incisors, one canine tooth, four premolars, and three molars.

It is important that dental charts be of sufficient size to be legible and allow for accurate placement of pathology. This is especially critical when document-

ing periodontal pockets. In addition, there must be incisal and lateral views of the teeth for accurate recording of pathology. The incisal view must have enough space to accommodate all six measurements. The minimum size for an acceptable dental chart is half a page, but most veterinary dentists utilize full-page charts (see Appendix C).

20.2.10 Step 10: Dental Radiographs

Dental radiographs should be taken of every area of pathology noted on the dental exam *at a minimum*. This includes any pathologic periodontal pockets, fractured teeth, masses, swellings, or missing teeth. In addition, numerous studies support taking full-mouth radiographs of all dental patients to reduce missed pathology (Verstraete et al. 1998a,b; Tsugawa and Verstraete 2000). A preliminary full-mouth series of six or seven radiographs, which can be performed by a well-trained nurse, will give the practitioner a good overview of what is going on in the oral cavity of a dog or cat (Figure 20.30).

Dental radiographs are critical to the evaluation of dental pathology and an essential complement to the clinical assessment, but they are *not* a substitute for clinical

(a)

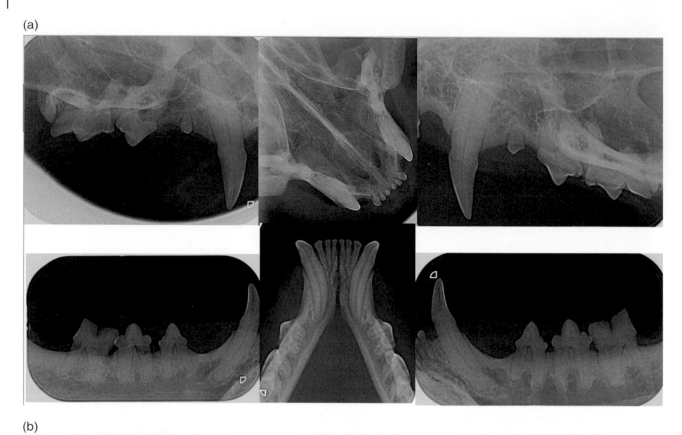

(b)

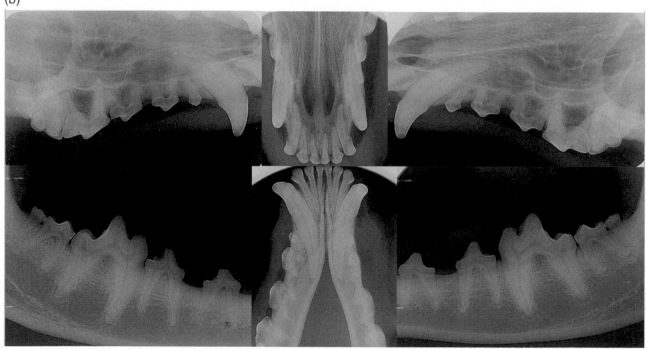

Figure 20.30   Preliminary radiographic assessment can fit in six radiographs: (a) cat; (b) dog.

examination, for several reasons (Tetradis et al., 2006; Niemiec, 2009):

- A change in radiographic exposure/technique (especially vertical angulation) can greatly affect the apparent level of alveolar bone (Tetradis et al. 2006; Niemiec 2010).
- The earliest stages of bone loss will not be seen radiographically (Ramadan and Mitchell 1962; Bender and Seltzer 2003a,b).
- Periodontal bone loss does not become radiographically evident until 30–50% of the mineralization is lost (Mulligan et al. 1998; Niemiec 2009).

Therefore, radiographic findings will always *underestimate* bone loss (Rees et al. 1971; Niemiec 2010). Help with radiographic interpretation is available via telemedicine review at www.vetdentalrad.com.

20.2.11 Step 11: Treatment Planning

Utilizing all available information (visual, tactile, and radiographic), any additional appropriate therapy should be determined. It is important to consider overall patient health, the owner's willingness to perform home care, and any necessary follow-up (Niemiec 2008). After forming an appropriate dental treatment plan, an estimate should be created and the client contacted for consent (see Chapter 17).

If a patient requires extensive treatment, or if the practitioner is unduly busy, rescheduling the remainder of the dental work is acceptable. Lengthy anesthesia is not recommended, as the two parameters that directly affect long-term morbidity and mortality in anesthetized patients are hypothermia and hypotension (Brodbelt et al. 2008; Torossian 2008), which become more pronounced with extended anesthesia. In fact, anesthetic length has been shown to increase the complication rate in both humans and animals (Tiret et al. 1986; Brodbelt et al. 2008). Hypothermia is especially a concern in smaller patients (Hall et al. 2001). However, if the patient is stable and all parameters (especially blood pressure and temperature) are normal, there is no universally recommended cut-off for anesthesia time.

20.2.12 Step 12: Application of a Barrier Sealant (Optional)

There are currently two plaque-reducing "sealers" commercially available. One is a waxy substance that is clinically proven to decrease plaque and calculus (Gengler et al. 2005). At the end of prophylaxis, the teeth are dried and the product is applied according to the manufacturer's directions. Continued applications are performed by the client on a weekly basis. This author has seen positive effects in clinical practice, but some veterinary dentists dispute the efficacy of the home-care product (Roudebush et al. 2005). Regardless, the professionally applied sealant is effective and provides a "bridge" to other forms of home care.

A newer sealant (Sanos) is purported to control plaque build-up for six months. This product is a good option for clients who cannot or will not perform *any* type of home care. It has been awarded the Veterinary Oral Health Council (VOHC) seal of approval.

20.2.13 Step 13: Client Education

Postsurgical discharge is an important step in periodontal therapy (Holmstrom et al. 1998a; Bellows 2004b). It provides an opportunity to review radiographs (and photographs) with the client. It also offers the chance to reinforce clinical findings, describe the treatments performed, and discuss periodontal disease in general. It is important to cover both immediate postoperative instructions and long-term periodontal care (including home care). It should be stressed that long-term success frequently hinges on the client's commitment to providing home care. In fact, professional therapy has been shown to be of little value without it (Needleman et al. 2005).

20.3 Key Points

- A complete dental prophylaxis is an involved procedure with numerous steps.
- All dental prophylactic procedures must be performed under general anesthesia.
- Each step must be properly performed to achieve a positive outcome.
- Sufficient time must be allotted for the procedure to have significant clinical benefit.
- *Sub*gingival scaling is the most important step in prophylaxis.
- A complete oral exam and charting is critical.

References

Al Maghlouth, A., Al Yousef, Y., and Al-Bagieh, N.H. (2007). Qualitative and quantitative analysis of microbial aerosols in selected areas within the College of Dentistry, King Saud University. *Quintessence Int.* 38 (5): e222–e228.

Arabaci, T., Çiçek, Y., and Canakçi, C.F. (2007a). Sonic and ultrasonic scalers in periodontal treatment: a review. *Int. J. Dent. Hyg.* 5 (1): 2–12.

Bellows, J. (2004a). Equipping the dental practice. In: *Small Animal Dental Equipment, Materials, and Techniques: A Primer* (ed. J. Bellows), 13–55. Ames, IA: Wiley-Blackwell.

Bellows, J. (2004b). Periodontal equipment, materials, and techniques. In: *Small Animal Dental Equipment, Materials, and Techniques: A Primer* (ed. J. Bellows), 115–173. Ames, IA: Wiley-Blackwell.

Bellows, J. (2004c). The dental operatory. In: *Small Animal Dental Equipment, Materials, and Techniques: A Primer* (ed. J. Bellows), 3–12. Ames, IA: Wiley-Blackwell.

Bellows, J. (2004d). *Small Animal Dental Equipment, Materials, and Techniques: A Primer*. Ames, IA: Wiley-Blackwell.

Bellows, J. (2010). Treatment of periodontal disease. In: *Feline Dentistry: Oral Assessment, Treatment, and Preventative Care* (ed. J. Bellows), 181–195. Ames, IA: Wiley-Blackwell.

Bender, I.B. and Seltzer, S. (2003a). Roentgenographic and direct observation of experimental lesions in bone: I. 1961. *J. Endod.* 29 (11): 702–706.

Bender, I.B. and Seltzer, S. (2003b). Roentgenographic and direct observation of experimental lesions in bone: II. 1961. *J. Endod.* 29 (11): 707–712.

Berglundh, T., Gotfredsen, K., Zitzmann, N.U. et al. (2007). Spontaneous progression of ligature induced peri-implantitis at implants with different surface roughness: an experimental study in dogs. *Clin. Oral Implants Res.* 18 (5): 655–661.

Beuchat, M., Busslinger, A., Schmidlin, P.R. et al. (2001). Clinical comparison of the effectiveness of novel sonic instruments and curettes for periodontal debridement after 2 months. *J. Clin. Periodontol.* 29 (7): 1145–1150.

Brägger, U., Schild, U., and Lang, N.P. (1994). Effect of chlorhexidine (0.12%) rinses on periodontal tissue healing after tooth extraction. (II). Radiographic parameters. *J. Clin. Periodontol.* 21 (6): 422–430.

Brine, E.J., Marretta, S.M., Pijanowski, G.J., and Siegel, A.M. (2000a). Comparison of the effects of four different power scalers on enamel tooth surface in the dog. *J. Vet. Dent.* 17 (1): 17–21.

Brodbelt, D.C., Pfeiffer, D.U., Young, L.E., and Wood, J.L.N. (2008). Results of the confidential enquiry into perioperative small animal fatalities regarding risk factors for anesthetic-related death in dogs. *J. Am. Vet. Med. Assoc.* 233 (7): 1096–1103.

Caffesse, R.G., Sweeney, P.L., and Smith, B.A. (1986). Scaling and root planing with and without periodontal flap surgery. *J. Clin. Periodontol.* 13 (3): 205–210.

Canis, M.F., Kramer, G.M., and Pameijer, C.M. (1979). Calculus attachment: review of the literature and findings. *J. Periodontol.* 50: 406.

Carranza, F.A. and Takei, H.H. (2006). Clinical diagnosis. In: *Carranza's Clinical Periodontology*, 10e (eds. F.A. Carranza, M.G. Newman, H.H. Takei and P.R. Klokkevold), 540–560. St. Louis, MO: W.B. Saunders.

Chang, Y.C., Huang, F.M., Tai, K.W., and Chou, M.Y. (2001). The effect of sodium hypochlorite and chlorhexidine on cultured human periodontal ligament cells. *Oral Surg. Oral Med. Oral Pathol. Oral Radiol. Endod.* 92 (4): 446–450.

Colmery, B. (2005). The gold standard of veterinary oral health care. *Vet. Clin. North Am.* 35 (4): 781–787.

Copulos, T.A., Low, S.B., Walker, C.B. et al. (1993). Comparative analysis between a modified ultrasonic tip and hand instruments on clinical parameters of periodontal disease. *J. Periodontol.* 64 (8): 694–700.

Daly, C.G., Mitchell, D.H., Highfield, J.E. et al. (2001). Bacteremia due to periodontal probing: a clinical and microbiological investigation. *J. Periodontol.* 72 (2): 210–214.

Day, C.J., Sandy, J.R., and Ireland, A.J. (2006). Aerosols and splatter in dentistry – a neglected menace? *Dent. Update* 33 (10): 601–602. 604–606.

Debowes, L.J. (2010). Problems with the gingiva. In: *Small Animal Dental, Oral and Maxillofacial Disease, a Color Handbook* (ed. B.A. Niemiec), 159–181. London: Manson.

Derdilopoulou, F.V., Nonhoff, J., Neumann, K., and Kielbassa, A.M. (2007). Microbiological findings after periodontal therapy using curettes, Er:YAG laser, sonic, and ultrasonic scalers. *J. Clin. Periodontol.* 34 (7): 588–598.

Drisko, C.H. (1998). Root instrumentation. Power-driven versus manual scalers, which one? *Dent. Clin. N. Am.* 42 (2): 229–244.

Felver, B., King, D.C., Lea, S.C. et al. (2009). Cavitation occurrence around ultrasonic dental scalers. *Ultrason. Sonochem.* 16 (5): 692–697.

Fichtel, T., Chra, M., Langerova, E., and Biberaur, G. (2008). Vla in M: observations on the effects of scaling and polishing methods on enamel. *J. Vet. Dent.* 25 (4): 231–235.

Fine, D.H., Mendieta, C., Barnett, M.L. et al. (1992). Efficacy of preprocedural rinsing with an antiseptic in reducing viable bacteria in dental aerosols. *J. Periodontol.* 63 (10): 821–824.

Fine, D.H., Yip, J., Furgang, D. et al. (1993). Reducing bacteria in dental aerosols: pre-procedural use of an antiseptic mouthrinse. *J. Am. Dent. Assoc.* 124 (5): 56–58.

Fischer, C., Wennberg, A., Fischer, Z.R.G., and Attstrom, R. (1991). Clinical evaluation of pulp and dentine sensitivity after supragingival and subgingival scaling. *Endod. Dent. Traumatol.* 7 (6): 259–265.

Floyd MR. The modified Triadan system: nomenclature for veterinary dentistry. J Vet Dent. 1991 Dec;8(4):18-9. PMID: 1815632.

Forner, L., Larsen, T., Kilian, M., and Holmstrup, P. (2006). Incidence of bacteremia after chewing, tooth brushing and scaling in individuals with periodontal inflammation. *J. Clin. Periodontol.* 33 (6): 401–407.

Gengler, W.R., Kunkle, B.N., Romano, D., and Larsen, D. (2005). Evaluation of a barrier sealant in dogs. *J. Vet. Dent.* 22 (3): 157–159.

Hall, L.W., Clarke, K.W., and Trim, C.M. (2001). *Veterinary Anesthesia*, 10e. London: W.B. Saunders.

Harrel, S.K. (2004). Airborne spread of disease – the implications for dentistry. *J. Calif. Dent. Assoc.* 32 (11): 901–906.

Harrel, S.K. and Molinari, J. (2004). Aerosols and splatter in dentistry: a brief review of the literature and infection control implications. *J. Am. Dent. Assoc.* 135 (4): 429–437.

Harrel, S.K., Barnes, J.B., and Rivera-Hildalgo, F. (1998). Aerosol and splatter contamination from the operative site during ultrasonic scaling. *J. Am. Dent. Assoc.* 129 (9): 1241–1249.

Hermann, J.S., Rieder, C., Rateitschak, K.H., and Hefti, A.F. (1995). Sonic and ultrasonic scalers in a clinical comparison. A study in non-instructed patients with gingivitis or slight adult periodontitis. *Schweiz. Monatsschr. Zahnmed.* 105 (2): 165–170.

Holmstrom, S.E., Frost, P., and Eisner, E.R. (1998a). Periodontal therapy and surgery. In: *Veterinary Dental Techniques*, 2e, 167–213. Philadelphia, PA: W.B. Saunders.

Holmstrom, S.E., Frost, P., and Eisner, E.R. (1998b). Ergonomics and general health safety in the dental workplace. In: *Veterinary Dental Techniques*, 2e, 497–506. Philadelphia, PA: W.B. Saunders.

Holmstrom, S.E., Frost, P., and Eisner, E.R. (1998c). Dental prophylaxis. In: *Veterinary Dental Techniques*, 2e, 133–166. Philadelphia, PA: W.B. Saunders.

Holmstrom, S.E., Frost, P., and Eisner, E.R. (2002a). Dental prophylaxis and periodontal disease stages. In: *Veterinary Dental Techniques*, 3e, 175–232. Philadelphia, PA: W.B. Saunders.

Holmstrom, S.E., Frost, P., and Eisner, E.R. (2002b). Dental equipment and care. In: *Veterinary Dental Techniques*, 3e, 31–106. Philadelphia, PA: W.B. Saunders.

Holmstrom, S.E., Frost, P., and Eisner, E.R. (2002c). General health safety and ergonomics in the veterinary dental workplace. In: *Veterinary Dental Techniques*, 3e, 637–664. Philadelphia, PA: W.B. Saunders.

Huffman, L.J. (2010). Oral examination. In: *Small Animal Dental, Oral and Maxillofacial Disease, a Color Handbook* (ed. B.A. Niemiec), 39–61. London: Manson.

Huntley, D.E. and Campbell, J. (1998). Bacterial contamination of scrub jackets during dental hygiene procedures. *J. Dent. Hyg.* 72 (3): 19–23.

Jacobson, L., Blomlöf, J., and Lindskog, S. (1994). Root surface texture after different scaling modalities. *Scand. J. Dent. Res.* 102 (3): 156–160.

Jahn, C.A. (2006a). Sonic and ultrasonic instrumentation. In: *Carranza's Clinical Periodontology*, 10e (eds. F.A. Carranza, M.G. Newman, H.H. Takei and P.R. Klokkevold), 828–835. St. Louis, MO: W.B. Saunders.

Jahn, C.A. (2006b). Supragingival and subgingival irricgation. In: *Carranza's Clinical Periodontology*, 10e (eds. F.A. Carranza, M.G. Newman, H.H. Takei and P.R. Klokkevold), 836–844. St. Louis, MO: W.B. Saunders.

Joubert, K.E. (2007). Pre-anesthetic screening of geriatric dogs. *J. S. Afr. Vet. Assoc.* 78 (1): 31–35.

Khambay, B.S. and Walmsley, A.D. (1999). Acoustic microstreaming: detection and measurement around ultrasonic scalers. *J. Periodontol.* 70: 626.

Klokkevold, P.R., Takei, H.H., and Carranza, F.A. (2006). General principals of periodontal surgery. In: *Carranza's Clinical Periodontology*, 10e (eds. F.A. Carranza, M.G. Newman, H.H. Takei and P.R. Klokkevold), 887–901. St. Louis, MO: W.B. Saunders.

Kocher, T., Rühling, A., Momsen, H., and Plagmann, H.C. (1997a). Effectiveness of subgingival instrumentation with power-driven instruments in the hands of experienced and inexperienced operators. A study on manikins. *J. Clin. Periodontol.* 24 (7): 498–504.

Kocher, T., Riedel, D., and Plagmann, H.C. (1997b). Debridement by operators with varying degrees of experience: a comparative study on manikins. *Quintessence Int.* 28 (3): 191–196.

Lafaurie, G.I., Mayorga-Fayad, I., Torres, M.F. et al. (2007). Periodontopathic microorganisms in peripheric blood after scaling and root planing. *J. Clin. Periodontol.* 34 (10): 873–879.

Lea, S.C., Felver, B., Landini, G., and Walmsley, A.D. (2009). Three-dimensional analyses of ultrasonic scaler oscillations. *J. Clin. Periodontol.* 36 (1): 44–50.

Leggat, P.A. and Kedjarune, U. (2001). Bacterial aerosols in the dental clinic: a review. *Int. Dent. J.* 51 (1): 39–44.

Legnani, P., Checchi, L., Pelliccioni, G.A., and D'Achille, C. (1994). Atmospheric contamination during dental procedures. *Quintessence Int.* 25 (6): 435–439.

Leon, L.E. and Vogel, R.I. (1987). A comparison of the effectiveness of hand scaling and ultrasonic debridement in furcations evaluated by differential dark field microscopy. *J. Periodontol.* 58 (2): 86–94.

Lie, T. and Leknes, K.N. (1985). Evaluation of the effect on root surfaces of air turbine scalers and ultrasonic instrumentation. *J. Periodontol.* 56 (9): 522–531.

Limeback, H. (1998). Implications of oral infections on systemic diseases in the institutionalized elderly with a special focus on pneumonia. *Ann. Periodontol.* 3 (1): 262–275.

Loose, B. and Kiger, R. (1987). An evaluation of basic periodontal therapy using sonic and ultrasonic scalers. *J Clin. Periodontol.* 14: 29–33.

Meiller, T.F., Depaola, L.G., Kelley, J.I. et al. (1999). Dental unit waterlines: biofilms, disinfection and recurrence. *J. Am. Dent. Assoc.* 130 (1): 65–72.

Mulligan, T.M., Aller, M.S., and Williams, C.E. (1998). Interpretation of periodontal discase. In: *Atlas of Canine and Feline Dental Radiography*, 104–123. Trenton, NJ: Veterinary Learning Systems.

Needleman, I., Suvan, J., Moles, D.R., and Pimlott, J. (2005). A systematic review of professional mechanical plaque removal for prevention of periodontal diseases. *J. Clin. Periodontol.* 32 (Suppl. 6): 229–282.

Nicoll, B.K. and Peters, R.J. (1998). Heat generation during ultrasonic instrumentation of dentin as affected by different irrigation methods. *J. Periodontol.* 69 (8): 884–888.

Niemiec, B.A. (2003). Professional teeth cleaning. *J. Vet. Dent.* 20 (3): 175–180.

Niemiec, B.A. (2008). Periodontal therapy. *Top. Companion Anim. Med.* 23 (2): 81–90.

Niemiec, B.A. (2009). Case based dental radiology. *Top. Companion Anim. Med.* 24 (1): 4–19.

Niemiec, B.A. (2010). Veterinary dental radiology. In: *Small Animal Dental, Oral and Maxillofacial Disease, a Color Handbook* (ed. B.A. Niemiec), 63–87. London: Manson.

Obeid, P.R., D'Hoore, W., and Bercy, P. (2004). Comparative clinical responses related to the use of various periodontal instrumentation. *J. Clin. Periodontol.* 31 (3): 193–199.

Okuda, M., Kaneko, Y., Ichinohe, T. et al. (2003). Reduction of potential respiratory pathogens by oral hygienic treatment in patients undergoing endotracheal anesthesia. *J. Anesth.* 17 (2): 84–91.

Osorio, R., Toledano, M., Liébana, J. et al. (1995). Environmental microbial contamination. Pilot study in a dental surgery. *Int. Dent. J.* 45 (6): 352–357.

Pattison, A.M. and Pattison, G.L. (2006). Scaling and root planing. In: *Carranza's Clinical Periodontology*, 10e (eds. F.A. Carranza, M.G. Newman, H.H. Takei and P.R. Klokkevold), 749–797. St. Louis, MO: W.B. Saunders.

Pederson, E.D., Stone, M.E., Ragain, J.C. Jr., and Simecek, J.W. (2002). Waterline biofilm and the dental treatment facility: a review. *Gen. Dent.* 50 (2): 190–195.

Quirynen, M., Mongardini, C., de Soete, M. et al. (2000). The rôle of chlorhexidine in the one-stage full-mouth disinfection treatment of patients with advanced adult periodontitis. Long-term clinical and microbiological observations. *J. Clin. Periodontol.* 27 (8): 578–589.

Ramadan, A.B. and Mitchell, D.F. (1962). A roentgenographic study of experimental bone destruction. *Oral Surg. Oral Med. Oral Pathol.* 15: 934–943.

Rees, T.D., Biggs, N.L., and Collings, C.K. (1971). Radiographic interpretation of periodontal osseous lesions. *Oral Surg. Oral Med. Oral Pathol.* 32 (1): 141–153.

Roudebush, P., Logan, E., and Hale, F.A. (2005). Evidence-based veterinary dentistry: a systematic review of homecare for prevention of periodontal disease in dogs and cats. *J. Vet. Dent.* 22 (1): 6–15.

Shearer, B.J. (1996). Biofilm and the dental office. *J. Am. Dent. Assoc.* 127: 181–189.

Silness, J. (1980). Fixed prosthodontics and periodontal health. *Dent. Clin. N. Am.* 24 (2): 317–329.

Spackman, S.S. and Bauer, J.G. (2006). Periodontal treatment for older adults. In: *Carranza's Clinical Periodontology*, 10e (eds. F.A. Carranza, M.G. Newman, H.H. Takei and P.R. Klokkevold), 675–692. St. Louis, MO: W.B. Saunders.

Szymańska, J. (2007). Dental bioaerosol as an occupational hazard in a dentist's workplace. *Ann. Agric. Environ. Med.* 14 (2): 203–207.

Tatnall, F.M., Leigh, I.M., and Gibson, J.R. (1990). Comparative study of antiseptic toxicity on basal keratinocytes, transformed human keratinocytes and fibroblasts. *Skin Pharmacol.* 3: 157–163.

Tetradis, S., Carranza, F.A., Fazio, R.C., and Takei, H.H. (2006). Radiographic aids in the diagnosis of periodontal disease. In: *Carranza's Clinical Periodontology*, 10e (eds. F.A. Carranza, M.G. Newman, H.H. Takei and P.R. Klokkevold), 561–578. St. Louis, MO: W.B. Saunders.

Thornton, S. and Garnick, J. (1982). Comparison of ultrasonic to hand instruments in the removal of subgingival plaque. *J. Periodontol.* 53 (1): 35–37.

Tiret, L., Desmonts, J.M., Hatton, F., and Vourc'h, G. (1986). Complications associated with anaesthesia – a prospective survey in France. *Can. Anaesth. Soc. J.* 33: 336–344.

Tomas, I., Alvarez, M., Limeres, J. et al. (2007). Effect of chlorhexidine mouthwash on the risk of post-extraction bacteremia. *Infect. Control Hosp. Epidemiol.* 28 (5): 577–582.

Torossian, A. (2008). Thermal management during anaesthesia and thermoregulation standards for the prevention of inadvertent perioperative hypothermia. *Best Pract. Res. Clin. Anaesthesiol.* 22 (4): 659–668.

Trenter, S.C., Landini, G., and Walmsley, A.D. (2003). Effect of loading on the vibration characteristics of thin magnetostrictive ultrasonic scaler inserts. *J. Periodontol.* 74 (9): 1308–1315.

Tsugawa, A.J. and Verstraete, F.J. (2000). How to obtain and interpret periodontal radiographs in dogs. *Clin. Tech. Small Anim. Pract.* 15 (4): 204–210.

Vérez-Fraguela, J.L., Vives Vallés, M.A., and Ezquerra Calvo, L.J. (2000). Effects of ultrasonic dental scaling on pulp vitality in dogs: an experimental study. *J. Vet. Dent.* 17 (2): 75–79.

Verstraete, F.J., Kass, P.H., and Terpak, C.H. (1998a). Diagnostic value of full-mouth radiography in cats. *Am. J. Vet. Res.* 59 (6): 692–695.

Verstraete, F.J., Kass, P.H., and Terpak, C.H. (1998b). Diagnostic value of full-mouth radiography in dogs. *Am. J. Vet. Res.* 59 (6): 686–691.

Von Troil, B., Needleman, I., and Sanz, M. (2002). A systemic review of the prevalence of root sensitivity following periodontal therapy. *J. Clin. Periodontol.* 29 (Suppl. 3): 173–177.

Walsley, A.D., Laird, W.R., and Williams, A.R. (1988). Dental plaque removal by cavitational activity during ultrasonic scaling. *J. Clin. Periodontol.* 15: 539.

Westfelt, E., Rylander, H., Dahlen, G., and Lindhe, J. (1998). The effect of supragingival plaque control on the progression of advanced periodontal disease. *J. Clin. Periodontol.* 25 (7): 536–541.

Wiggs, R.B. and Lobprise, H.B. (1997a). Periodontology. In: *Veterinary Dentistry: Principles and Practice* (eds. R.B. Wiggs and H.B. Lobprise), 186–231. Philadelphia, PA: Lippincott-Raven.

Wiggs, R.B. and Lobprise, H.B. (1997b). Dental equipment. In: *Veterinary Dentistry: Principles and Practice* (eds. R.B. Wiggs and H.B. Lobprise), 1–28. Philadelphia, PA: Lippincott-Raven.

Wiggs, R.B. and Lobprise, H.B. (1997c). Oral exam and diagnosis. In: *Veterinary Dentistry, Principals and Practice* (eds. R.B. Wiggs and H.B. Lobprise), 87–103. Philadelphia, PA: Lippincott-Raven.

Wirthlin, M.R., Marshall, G.W. Jr., and Rowland, R.W. (2003). Formation and decontamination of biofilms in dental unit waterlines. *J. Periodontol.* 74 (11): 1595–1609.

Zander, H.A. (1953). The attachment of calculus to root surfaces. *J. Periodontol.* 24: 16.

21

Oral and Maxillofacial Surgery

What's the Difference?

Jerzy Gawor

Veterinary Clinic Arka, Kraków, Poland

General motto: "Tooth is not bone, gum is not skin."

21.1 Introduction

Standardization plays an important role in medicine. Standards for techniques, instruments, and materials utilized in oral and maxillofacial surgery help avoid complications due to medical errors.

Oral and maxillofacial surgery includes numerous procedures with differing levels of difficulty and requirements. Within this group, the following categories exist: extraction, periodontal surgery, palatal surgery, soft-tissue surgery, oncologic surgery, fracture repair, temporomandibular joint surgery, and surgical endodontics. Regardless of the category, however, the principles are the same and must always be fulfilled. General standards refer to the following aspects of the surgical procedure: pain management, infection control, planning, respect for structures and anatomy, specific techniques, tactile handling of the tissue, and good closure. Of course, these standards relate to all surgical procedures, but since the head and oral cavities are unique environments, the number of factors affecting the final outcome in oral and maxillofacial surgery is larger.

Numerous strains of microorganisms exist in equilibrium with normally functioning anatomic structures within the oral cavity. Sterility can be strongly compromised and vascularity and innervation are very rich. In animals, the oral cavity and face do not play an important and emotional role as in humans, where they form part of the identity and enable expression via the voice. Nonetheless, these structures are still important in animal communication and behavior.

A growing number of oral tumors, in combination with advances in oncologic treatment and diagnostic modalities, provide additional need for improvements in oral and oral-reconstructive surgery.

21.2 Pain Management

The head – and especially the oral cavity – is very well innervated, and thus pain sensation is particularly intense from this site. Pain affects recovery and requires serious and efficient management. In dentistry and maxillofacial surgery, pain control is the gold standard for all procedures and always starts in the preoperative phase, continues through surgery, and lasts until full recovery of all oral organ functions is achieved. This part of veterinary dental patient care is described in detail in Chapter 11.

21.3 Infection Control

Overuse of antibiotics and contraindication for the empiric use of antibiotics are of concern, but *all* oral diseases are either started or complicated by infection. The benefits of antibiotic administration usually come from anaerobic infection control (deep wounds, periodontal abscesses, periapical periodontitis, contaminated oral injuries) and prevention of the dissemination and treatment of local and regional complications of oral problems, as well as the management of systemic complications. Some antibiotics (e.g., doxycycline) have additional features that may be used in immunomodulation of the host response. Due to the very important character of this subject, it is covered in detail in Chapter 7.

The Veterinary Dental Patient: A Multidisciplinary Approach, First Edition. Edited by Jerzy Gawor and Brook Niemiec.
© 2021 John Wiley & Sons Ltd. Published 2021 by John Wiley & Sons Ltd.
Companion website: www.wiley.com/go/gawor/veterinary-dental-patient

21.4 Treatment Planning

Many oral surgeries have their best outcome on the first attempt. Because of the presence of numerous structures that influence functionality and quality of life (QOL), a thorough knowledge of oral and maxillofacial anatomy is required prior to commencing surgery. Further, a detailed plan of the procedure is mandatory, which should include incisions, possible access to deeper structures, required flaps, resective margins in oncologic surgery, and closure of the wound with a plan for immediate use of surgical sites in regular life. Using a tissue marker is recommended, particularly in reconstructive and oncologic surgery (Figure 21.1).

3D reconstruction and well-documented diagnostics can be very helpful in preoperative considerations and the planning of surgical access (Figure 21.2). Good preparation of the operating field, materials, and instruments, as well as the position of the patient, will improve surgical comfort and outcome.

For many practitioners, including specialists, it is best to practice difficult or rarely performed procedures in a cadaver before proceeding to the live patient.

21.5 Four-Handed Surgery

Employing an assistant in oral surgery not only makes work more comfortable but also provides necessary visualization and access to the area of interest. In addition, an assistant is imperative to performing some procedures that otherwise would be impossible.

When four-handed dentistry is performed, the following requirements must still be met:

- An ergonomically designed facility, to minimize unnecessary motion.
- A comfortable position of the operator and recumbency of the patient.
- Utilization of a surgical kit relevant to the procedure.
- Agreement on the procedure plan prior to initiation, including any possible variations.
- Exposure of the operatory field, suction, cleaning, and illumination, in order to reduce surgical and anesthesia time (Figure 21.3).

Communication and cooperation between the surgeon and assistant is vital for the success of the procedure.

21.6 Structures and Anatomy

Proper orientation and a thorough knowledge of normal anatomy are obviously necessary for any surgery. Without this knowledge, and a certain amount of experience, performing a procedure is simply unethical. In oral and maxillofacial procedures, one has to take into account the many variations linked to different breeds and head types, as well as the possibility that any abnormalities and pathologies may change the presence and location of teeth and other structures. Innervation and vascularization cannot be compromised by inappropriate or aggressive dissection. It has been reported that the most common complication during maxillectomy is massive hemorrhage, and it is even recommended that temporary ligation of the carotid artery be carried out in order to avoid this (Lantz 2012). If a large maxillofacial surgery is planned, it is reasonable to prepare for a blood transfusion in case of significant hemorrhage. However, good anatomical orientation and appropriate techniques should be sufficient to avoid this life-threatening complication.

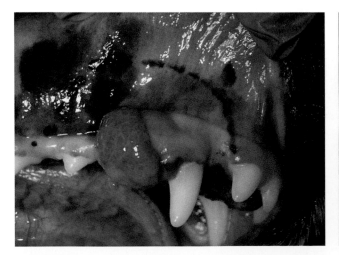
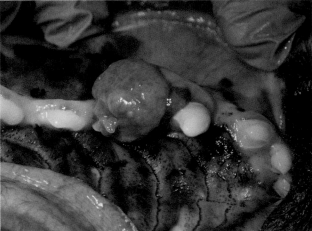

Figure 21.1   Use of a tissue marker helps the surgeon follow section margins during resective treatment of tumors.

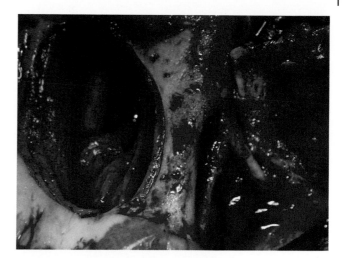

Figure 21.3 It is essential to be able to see the structures during oral surgery and identify them during dissection.

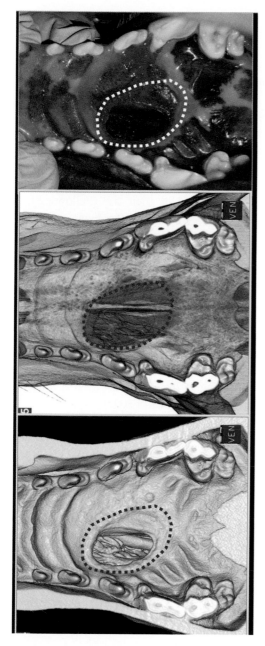

Figure 21.2 3D reconstruction utilized after CT scan helps in planning surgery and determining the extent of defects.

During the procedure, it may help to have continuous visualization of the preoperative 3D reconstruction, or at least to a dry skull of similar size/type to the patient.

In oncologic surgery, it is very common for vital structures present within surgical margins require excision. Eye enucleation and salivary gland or nasal turbinate excision are quite common. Appropriate techniques must be used to avoid neurological or functional complications following an operation, such as emphysema, blindness, or sialocoele.

21.7 Techniques, Instruments, and Materials

While the instrumentation will always be organized according to the personal preference of the operator, the general requirement is to have clean, autoclaved, and sharp instruments, ideally with at least one spare kit ready to use. The wide range of breeds, sizes, and anatomic features within dogs and cats requires different surgical kits for different individuals. Usually, feline surgery or extraction kits are different than canine ones. Some specific procedures are well described in journals and atlases of procedures, with suggestions that certain types or sizes of instruments be used.

It is a good idea to practice the uncommon procedures in a cadaver from time to time regardless of whether they are on the schedule.

Before a procedure, the correct instrumentation and materials for the most common complications and scenarios must be prepared. The most important factor in any oral surgery is correct magnification of the operating field, which in most cases comes alongside proper illumination. Dental loupes offer from 2.5× to 3.5× or more magnification and are the standard in veterinary operating theaters (not just for dentistry). Their use significantly helps with viewing small structures in appreciate detail and achieving good outcomes. For particularly small areas, as in prosthodontics, restorations, and endodontics, the use of operating microscopy is also possible (Zeiss et al. 2005) (Figure 21.4). Moreover, both magnification modalities provide the option to take a picture and transfer it to a presentation screen (Figure 21.5).

21.7.1 Surgical Techniques: Cold Steel, Scissors, Radiosurgery, Laser Surgery, Piezosurgery

Cold steel scalpel blades and other instruments are minimally invasive and very precise. Blades in sizes 11, 15, and 15C are designed for use in the oral cavity and difficult-to-reach areas. Healing of surgical wounds in the oral cavity is fast if the closure is performed in a tension-free manner and sutures are placed according to standards. The area may appeared scarred, but its elasticity will be the same as in adjacent tissues (Figure 21.6).

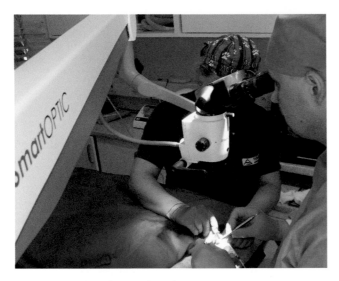

Figure 21.4   Use of operating microscopy.

Lasers have become a popular tool in veterinary practice, particularly the carbon dioxide (CO2) type. In humans, CO_2 lasers are used most commonly in oral and maxillofacial soft-tissue surgery due to their favorable interactions with oral soft tissues. They have features including hemostasis control, the ability to reach difficult areas, and reduced pain, which make them suitable for oral surgery (Peavy and Wilder-Smith, 2012). Periodontal pocket surgery, gingivectomy, gingivoplasty, gingival hyperplasia, operculectomy, tongue surgery, oropharyngeal inflammation therapy, oral mass surgery, and frenectomy are the most common indications for their use (Bellows 2013) (Figure 21.7). The list of applications includes maxillofacial surgeries in the nasal plane and nasal passages, elongated soft-palate correction, tonsillectomy, and access to the nasal cavity. In such cases, a laser is efficient, allows for rapid healing, and has hemostatic and bactericidal effects. Moreover, postoperative patient comfort is increased due to the less painful and harmful character of laser surgery as compared to traditional (cold steel) methods (Peavy and Wilder-Smith 2012). The critical point when using a cutting mode in a laser is to gently remove any charcoal substance prior to suturing, as leaving it may delay healing or cause dehiscense (Taney and Smith 2009).

Electrosurgery uses a controlled high-frequency electrical current at between 1.5 and 7.5 MHz (Figure 21.8). There are three basic types of functional instrument tips: single-wire electrodes for incising or excising; loop electrodes for planing; and flat or round electrodes for

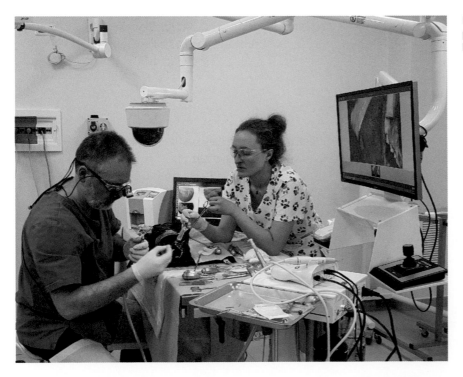

Figure 21.5   Live presentation of a procedure on a display screen, which was being recorded.

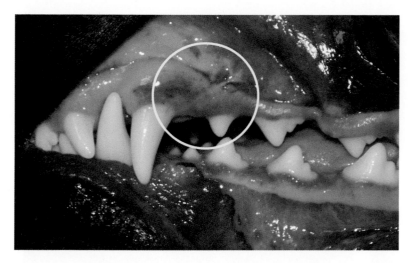

Figure 21.6 Scar tissue (circle) in the oral cavity is elastic and functional with proper healing.

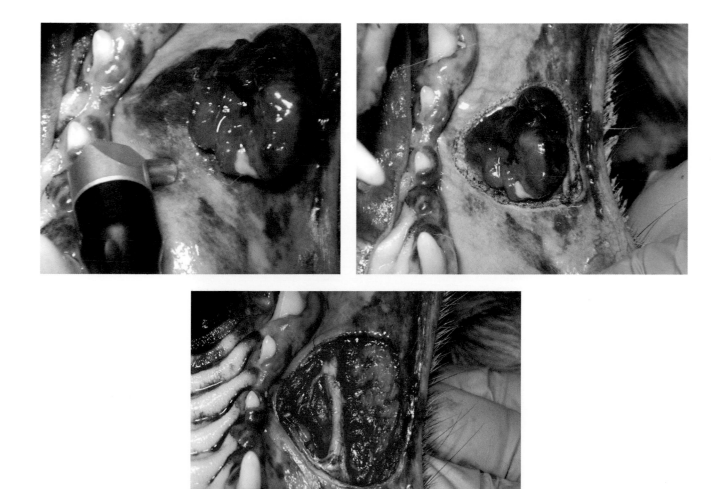

Figure 21.7 Application of laser surgery during excisional biopsy.

(a) (b)

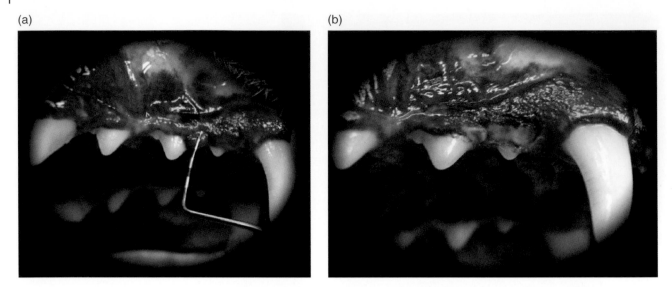

Figure 21.8   Application of electrosurgery with radio frequency: (a) gingival enlargement; (b) result. *Source:* Jan Schreyer.

(a) (b)

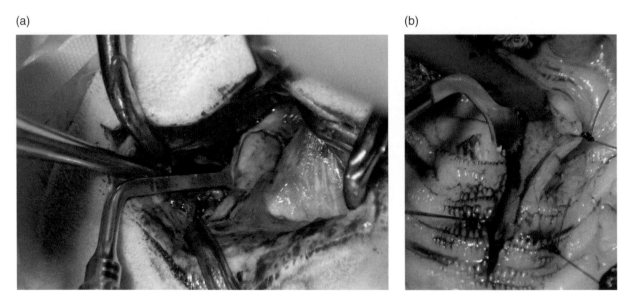

Figure 21.9   Application of piezosurgery in (a) TMJ arthroplasty in a cat (b) Performing palatal access to nasal cavity in a cat.

electrocoagulation. One of the most important guidelines for the use of electrosurgery is to always keep the electrode tip moving (Force and Niemiec 2009).

Piezoelectric bone surgery constitutes a new and exciting field in veterinary oral and maxillofacial surgery. It provides major advantages over hand instruments, a surgical bur, or an oscillating saw in a surgical field with limited access or one close to major neurovascular structures. Piezoelectric bone cutting does not require a high force, reducing the risks of collateral damage (Hennet 2015). With piezosurgery, the surgery on the temporomandibular joint (TMJ) (Figure 21.9), ostectomy, oncologic surgery, and endodontic or periodontal tissue (alveolar bone) surgery is safer and faster, and soft-tissue friendly. Its major advantages are precision of use and the reduction of trauma to the surrounding soft tissue, resulting in low bleeding, improved healing, less pain for the patient, and minimal necrosis of the operated area.

21.7.2   Gentle Tissue Handling

The delicate handling of tissues will improve the healing process and decrease the risk of dehiscense. The area of interest in the oral cavity is normally small, and it requires continuous effort to maintain visibility for the operator. Comfortable access and good visibility of the surgical site can be achieved when the positions of the surgical light and both the operator and the patient are optimal.

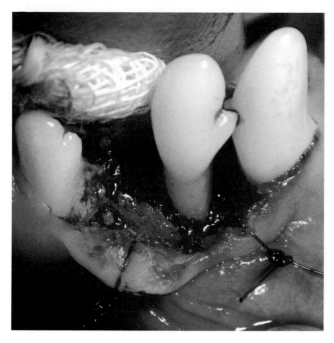

Figure 21.10 The use of stay sutures preserves the wound margins.

Additionally, there are methods that can improve comfort of work and quality of access, such as retracting the tissues and applying stay sutures.

Handling can be performed with tissue forceps (Addson Brown 7×7) for brief periods (e.g., while suturing), but if longer manipulation is required, it is better to use stay sutures or retraction, in order to avoid fatigue of the wound margins (Figure 21.10).

During surgery, it is very important not to allow the tissue to become dry. This can be accomplished by frequent use of a moistened gauze. It is also important to protect the tissues and structures adjacent to the operated area from damage and contamination. Retractors, mouth props, and covers can be used to isolate them from cooling water and any other contaminating substances. Prior to closure, a lactated ringers solution flush must be applied and the operated area cleaned. Force is rarely indicated in any surgery, and almost never used in dentistry. Appropriate sharpening and maintenance of instruments, working tips, and surfaces is necessary in order to allow them to be employed with the correct technique and without force. Dull and damaged instruments negatively affect the quality of surgery.

Minimally invasive surgery is currently preferred, and many techniques, instruments, anesthesia regimes, and supportive medical treatments are thus adapted to its requirements.

21.7.3 Hemostasic Techniques

The head, face, and oral cavity are very rich in vascularity. There are numerous small blood vessels and capillaries originating from several major arteries. Bleeding can be capillary, arterial, or venous; the former can be controlled by gentle pressure or the use of surgical techniques (e.g., electrosurgery, laser), while the latter two other are best avoided or predicted, if possible, and ligating is the ideal method of therapy.

Hemostasis is an important point of oral surgery, as having good visibility of the operating field helps decrease medical errors and consequent complications. A wide range of operating modalities are available to reduce bleeding. Applications of laser surgery, radiosurgery, piezosurgery, harmonic scalpel, or water jet are described in review articles and have become more and more common in veterinary maxillofacial, head, and neck surgery (Sherman and Davies 2000; Gasinski et al. 2009; Bellows 2013; Hennet 2015). The choice of hemostatic method is always based on personal preference, and there is currently no evidence that any single technique is significantly superior to any others in all procedures.

Blood vessels in the area of the head very often run in canals or in areas with challenging access. When it is necessary to ligate them, it is important to do so in a comfortable and planned way. Once the vessels are cut, it can be very difficult to identify them, and it is potentially dangerous to find and ligate them blindly. This applies especially to blood vessels in the mandibular canal during partial or total mandibulectomy, in the maxillary artery during caudal maxillectomy, and in the palatal blood vessels during palatal surgeries (Figure 21.11, 21.12). Preserving these vessels when during surgery planned operations is very important to their success. Ligation of larger blood vessels requires the use of a 3/0 or 2/0 suture. In general, the suture must be at least as strong as the tissue being apposed.

The oral and maxillofacial structures as well as the dentition create a unique environment when repairing fractures. Knowledge of the presence of anatomical structures and attempts to preserve their integrity are essential for surgical success.

This author's recommendation is to seek the opportunity to test different technologies at hands-on training courses and to determine the optimal technology for the particular needs and character of the surgery performed at your clinic. Having too many devices available is an unnecessary expense and will not allow you to become an expert in the use of any of them. One important factor in selecting a technique is adapting its use to your clinic. Laser and electrosurgery require a good air-conditioning system to avoid build-up of smoke, while other techniques may require good recycling of water.

(a)   (b)

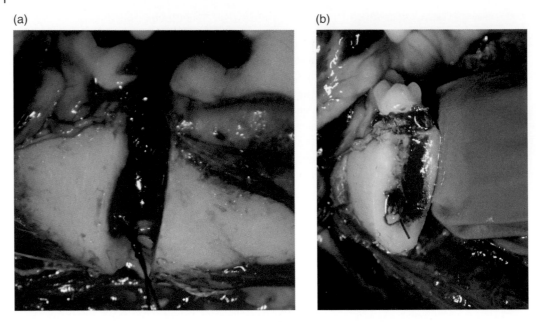

Figure 21.11   During segmental mandibulectomy, it is important first to (a) identify mandibular canal structures and then (b) ligate them.

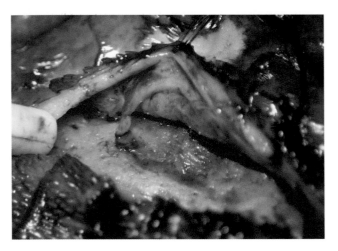

Figure 21.12   It is important to identify the palatal artery when doing palatal surgery in order to preserve its integrity.

An important part of hemostasis is performing laboratory tests to ensure adequate coagulation. This includes identification of any factors that might cause hemorrhage (e.g., current medications, existing systemic diseases). To avoid bleeding, the incision lines should be planned away from major blood vessels; if this is not possible, the vessel should be ligated to avoid its being incidentally damaged. For example, it is particularly important when doing palatal surgery to identify and ligate the palatal arteries when performing a double-flap technique on closure of the oronasal fistulas, the maxillary arteries when performing maxillectomies, and the mandibular arteries when performing mandibulectomy.

Incidental damage of the arteries can cause massive bleeding and difficulties in their ligation. Moreover, employing hemostatic forceps blind when hemorrhage occurs can result in damage of adjacent structures (e.g., nerves). After major surgery, the resultant large empty space can cause a large hematoma due to capillary bleeding if left unattended. To prevent this problem, the empty space can be augmented with hemostatic absorbable material. A broad variety of hemostatic agents have been developed in recent decades, including vegetal-origin sealants (Surgicel, Tabotamp, Hemostase), fibrin sealants (Tachosil, Tisseel), sponge products composed of gelatine (Gelfoam), and specific techniques such as polyvinyl alcohol sponge (Merocel) and infrared-sapphire coagulation, which involves the conversion of light into thermal energy, causing coagulation and hemostasis (Echave et al. 2014).

21.7.4   Line Angles, Access Flaps, and Fenestration of the Periosteum

A flap is raised to provide access to an area requiring debridement or removal, or to cover large tissue deficits. Full flaps must have slightly wider bases in order to maintain blood supply and should never begin in the middle of the crown, but rather at the line angle of the adjacent tooth, or at the diastema if it exists. The line angle is the junction of perpendicular surfaces of the tooth (e.g., mesio-lingual, disto-buccal) (Tutt 2006). To make an envelope flap, the interdental gingival attachment is incised and the flap is

(a)

(b)

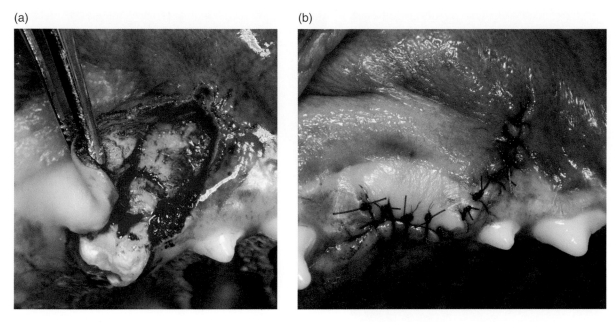

Figure 21.13 A triangle flap is created by making a vertical incision at one end of an envelope flap (a) during preparation and (b) after closure.

raised with a periosteal elevator. The longer the envelope flap, the better the access to the alveolar bone – but there is no reason to create an especially long one. When more visibility is needed, vertical releasing incisions can be made at one or both ends of the envelope flap (the choice depends on where the least damage of underlying tissues will occur and where the fewest blood vessels are located); one incision creates a triangle flap, while two (one at each end) create a trapezoidal (or full) flap (Figure 21.13).

Full-thickness flaps consist of a mucoperiosteal flap comprising mucosa and underlying periosteum. The latter is a connective-tissue membrane that covers the alveolar bone, limiting pliability of the flap. Therefore, to make the flap larger, the periosteum must be incised (this is known as "fenestration") (Figure 21.14).

Another type of flap is the partial-thickness flap, which is utilized in some periodontal surgery techniques (e.g., lateral sliding flaps in the treatment of gingival clefts; Figure 21.15).

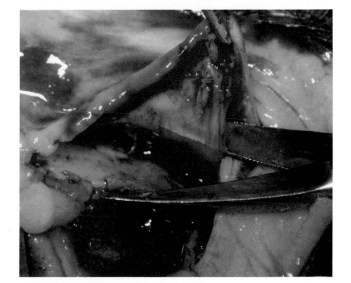

Figure 21.14 Fenestration involves cutting the periosteum to extend the flap.

21.8 Wound Closure

Any wounds occurring during the surgical procedure eventually must be closed. Standards referring to suturing help in avoiding dehiscence and necrosis of wounds in the oral cavity and enhance the healing process. Tension-free suturing and an appropriate shape and size of flap are key. The flaps used to cover and close certain areas must be larger (by approximately 50%) than the defect, due to postoperative shrinkage. Wound margins should be even and regular

and without rectangles, and the underlying bone must be smoothed and adapted to the shape of the defect.

The specific character of the oral tissues and their function and shape should be taken into account when apposing the wound margins. It is important in palatal surgery to follow the shape of the palatine rugae and in periodontal surgery to mind the mucogingival junction and attached gingiva. The oral mucosa will not replace the attached gingiva, and lack of attached gingiva is considered a limiting factor in periodontal flap surgery for the management of

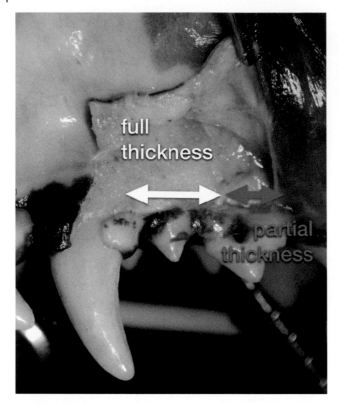

Figure 21.15 A partial-thickness flap is created during pedicle sliding flap to repair a gingival cleft.

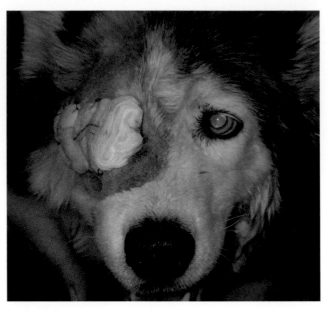

Figure 21.16 Suturing a dressing to the skin to provide compression is indicated after major maxillofacial surgery to avoid emphysema.

gingival defects. When closure of the oral mucosa is performed, the connective submucosal tissue should contact the same tissue from the other side of the wound, and infolding of the wound margin must be avoided when primary closure is critical for the outcome (e.g., in palatal surgery or oronasal communication management).

In major surgeries of the maxilla, when the nasal cavity is opened, emphysema may occur. To limit this, compression by appropriate dressing is recommended for the first five to seven days (Figure 21.16).

The most recommended suturing material for use intraorally is Polyglecaprone 25, which is an absorbable monofilament 5/0 (cats and small dogs) or 4/0 (all other dogs) with a taper cut or reverse cutting needle (Tsugawa and Verstraete 2012). For many dentists, catgut is the preferred choice in terms of size and needle type, but this material is not available everywhere.

Suture needles for oral surgery must be swaged-on. Needle curvature is either 3/8 or 1/2, with the latter more indicated in the caudal part of the oral cavity. A reverse-cutting needle is best for suturing the gingiva and mucosa, but for delicate or inflamed mucosa, a taper point may be better (Dominick 2014). The needle should be inserted into the tissue perpendicularly in order to make the smallest possible entry and avoid tearing the mucosa (Figure 21.17)

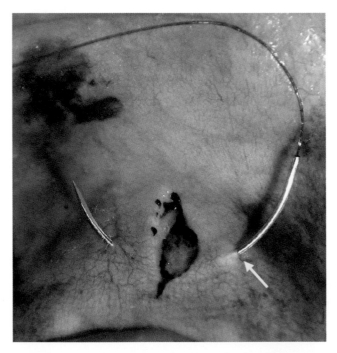

Figure 21.17 Perpendicular piercing reduces the amount of damage caused, while attempts to suture with a single pierce can increase it (arrow).

When gingival and/or palatal tissues are firmly bound down to bone the sutured portion of them should be gently detached from the bone to avoid bending or breaking the needle.

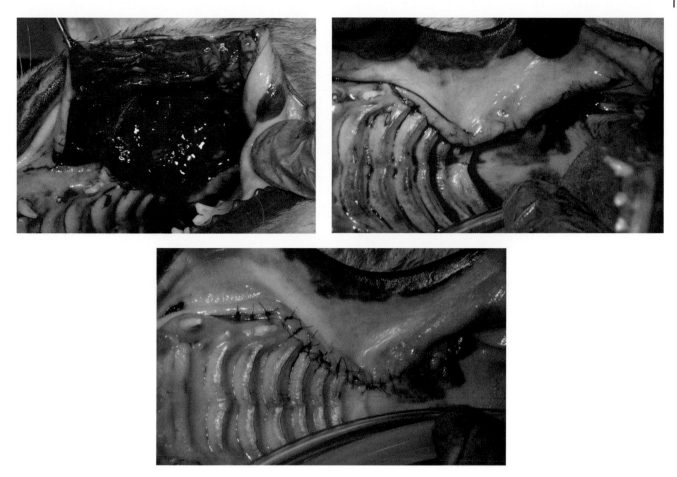

Figure 21.18 Double-layer suturing in major oral surgery (e.g., maxillectomy) helps avoid dehiscense.

(a)   (b)

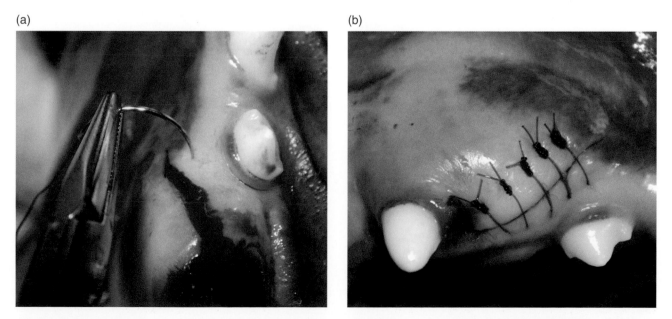

Figure 21.19 (a) A distance of 2–3 mm should be kept between the wound edge and the suture entry point, and another 2–3 mm between interrupted sutures. (b) The knots should not be placed over the wound.

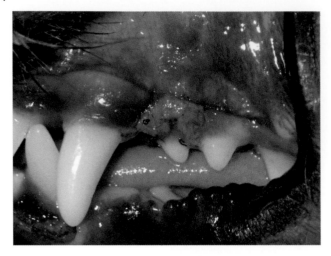

Figure 21.20 Standard interrupted sutures are often associated with irritation and debris entrapment.

Double-layer suturing in major surgical procedures is better than single-layer (Figure 21.18). Whenever possible, it is recommened to apply a submucosal layer. It is important to keep a 2–3 mm distance between the wound edge and the suture access, and 2–3 mm between interrupted sutures (Figure 21.19). In general, a simple interrupted suture is recommended in most oral procedures. Some authors suggest that a simple continuous suture be used after full-mouth extraction in stomatitis patients to reduce the time of closure and decrease anesthesia time, but this author still prefers simple interrupted buried knot sutures. No area of denuded bone should be left uncovered by soft tissue, and the suture line should not be over a defect – but the most important thing is a tension-free incision line (Wiggs 1997).

Depending on the material, the number of throws should be sufficient to provide a firm knot, but there should not be so many that it increases the amount of suture material required for degradation, which will in turn increase the inflammatory response.

The length of the suture should be sufficient that the knot cannot become released. In some places, short knots are reported to cause more irritation to adjacent tissues (Figure 21.20). The suture material can be impregnated with triclosan, which has an antiseptic character, but there is not yet evidence for its use.

The general rule of tension free closure applies to any suture in the oral cavity. To avoid compromise of blood supply, mattress sutures should avoided. Continuous sutures are also not recommended due to the complete failure of closure that will occur if even a part of them is broken.

The following tips apply to sutures in the oral cavity:

1) The needle should pierce the tissue perpendicularly. When gingival and palatal tissues are firmly bound down to bone, it is possible to either detach the sutured margin form the bone or to rotate the needle from the vertical position to a horizontal direction so that it can be slid along the surface of the bone.
2) Double-layer suturing is better than single-layer in major surgical procedures.
3) A distance of 2–3 mm should be kept between the wound edge and the suture entry point.
4) A distance of 2–3 mm should be kept between interrupted sutures.
5) The knot should not be placed directly over the incision.
6) The aposed wound margins should have the support of the bone, rather than being placed over empty space.
7) The average number of throws in monofilament 4/0 or 5/0 should be 4×.
8) In some locations, free ends of suture may irritate or entrap foreign material.

21.9 Biopsy

The clinical appearance of an oral mass is never sufficient to assess its character and prognosis. Any growth must be diagnosed through biopsy. Though fine-needle aspiration (FNA) techniques are convenient and easy to perform, with a low risk of bleeding, and in certain lesions the correlation between cytology and histopathology is very high, histopathology is required for a definite diagnosis (Ehrhart and Withrow 2007; Bonfanti et al. 2015).

Punch-biopsy instruments like trephines work well for superficial, flat tumors (Figure 21.21). Incisional biopsies should be utilized in the case of large ulcerated or necrotic-appearing lesions, or as a follow-up to an unsuccessful needle biopsy (Ehrhart and Withrow 2007).

When planning an incisional biopsy, the removal should be placed as close as possible to the edge. Laser or electrosurgery allows bleeding control, but the size of the tissue sample must be sufficient to avoid submitting only coagulated material.

Regional lymph nodes should also be sampled (FNA cytology or surgical biopsy) (Smith 1995).

21.10 Conclusion

Following oral surgical procedures, the oral and maxillofacial structures must be ready to perform regular functions like chewing, swallowing, and very rapid breathing.

(a)

(b)

(c)

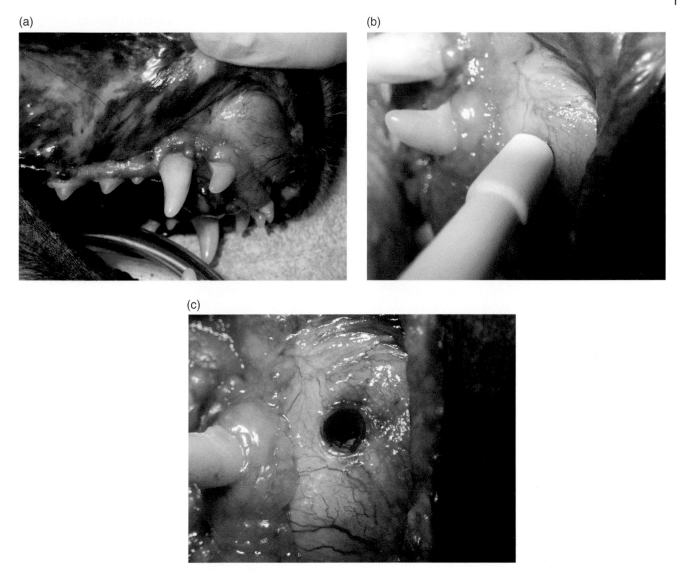

Figure 21.21 Incisional biopsy with the use of trephine should be performed in flat superficial masses. (a–c) Small-wound after biopsy is easy to close with a single suture.

Therefore, the wound shape must allow for full functioning and the patient must be kept comfortable. In certain extreme situations, nutrition may be compromised following surgery, in which case the employment of esophagostomy feeding tubes is warranted.

Oral and maxillofacial surgical techniques differ from those applied elsewhere, and as such require different skills and experiences. The use of dedicated oral surgery materials will enhance procedure quality, accelerate healing, and help avoid complications.

References

Bellows, J. (2013). Laser and radiosurgery in veterinary dentistry. *Vet. Clin. North Am. Small Anim. Pract.* 43 (3): 651–668.

Bonfanti, U., Bertazzolo, W., Gracis, M. et al. (2015). Diagnostic value of cytological analysis of tumours and tumour-like lesions of the oral cavity in dogs and cats: a prospective study on 114 cases. *Vet. J.* 205 (2): 322–327.

Dominick, E.D. (2014). Suture material and needle options in oral and periodontal surgery. *J. Vet. Dent.* 31 (3): 204–211.

Echave, M., Oyagüez, I., and Casado, M.A. (2014). Use of Floseal, a human gelatine-thrombin matrix sealant, in surgery: a systematic review. *BMC Surgery* 14: 111.

Ehrhart, N.P. and Withrow, S.J. (2007). Biopsy principles. In: *Small Animal Clinical Oncology* (eds. S.J. Withrow and D.M. Vail), 147–153. St. Louis, MO: W.B. Saunders.

Force, J. and Niemiec, B. (2009). Gingivectomy and gingivoplasty for gingival enlargement. *J. Vet. Dent.* 26 (2): 132–137.

Gasinski, M., Modrzejewski, M., Cenda, P. et al. (2009). Application of water jet ERBEJET 2 in salivary glands surgery. *Otolaryngol. Pol.* 63 (7): 47–49.

Hennet, P. (2015). Piezoelectric bone surgery: a review of the literature and potential applications in veterinary oromaxillofacial surgery. *Front. Vet. Sci.* 2: 8.

Lantz, G. (2012). Maxillectomy techniques. In: *Oral and Maxillofacial Surgery in Dogs and Cats* (eds. F.J.M. Verstraete and M.J. Lommer), 451–465. Philadelphia, PA: Elsevier.

Peavy, G.M. and Wilder-Smith, P.E. (2012). Laser surgery. In: *Oral and Maxillofacial Surgery in Dogs and Cats* (eds. F.J.M. Verstraete and M.J. Lommer), 79–89. Philadelphia, PA: Elsevier.

Sherman, J.A. and Davies, H.T. (2000). Ultrasonic: the harmonic scalpel and its possible uses in maxillofacial surgery. *Br. J. Oral Maxillofac. Surg.* 38: 530–532.

Smith, M.M. (1995). Surgical approach for lymph node staging of oral and maxillofacial neoplasms in dogs. *J. Am. Anim. Hosp. Assoc.* 31: 514–518.

Taney, K. and Smith, M.M. (2009). Resection of mast cell tumor of the lip in a dog. *J. Vet. Dent.* 26 (1): 28–34.

Tsugawa, A.J. and Verstraete, F.J.M. (2012). Suture materials and biomaterials. In: *Oral and Maxillofacial Surgery in Dogs and Cats* (eds. F.J.M. Verstraete and M.J. Lommer), 69–78. Philadelphia, PA: Elsevier.

Tutt, C. (2006). *Exodontics in Small Animal Dentistry: A Manual of Techniques*, 132–171. New York: Blackwell.

Wiggs, B. (1997). *Oral Surgery in Veterinary Dentistry Principles and Practice*, 232–258. Philadelphia, PA: Lippincott-Raven.

Zeiss, A., Lin, S., and Fuss, Z. (2005). Endodontic surgery (apicoectomy) – success rate of more than 90% using dental operating microscope and ultrasonic tips. *Refuat Hapeh Vehashinayim* 22 (1): 33–41. 86.

22

Extraction Techniques and Equipment
Brook Niemiec

Veterinary Dental Specialties and Oral Surgery, San Diego, CA USA

22.1   Introduction

Dental extractions are an exceedingly common surgical procedure, performed virtually daily in almost every veterinary practice. However, they are *not* a simple undertaking. They should be approached with the same level of care as any other surgical procedure.

Extractions are typically performed to remove infected or painful teeth. Indications include, but are not limited to endodontic disease (i.e., fractured or intrinsically stained teeth), severe periodontal disease, traumatic malocclusion, persistent or infected deciduous teeth, tooth resorption, abscessed teeth, caudal stomatitis, and unerupted teeth (Wiggs and Lobprise 1997; Niemiec 2012). It must be noted, however, that options such as root canal therapy and periodontal surgery can effectively save many of these teeth and therefore should be offered prior to considering extraction (Holmstrom et al. 1998 and Niemiec 2012).

Complete extraction of the diseased tooth almost invariably resolves the pain or infection. However, if extractions are improperly performed, even simple procedures can result in iatrogenic complications, including hemorrhage, osteomyelitis, oronasal fistula, forcing of a root tip into the mandibular canal or nasal cavity, jaw fracture, and ocular damage (Harvey and Emily 1993; Holmstrom et al. 1998; Taylor et al. 2004). By far the most common iatrogenic complication is retained tooth roots (Holmstrom et al. 1998; Smith 1998; Woodward 2006), which results in continued infection in and around the root site (Wiggs and Lobprise 1997; Smith 1998; Woodward 2006). It is rare for animal patients to show obvious clinical signs, but they suffer regardless. Occasionally, this problem causes a draining tract from the retained roots, which can result in a malpractice claim (Holmstrom et al. 1998).

Single-root extractions are performed via the nine steps outlined in the next section (Niemiec 2012). Multiroot teeth require sectioning into single-rooted pieces, which are then each treated as single-root extractions. Large teeth or any difficult/complicated presentations (due to root malformations or ankylosis) are best extracted via an open technique (i.e., the creation of gingival flaps and removal of buccal cortical bone).

22.2   Nonsurgical (Closed) Extractions

22.2.1   Step 1: Consent

Never extract a tooth without prior owner consent, no matter how advanced the problem or how obvious it is that extraction is the proper therapy (Shipp and Fahrenkrug 1992; Holmstrom et al. 1998; Niemiec 2008). Consent should preferably be written, but verbal consent is acceptable. It is reasonable to ask the owner whether they want to keep the extracted teeth.

22.2.2   Step 2: Preoperative Dental Radiographs

Dental radiographs should be made of all teeth prior to extraction (Holmstrom et al. 1998; Blazejewski et al. 2006; Niemiec 2009; Niemiec 2012). These are invaluable resources for guiding the practitioner through the extraction process, showing the amount of disease present, any root abnormalities (Figure 22.1a), and any resorption or ankylosis (Holmstrom et al. 1998; Blazejewski et al. 2006) (Figure 22.1b). Approximately 10% of feline maxillary third premolars have a third root (Verstraete and Terpak 1997) (Figure 22.1c). Significant mandibular alveolar bone loss

The Veterinary Dental Patient: A Multidisciplinary Approach, First Edition. Edited by Jerzy Gawor and Brook Niemiec.
© 2021 John Wiley & Sons Ltd. Published 2021 by John Wiley & Sons Ltd.
Companion website: www.wiley.com/go/gawor/veterinary-dental-patient

(a)

(b)

(c)

(d)

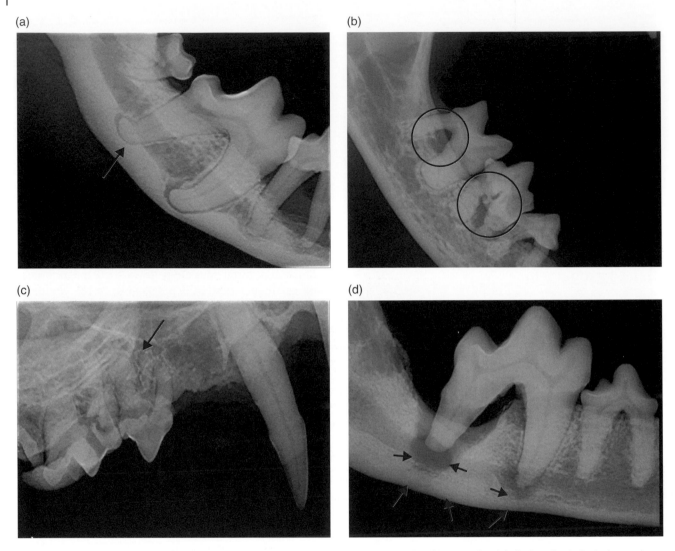

Figure 22.1 Preoperative radiographs allow visualization of (a) tooth abnormalities, (b) resorption (circles) and ankylosis (arrows), and (c) supernumerary roots. They also help assess (d) the amount of alveolar bone in the extraction site.

secondary to periodontal disease weakens the bone and predisposes the patient to an iatrogenic pathologic fracture (Mulligan et al. 1998; Niemiec 2012) (Figure 22.1d). This is most common with the canine and first molar teeth in small- and toy-breed dogs, due to the proportionally larger root size of these teeth compared to the jaw (Gioso et al. 2001). Dentoalveolar ankylosis makes extraction by traditional elevation practically impossible (Niemiec 2012). In short, dental radiographs provide critical information for treatment planning and the successful outcome of dental extraction procedures.

22.2.3 Step 3: Pain Management

Extractions are moderately to severely painful procedures. A multimodal approach typically provides superior analgesia and safety (Kelly et al. 2001a, b; Lanz 2003;

Woodward 2008). This should include regional anesthesia (Niemiec 2012) (see Chapter 11).

22.2.4 Step 4: Cutting of the Gingival Attachment

This is important because the gingival attachment contributes approximately 15% of the retention of the periodontal apparatus (Niemiec 2012). More importantly, however, it helps avoid tearing the gingiva during extraction. Gingival tearing can cause defects that require closure or can make a planned closure more difficult.

This procedure may be performed with a scalpel blade (#11 or 15), but this author prefers a periosteal or luxating elevator (Niemiec 2012). Here, the instrument is placed into the gingival sulcus with the tip of the blade angled slightly (10–20°) toward the tooth (to help avoid slippage)

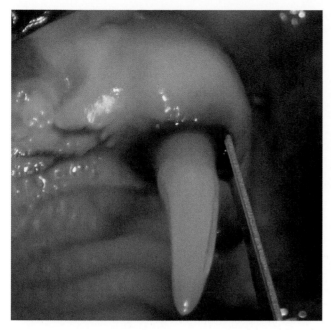

Figure 22.2   The first step in extraction is to cut the gingival attachment. The scalpel blade is placed approximately 10–20° toward the tooth to avoid slippage. The same goes for insertion of the luxator or elevator into the periodontal ligament space.

(Figure 22.2). The blade is then advanced apically to the level of the alveolar bone and carefully worked around the entire tooth circumference.

22.2.5   Step 5: Luxation and Elevation

22.2.5.1   Instrument Selection
Numerous instruments are available for elevation, including the classic elevator and the luxating and winged types. Classic and winged elevators are used in an "insert and twist" motion to tear the periodontal ligament, whereas luxators are used in a rocking motion during insertion to fatigue and cut the periodontal ligament. Luxators may be *gently* twisted, but they are not designed for this and can be easily damaged when used in this manner (Niemiec 2012). It is important to select an instrument that approximates the curvature and size of the root (Woodward 2006). In general, "go small," as this results in less pressure and bone/tooth damage. Elevators larger than 3 mm are rarely indicated; generally, sizes of 1–2 mm work well for cats and of 2–3 mm for dogs (Niemiec 2012).

22.2.5.2   Safety
Elevation can be dangerous, as elevators are sharp surgical instruments that are used in close proximity to numerous critical and delicate structures (Niemiec 2012). There are many reports of eyes that have been gouged, and at least

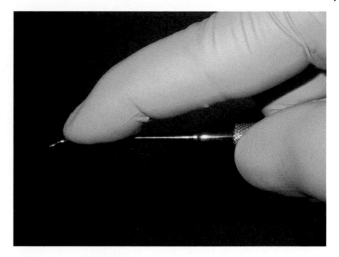

Figure 22.3   The index finger should be placed near the tip when using an elevator.

one confirmed fatality due to an elevator puncturing a patient's brain (Smith et al. 2003). To help avoid causing iatrogenic trauma in the event of slippage, the index finger should be placed near the tip of the instrument (Harvey and Emily 1993; Wiggs and Lobprise 1997; Blazejewski et al. 2006; Niemiec 2008) (Figure 22.3).

22.2.5.3   Technique
Elevation is initiated by inserting the instrument firmly yet gently into the periodontal ligament space (between the tooth and the alveolar bone) (Wiggs and Lobprise 1997; Niemiec 2012). The insertion should be performed while keeping the instrument at a 10–20° angle toward the tooth, to avoid slippage (Harvey and Emily 1993; Niemiec 2012).

Once in the space between the bone and the tooth, the instrument is *gently* twisted with two-finger pressure (Wiggs and Lobprise 1997). This is not to say that the instrument should be actually held with two fingers, but it should be twisted only with the force that two fingers could generate (Niemiec 2012). The tooth is held in the slightly displaced position for 10–30 seconds in order to fatigue and tear the periodontal ligament (Harvey and Emily 1993; Holmstrom et al. 1998; Woodward 2006). It should move at least slightly during elevation; if not, no damage is being done to the periodontal ligament (Figure 22.4). This may be due to improper technique, or the tooth may be ankylosed.

The periodontal ligament is very effective in resisting short, intense forces (Proffit and Fields 2000). Thus, only by the exertion of prolonged force (10–30 seconds) will it become weakened (Niemiec 2012). Increased pressure will transfer the excess force to the alveolar bone and tooth, which can result in the fracture of one of these structures (Niemiec 2012).

(a)

(b)

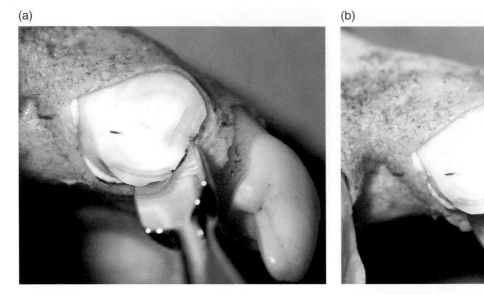

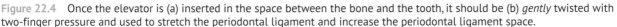

Figure 22.4   Once the elevator is (a) inserted in the space between the bone and the tooth, it should be (b) *gently* twisted with two-finger pressure and used to stretch the periodontal ligament and increase the periodontal ligament space.

After holding for 10–30 seconds, the instrument is repositioned approximately one-eighth of the way around the tooth and the procedure is repeated (Niemiec 2012). This is continued 360° around the tooth, each time moving the elevator apically as much as possible. Depending on the level of disease and the size of the tooth, a few to several rotations of the tooth may be necessary.

The key to successful elevation is patience (Blazejewski et al. 2006; Niemiec 2008). Only slow, consistent elevation will loosen the root without breaking it. Remember, it's easier to extract an intact root than to remove fractured root tips (Woodward 2006).

Elevation should create tooth mobility in a fairly short period of time; if not, faulty extraction technique or, more likely, an area of dentoalveolar ankylosis should be suspected (Niemiec 2012). Technique should be reviewed, making sure the elevator is between the tooth and the bone. If the technique is proper, the dental radiographs should be checked for signs of ankylosis, in which case a surgical (open) approach should be employed. Regardless of radiographic signs, if the extraction is not progressing, a surgical approach should be considered.

22.2.5.4   New Mechanical Technique

A new mechanical extraction device (iM3 Vet-Tome) has recently been introduced. This device has a mechanically driven blade of two sizes (narrow and wide) that passes along the periodontal ligament space, luxating and loosening the tooth without the need for buccal or lingual alveolar bone removal (though this may be required to achieve primary closure post-extraction). The outcome is a less

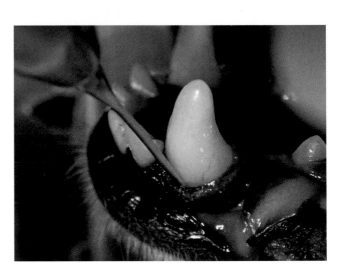

Figure 22.5   Initial insertion of an iM3 Vet-Tome blade into the periodontal ligament space.

traumatic and less invasive tooth extraction, due to the limited alveolar bone damage, which will likely allow for less postoperative pain and quicker healing of the extraction site.

The instrument is mechanically driven, with a power setting of 1–10. It is initially introduced at about 45° to the root surface on the mesial or distal surfaces of the tooth (Figure 22.5). It uses a side-sweeping action in short bursts of up to 10 seconds to cut along the periodontal ligament to close to the apex of the tooth, eventually going 360° around it, normally without the need to raise a mucoperiosteal flap or remove any bone. The different blade sizes can be matched to the size of the tooth. Once the tooth has become

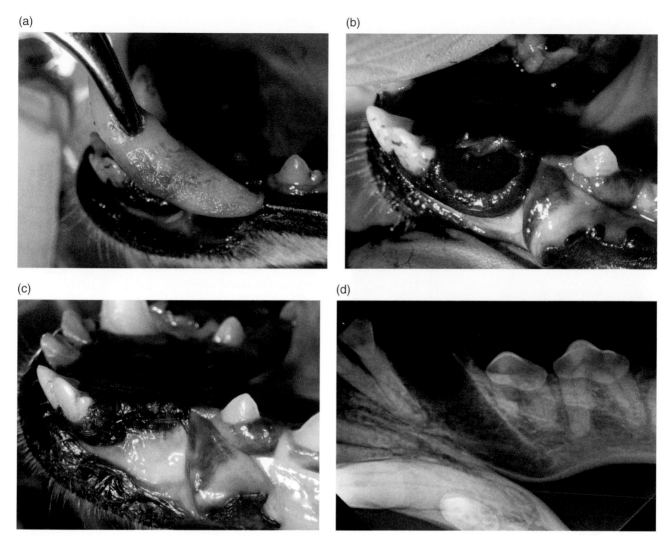

Figure 22.6 Further steps in extraction with iM3 Vet-Tome lead to (a) pulling out of the tooth without damage of the alveolar bone, then (b) the empty alveolus is closed by (c) single interrupted sutures and (d) a postoperative radiograph is exposed.

loose, dental elevators can be used to further loosen it, following the path created by the iM3 Vet-Tome. Finally, with the use of extraction forceps, the tooth can be extracted. The alveolus or socket can then be sutured, while maintaining the four bony walls of the socket. If primary closure cannot be performed, a small envelope flap is raised, labial or buccal bone is removed, a periosteal release with scalpel and scissors is carried out, and suturing is used to close the alveolus and preserve the developing blood clot (Figure 22.6).

22.2.6 Step 6: Extraction

Removal of the tooth should only be attempted when it is very loose (Harvey and Emily 1993; Wiggs and Lobprise 1997). The tooth is grasped with the extraction forceps near the gingival margin and gently pulled from the alveolus (Niemiec 2008) (Figure 22.7). Undue pressure must *not* be applied as this may result in root fracture (Wiggs and Lobprise 1997). If the tooth does not come out easily, more elevation is necessary. More experienced operators can apply gentle pressure and twist the extracted root till it meets resistance then holding for 10 seconds to one then another direction, in order to help tear the ligaments.

22.2.7 Step 7: Debridement, Alveoloplasty, and Augmentation of the Alveolus

This is done to remove diseased tissue and smooth any rough bony edges that might irritate the gingiva and delay healing (Holmstrom et al. 1998; Smith 1998; Carmichael 2002; Blazejewski et al. 2006). Diseased tissue can be removed by hand with a curette. Bone removal and smoothing is best performed with a coarse diamond bur on a water-cooled

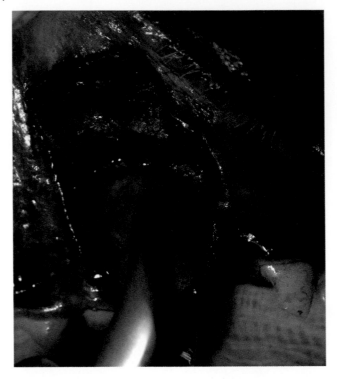

Figure 22.7 Use of extraction forceps to pull out a loosened tooth.

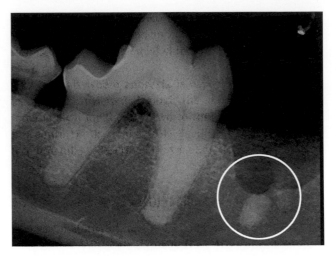

Figure 22.8 Retained roots are a very common complication associated with dental extractions.

high-speed air-driven handpiece (Harvey and Emily 1993; Holmstrom et al. 1998; Carmichael 2002; Frost Fitch 2003; Blazejewski et al. 2006). Next, the alveolus should be gently flushed with sterile tissue-friendly fluid (Ringers solution) to decrease bacterial contamination and reduce the harmful influence of demineralized water (Smith 1998; Manfra Marretta 2002; Blazejewski et al. 2006; Taney and Smith 2006). After the alveolus is cleaned, it may be packed with an osseopromotive substance (Periomix, Veterinary Transplant Services) (Manfra Marretta 2002; Blazejewski et al. 2006; Taney and Smith 2006).

22.2.8 Step 8: Postoperative Dental Radiographs

Dental radiographs must be exposed post-extraction in order to document complete removal of the root(s) (Holmstrom et al. 1998; Niemiec 2009; Niemiec 2012). Retained roots are a very common complication (Figure 22.8). In fact, a recent study reported that 92% of extracted carnassial teeth in dogs and cats have retained roots (Moore and Niemiec 2014). A retained root tip may become infected, or more commonly it may act as a foreign body, creating significant inflammation (Wiggs and Lobprise 1997; Ulbricht et al. 2003; Niemiec 2012). There are rarely any clinical signs with this complication, but occasionally retained roots do create an abscess. The postoperative radiograph can also on occasion reveal the presence of radiopaque debris contaminating the alveolus.

22.2.9 Step 9: Closure of the Extraction Site

Closure of the extraction site promotes hemostasis and improves postoperative comfort and esthetics (Harvey and Emily 1993; Niemiec 2012). Prior to suturing it is imperative to assure that the closure will be tension-free. To achieve it the sutured marging are to be free form the bone and sometimes fenestration of the periosteum is required. It is always indicated in cases of larger teeth or any time a gingival flap is utilized, but this author tends to close *all* extraction sites (Holmstrom et al. 1998; Frost Fitch 2003). However, primary (edge to edge) closure is not necessary if no flap has been created nor fistula present. This is best accomplished with size 4/0 to 5/0 absorbable sutures (e.g., chromic gut, monocryl) on a reverse cutting needle (Wiggs and Lobprise 1997; Holmstrom et al. 1998; Carmichael 2002; Taney and Smith 2006). A simple interrupted pattern should be employed, placing the sutures 2–3 mm apart (Holmstrom et al. 1998; Smith 1998; Carmichael 2002; Frost Fitch 2003; Blazejewski et al. 2006; Taney and Smith 2006) (Figure 22.9). Additionally, it is best to utilize one additional throw over the manufacturer's recommendation in order to counteract tongue action.(Niemiec 2012).

There are several key points associated with successful healing of flaps (Wiggs and Lobprise 1997; Niemiec 2012). Primarily, there must be *no tension* on the incision line (Carmichael 2002; Frost Fitch 2003; Blazejewski et al. 2006). Tension can be removed by fenestrating the periosteum or creating a gingival flap (see later) (Carmichael 2002; Manfra Marretta 2002; Frost Fitch 2003; Blazejewski et al. 2006). Ideally, suturing should be done from the unattached to the attached tissue, in order to avoid tearing the flap as the needle dulls (Blazejewski et al. 2006). Finally, it should be ensured that all tissue edges have been thoroughly debrided, if epithelilized as intact epithelial tissues will not heal (Blazejewski et al. 2006).

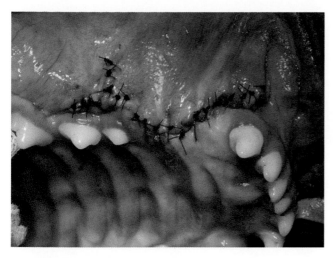

Figure 22.9 Closure is best performed with a simple interrupted pattern, placing sutures 2–3 mm apart.

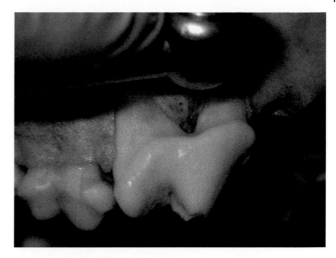

Figure 22.10 When sectioning teeth, if possible start at the furcation and work toward the crown.

22.3 Extraction of Multirooted Teeth

All multirooted teeth should be sectioned into single-rooted pieces (Holmstrom et al. 1998; Smith 1998; Carmichael 2002). This is important, as the roots of most multirooted teeth are divergent, and thus the root tips will break if extractions are attempted in one go (Wiggs and Lobprise 1997; Manfra Marretta 2002; Niemiec 2008). Root fracture can occur even if a tooth is relatively mobile at first.

The best tool for sectioning teeth is a bur on a high-speed air-driven handpiece (Holmstrom et al. 1998; Carmichael 2002; Blazejewski et al. 2006). In addition to being the most efficient technique, it also has air and water coolant to help avoid overheating the tooth and bone (Niemiec 2012). Many different styles of burs are available, but this author prefers a cross-cut taper-fissure bur (Niemiec 2012). Number 699 is ideal for cats and small dogs, 701 for medium dogs, and 702 for large breeds (Harvey and Emily 1993; Wiggs and Lobprise 1997; Smith 1998; Carmichael 2002; Blazejewski et al. 2006; Niemiec 2008).

When sectioning teeth, if possible start at the furcation and work toward the crown (Wiggs and Lobprise 1997; Blazejewski et al. 2006) (Figure 22.10). This prevents missing the furcation and cutting down into a root or cutting through the tooth and damaging the gingiva or bone (Smith 1998). If the furcation is not already exposed due to gingival recession, a periosteal elevator should be used to carefully raise a small gingival flap (Niemiec 2012).

Two-rooted teeth are generally sectioned in the middle to separate them into halves. The mandibular first molar in cats is an exception, due to its disproportionate roots (Niemiec 2012). Proper sectioning of a three-rooted molar

tooth in a dog is performed by cutting between the buccal cusp tips and then just palatal to them.

After the tooth has been properly sectioned, follow the previous set of steps for each single-rooted piece. In some cases, the individual tooth pieces can be carefully elevated against one another to gain purchase (Holmstrom et al. 1998; Manfra Marretta 2002; Blazejewski et al. 2006).

Crown resection may be used prior to sectioning into single-rooted fragments (Figure 22.11). This technique can allow for easier design of the envelope flap and easier identification of where to section the tooth.

22.4 Surgical (Open) Extractions

Difficult extractions are best performed via an open approach (Niemiec 2008, 2012). While this typically involves the canine and carnassial teeth, it may also be beneficial in teeth with root malformations (curves), pathology (e.g., ankylosis), or retained roots (Holmstrom et al. 1998; Manfra Marretta 2002; Frost Fitch 2003; Blazejewski et al. 2006; Woodward 2006).

Surgical extractions are initiated by creating a gingival flap. The two options are a horizontal incision along the arcade to create an envelope flap and vertical releasing incision(s) to create a full flap (Holmstrom et al. 1998; Frost Fitch 2003; Blazejewski et al. 2006).

An **envelope flap** (Grant et al. 1988) is made by releasing the gingival attachment along the arcade, including one to several teeth on either side of the tooth or teeth to be extracted (Niemiec 2008, 2012) (Figure 22.12). The flap is initiated by incising the interdental gingiva along the arcade and then releasing the tissue to or below the level of

(a)

(b)

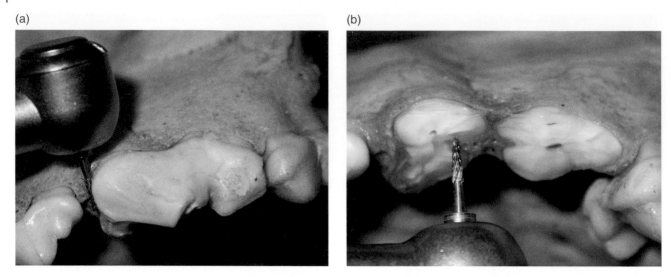

Figure 22.11   In multirooted teeth, (a) crown resection may be used prior to (b) sectioning into single-rooted fragments.

(a)

(b)

(c)

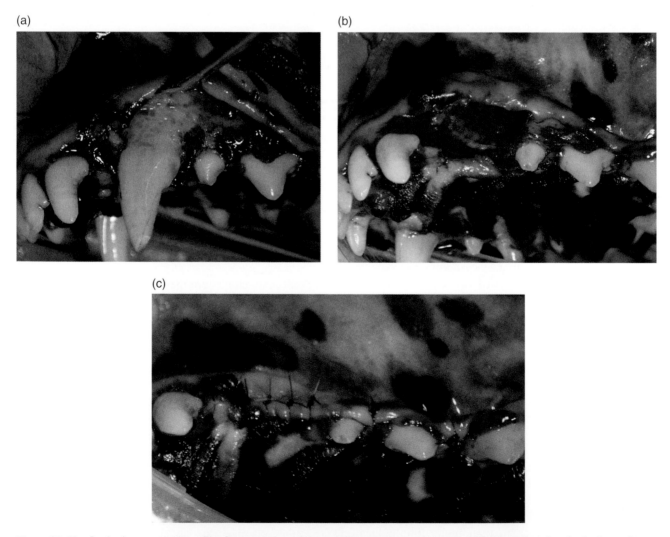

Figure 22.12   Designing an envelope flap for extraction of the maxillary canine tooth starts with (a) cutting the gingival attachment and elevation of the full-thickness flap containing periosteum and mucosa. After extraction, (b) the alveolar bone is smoothed and tension is released via fenestration of the periosteum in preparation for a closure and (c) the flap margins are closed by single interrupted sutures.

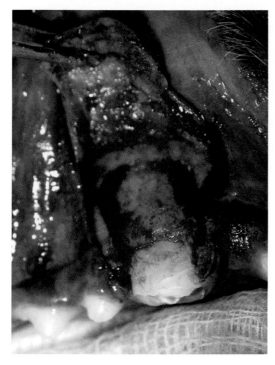

Figure 22.13   A full flap includes two vertical releasing incisions, which should be made *slightly* apically divergent (wider at the base than at the gingival margin).

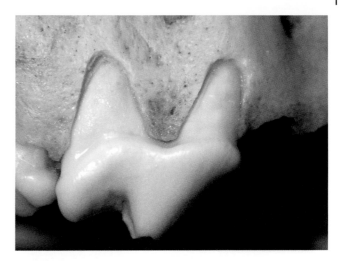

Figure 22.14   Removal of the buccal alveolar bone helps in providing superior access to the extracted tooth roots.

the mucogingival junction (MGJ) with a periosteal elevator. Using this type of flap does not interrupt the blood supply and requires less suturing. This author uses this flap in most cases.

The **full flap**, which is favored by many dentists, includes one or two vertical releasing incisions (Harvey and Emily 1993; Holmstrom et al. 1998; Manfra Marretta 2002) (Figure 22.13). This allows for a much larger flap to be created, so that larger defects can be covered. Classically, the vertical incisions were made at the line angle of the target tooth (its theoretic edge), or one tooth mesial and distal to it (Smith 1998; Carmichael 2002; Manfra Marretta 2002; Smith 2003). However, if there is space between the teeth (either a naturally occurring diastema or due to previous extraction), the incision can be made here rather than extending to a healthy tooth (Niemiec 2012).

The vertical incisions for a full flap should be made *slightly* apically divergent (wider at the base than at the gingival margin) (Holmstrom et al. 1998; Carmichael 2002; Manfra Marretta 2002; Frost Fitch 2003). It is critical that full-thickness incisions be made in one single motion (rather than slowly and choppily). A full-thickness incision is created by incising all the way to the bone, thereby keeping the periosteum with the flap (Carmichael 2002; Frost Fitch 2003). Once created, the entire flap is *gently* reflected with a periosteal elevator. Gentle handling is necessary to

avoid tearing the flap, especially in cats or at the location of the MGJ.

Following flap elevation, buccal bone can be removed (Figure 22.14). This author favors a cross-cut taper-fissure bur. The amount of buccal bone that should be removed is controversial, with some dentists removing the entire buccal covering. This author prefers to maintain as much buccal bone as possible, starting with removal of an amount equal to one-third of the root length of the target tooth on the mandible, or one-half for maxillary teeth (Smith 1998; Frost Fitch 2003). If this does not allow for mobility in a short amount of time, more can be removed; if ankylosis is present, a significant amount of removal may be required. Bone removal should only be performed on the buccal side.

In this author's experience, there is an association between the amount of alveolar bone removal required and the anatomic features of the extracted tooth. These features can be assessed at the preoperative radiograph, and the decision about surgical access to the root can then be made (Table 22.1).

Following bone removal, the multirooted tooth should be sectioned, and each piece should be removed as in the steps outlined for single-root extractions (Niemiec 2008). Flap closure is typically initiated with an important step called "fenestrating the periosteum." The periosteum is a very thin fibrous tissue that attaches the buccal mucosa to the underlying bone (Grant et al. 1988; Smith 2003). Since the periosteum is fibrotic, it is inflexible and therefore interferes with the ability to close the defect *without* tension. The buccal mucosa however, is flexible, and will stretch to cover large defects. Incising the periosteum takes advantage of this attribute, making the flap more flexible. Fenestration should be performed at the base of the flap, and must be below the MGJ. Careful attention is required

Table 22.1 Amount of alveolar bone to be removed in different clinical situations.

Amount of bone removed	Size of tooth	Age of patient	Periodontal ligament space	Tooth mobility	Shape of tooth	TR type 1 presence and stage	Other radiographic features
30%	Small	Young	Wide	Normal	Straight and regular	No TR	Periodontal disease
50%	Medium	Mature	Normal	Limited	Angulated in one plane	TR1, TR2	Developmental grooves
75%	Large	Old	Narrow	No mobility	Angulated in two planes	TR3	Apical area bulge
>75%			Ankylosis	Ankylosis	Malformed	TR4a,b,c	Dilaceration

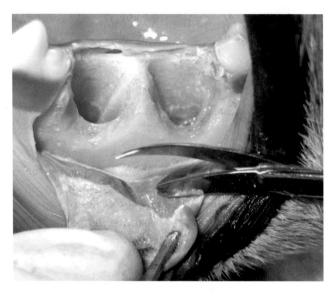

Figure 22.15 Fenestration releases tension and extends the flap before closure.

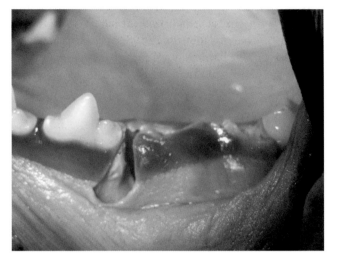

Figure 22.16 Tension-free flap covering surgical access.

in order to avoid cutting through (or off) the entire flap. This procedure can be performed with a scalpel blade, but a LaGrange scissor allows superior control (Niemiec 2012) (Figure 22.15).

Following adequate fenestration, the mucogingival flap should stay in the desired position without sutures (Figure 22.16). If the flap does not remain in position, tension is still present and further release is necessary. Once adequate release is accomplished, the flap is closed (as described for Step 9 of the single-root extraction).

22.4.1 Instrumentation

22.4.1.1 Hand Instruments

There are a plethora of equipment options for veterinary extractions. Ideally, separate sterilized surgical packs should be used for each patient. The minimum supply of hand instruments should include (Niemiec 2012):

- Various sizes of elevators.
- A periosteal elevator.
- Small breed-sized extraction forceps.

- Small scissors.
- Brown–Adson forceps.
- Small needle holders.
- Scalpel handle.

Elevators come in many types and sizes. Some veterinary dentists recommend winged elevators, but this author prefers luxating ones (Figure 22.17). A variety of sizes is essential, with 2, 3, and 5 mm ones recommended as a minimum. Additionally, a 1 mm elevator can be beneficial for feline extractions.

There are also numerous types of periosteal elevators, all of which are acceptable. This author prefers a Molt 2-4.

This author recommends that only small breed-sized extraction forceps be used (Figure 22.18). Those designed for human dentistry do not work well in veterinary patients, and large-sized forceps place too much force on the tooth.

Many varieties of surgical scissors are available, but this author prefers LaGrange ones (Figure 22.19).

The choice of forceps for use in dental/oral surgery is important, as 1 × 2 (rat tooth) forceps are too traumatic to the delicate gingiva. Brown–Adson (7 × 7) thumb forceps are recommended. Any type of needle holder can be used, but small-sized instruments are preferred. Olsen–Hager and Castroviejo are typical choices.

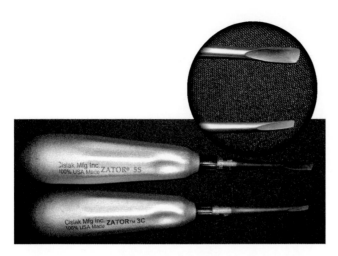

Figure 22.17 Luxating elevators.

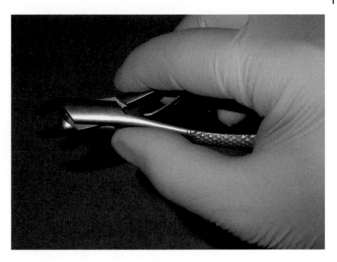

Figure 22.18 Small-sized extraction forceps are convenient for use in the mouths of cats and small dogs.

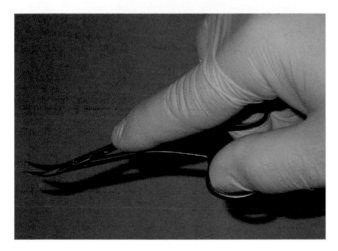

Figure 22.19 LaGrange tissue scissors.

The recommended instruments listed here are combined in commercially available kits, which include sharpening equipment and a sterilization cassette: the Niemiec Extraction Kit (Intregra-Miltex, York, PA) and the Diplomate Extraction Kit (Dentalaire Products, Fountain Valley, CA) (Figure 22.20a,b).

22.4.1.2 Power Instruments

Powered equipment is required for sectioning, buccal cortical bone removal, and bone smoothing/alveoloplasty. An air-driven high-speed delivery unit is strongly recommended (Niemiec 2012). It should be equipped with a high-speed, low-speed, and air-water syringe.

(a)

(b)

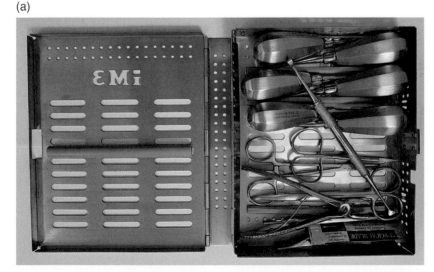

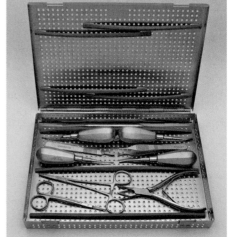

Figure 22.20a,b Two different extraction kits organized in an autoclavable cassette.

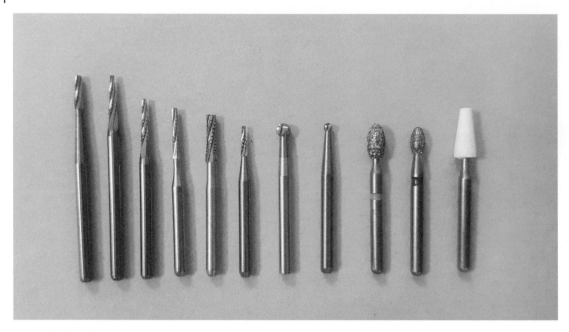

Figure 22.21   Selection of burs recommended for surgical extraction. Source: Emilia Klim.

Dental burs are available in various types and sizes. This author recommends carbide cross-cut taper-fissure burs for sectioning and bone removal, but many other dentists recommend round burs (Niemiec 2012). Cross-cut taper-fissure burs come in various sizes, with 699 being the smallest and 703 the largest (Figure 22.21). All are useful. In addition, sizes 701 and 702 come in surgical lengths, which provide an increased surface area for cutting, and therefore speed the sectioning/bone removal procedure. It is very important to note that dental burs are *disposable* (Niemiec 2012). Moreover, they begin to dull after a very short period of time (10 seconds). Once burs dull even a little, their cutting ability decreases, which increases cutting time as well as thermal damage to the tooth and bone. Therefore, this author recommends using a new bur for every patient. Coarse diamond burs are used for bone smoothing and alveoloplasty, and are available in flame or cylindrical options (Figure 22.21). They are still disposable, but last longer than carbide burs.

References

Blazejewski, S., Lewis, J.R., and Reiter, A.M. (2006). Mucoperiosteal flap for extraction of multiple teeth in the maxillary quadrant of the cat. *J. Vet. Dent.* 23 (3): 200–205.

Carmichael, D.T. (2002). Surgical extraction of the maxillary fourth premolar tooth in the dog. *J. Vet. Dent.* 19 (4): 231–233.

Frost Fitch, P. (2003). Surgical extraction of the maxillary canine tooth. *J. Vet. Dent.* 20 (1): 55–58.

Gioso, M.A., Shofer, F., Barros, P.S., and Harvey, C.E. (2001). Mandible and mandibular first molar tooth measurements in dogs: relationship of radiographic height to body weight. *J. Vet. Dent.* 18 (2): 65–68.

Grant, D.A., Stern, I.B., and Listgarten, M.A. (1988). Periodontal flap. In: *Periodontics in the tradition of Gottlieb and Orban*, 6e (eds. D.A. Grant, I.B. Stern, M.A. Listgarten, et al.), 786–822. St. Louis, MO: C.V. Mosby.

Harvey, C.E. and Emily, P.P. (1993). Oral surgery. In: *Small Animal Dentistry* (eds. C.E. Harvey and P. Emily), 213–265. St. Louis, MO: C.V. Mosby.

Holmstrom, S.E., Frost, P., and Eisner, E.R. (1998). Exodontics. In: *Veterinary Dental Techniques for the Small Animal Practitioner*, 2e (eds. S.E. Holmstrom, P. Frost Fitch and E.R. Eisner), 238–242. Philadelphia, PA: W.B. Saunders.

Holmstrom, S.E., Bellows, J., Colmrey, B. et al. (2005). AAHA dental care guidelines for dogs and cats. *J. Am. Anim. Hosp. Assoc.* 41 (5): 277–283.

Kelly, D.J., Ahmad, M., and Brull, S.J. (2001a). Preemptive analgesia I: physiological pathways and pharmacological modalities. *Can. J. Anesth.* 48 (10): 1000–1010.

Kelly, D.J., Ahmad, M., and Brull, S.J. (2001b). Preemptive analgesia II: recent advances and current trends. *Can. J. Anesth.* 48 (11): 1091–1101.

Lanz, G.C. (2003). Regional anesthesia for dentistry and oral surgery. *J. Vet. Dent.* 20 (3): 181–186.

Manfra Marretta, S. (2002). Surgical extraction of the mandibular first molar tooth in the dog. *J. Vet. Dent.* 19 (1): 46–50.

Moore, J.I. and Niemiec, B. (2014). Evaluation of extraction sites for evidence of retained tooth roots and periapical pathology. *J. Am. Anim. Hosp. Assoc.* 50 (2): 77–82.

Mulligan, T., Aller, S., and Williams, C. (1998). *Atlas of Canine and Feline Dental Radiography*, 176–183. Trenton, NJ: Veterinary Learning Systems.

Niemiec, B.A. (2008). Extraction techniques. *Top. Companion Anim. Med.* 23 (2): 97–105.

Niemiec, B.A. (2009). Case based dental radiology. *Top. Companion Anim. Med.* 24 (1): 4–19.

Niemiec, B.A. (2012). *Dental extractions made easier*. Tustin, CA: Practical Veterinary Publishing.

Proffit, W.R. and Fields, H.W. (2000). *Contemporary Orthodontics*, 3e, 297–306. St. Louis, MO: W.R. Mosby.

Shipp, A.D. and Fahrenkrug, P. (1992). Exodontics. In: *Practitioner's Guide to Veterinary Dentistry* (ed. A.D. Shipp), 60–65. Beverly Hills, CA: Dr. Shipp's Laboratories.

Smith, M.M. (1998). Exodontics. *Vet. Clin. N. Am. Sm. Anim. Pract* 28 (5): 1297–1319.

Smith, M.M. (2003). Line angle incisions. *J. Vet. Dent.* 20 (4): 241–244.

Smith, M.M., Smith, E.M., La Croix, N., and Mould, J. (2003). Orbital penetration associated with tooth extraction. *J. Vet. Dent.* 20 (1): 8–17.

Taney, K.G. and Smith, M.M. (2006). Surgical extraction of impacted teeth in a dog. *J. Vet. Dent.* 23 (3): 168–177.

Taylor, T.N., Smith, M.M., and Snyder, L. (2004). Nasal displacement of a tooth root in a dog. *J. Vet. Dent.* 21 (4): 222–225.

Ulbricht, R.D., Marretta, S.M., and Klippert, L.S. (2003). Surgical extraction of a fractured, nonvital deciduous tooth in a Tiger. *J. Vet. Dent.* 20 (4): 209–212.

Verstraete, F.J. and Terpak, C.H. (1997). Anatomical variation in the dentition of the domestic cat. *J. Vet. Dent.* 14 (4): 137–140.

Wiggs, R.B. and Lobprise, H.B. (1997). Oral surgery. In: *Veterinary Dentistry, Principles and Practice* (eds. R.B. Wiggs and H.B. Lobprise), 312–377. Philadelphia, PA: Lippincott-Raven.

Woodward, T.M. (2006). Extraction of fractured tooth roots. *J. Vet. Dent.* 23 (2): 126–129.

Woodward, T.M. (2008). Pain management and regional anesthesia for the dental patient. *Top. Companion Anim. Med.* 23 (2): 106–114.

23

Oral Emergencies
Jerzy Gawor

Veterinary Clinic Arka, Kraków, Poland

23.1 Introduction

The patient who presents in an emergency situation always requires immediate and accurate action. Oral emergencies are not generally life-threatening, and quite often are associated with other, more serious conditions (Figure 23.1). Nonetheless, their management should not be delayed, if at all possible (Gorrel et al. 1993). Before referring such patients to the dental specialist (or other qualified surgeon or practitioner), first aid must be provided. This may include the use of various temporary measures (e.g., a tape muzzle), so long as they will not hinder definitive care.

Emergency referrals are categorized according to the following criteria:

1) Anatomic location of problem (soft tissue, dentition, orofacial structures, temporomandibular joint [TMJ]).
2) Time of veterinary action (first aid, treatment plan, consequences of trauma or complications).
3) Character of emergency (traumatic or infectious).

There are thus many variations on conditions and situations, but the management protocol will always remain the same:

- patient stabilization
- diagnosis
- treatment plan
- therapy
- follow-up
- resolving possible future complications

Stabilization of the injured or acutely ill patient is the number one priority in all emergency situations. This starts with a general examination of the airway, central nervous system (CNS), cardiac system, thorax, and locomotory system. A stabilized patient is a patient whose airway is secured, hemorrhage is controlled, shock is treated, and fractures are immobilized. In dentistry, that last item is not a part of the stabilization process because in order to immobilize a fracture, diagnosis is needed, and therefore intraoral radiographs or other imaging technique must be employed first. Simultaneously, the pain-control and antimicrobial administration should be initiated and a preanesthetic examination performed, including a complete chemistry panel and complete blood count (CBC). General anesthesia for diagnostic purposes should be considered, if necessary (Dewhurst et al. 1998; Gaynor et al. 2006).

After the patient is stabilized, the diagnostic procedures begin. A physical oral examination followed by maxillofacial and dental radiography is the main basis of diagnosis and decision making. The results of the oral and dental assessment determine the treatment plan.

Emergency situations typically require fast action, but the treatment options must still be discussed and accepted by the owner prior to therapy. The range of options for discussion depends on several factors, with the level of competence of the veterinarian and their access to dental equipment and materials being the most important. Whatever management option is selected, it must respect the normal functional, physiological, and ethical rules. The treatment plan should include knowledge of the need for anesthetia, treatment costs, and possible complications. If the client declines optimal repair and opts for the easiest or cheapest treatment, make sure an against medical advice (AMA) form is signed.

Surgical or conservative management procedures should start as soon as the general status of the patient allows. If the animal is already anesthetized for the diagnostic procedures, it is reasonable to proceed with the repair at the same time. A part of patient management is a consideration of providing nutrition. Cats in particular require a precise plan regarding postoperative nutrition. In cases where

The Veterinary Dental Patient: A Multidisciplinary Approach, First Edition. Edited by Jerzy Gawor and Brook Niemiec.
© 2021 John Wiley & Sons Ltd. Published 2021 by John Wiley & Sons Ltd.
Companion website: www.wiley.com/go/gawor/veterinary-dental-patient

problems with eating can be expected, the use of an esophageal or gastric feeding tube should be considered (Zoran 2006; DeBowes 2007). The nutritional challenges in post-traumatic patients are discussed in Appendix F.

Another very important part of the treatment plan is a precise schedule for the follow-up and postoperative protocol. In particular, the owner must be made aware that the follow-up is almost as important as the surgery itself. A good way to convince them to show up for recheck is to offer it free of charge.

Distant complications can always occur despite all best efforts. The more complex the case, the more important it is to discuss all possible complications with the owner *before* initiating treatment. Some complications can be really severe, such as TMJ ankylosis, periapical abscess, and bone sequestrum (Figure 23.2). These may occur despite

proper therapy being performed and all standards being followed. Proper imaging provides the most accurate information about the healing process and must be obtained.

23.2 Selected Topics Related to Oral Emergencies and Maxillofacial Surgery

23.2.1 Management of Trauma and First Aid in Oro-Maxillary Injuries

Resuscitation, fluid therapy, heart and respiratory system control, and the general medical protocol are not covered in this chapter.

Foreign bodies belong to a particular category of emergency. Some are just irritating, but occasionally they may create a life-threatening situation.

Emergency situations always require quick decisions. Regardless of whether you are dealing with luxation, acute inflammation, or fracture, you must control the pain and infection and respect all systemic aspects of anesthesia and surgical procedures. Analgesics and fast-acting antibiotics (if required) will provide the necessary protection before diagnostic procedures are initiated. The list of recommended medications is covered in many papers, and there is not any one specific drug that provides extraordinary pain control in all circumstances. Acute, moderate pain can be controlled with the use metadone or butorfanol at a dose of 0.01 mg/kg, which lasts for one to two hours (WSAVA 2014). Additional pain-control can include carprofen 4 mg/kg, ketoprofen 1 mg/kg, fluniksin 0.1 mg/kg, or meloxicam 0.1 mg/kg (Gaynor et al. 2006). However, the gold standard in pain relief and protection in dentistry is a local nerve block performed before any painful procedure

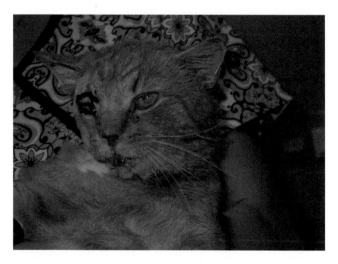

Figure 23.1 Oral injuries are very often the result of head injury, which may be significant for all vital organs.

(a)

(b)

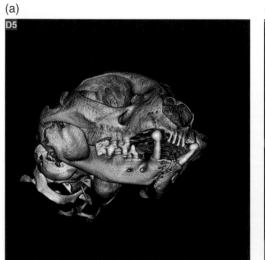

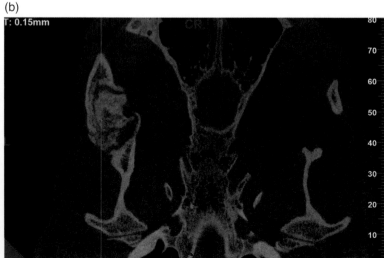

Figure 23.2 Distant complications of head injury: (a) TMJ ankylosis of the right joint; (b) pseudoankylosis affecting the left zygomatic arch and mandible.

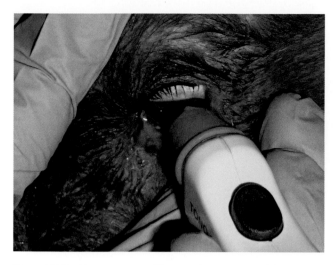

Figure 23.3   Measurement of intraocular pressure with a tonometer provides indirect information on intracranial pressure.

as an imperative part of a multimodal analgesic protocol, but it cannot be applied in the awake patient.

Stress release, medical oxygen delivery, and fluid therapy are the next steps; these all require the use of an oxygen mask or kennel and placement of intravenous catheter. While catheterization is performed, it is reasonable to take a blood sample for a basic blood test. Assessment of electrolytes allows for optimal selection of fluid. At this point, in patients with head injury, it is important to diagnose any brain injury signalments and implement adequate treatment. As there is an association between intracranial pressure and intraocular pressure, the easiest diagnostic method is to use a tonometer to measure the latter (Figure 23.3).

High-rise syndrome is the term used when cats fall from balconies or windows of high-rise buildings in urban areas, the minimal height of the fall being the second story (Vnuk et al. 2004). Possible orofacial findings include epistaxis, abrasions, jaw fractures, symphyseal separation, hard-palate fractures, tooth fractures, and temporomadibular luxation (Bonner et al. 2012). Apart from the orofacial injuries, many other organ systems may be affected, including the orthopedic, thoracic, neurological, abdominal, and other soft tissues (Baines and Langley-Hobbs n.d.; Whithey and Mehlhaff 1987; Pratschke and Kirby 2002; Cruz-Arambulo and Nykamp 2012; Liehmann et al. 2012).

Challenges in high-rise syndrome injury management begin with emergency care and stabilization. Dealing with life-threatening conditions such as shock as well as thoracic and neurologic trauma is the first priority. Very few patients require immediate dental or maxillofacial diagnostic and surgical procedures. Even when they do, repair may be postponed until the patient has been stabilized. For the anesthetic protocol and during anesthesia, particular attention should be paid to providing appropriate vascular action in the head and neck, avoiding drugs that may increase intracranial pressure

and sudden changes in cardiovascular system, and precise monitoring for renal sufficiency (Scott and Timmermann 2004; Khandelwal et al. 2019).

Some patients are referred to a dental specialist once they have been stabilized, but for the first-contact veterinarian, a full range of emergency and post-traumatic procedures is required (Adamantos and Garosi 2011). First aid may in some cases also be definitive care, but if there is a lack of experience or skill, it is better to provide a temporary therapy and refer the case to the specialist. Sometimes, the character of the injury and the time interval from injury to presentation may determine the outcome. This is always the case with tooth avulsion, and it may affect the treatment of complicated fractures as well. With dental avulsions, the question is always whether to try to save the tooth. With fractured teeth, timing is of less concern, as it only affects the decision if vital pulp therapy is necessary.

All other dental emergencies may be postponed until after proper first aid is performed and stabilization is achieved. All small-animal veterinarians should be able to perform some basic first-aid procedures, depending on the available instrumentation and materials, as well as their own skills. Hands-on workshops offered and supervised by specialists are much more valuable than the best books or didactic lectures. Therefore, this chapter will describe only those procedures that every veterinarian should be familiar with.

In sum, trauma management should include:

1) Proper diagnostic imaging procedures:
   a) 3D imaging – cone beam computed tomography (CBCT), computed tomography (CT), or magnetic resonance imaging (MRI). CT scans demonstrate 1.6 times more maxillofacial injuries for dogs and 2.0 times more for cats than conventional radiographs. The average number of maxillofacial traumatic injuries per animal by radiograph and CT scan is 4.8 and 7.6 in dogs and 3.8 and 7.7 in cats, respectively. 81.5% more findings in traumatic injury cases are identified by CT than by radiograph, though a significant difference is found for only 29.6% (Bar-Am et al. 2008).
   b) Standard 2D radiography for an overview of the skull, which allows for orientation of the damages. At least three projections should be made:
      i) Left lateral oblique.
      ii) Right lateral oblique. These provide a general view of the left and right canine, premolars, and molars, TMJ, and mandibular body.
      iii) Dorso-ventral projection. This shows the symmetry of the TMJ, mandibular body, and incisors. If the problem relates to a specific tooth or area, it is better to expose an intraoral dental film (Figure 23.4).
   c) Full mouth radiography assessing entire dentition and surrounding structures.

(a)

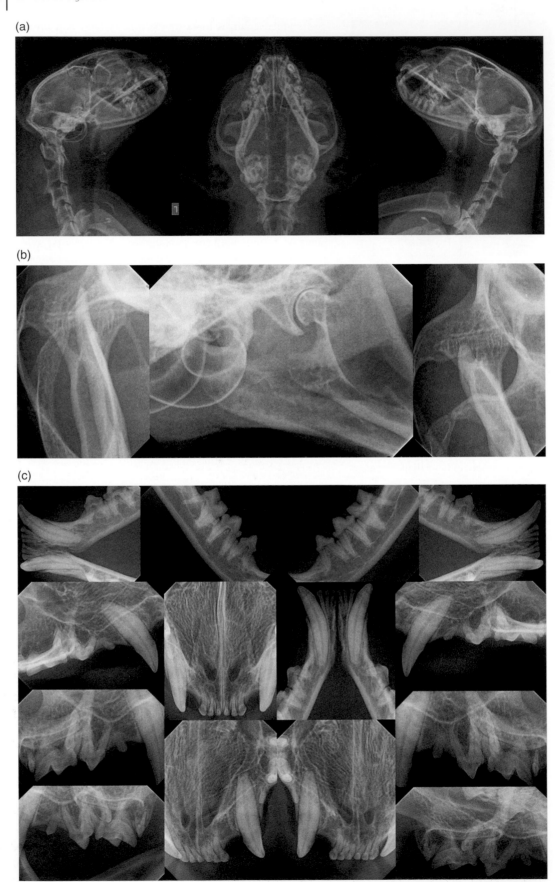

(b)

(c)

Figure 23.4 Example standard 2D imaging of the feline head (a) feline TMJs (b) and feline dentition (c).

(a)

(b)

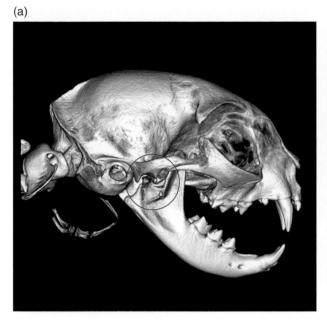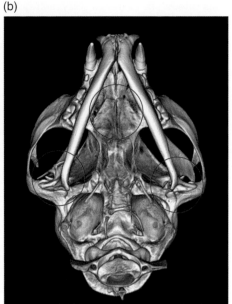

Figure 23.5 3D imaging allows for detailed information about the structures most often affected with orofacial injuries. Circles show damaged areas in this cat after high rise syndrome.

2) Pain management (see Chapter 11).
3) Suturing of oral wounds (see Chapter 21).
4) Tape muzzle or nylon muzzle. These are the simplest methods for the stabilization of maxillofacial fractures and luxations. The muzzle must not compromise breathing of the patient.

Only stable patients may undergo diagnostic procedures followed by preliminary or definitive treatment.

23.2.2 Diagnosis: Physical Examination and Imaging – Establishing the Treatment Plan

The key thing in an emergency is to obtain a quick and reliable diagnosis, which will provide the basis for treatment planning. Pain and many other factors make examination in a conscious dog or cat rarely possible. A general examination with palpation, delicate movement of the jaw, and inspection of the oral cavity may be accepted, but to get the full range of information, sedation or anesthesia is necessary. The time from the moment of injury to the induction of anesthesia is not always easily defined. On one hand, the patient must be stable, and the sedation cannot be hazardous; on the other, any unnecessary prolongation of pain and suffering should be avoided.

Clinical assessment is important and delivers significant information if performed accurately. Studies show that it plays a role whether the oral cavity is assessed by someone skilled in dentistry or not (Bonner et al. 2012; Gawor 2017).

The soft tissue and dental lesions can suggest the location of skeletal damage. Full-mouth dental radiography and three extra-oral projections of the head are the minimum required to evaluate maxillofacial and dental pathologies following injury. 3D imaging (CT or CBCT), if available, provides superior information (Bar-Am et al. 2008) (Figure 23.5).

Before the treatment plan is created, each case must be analyzed individually. The type, size, and shape of the patient's skull are all important considerations, as are the patient's age, activity level, temperament, and character. If the patient is uncooperative, the method of repair must take this into account. It is reasonable to discuss the habits and character of the animal with the owner before the final treatment plan is devised. Some protection of fixation or sutures can be obtained with the use of an "Elizabethan collar". An additional consideration is postoperative pain control. This should include regional anesthesia (nerve block), which provides the patient comfort upon recovery from anesthesia and blunts the first shock related to it.

Not all fractures require surgical correction. The first attempt should utilize a more "dental" or conservative approach, as this is typically less invasive and does not cause irreversible consequences (e.g., holes in tooth roots). At this point, screws, plates, and pins are rarely indicated, and interdental wiring, acrylic splints, and tape or nylon muzzles are preferred.

After a head injury, long anesthesia can be a concern. Reducing its duration by performing temporary solutions like pulp capping rather than endodontic treatment is a reasonable concept. Moreover, weakened or damaged maxillofacial structures should be handled very gently. Therefore, extractions should be postponed if possible, especially if significant force is required. During this time, adequate pain management is mandatory.

It is important to know one's own ability and skills. The best plan is the one that will work on the first attempt.

23.2.3 Fractures of Orofacial Hard Structures

Fractures typically occur due to traumatic injury, and the mandible is the most commonly fractured oro/maxillofacial bone. When discussing mandibular fractures, one has to remember that the mandibular symphysis should be treated as a joint, and therefore a symphyseal separation is not a true fracture. In fact, it is the most common site of mandibular damage in cats, whereas in dogs that is the mandibular body.

The location of a fracture is very important in both management and prognosis. The two major categories were previously favorable and nonfavorable fractures, but today the terms "stable" and "nonstable" are used (Figure 23.6). The former includes those injuries that are positively influenced by the action of the masticatory muscle, which through natural forces and the location of the muscle attachments places compression on the fracture line which runs rostroventrally. The latter group represents the fact that the fracture line, that runs caudoventral is distracted by the same forces. These cases always require specialist intervention to provide proper reduction, good contact of the bone ends, effective stabilization, and a natural occlusion. The golden rule when undertaking a reduction is that the occlusion should be as close to natural and functional as possible. Fractures in the oral cavity – particularly the mandible – are typically open and complicated, so the

first step in repair is to close the ruptured oral mucosa. Single interrupted simple sutures placed 2–3 mm apart provide an adequate seal and complete closure.

In minimally displaced and mostly stable fractures, the simplest method is to reduce the mobility of the jaws by applying a tape muzzle. Mesaticephalic and dolichocephalic dogs are good candidates for this, but brachycephalic breeds are not, due to poor occlusion and breathing issues. The muzzle should not be too tight, as the dog must be able to drink and eat unaided. Sometimes, because of swelling slightly uncomfortable occlusion can be present for a couple of days after the fixation is removed. This should be allowed to resolve before performing another surgery.

A **pathologic fracture** (also called an **insufficiency fracture**) is a bone fracture caused by a disease that weakens the bone structure. A retrospective study of 100 canine patients with maxillofacial fractures revealed that 13% were associated with periodontal diseases, neoplasms, or an iatrogenic background (Lopes et al. 2005). Pathologic fractures can present as an emergency or as an iatrogenic jaw fracture occurring during an extraction attempt. This normally results from a lack of preoperative radiographs. An exception is when the bone is weakened by a neoplasm, which can predispose to a pathologic fracture. Periapical pathology and alveolar bone loss are always risk factors because they weaken the bone. This is particularly important in the mandibular dentition, as most pathologic iatrogenic fractures happen in the mandible. The area of the first mandibular molars in small and toy breeds is specifically predisposed to pathologic fracture associated with periodontal disease due to the very unfavorable ratio between the size of the tooth (M1) and the bone surrounding it, which makes the bone prone to fracture (Gioso et al. 2001) (Figure 23.7).

(a)

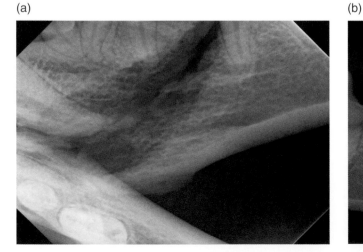

(b)

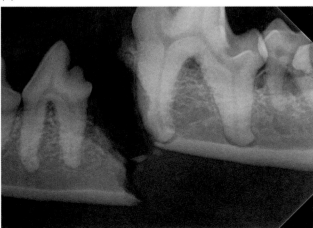

Figure 23.6 (a) Stable (fracture that runs in rostroventral direction) and (b) nonstable (fracture that runs in caudoventral direction) fractures of the mandible.

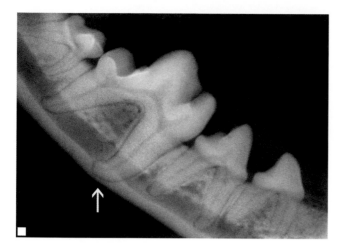

Figure 23.7 Predisposition to pathologic fracture at the mandibular first molar.

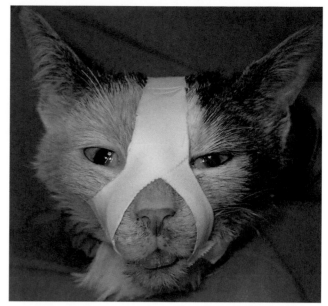

Figure 23.8 Tape muzzle on a cat.

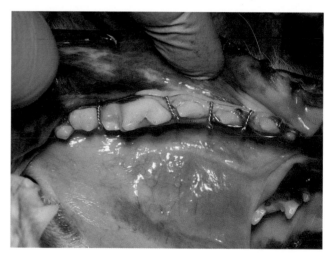

Figure 23.9 Stout multiple-loop interdental wiring can be applied for a mandibular fracture in the 307/308 area. The interdental wiring should be complemented with acrylic splint to provide optimal stabilisation.

In these cases, the fracture line is surrounded by infection. Therefore, in order to provide a proper environment for healing, it is necessary to remove the infected tooth/root or surrounding tissues. On occasion, resection of the tooth and extraction of the infected part present in the fracture line via endodontic therapy of the other root is sufficient. This allows for preservation of part of the tooth, and should be particularly considered in strategic teeth (like the mandibular M1) where it may help improve interdental stabilization. Both procedures (partial resection of the tooth followed by endodontic treatment and interdental wiring) require good skills and access to specific materials and instrumentation.

Pathologic fractures should always be referred to the dental specialist.

The first attempt at oromaxillary fracture repair should be the least invasive.

Stabilization methods include (Verstraete 2004):

1) tape muzzle (Figure 23.8)
2) intraoral acrylic fixation (Figure 23.12)
3) interdental wiring (Figure 23.9)
4) maxillary/mandibular fixation (Figure 23.10)
5) interosseous wiring (Figure 23.11)
6) variations on points 1–5 (Figure 23.12)
7) use of microplates and screws (Figure 23.13)
8) external fixation

For the general practitioner, and even for specialists in small-animal medicine, the most affordable method is a tape muzzle. All the other options require experience, skills, and access to specific materials, equipment, and instrumentation. Step-by-step procedures may be found in Verstraete and Lommer (2013) and the page of the *Journal of Veterinary Dentistry*.

Tape muzzle fixation in favorable fractures may be the final fixation method, particularly in young animals. In all other fractures, it can be used as a temporary or adjunct method. The muzzle should hold the jaws in occlusion to allow for healing, while at the same time enabling the use of the mouth for drinking and for eating liquid food. Depending on the fracture and the condition and activity of the animal, it can be placed for three to six weeks. After that time, further decisions should be made based on radiographic recheck results. Alternatively, nylon muzzles may be used, though these must be periodically swapped out to keep them clean.

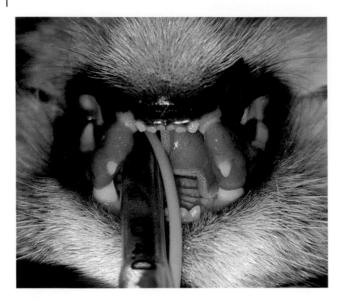

Figure 23.10 Maxillary/mandibular fixation in a cat. Source: Emilia Klim.

Tape muzzles are difficult or impossible to apply in brachycephalic dogs and in cats. Another contraindication is damage of the facial skin (wounds, inflammation, etc.).

In animals where anorexia is expected, an esophageal feeding tube inserted through the skin after pharyngostomy is ideal for the first two to three weeks following a procedure (Fink et al. 2014) Feeding the patients with feeeding tube is described in Appendix F.

23.2.4 Damage to the Oral Soft Tissues

The vast majority of maxillofacial bone fractures are associated with soft-tissue damage (i.e., exposure of submucosal structures). For this reason, such fractures are termed "complicated." In addition, traumatic injuries such as falls from a height, car accidents, hits, bites, and fights very often cause wounds, lacerations, or erosions of the lips,

(a)

(b)

(c)

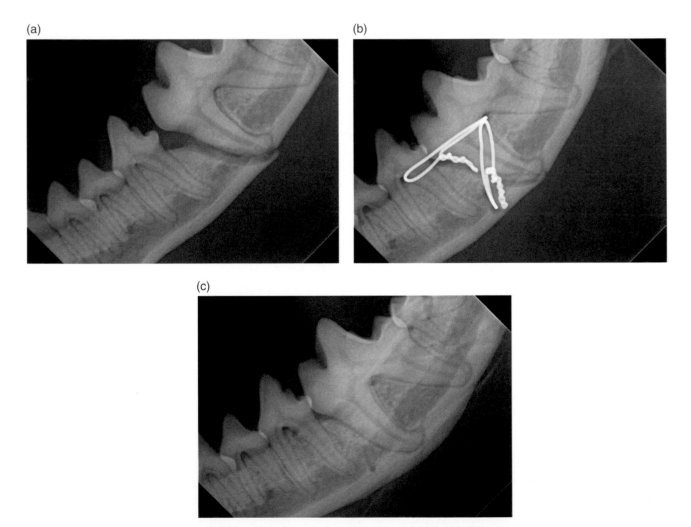

Figure 23.11 (a) Nonstable fracture of the left mandible. (b) Stabilization by interfragmentary fixation. (c) Proper healing after eight weeks. *Source:* Emilia Klim.

(a)

(b)

(c)

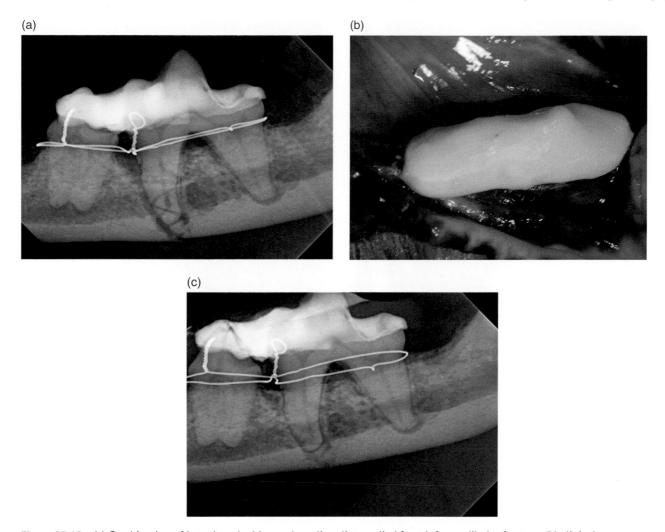

Figure 23.12 (a) Combination of interdental wiring and acrylic splint applied for a left mandibular fracture: (b) clinical appearance and (c) radiographic control after six weeks. The dog had no dentition rostrally from the left mandibular fourth premolar (308).

cheeks, tongue palate, and oral mucosa. Sometimes, there are no mucosal tears, and the only signalment of soft-tissue damage is a bruise. Because of the rich innervation of the oral cavity, any damage is very painful and affects normal functions of oral cavity (Figure 23.14).

Further soft-tissue damage can be caused by fractured teeth, as their sharp edges can damage the oral mucosa and make the situation worse. Therefore, prior to stabilization or placing the intraoral splint, it is important to close any open wounds.

23.2.5 Acute and Chronic Problems with Jaw Motion: TMJ Traumatic Problems

Acute jaw-motion disorders are typically caused by one of three conditions:

1) TMJ luxation (Figure 23.15)
2) TMJ fracture (Figure 23.16)
3) jaw-locking syndrome

All three require therapy and must be diagnosed and treated under general anesthesia. Luxation of the TMJ is easily visible, as the animal cannot close its mouth and, in most cases, has an obviously visible malocclusion. Pain occurs upon palpation and manipulation of the jaws. Additional signalments include hemorrhage or bruising of the palatal mucosa. There is no well-defined method for obtaining good-quality TMJ radiographs in cats. However, a series of lateral, lateral/oblique, and dorsoventral projections eventually show good images of the joint. The best way to evaluate the caudal mandibular area and TMJ is to follow the dense ventral cortex of the mandible and evaluate its integrity. 3D imaging provides a much more precise and superior image.

Two types of TMJ luxation may occur: rostrodorsal and caudoventral. The latter is typically associated with fracture of the retroarticular process of the temporal bone (Figure 23.17). The former is more common.

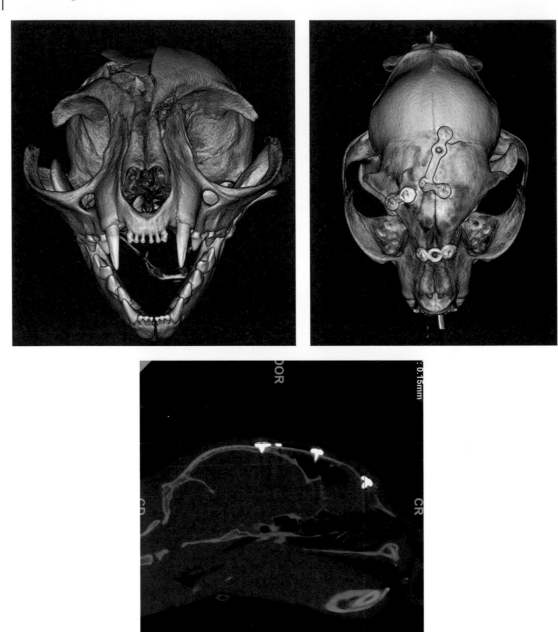

Figure 23.13 Microplate application in multiple maxillofacial and cranial fractures in a cat.

Rostrodorsal luxation can be either unilateral or bilateral. Unilateral rostrodorsal luxation causes a shift of the rostral portion of the mandible laterally to the opposite side from the luxated joint. In bilateral rostrodorsal luxation, on the other hand, the mandible is positioned as in class III malocclusion. Reduction of this type of luxation can be performed manually by forcing the mandible in the ventrocaudal direction. Alternatively, a wooden stick (pencil) can be placed between the jaws at the level of the caudal cheek teeth, which acts as a fulcrum as the rostral part of the mandible is gently pressed, causing the stick to slowly rotate caudally.

Success in the reduction of a luxated TMJ largely depends on the time between injury and therapy. If conservative reduction is not possible, a surgical approach can be performed, as visualizing the joint makes reduction easier. Finally, coronoid process resection may be considered to enable complete closure of the jaws and return to function.

Caudoventral luxation can likewise be either unilateral or bilateral. In unilateral luxation, the rostral part of the mandible is shifted in the same direction as the affected joint. In bilateral luxation, the jaws are positioned as in a class II malocclusion.

(a)   (b)

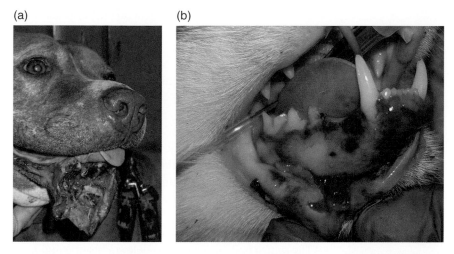

Figure 23.14   Lower-lip avulsion in a (a) dog and (b) a cat. Source (Figure b): Emilia Klim.

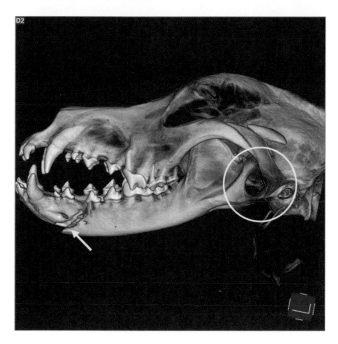

Figure 23.15   Dorsorostral left TMJ luxation (circle) associated with left mandibular fracture (arrow).

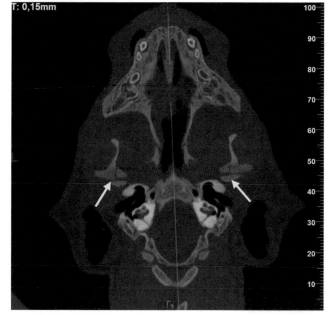

Figure 23.16   Intracapsular bilateral TMJ fracture (arrows).

It is virtually impossible to determine the type of TMJ luxation based solely on clinical assessment. Precise diagnostic imaging is mandatory prior to treatment.

If TMJ fractures occur without damage of the TMJ capsule or creation of a malocclusion, they can be managed by limiting mobility of the jaws (e.g., tape muzzle) or through adequate (in terms of strength and time) pain management. Nondisplaced condylar fractures can heal well. Fractures that create malocclusion should be managed by a specialist.

Distant, chronic consequences of TMJ and jaw injury include arthritis and both real and pseudoankylosis of the

TMJ. Post-traumatic ankylosis of the TMJ is a potential complication. It typically occurs as a result of insufficient postoperative care or a complete lack of treatment, possibly due to an improper primary diagnosis. An ankylotic TMJ may create an emergency whereby the patient cannot pant and thus suffers an increase in internal temperature. It is important to determine whether the limitations on jaw movement are caused inside the TMJ (true ankylosis) or outside it (pseudoankylosis). In ankylotic arthritis, local intracapsular administration of bethamethasone may improve the mobility and function of the joint. Surgical removal of the ankylosed tissue may be also considered, which often requires either unilateral or bilateral

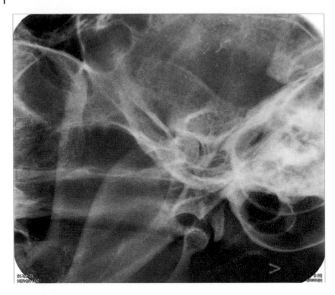

Figure 23.17 Extraoral radiograph of Caudoventral TMJ luxation in a cat.

condylectomy of all involved structures. Prior to surgery, it is necessary to properly identify the parts to be resected.

Problems with jaw motion can include conditions that have no traumatic background, which should be taken into account in the differential diagnosis (Taney and Smith 2010):

1) neoplasms of the TMJ
2) masticatory muscle myositis (MMM)
3) mandibular neurapraxia

23.2.6 Oral and Maxillofacial Complications and Consequences of Head Injury

The list of complications or consequences of head injury that may present to the first-contact practitioner or small-animal specialist includes malocclusion, osteomyelitis, bone sequestration, facial deformities, oronasal fistulas, and various forms of dental abnormalities.

Malocclusions that occur as a result of head injuries are managed by interceptive or corrective methods. Postoperative malocclusions that create soft-tissue or tooth-on-tooth trauma require interceptive extractions or crown height reduction followed by endodontic therapy of the offending tooth.

Osteomyelitis requires a surgical approach and long-term pharmacologic treatment. Because radiographic features of osteomyelitis like osteolysis, osteosclerosis, and proliferation of periosteal new bone can mimic neoplastic lesions, the final diagnosis is always based on histopathologic assessment. Excision of the sequestra, debridement, and drainage of the infected bone represents the surgical aspect of therapy. An additional aspect is the use of antimicrobials according to the general health status of the patient and culture/sensitivity testing.

Osteomyelitis and bone sequestration may occur following jaw fractures, but also due to periodontal disease and pulp infections. An essential aspect of therapy is thus determining the inciting cause of the problem and removing it.

Acquired palatal defects can be surgically repaired with a flap or by the use of prosthetic devices that close the oronasal communication, depending on the size of the defect and its relation to the total amount of tissue. When planning surgery, it is very important that the first attempt be a quality one, as it has the best chance for success; therefore, it must be performed by a competent surgeon.

The same challenges apply to delayed healing and nonunion of the fractured facial bones. Referral to a specialist for the use of more advanced repair methods is the best solution.

TMJ ankylosis, palatal defects, endodontic problems, and many other conditions that require accurate advanced imaging necessitate good preparation, occasional staging of treatment, and – often – referral to a specialist.

Luxated and avulsed teeth, even when properly treated, must be monitored for the occurrence of ankylosis or root resorption. Ankylosis of the periodontal ligament will increase the risk of fracture of the affected tooth.

Functional disorders can result from post-traumatic conditions, even after many surgical attempts. In extreme cases, it may be necessary to resect a nonfunctional or compromised part of the face. It is up to the client to accept this situation. The vast majority of patients fully accept the lack of a mandible, lip, and other parts of the face.

23.3 Most Common Emergency Procedures

23.3.1 Tape Muzzle Placement

This is contraindicated in brachycephalic breeds and all patients with significant problems with breathing (pharyngeal swelling or pulmonary trauma), as well as in vomiting patients.

The main indications for this technique are fractures with minimal displacement (e.g., unilateral) in young individuals and situations that require first aid. In cats, a major indication in this author's experience is a nonstabile reduction of the TMJ rostrodorsal luxation.

The muzzle must simultaneously be tight enough to allow large lateral movement and keep the occlusion in place and loose enough to enable water and liquid food drinking. Fabric muzzles can be used, but custom-made tape muzzles may better accommodate the purposes of such conservative stabilization.

(1)
(2)
(3)
(4)

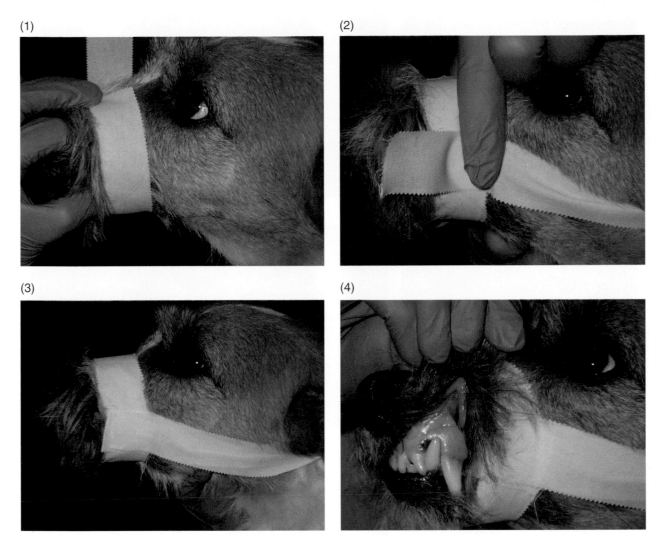

Figure 23.18 Tape muzzle application in a dog, step by step.

23.3.1.1 Dogs

Placement in a dog requires the use of tape and at least sedation – if not general anesthesia – of the animal (Figure 23.18).

1) The first wrap around the muzzle should be made with the sticky side out, which allows the patient to open their jaws 0.5–0.8 cm. It is very important to check the occlusion after placement. The second wrap should be made with sticky side to sticky side

2) Next, a head loop is created. This can done either with the muzzle on the face or after it is removed from the head. The first loop is again made with sticky side out, around the head and over the ears, and the second loop once more is sticky side to sticky side.

3) Adjustment is made as necessary to reduce the tape size near the eyes and mouth. The muzzle may become loose after a couple of days, once the swelling resolves, so follow-up is necessary to check whether a new one is required.

23.3.1.2 Cats

Cats are much better at removing strange materials from their body than dogs, so an Elizabethan collar is necessary to prevent pawing (Figure 23.19). An additional piece of tape between the eyes will also improve retention, but it is imperative to cut off any excess and adjust it such that it does not disturb the eyes or nose.

23.3.2 Dentinal Bonding

23.3.2.1 Indications

Enamel and enamel/dentin crown fractures with distance to pulp chamber >0.5 mm (Theuns and Niemiec 2011) (Figure 23.20a).

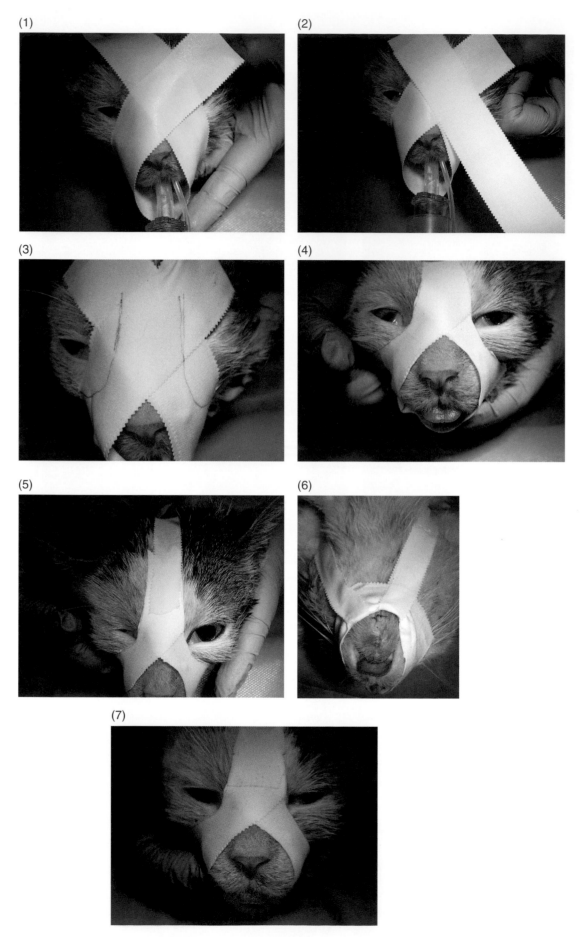

Figure 23.19   Tape muzzle application in a cat, step by step.

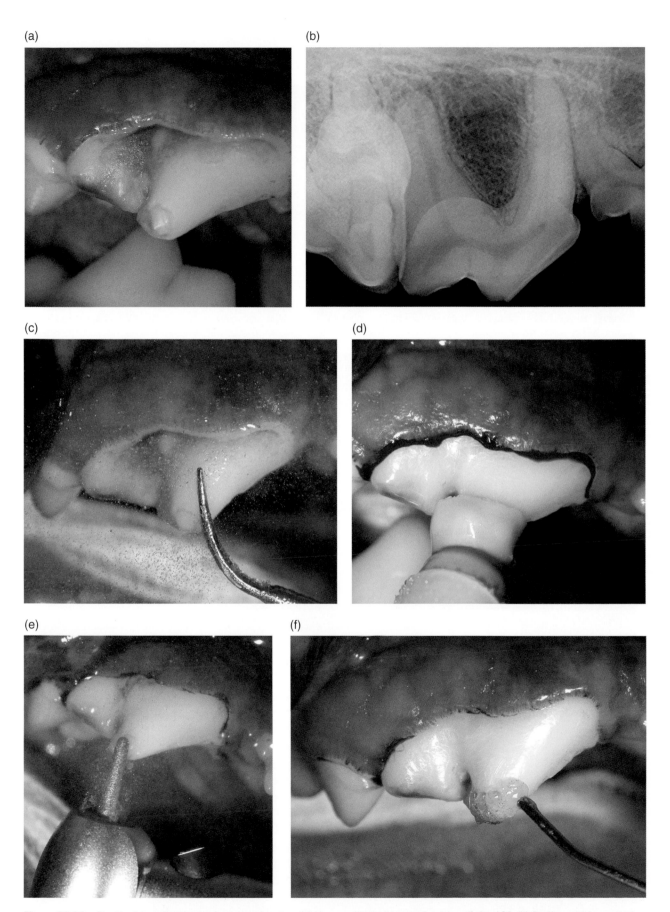

Figure 23.20 Dentinal bonding procedure, step by step: (a) Uncomplicated crown fracture of the 108. (b) Radiographic control. (c) Affected tooth descaling. (d) Polishing. (e) Smoothing of the sharp edge of the fracture line with a diamond fissure bur. (f) Acid etch application. (g) Flushing out of the acid etch with copious amount of water, followed by drying. (h) Application of dentinal bonding agent. (i) Lightcure of the applied bond. (j) Final outcome.

(g)

(h)

(i)

(j)

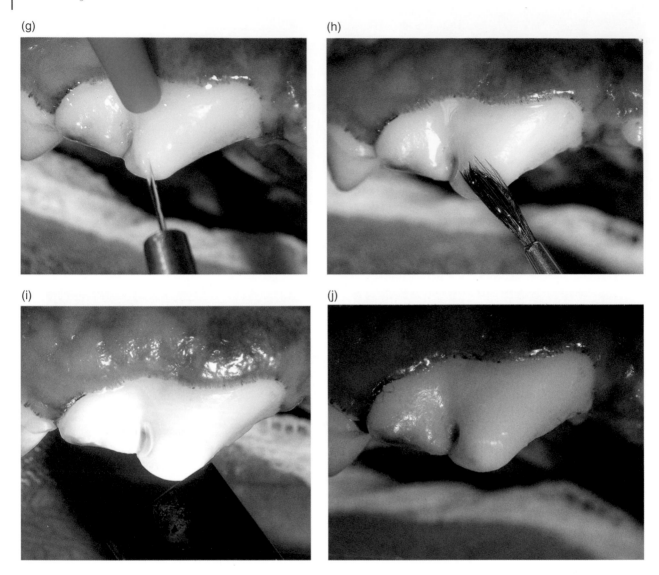

Figure 23.20 (Continued)

23.3.2.2 Purpose
Sealing of dentinal tubules. A bonding system should be used that seals the tubules to a depth of 200–400 μm. Lack of therapy of noncomplicated crown fracture may result in eventual pulp necrosis (DuPont 2010).

23.3.2.3 Steps

1) Radiograph of the damaged tooth to rule out any signs of other injuries or the presence of periapical pathology, and to determine the condition of the hard dental tissues (Figure 23.20 b)
2) Teeth scaling and polishing with polishing paste that does *not* contain fluoride (Figure 23.20c,d)
3) Smoothing of the sharp edges with a white stone, sanding disc, or fine diamond abrasive bur (Figure 23.20e)
4) Rinsing of the crown to remove debris, followed by drying.

5) Application of acid-etch gel to the enamel and dentin. This process normally lasts approximately 20 seconds, but it should be shorter if the fracture line is close to the pulp chamber. If the fracture is closer than 0.5 mm, the indirect pulp dressing should be considered for endodontic treatment (Figure 23.20f)
6) Copious flush with water to completely remove of the acid-etch gel (Figure 23.20g).
7) Drying (but not overdrying) of the tooth. The etched area will appear chalky.
8) Application of the bonding agent (a class V single-agent system is preferred as it is simple and efficient) with the use of a disposal brush (Figure 23.20h)
9) Gentle drying of the bonded surface to remove any excess bonding agent and thin the restoration.

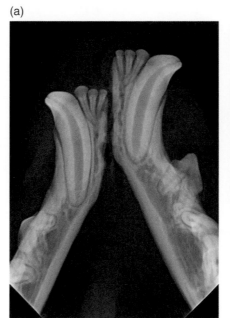
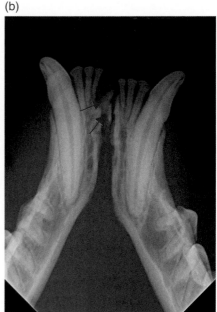

Figure 23.21 Radiographs of (a) symphyseal separation and (b) symphyseal separation combined with parasymphyseal fracture (arrowed).

10) Light curing of the surface for 10–15 seconds (utilizing a lightcure gun, 1700 W) followed by application of a thin layer of unfilled resin and second lightcure (Figure 23.20i).

23.3.2.4 Follow-up

Despite preservation of the exposed dentinal tubules (Figure 23.20j), it is important to recheck the treated tooth after six months and evaluate the periapical area, as some pathologies may not be detectable at the time of therapy.

23.3.3 Mandibular Symphyseal Separation Management

The clinical signalments of symphyseal separation and parasymphyseal fracture are very similar. Often, the two problems are combined. The diagnosis should therefore be based on dental radiology (Figure 23.21). In cases of typical symphyseal separation, reduction and fixation are stable. In this situation, a simple cerclage wire tightened either in the ventral intermandibular space subcutaneously or laterally behind the canine teeth is sufficient (Figure 23.22). The lateral placement of tightened cerclage endings is easier to remove and can be performed under much shorter general anesthesia, and is also significantly less invasive than other methods (Mulherin et al. 2012).

When a part of the symphyseal structure is damaged or the injury is associated with parasymphyseal fracture of the mandible, the reduction is more difficult and often requires more than just a cerclage wire. Additional stabilization of the rostral mandible can be provided via a figure-eight loop around the canine teeth, which can

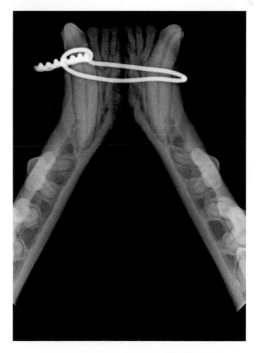

Figure 23.22 Often, a simple symphyseal separation can be stabilized by a single cerclage tightened either at the ventral or the lateral part of the mandibles. It is important to secure the sharp edges of the wire by bending them towards the mandible and or covering with composite material.

optionally be designed in such a way as to reduce occlusal interference (Figure 23.23a). The wire reduction can finally be covered by composite to maintain proper canine teeth position (Figure 23.23b,c). The cerclage wire diameter could be thicker (0.3–0.4 mm), while the figure-eight wire should be thinner (0.2 mm).

(a)

(b)

(c)

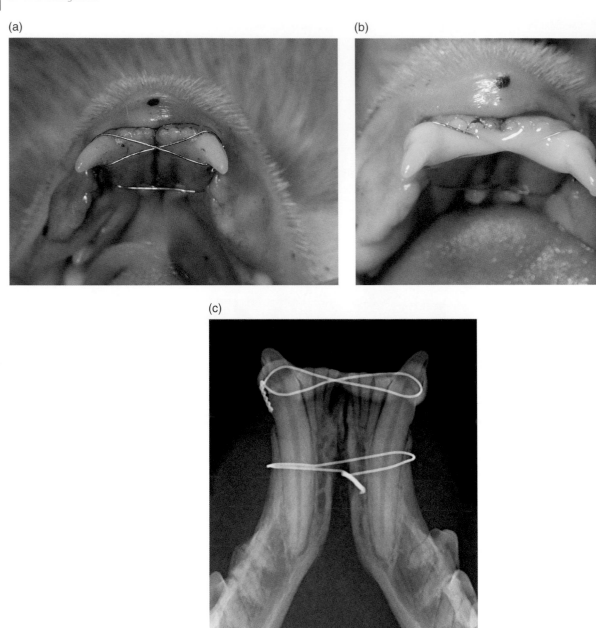

Figure 23.23 More complicated symphyseal injuries must be stabilized with both (a) cerclage and an additional figure-eight loop, (b) strengthened with an acrylic splint. (c) Radiography allows evaluation of correct reduction of separation.

References

Adamantos, S. and Garosi, L. (2011). Head trauma in the act. 1. Assessment and management of craniofacial injury. *J. Feline Med. Surg.* 13: 806–814.

Baines, S.J. and Langley-Hobbs, S. Horner's syndrome associated with a mandibular symphyseal fracture and bilateral temporomandibular luxation. *J. Small Anim. Pract.* 42 (12): 607–610.

Bar-Am, Y., Pollard, R.E., Kass, P.H., and Verstraete, F.J.M. (2008). The diagnostic yield of conventional radiographs and computed tomography in dogs and cats with maxillofacial trauma. *Vet. Surg.* 37: 294–299.

Bonner, S.E., Reiter, A.M., and Lewis, J.R. (2012). Orofacial manifestations of high-rise syndrome in cats: a retrospective study of 84 cases. *J. Vet. Dent.* 29 (1): 10–18.

Cruz-Arambulo, R. and Nykamp, S. (2012). Acute intraparenchymal spinal cord injury in a cat due to high-rise syndrome. *Can. Vet. J.* 53 (3): 274–278.

DeBowes, L.J. (2007). Use of esophageal feeding tube after oral surgery. *Pesquisa Veterinária Brasileira* 27 (Suppl).

Dewhurst, S.N., Mason, C., and Roberts, G.J. (1998). Emergency treatment of orodental injuries: a review. *Brit. J. Oral Maxillofacial Surg.* 36: 165–175.

DuPont, G. (2010). Pathologies of the dental hard tissues. In: *A Color Handbook of Small Animal Dental Oral and Maxxillofacial Disease* (ed. B. Niemiec), 128–156. Totnes: Manson.

Fink, L., Jennings, M., and Reiter, A. (2014). Esophagostomy feeding tube placement in the dog and cat. *J. Vet. Dent.* 31 (2): 133–138.

Gawor, J. (2017). Diagnozowanie urazów trzewioczaszki kotów w syndromie upadku z wysokości. *Weterynaria w Praktyce.* 11 (/12): 41–49.

Gaynor, J.S., Short, C., Tranquilli, W., et al. (2006). The Essential Guide to Pain Management: A Complete Resource for Veterinary Pain Management. The Companion Animal Pain Management Consortium, pp. 2–42.

Gioso, M., Shofer, P., Barros, P., and Harvey, C.E. (2001). Mandible and mandibular first molar tooth measurements in dogs: relationship of radiographic height to body weight. *J. Vet. Dent.* 18 (2): 65–68.

Gorrel, C., Penman, S., and Emily, P. (1993). *Handbook of Small Animal Oral Emergencies.* Oxford: Pergamon.

Khandelwal, A., Bithal, P.K., and Rath, G.P. (2019). Anesthetic considerations for extracranial injuries in patients with associated brain trauma. *J. Anaesthesiol. Clin. Pharmacol.* 35 (3): 302–311.

Liehmann, L.M., Dorner, J., Hittmair, K.M. et al. (2012). Pancreatic rupture in four cats with high-rise syndrome. *J. Feline Med. Surg.* 14 (2): 131–137.

Lopes, F.M., Gioso, M.A., Ferro, D. et al. (2005). Oral fractures in dogs of Brazil – a retrospective studies. *J. Vet. Dent.* 22 (2): 86–90.

Mulherin, B.L., Snyder, C.J., and Soukup, J.W. (2012). An alternative symphyseal wiring technique. *J. Vet. Dent.* 29 (3): 176–184.

Pratschke, K.M. and Kirby, B.M. (2002). High rise syndrome with impalement in three cats. *J. Small Anim. Pract.* 43 (6): 261–264.

Scott, P. and Timmermann, C. (2004). Stroke, transient ischaemic attack, and other central focal conditions. In: *Emergency Medicine*, 6e (eds. J. Tintinalli, G. Kelen and S. Stapczynski), 1382–1390. New York: McGraw-Hill.

Taney, K. and Smith, M. (2010). Problems with muscles, bones and joints. In: *A Color Handbook of Small Animal Dental Oral and Maxxillofacial Disease* (ed. B. Niemiec), 200–224. Totnes: Manson.

Theuns, P. and Niemiec, B.A. (2011). Bonded sealants for uncomplicated crown fractures. *J. Vet. Dent.* 28 (2): 130–132.

Verstraete, F.J.M. (2004). Maxillofacial fractures. In: *Veterinary Dental Techniques for the Small Animal Practitioner*, 3e (eds. S. Holmstrom, P. Frost and E. Eisner), 559–600. St Louis, MO: W.B. Saunders.

Verstraete, F.J.M. and Lommer, M. (2013). *Oral and Maxillofacial Surgery in Dogs and Cats.* St Louis, MO: W.B. Saunders.

Vnuk, D., Pirkic, B., Maticic, D. et al. (2004). Feline high-rise syndrome: 119 cases (1998–2001). *J. Feline Med. Surg.* 6 (5): 305–312.

Wlithey, W.O. and Mehlhaff, C.J. (1987). High-rise syndrome in cats. *J. Am. Vet. Med. Assoc.* 191 (11): 1399–1403.

WSAVA. (2014). Global Pain Council Guidelines. Available from https://wsava.org/global-guidelines/global-pain-council-guidelines/ (accessed July 5, 2020).

Zoran, D.L. (2006). Nutrition for anorectic, critically ill or injured cats. In: *Consultations in Feline Internal Medicine* (ed. J.R. August), 145–149. St Louis, MO: Saunders-Elsevier.

24

Feline Dentistry

Jerzy Gawor[1] and Brook Niemiec[2]

[1] *Veterinary Clinic Arka, Kraków, Poland*
[2] *Veterinary Dental Specialties and Oral Surgery, San Diego, CA, USA*

24.1   Introduction

It is important to have a separate feline chapter because there are several conditions that are only seen in cats. Despite some interspecies similarities, cats are definitely not small dogs. Feline medicine is increasingly popular and cat-friendly or exclusively feline clinics are becoming more and more common. Cat owners often have quite different personalities from dog owners, and many demand detailed, quality knowledge and information from their veterinarian. They look at Internet resources and participate in discussion groups. They want to be well informed about any planned treatment, including all its pros and cons.

On top of that, cats have significantly different behavior compared to dogs. Veterinarians must understand this behavior and respect specific signalments of cats in order to be able to perform oral examinations and cooperate with their feline patients (Figure 24.1).

Three major problems affect most feline dental patients: periodontal diseases, caudal stomatitis, and tooth resorption. Additionally, many other maladies may be encountered, and it is very common for several to exist concurrently in the oral cavity. Because it is difficult to provide home care for cats suffering from oral pain, many are diagnosed at an advanced stage. Further, many feline oral conditions have an ethology or treatment that is either very complex or unknown. Quite often, therefore, cats are treated via selective or total extraction of affected teeth. One recently described condition is feline oral pain syndrome (FOPS) (Rusbridge et al. 2010), while a growing clinical challenge is juvenile periodontal disease.

The first part of the management of oral disease is a thorough clinical and radiographic assessment. Full-mouth radiography is recommended in every feline patient regardless of age, sex, and breed, presenting complaint, or preliminary treatment plan. Studies show that full-mouth radiography in cats reveals more pathology than in dogs (Verstraete et al. 1998) (Figure 24.2).

It is very common for feline patients with oral inflammatory disease to have undergone empiric treatment performed by first-contact vets. From the specialist perspective, it is very frustrating to hear about all the inappropriate medical treatment performed, such as antibiotic and corticosteroid administration prior to diagnosis. The correct dental approach is proper diagnosis followed by definitive treatment and prevention by established, regular plaque control with regular rechecks, but this is rare and not well understood. Therefore, the first consultation in a specialty clinic is spent mostly on explaining the mechanisms of inflammatory process in cats, the role of pain, the pathogenesis of tooth resorption, and how to implement the treatment strategy. Often, it is too late to implement a prophylactic plan because inflammation has already caused irreversible changes in periodontal or dental tissue.

24.2   Preoperative Actions

Not every feline patient will allow for a thorough oral inspection without sedation. However, sedation decreases peripheral perfusion (particularly with the use of medetomidine) (Figure 24.3), which decreases the level of gingival inflammation, potentially leading to a misdiagnosis of a benign condition.

Basic information such as the level of dental deposits and mandibular lymph node status can be obtained even with nervous or fractious cats. The point is to perform the examination in a delicate and patient manner. A finger protector can be used to gently aid in oral inspection

The Veterinary Dental Patient: A Multidisciplinary Approach, First Edition. Edited by Jerzy Gawor and Brook Niemiec.
© 2021 John Wiley & Sons Ltd. Published 2021 by John Wiley & Sons Ltd.
Companion website: www.wiley.com/go/gawor/veterinary-dental-patient

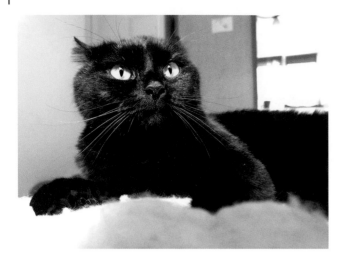

Figure 24.1 Before oral cavity inspection in a cat, it is worth looking at its body language to avoid stress and conflict. Source: Dr Pille Saar.

(see Figure 1.7, Chapter 1), but in this author's experience, if a cat is not willing to cooperate, it is better to sedate it rather than perform the examination by force.

Numerous videos and PowerPoint presentations showing correct inspection procedures are available through the website of the International Society of Feline Medicine (ISFM) and elsewhere on the Internet.

24.3 Perianesthetic Hazards

Hypotension can be a cause of acute renal failure in cats (Gaynor et al. 1999). It may result from many factors, including overdose of anesthesia medications or inadequate fluid therapy under anesthesia. In older cats, renal and thyroid conditions require very precise qualification for anesthesia. The anatomy of the trachea in cats makes intubation a procedure that must be performed with caution, including appropriate selection of the endotracheal tube size and careful filling of the cuff (Figure 24.4). The total dose of local analgesic administered in nerve blocks, vocal cord anesthesia, and lubrication gel on the e-tube must be precisely calculated to not exceed the toxic level. The estimated total safe dose of lidocaine when administered in nerve blocks is 1 mg/kg, while the toxic dose when administered intravenously is 10 mg/kg (Aguiar et al. 2015).

24.4 Surgery

The correct instrumentation will respect the fragile feline structures and the small space in oral cavity. Furthermore, the mouth cannot be extensively opened by mouth gags as

they may compromise blood delivery, leading to cortical blindness (Reiter 2014) (Figure 24.5). The infraorbital canal is very short, so infraorbital nerve block must be performed with caution (Perry 2015) (Figure 24.6).

The specific character of feline pathology predisposes to several complications: resorption and ankylosis increase the likelihood of the root fracture; inflammation creates bleeding; alveolar bone expansion requires adequate tissue preparation for tissue reapposition with closure; and tight occlusion can create lip trauma when maxillary canines are extracted, or traumatization of the periodontium when mandibular first molars are removed (Niemiec 2016).

24.5 Postoperative Challenges

These include anorexia, difficulty eating, food considerations, and pain management, especially due to the limited drug availability in cats and the difficulty of oral administration. For these reasons, it may be a good idea to place feeding tubes after surgery, in order to provide adequate nutrition (Fink et al. 2014) (Figure 24.7). The inflammatory character of lesions often requires medical treatment after surgery, which must be in line with the overall health status of the cat. For example, diabetic cats cannot tolerate steroids, and patients with renal failure or pancreatitis cannot take nonsteroidal anti-inflammatory drugs (NSAIDs).

24.6 Imaging and Radiography

Proper diagnosis is crucial for the determination of effective treatment. The most common dilemma is whether extraction or crown amputation is indicated for a tooth affected by resorption. Dental radiography is not always diagnostic (e.g., the radiographic and clinical appearance of osteomyelitis in cats can mimic malignancy; Figure 24.8), so biopsy is mandatory for final diagnosis and treatment (Gawor 2017). Increasing access to 3D imaging allows for its use in traumatic and oncologic conditions, where it is superior to standard 2D radiography (Bar-Am et al. 2008; Roza et al. 2011).

24.7 Brachycephalic Breeds

These breeds can have a predilection to periodontal disease due to teeth crowding (Millela 2015) and mouth breathing, as well as other problems. In brachycephalic breeds, skull asymmetry can be seen in association with skeletal malocclusion and masticatory apparatus dysfunctions (Emily 1992).

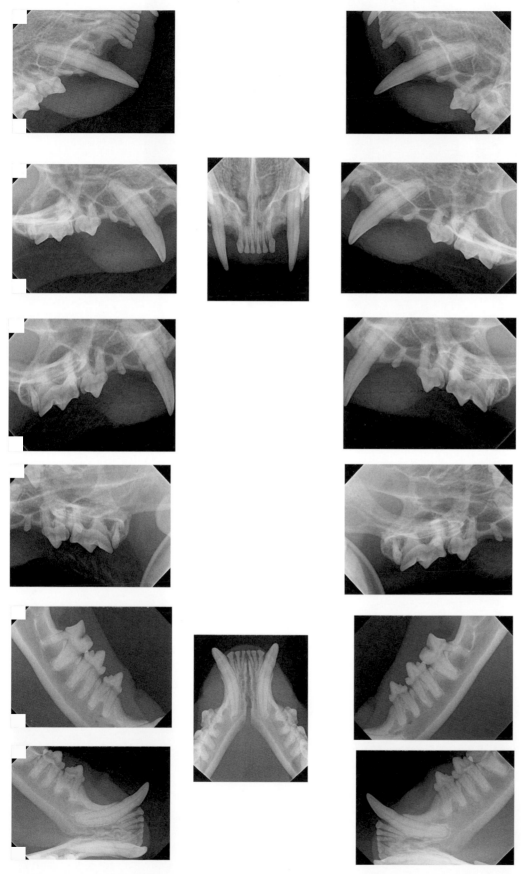

Figure 24.2 Full-mouth radiography is the gold standard in feline oral diagnostics. Source: Emilia Klim.

(a) (b)

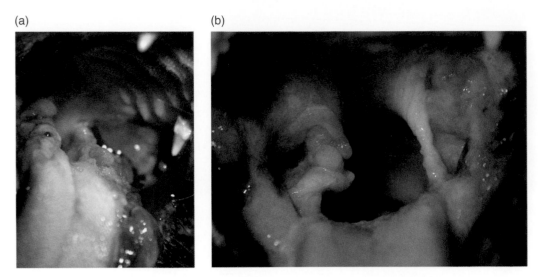

Figure 24.3   Some drugs used in sedation (e.g., medetomidine) can affect vascularization of the mouth and cause different appearances of the same oral lesions. (a) Conscious patient and (b) sedated with the use of medetomidine.

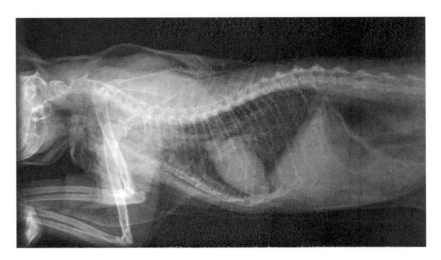

Figure 24.4   Subcutaneous emphysema associated with tracheal rupture caused by excessive and careless filling of the endotracheal cuff.

(a)   (b)

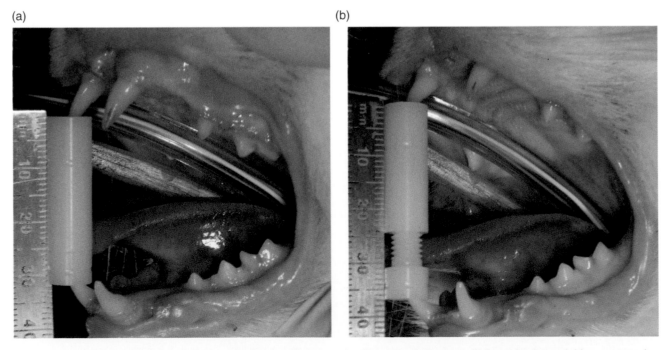

Figure 24.5   (a) Approximately 2.5–3 cm jaw extension is sufficient to visualize the oral structures. (b) Extension beyond this causes tension of the cheek and lips, limits visibility, and applies forces to the temporomandibular joints and muscles and can compromise blood supply.

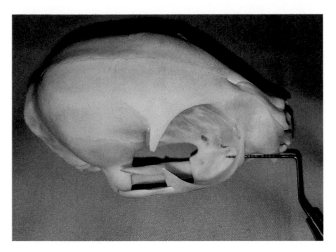

Figure 24.6 The short infraorbital canal in cats requires careful performance of infraorbital nerve block.

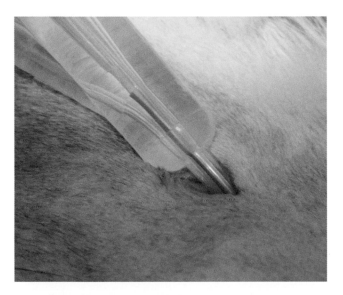

Figure 24.7 Placement of a feeding tube is important in order to maintain nutrition in an anorexic cat.

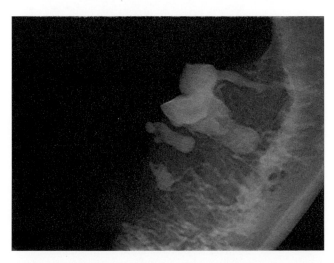

Figure 24.8 The radiographic appearance of feline osteomyelitis can mimic malignacy.

24.8 Oral Neoplasms

Oral tumors in cats are less prevalent than in dogs, but most are malignant, with approximately 70% being squamous cell carcinoma (SCC) (Stebbins et al. 1989).

24.9 High-Rise Syndrome

This is a group of post-traumatic pathologies that accompany falls from heights in cats, including injuries to the thorax and extremities as well as oral injuries. Studies show that the incidence of oral injuries in high-rise syndrome depends on who is examining the injured patient: a dental specialist will diagnose many more maxillofacial issues than a first-contact veterinarian or surgeon (Vnuk et al. 2004; Bonner et al. 2012). Additionally, 3D imaging in cats reveals twice the number of findings than are demonstrated with conventional radiography (Bar-Am et al. 2008).

24.10 The Cat-Friendly Clinic

The guidelines on cat-friendly clinics include many instructions specifically for dentistry, showing its importance in feline medicine (FAB 2008) (Figure 24.9). Many cats suffer with dental disease, and it is essential that suitable dental equipment be available and maintained so that procedures can be carried out to a high standard.

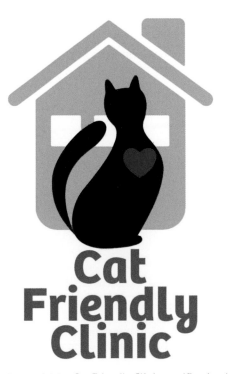

Figure 24.9 Cat Friendly Clinic certification logo.

Proper dental care should involve:

- Good client education, so that the importance of dental and oral care is recognized.
- A thorough oral examination as part of every physical exam.
- A full dental examination under anesthesia, when indicated (e.g., when abnormalities are identified on routine conscious evaluation, or if signalments suggest oral pathology).
- The ability to make dental radiographs (ideally, this should include digital systems or intraoral non-screen radiographs).
- Proper dental records and charts

Available dental tools should include:

- A selection of scalers, curettes, periodontal probes, elevators, and luxators (e.g., Superslim elevator, Couplands #1 elevator, Extraction forceps pattern 76 N). Instruments should be sharp and properly maintained.
- Protective equipment, including aprons, masks, goggles, and disposable gloves.
- Facilities for mechanically scaling and polishing teeth, sectioning teeth, and performing extractions. Cooling water must be available at the operative site. High-speed air-driven dental units are recommended. Small, round friction-grip burs #1 or 2 or cross-cut taper-fissures #699 are typically recommended.

All dental equipment should be properly cleaned and disinfected/sterilized between patients, in order to avoid transmission of infectious diseases (Figure 24.10).

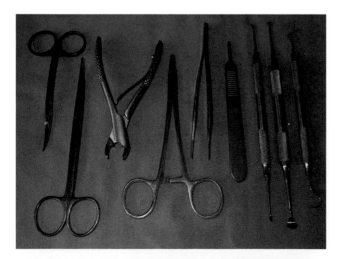

Figure 24.10 The feline dental kit may include (from left): LaGrange tissue scissors, suture scissors, extraction forceps, needle holder, tissue forceps, scalpel blade holder, two different-sized double-sided periosteal elevators, and a probe with explorer.

24.11 Caudal Stomatitis

Caudal stomatitis is a severe inflammatory reaction of the oral tissues of cats. It is a clinical diagnosis of inflammation and proliferation of the gingiva and oral mucosa. Specifically, it is inflammation associated with the caudal part of the oral mucosa (mucositis), which includes the pharynx, soft palate, glossopalatal folds, and tonsils, and very often extends to the sublingual, lingual, and buccal mucosa.

24.11.1 Etiology

The etiology of this disease process is currently unknown. Multiple etiologies may exist that, either singly or in combination, create the inflammation. Possible causative agents include an inflammatory response to bacterial plaque, viruses (in particular calicivirus), *Bartonella henselae* infection, and altered immune status (coexisting infection of feline leukemia virus [FeLV] or feline immunodeficiency virus [FIV]).

24.11.2 Clinical Signs

In cases of caudal stomatitis, the history typically includes halitosis, dysphagia, pawing at the mouth, reluctance to eat, anorexia (complete or partial), crying out in pain when eating or yawning, weight loss, decreased grooming (which results in an unkempt appearance), and drooling (pseudoptyalism) (Figure 24.11).

The affected gingiva and oral mucosa have varying amounts of inflammation, proliferation, and ulceration. The inflammation is typically – but not always – bilaterally symmetrical, with friable oral tissues that bleed easily.

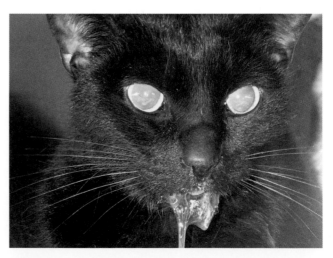

Figure 24.11 Drooling very often indicates oral problems in cats.

In certain breeds (Maine coon), juvenile gingivitis tends to progress into caudal stomatitis if left untreated (Figure 24.12).

24.11.3 Diagnostics

Caudal stomatitis is a clinical syndrome and does not indicate a specific etiology or diagnosis. Diagnosis is made by visual inspection of the oral cavity and analysis of clinical history. Diagnostic tests to further define the disease should include at a minimum: dental radiographs, a minimum database (CBC, chemistry panel, T4, U/A) to evaluate for underlying and concurrent systemic health problems, and evaluation of FeLV/FIV status. A biopsy

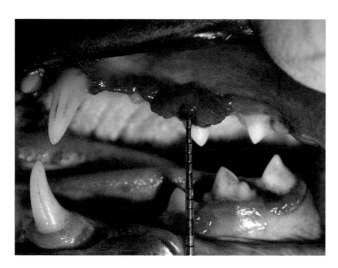

Figure 24.12 Juvenile proliferative gingivitis in a cat can turn into periodontitis if not treated.

can be taken and submitted for histopathology, especially if the inflammation is asymmetrical or otherwise atypical, or if radiographic findings are suspicious for neoplasia.

24.11.4 Management

The goal of therapy for this disease process is to completely eradicate the oral inflammation. However, maintaining a state of decreased inflammation is sometimes the best that can be achieved. Several treatments have been suggested, including extraction of all premolars and molars, full-mouth extraction, chronic immune-suppressive treatment, anti-inflammatory treatment, interferon, and antibiotics. Any chronic ulceration – particularly unilateral – should be biopsied to rule out malignancy.

24.11.5 Surgical Therapy

Controlling inflammation is key to the management of this disease process. Therefore, any tooth affected with inflammation from any cause should be extracted, and all remaining teeth should receive strict home care and routine professional cleanings to keep further inflammation at bay. However, since the majority of patients have widespread inflammation, the most successful long-term treatment for cats with chronic gingivostomatitis is complete extraction of all premolars and molars, as well as smoothing of the alveolar bone. An additional step taken by many veterinary dentists is to perform a careful alveloplasty to remove periodontal ligament remnants, which has anecdotally improved success rates (Figure 24.13).

(a)

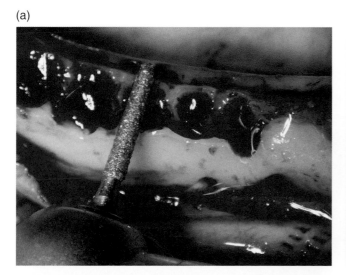

(b)

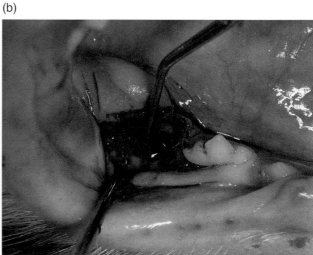

Figure 24.13 (a) Alveolar bone smoothing and (b) gentle removal of granulation tissue with the use of currette enhance recovery and decrease stomatitis.

Extraction of the canine and incisor teeth is indicated when the inflammation extends to include the surrounding gingiva. Many veterinary dentists prefer to leave the canines and incisors if at all possible, but these authors favors full-mouth extraction. Postoperative dental radiographs *must* be exposed to document complete extraction of all tooth roots. The majority of cats have an excellent response to this treatment. If the canines and incisors are not extracted, owners must provide meticulous home care for these teeth.

Regardless of the quality of extractions, some cats have only partial improvement and require long-term medical management, albeit typically at much lower doses than prior to surgery. If extraction therapy does not prove to be effective, it is usually due to incomplete extractions. In rare cases, however, properly performed extractions may have only an incomplete therapeutic effect, and in these cases, the patient will require long-term medical management. The patients that have the least response to extraction therapy are typically those that have had longstanding, chronic inflammation that has been treated with repeated high doses of glucocorticoids. It is important to note that generally, the earlier the teeth are extracted, the better the outcome. In recent studies, complete resolution of clinical signs after total or subtotal extraction was seen in 28.4% of cats (n = 95). In 68.85% of these patients, additional medical therapy was necessary (Jennings et al. 2015) (Figure 24.14).

24.11.6 Medical Therapy

In cases where owners are reluctant to have multiple extractions performed early in the course of treatment, medical management may be attempted to reduce bacterial load and inflammation. The majority of the products utilized are oral medications, which require daily to twice daily administration. This is difficult to achieve in cats in general, and the oral pain and inflammation only serves to complicate matters. Many of these products also have significant side effects.

Clients should be informed that medical therapy is almost invariably a lifelong process with numerous side effects. In addition, there are no medical protocols that have been shown to be completely effective; rather, they just temporarily reduce the clinical signs. Therefore, clients should be counseled that delaying extraction therapy often results in a decreased response, possibly yet again necessitating long-term medical therapy.

24.11.6.1 Antibiotics/Antiseptics

Systemic antibiotics *may* result in some improvement in the amount of oral inflammation. However, this is generally temporary at best, and most patients will relapse even during the course of therapy. Rinsing with a 0.12% chlorhexidine (CHX) gluconate solution or using an adhesive 0.2% gel with CHX may also be beneficial in some cases. In cats with compromised immunity, antibiotic therapy can be used as part of a complex treatment. Doxycycline and clindamycin had a positive impact on local immunomodulation in some studies, but the use of antibiotics as an exclusive therapy is contraindicated.

24.11.6.2 Anti-Inflammatories

Corticosteroids are by far the most commonly used and effective drugs for immune modulation. However, long-term use of corticosteroids may have detrimental effects, such as the induction of diabetes mellitus, other endocrine problems, or opportunistic infections. Moreover, as viral infection is often a part of the etiology in caudal stomatitis,

(a)

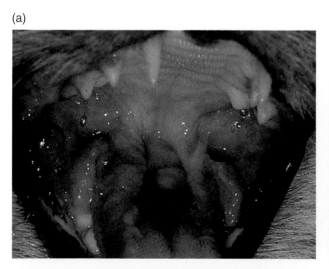

(b)

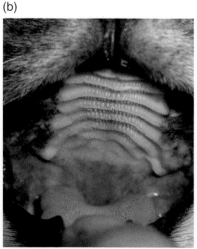

Figure 24.14 Extraction of the entire dentition or cheek teeth results in total improvement in 28.4% of cases: (a) prior to operation; (b) six weeks after operation.

corticosteroids may be contraindicated. When this treatment modality is selected, use the lowest effective dose and monitor biochemical values on a regular basis. Injectable treatment (methylprednisone 10–20 mg SC) is usually recommended initially, due to the degree of oral pain. This typically results in clinical improvement within 24–48 hours, and lasts for 3–6 weeks. However, these intervals tend to progressively shorten the longer the injections are continued. For all these reasons, chronic corticosteroid therapy should only be performed as a last resort when an owner will not allow extractions or in edentulous cats that still have significant oral inflammation where tests for the presence of viral infections are negative. Whenever chronic corticosteroid therapy is performed, it is reasonable to use drugs to protect the alimentary-tract mucosa.

24.11.6.3 Cyclosporine

Cyclosporine A has been suggested as an immunosuppressive drug for cats with chronic gingivostomatitis. Some veterinarians have promoted it as an alternative to extractions, in order to avoid the use of glucocorticoids. However, these authors prefers to withhold its use to those cases where additional medical management is necessary following extractions.

The benefits of the use of cyclosporine have been published, and a dose of 2.5–5.0 mg/kg has shown improvement. Side effects include diarrhea and vomiting (Lommer 2013). It may provide an alternative to long-term steroid therapy, but it must be used with caution in cats with hepatic or renal disease, and there are reports of fatal opportunistic infections (fungal) associated with it.

The bioavailability of the three forms of cyclosporine is quite variable, so dosing depends on which is used. Ideally, serum cyclosporine levels should be evaluated within 24–48 hours of beginning therapy and then monitored weekly for a month and monthly thereafter, to maintain concentrations within the therapeutic range and avoid toxic levels. Cats with cyclosporine levels in serum above 300 ng/mL showed improvement >70%, while those with levels below 300 ng/mL showed only 28% improvement. In addition to monitoring cyclosporine levels, standard biochemical tests should be routinely performed as surveillance for deleterious side effects.

24.11.6.4 Feline Interferon Omega

There is currently significant interest in the use of this product for caudal stomatitis. It is reported to provide not only an antiviral effect, but also an immunomodulatory one, and to bring about a return to normal local immune response. Because of its antiviral indication, it is important to perform a feline calicivirus (FCV) test prior to administration of interferon. Several studies have shown efficacy in resistant cases, but as of yet, no evidence exists to show that it works as a primary treatment. There are several options for therapy, including intralesional injection and oral versus injectable systemic treatment. The preferred method at present is to inject 5 MU intralesional (often at the time of extractions) and follow this up with the remainder of the vial (5 MU) diluted into 100 cc of sterile saline and administered per os by the owner at a dose of 1 mL once daily for 100 days (Figure 24.15) (Hennet at al , 2011).

24.11.6.5 Other Treatment Options

Finally, lactoferrin (topically at 40 mg/kg), gold salts (1–2 mg weekly for eight weeks and monthly thereafter), levamisole (2–5 mg/kg PO three times weekly), doxycycline

(a)

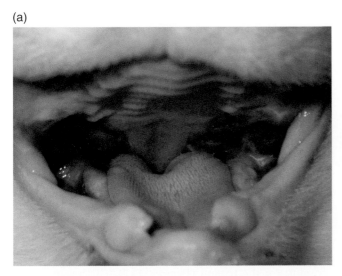

(b)

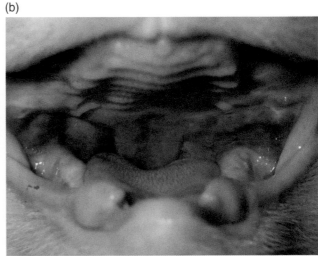

Figure 24.15 Use of medical treatment (in this case, Interferon Omega [Virbagen, Virbac]) in edentulous cats can improve oral health in a long-term protocol. (a) Prior to treatment and (b) after 2 months of Interferon Omega treatment.

(a) (b)

(c) (d)

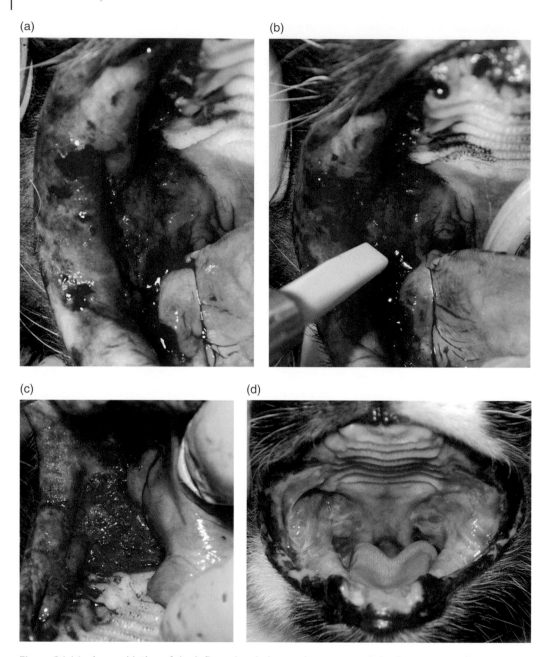

Figure 24.16   Laser ablation of the inflamed and ulcerated mucosa can bring improvement in some cases.

(2 mg/kg BID, with decreasing doses if effective), and coenzyme Q10 (30–60 mg daily) have also been used with occasional success. However, none of these is recommended at this time (Winer et al. 2016). Laser ablation of the ulcerated areas, with its antimicrobial effect and healing influence, has been considered and published as an additional method of managing caudal stomatitis unsolved by extractions (Lewis et al. 2007) (Figure 24.16). Another suggestion is the use of stem cells, which results in immunomodulation (Arzi et al. 2017).

In conclusion, at the time of this writing, surgical extraction therapy is the preferred treatment and should be

performed as soon as possible. Medical therapy should be reserved for those cases where clients will not allow (or cannot afford) extraction therapy.

24.12   Tooth Resorption

24.12.1   Clinical Features

Completely subgingival resorptions (those that have not progressed to the crown of the tooth) likely cause no discomfort for the patient (Figure 24.17). This presumption is based on the fact that similar lesions in humans are

(a)   (b)

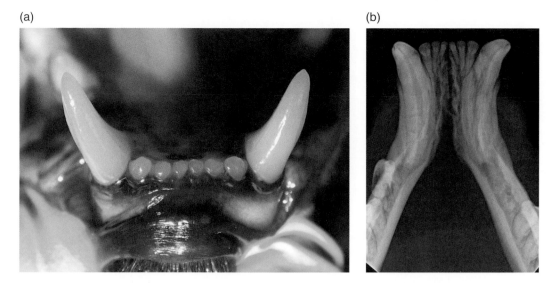

Figure 24.17   Subgingival tooth resorption can occur without symptoms and often is revealed incidentally (a) Clinical appearance of the mandibular rostral dentition. (b) Radiography revealed both canine teeth affected by TR.

(a)   (b)

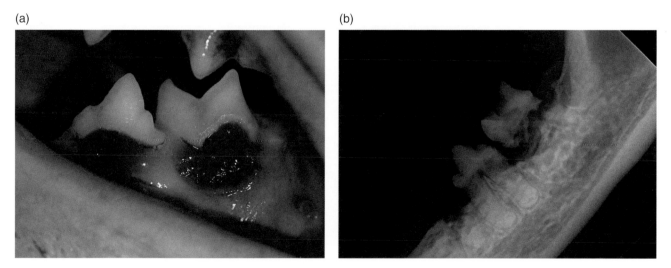

Figure 24.18   Type 1 resorption is associated with (a) surrounding tissue inflammation, including of the (b) osteomyelitis of the alveolar bone.

nonpainful. Once lesions progress to the crown, however, they are typically very painful, but cats rarely show overt clinical signs. It is possible that the tissue filling the defect may provide some protection from sensitivity.

Most tooth resorptions are quite large before they become clinically evident. Therefore, it is very important to perform a thorough oral exam on all cats. Visualization of a resorptive defect near the gingival margin is almost diagnostic for a tooth resorption. The vast majority of feline patients afflicted with resorptions will show no outward clinical signs. However, patients may present for oral pain, anorexia, ptyalism, lethargy, depression, dysphagia, or halitosis.

24.12.1.1   Type 1

The lesions are first clinically evident on the crown at the gingival margin when the internal resorption reaches the coronal dentine. The gingiva surrounding teeth with type 1 lesions is usually affected by a significant inflammatory problem such as caudal stomatitis or periodontal disease. In cases of periodontal disease, it is very common to have calculus covering the lesion, which must be removed to properly diagnose it. The clinically visible defect typically indicates a much larger subgingival one. In addition, the defect is often covered by hyperplastic gingiva. Type I resorption is proven to be associated with inflammation in surrounding tissues (Gorrel 2015) (Figure 24.18).

(a)

(b)

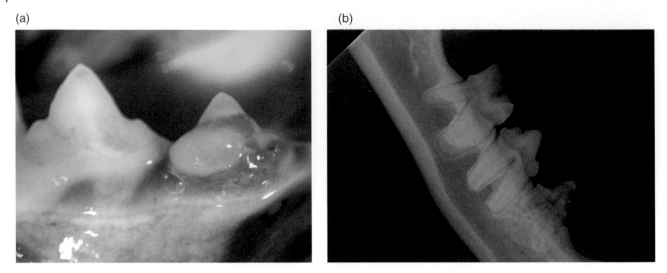

Figure 24.19   Type 2 resorption of 407: (a) clinical and (b) radiographic appearance.

(a)

(b)

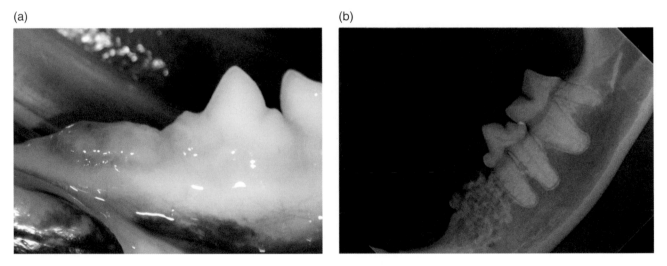

Figure 24.20   (a) A bump above the gingival margin indicates stage V resorption. (b) Radiographic appearance of the stage V resorption.

24.12.1.2 Type 2

Type 2 resorptions are usually associated with only local-ized gingivitis on oral exam, in contrast to the more severe inflammation due to periodontal disease or caudal stomati-tis seen with type 1. They often begin just below the gingi-val surface near the cemento-enamel junction close to the gingival margin, or the "neck" of the tooth. Visualization of a defect on the tooth surface or of gingival hyperplasia on the crown surface is indicative of a tooth resorption. The lower third premolar is commonly the first tooth affected in such cases, though canines can also be affected without other teeth being involved. Cats with a type 2 resorption will generally have more than one lesion and are at increased risk for developing additional ones. Early

lesions may appear only as localized marginal gingivitis in a mouth that has very little inflammation.

Tooth resorptions can be differentiated from a normal fur-cation damage or periodontal pocket with a dental explorer. This instrument catches on the edge of the defect, which feels rough, in distinction to the smoothness of a furcation. Larger lesions are seen extending above the gingival margin on to the crown of the tooth (Figure 24.19). Advanced type 2 lesions often have gingiva or inflamed granulation tissue growing up on to the crown. In end-stage lesions, the tooth fractures and gingiva grow over the area, developing a firm "bump" around the missing tooth. This bump distinguishes these lesions from tooth loss caused by periodontal disease or previously performed extraction (Figure 24.20).

24.12.2 Diagnosis

Determination of whether a lesion is type 1 or type 2 requires a dental radiograph.

Type 1 lesions have normal root density (as compared to the surrounding teeth) and a well-defined periodontal space in some areas. These teeth often have a definable root canal in the intact part. Additionally, type 1 lesions are generally associated with periodontal bone loss (either horizontal or vertical) (Figure 24.21).

The radiographic appearance of type 2 lesions is that of teeth with an abnormal radiographic density (as compared to the surrounding teeth), as they have undergone significant replacement resorption. Radiographic findings will include areas with no discernable periodontal ligament space (dentoalveolar ankylosis) or root canal, and in late stages there will be little discernable root structure (ghost roots) (Figure 24.22).

Tooth extrusion and alveolar bone expansion are also signs of tooth resorption in cats (Lewis et al. 2008; Bell and Soukup 2015) (Figure 24.23 and Figure 18.19).

Missing teeth should prompt radiographic investigation. Inflammation on the surface of a tooth that is incompatible with the degree of periodontal disease or markedly different from the remainder of the teeth is suspect for a lesion. In such cases, the prudent clinician will run a dental explorer across the area to feel for roughness, which is diagnostic of a tooth resorption.

24.12.3 Management

Restoration of any tooth resorption carries a very poor prognosis, because the odontoclasts remain present under the restoration, and so the resorptive process continues. Within around six months, the restoration will typically be lost and the pain and inflammation will recur. In addition, the visible lesion normally represents only a small part of the actual pathology (i.e., it is the tip of the iceberg).

The treatment of choice for teeth with resorption is extraction. Recently, crown amputation has been suggested as an acceptable treatment option for advanced type 2 lesions. This results in significantly less trauma to the patient, with faster healing than complete extraction. Though widely accepted, however, this procedure is somewhat controversial. Most veterinary dentists do employ it, but in widely varying frequencies. Veterinary dentists typically use it only when there is significant or complete root replacement by bone. Unfortunately, the majority of general practitioners turn to it far too often. Crown amputation

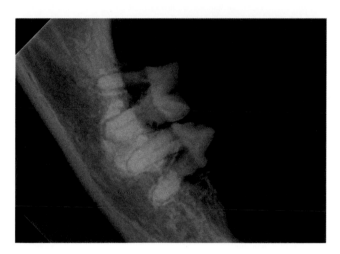

Figure 24.21 Type 1 resorptive lesions are often associated with alveolar bone loss (horizontal or vertical, or both).

(a)

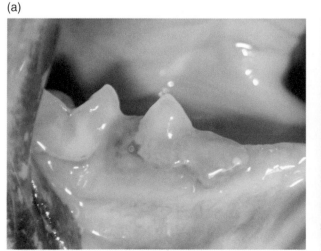

(b)

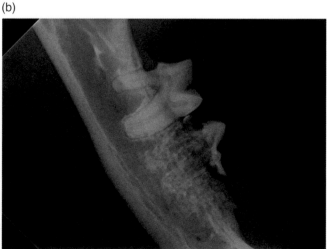

Figure 24.22 "Ghost roots" indicate an advanced stage of tooth resorption: (a) clinical and (b) radiographic appearance.

(a) (b)

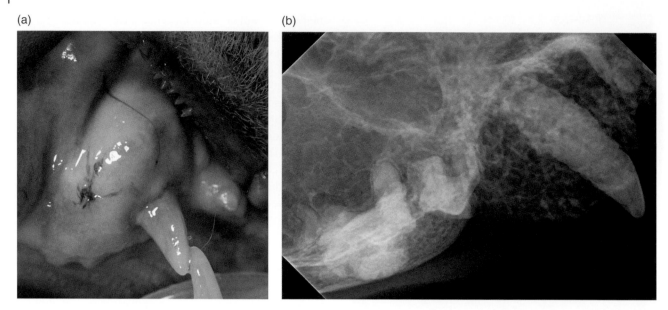

Figure 24.23 Alveolar bone expansion like (a) that in the area of 104 can be associated with (b) osteomyelitis and tooth resorption.

can only be performed on teeth with radiographically confirmed type 2 resorptions that show no periapical or periodontal bone loss, and that have roots that are being completely resorbed. It should not be performed in teeth with type 1 resorptions, radiographic or clinical evidence of endodontic or periodontal pathology, inflammation, or infection. It should also not be performed in patients that have any evidence of inflammation in the caudal tissues between the upper and lower molar teeth or that are known to be positive for retrovirus. Those practitioners without dental radiology capability *should not* perform crown amputation. Instead, either the teeth should be fully extracted or the patient should be referred to a facility with dental radiology.

In teeth with alveolar bone expansion, preventive action with osseous surgery is possible (Beebe and Gengler 2007).

24.13 Feline Orofacial Pain Syndrome (FOPS)

FOPS is a pain disorder of cats with behavioral signs of oral discomfort and tongue mutilation. It is suspected to be a neuropathic pain disorder, and its predominance within the Burmese cat breed suggests an inherited condition, possibly involving central or ganglion processing of sensory trigeminal information. The disease is characterized by an episodic, typically unilateral discomfort with pain-free intervals; the discomfort is in many cases triggered by mouth movements. The disease is often recurrent, and with time may become unremitting – 12% of cases in one

study were euthanized as a consequence of the condition (Rusbridge et al. 2010). Sensitization of trigeminal nerve endings as a consequence of oral disease or tooth eruption appears to be an important factor in the etiology: 63% of cases had a history of oral lesions, and at least 16% experienced their first sign of discomfort during eruption of permanent teeth. External factors can also influence the disease as FOPS events can be directly linked to a situation causing anxiety in 20% of cats. FOPS can be resistant to traditional analgesics, and in some cases successful management requires anticonvulsants with an analgesic effect (Rusbridge et al. 2010).

24.14 Juvenile Periodontal Diseases

Juvenile periodontal disease is a fairly common oral problem in kittens aged up to 12 months (Clarke and Caiafa 2014). Depending on the stage of the disease, as well as the clinical and radiographic appearance, it is possible to distinguish three major types: juvenile early-onset gingivitis, juvenile hyperplastic gingivitis, and juvenile-onset gingivitis–periodontitis (Perry and Tutt 2015). All these conditions are commonly mistaken for caudal stomatitis; the difference is that in these cases, there is no caudal inflammation.

Juvenile gingivitis occurs in young cats around the time of permanent teeth eruption and is associated with circumferential marginal and free gingiva inflammation. This is inflammation of the gingiva during and just after tooth eruption and it may be accompanied by persistent deciduous

(a)

(b)

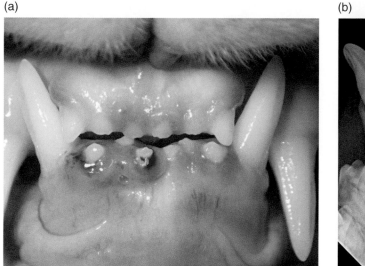
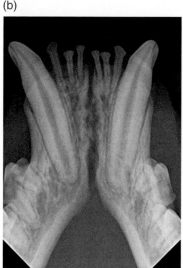

Figure 24.24 Juvenile periodontitis in a 12-month-old Maine coon cat, requiring extraction of the mandibular incisors: (a) clinical and (b) radiographic appearance.

dentition. The gingival bleeding index is II or III, meaning bleeding may occur on probing or spontaneously. Thick plaque deposition is present, but gingival probing depth does not necessarily exceed 1 mm. It is self-limiting in most cases, but home care (brushing or CHX rinses) is recommended to decrease the inflammation. If the condition does not resolve within a short period of time, additional diagnostics and therapy are recommended as it could progress into juvenile periodontitis (Figure 24.24).

Juvenile hyperplastic gingivitis is also diagnosed in young cats under nine months of age. Often, these cats have had previous problems with eruption and suffered from juvenile gingivitis. The free gingiva may become very inflamed and enlarged, particularly over the maxillary fourth premolars, mandibular molars, and canine teeth. Due to hypertrophy of the gingiva, pseudopockets are present at a probing depth of 2–4 mm, without alveolar bone loss. This must be confirmed radiographically. Treatment involves gingivectomy/gingivoplasty performed with the use of radiosurgery, laser surgery, dental bur trimming, or cold steel techniques. It is very important to perform professional periodontal therapy at the same time, followed by thorough and consistent oral home care. The duration of home care is not defined, but some resources suggest a minimum of two years, at which point the condition may settle.

Juvenile periodontitis may be seen as a rapidly progressive condition in young cats, with predilection in Siamese and Maine coon breeds (Wiggs and Lobprise 1997), and in this author's experience also in British shorthairs. Apart from fast-progressing gingivitis, alveolar bone loss is

visible radiographically. Therapy is strict plaque control, which consists of early 9–12 months) and regular (q 9–12 months) professional cleanings and mandatory thorough and consistent oral home care. The treatment also includes extraction of periodontally affected teeth, and gingivoplasty/gingivectomy when indicated. Without a commitment to long-term consistent therapy, the disease will progress and further tooth loss will occur (Figure 24.24).

24.15 Eosinophilic Granuloma Complex

Eosinophilic granuloma complex (EGC) is a group of conditions that share a common etiology, as well as some histopathological features. While these lesions have been reported in dogs (especially Siberian huskies, Malamutes, and cavaliers), they are much more common in cats.

The true etiology of these conditions is unknown. Local accumulation of eosinophils (and their release of inflammatory agents) is thought to initiate inflammation and necrosis. The presence of eosinophils suggests that these lesions are secondary to an immune-mediated or hypersensitivity reaction. This reaction may result from a local (food) or systemic (flea or atopy) allergy, or from parasitic conditions (Lommer 2013), though these lesions have been seen in cases where allergic and infectious disease have been ruled out. Additional causes may include a response to irritation, such as chronic grooming, or a traumatic malocclusion. Finally, there appears to be a genetic predisposition to EGC.

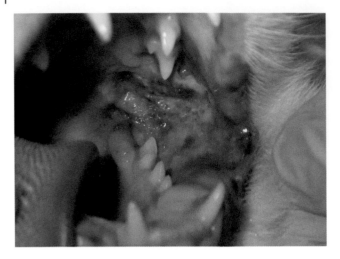

Figure 24.25   EGC can appear as indolent ulcers.

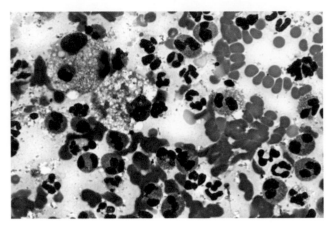

Figure 24.26   Cytology of an oral lesion from a cat showing mixed inflammation with a prominent eosinophilic component (typical of EGC). Hemacolor stain, 50× objective. Source: Courtesy of Dr. Maciej Guzera Laboklin.

24.15.1   Clinical Features

There are several different clinical syndromes in this category, all of which may have oral manifestations. There may also be concurrent dermatologic manifestations.

The most common oral manifestation in cats is indolent ulcers (Figure 24.25). These appear as red-brown lesions on the upper lip, at the philtrum, or around the maxillary canine teeth. Eosinophilic ulcers on the upper lip usually have a carved-out, depressed appearance with a yellowish center. These lesions are typically not painful and not pruritic.

Plaques are usually raised, with an overall red appearance. They tend to be more painful and may be pruritic. Lesions can be unilateral or bilateral. Females are two to three times more likely to be affected than males. Some texts report that young cats are overrepresented, while others report that older to middle aged cats are predisposed. CBC may reveal peripheral eosinophilia, but this finding is not always present. Biochemical profiles are usually normal, and FeLV and FIV tests are usually negative. The lesions of eosinophilic ulcer on the upper lip are classic in appearance and are rarely confused with anything else. EGC lesions in other locations, however, can be confusing, and biopsy is required for definitive diagnosis. Cytology may be useful if superficial material is removed from the lesion prior to scraping or imprint so that the eosinophilic infiltrate can be detected (Figure 24.26).

24.15.2   Management

The acute disease process is best treated with corticosteroids. However, corticosteroids should not be used for long-term disease control, due to their significant systemic side effects. The typical initial protocol is prednisone 2 mg/kg q 12 hours for three to four weeks. Other corticosteroid options include intralesional triamcinalone (3 mg weekly)

and methyl prednisone injections (20 mg q two weeks). This author prefers bethamethasone (Diprophos MSD) injection 1 mg per affected side into the submucosa (0.2 mL OD). Antibiotic therapy is required in some cases to induce remission or to treat secondary infection. In addition, there are cases that appear to respond to antibiotic therapy alone, such as doxycycline at 10 mg/kg PO q 24 hours.

It is routine in our practices to treat mild cases initially with antibiotics alone and more severe cases with a combination of antibiotics and corticosteroid medications. Thorough allergy testing should be performed, especially in nonresponsive or recurrent cases. If an underlying allergic component is found, specific treatment can be instituted, with a good rate of success. Many cases remain idiopathic and require lifelong therapy. Cyclosporine has recently been introduced as a veterinary labeled product for atopy and appears as effective as corticosteroids for atopic dermatitis in dogs and cats. Cats should be treated for 60 days with 25 mg (4.9–12.5 mg/kg) given two hours before a meal. This has also been proven to be an effective medication for long-term therapy of oral eosinophilic diseases. In addition, a lower incidence of severe side effects may be expected in comparison to steroids, which is especially valuable in cases requiring long-term therapy. Consequently, many dermatologists use this medication rather than corticosteroids for inflammatory skin diseases, including EGC. When treating larger patients long-term, the addition of ketoconazole may lower the necessary dosage of cyclosporine, and thus the cost to the client. It is important to note that cyclosporine is currently not approved in cats and that there are reports of opportunistic fungal and fatal protozoal infections associated with its chronic use. Therefore, using the lowest effective dose (by tapering) and performing regular therapeutic levels and routine blood testing is recommended.

Hormonal therapy is another medical option for treating these lesions, but the significant potential side effects should make it the last option. Additional therapies that may benefit some cats include antihistamines, chlorambucil (more effective on lymphocytes), and gold salts. One practitioner has had success using Prozac in a patient with oral EGC that was refractory to all other treatments.

Surgical removal of these lesions has been performed with some success, including laser and cryosurgery. Finally, radiation treatment has been used effectively in some cases.

24.16 Pyogranuloma Secondary to Traumatic Dental Occlusion

This is an inflammatory lesion that develops at the contact point of the premolar and molar teeth of the opposite arcade and forms due to impingement of the mucosa. It appear as a gingival cleft, granulation, or ulceration. Biopsy is indicated to rule out malignancy. Immediate resolution of symptoms can be observed after either coronal reduction or extraction of the offending tooth (Gracis et al. 2015) (Figure 24.27).

24.17 Common Procedures

Crown amputation is a procedure for the management of advanced type 2 resorption. This procedure is possible only after radiographic confirmation of dentoalveolar ankylosis and advanced root replacement resorption (DuPont 2002). It involves creating a small gingival flap and then using a high-speed bur to remove the entire crown to the level of the alveolar bone. Following radiographic conformation that the tooth is removed to at least the level of the bone (and that the resulting bone is smooth), the gingiva is sutured over the defect (Figure 24.28). Some specialists advice further reduction of the root with a round diamond bur by additional 1-2mm below the level of alveolar margin.

Odontoplasty of the canine or 108, 107 can be performed to resolve the traumatizing relations of cheek teeth causing pyogranuloma at an early stage of this problem. It involves coronal reduction of the tooth/teeth in occlusal contact with the lesion through the use of aluminum oxide abrasive or diamond burs. This odontoplasty will typically expose dentin, and therefore a mandatory part of the procedure should be dentinal bonding with unfilled resin (Figure 24.29). Extraction of the tooth/teethis performed in cases where coronal reduction would cause pulp exposure or where odontoplasty does not bring remission of the problem (Gracis et al. 2015).

Composite application in mandibular canines after extraction of maxillary canines reduces the risk of upper-lip entrapment and impingement by the lower canine after maxillary canine extraction (Figure 24.30). Applying a round-shaped composite to the crown so that it does not become longer can prevent traumatization after extraction. Cases that still have contact of the mandibular canine teeth require crown height reduction followed by vital pulp therapy or standard endodontic therapy. Composite application consists of three steps:

1) **Acid etching:** This is performed with a 37% phosphoric acid. The aim is to remove all impurities from the tooth surface and slightly demineralize it, producing an increased surface area for bonding and strengthening

(a)

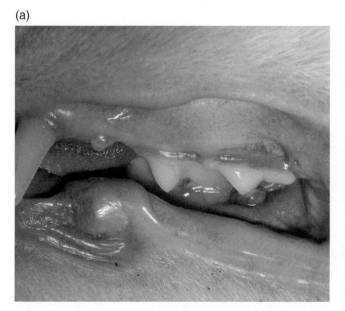

(b)

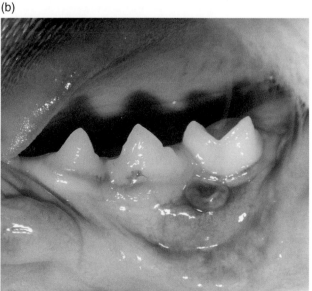

Figure 24.27 Pyogranuloma caused by traumatic occlusion of the cheek dentition in a young British shorthairted cat. Clinical presentation with (a) jaws closed and (b) with mouth open.

the mechanical bond of the resin. The acid etch gel is left on the enamel for 10–30 seconds, before being rinsed with copious amounts of water for 20 seconds to remove it entirely from the tooth structure. Any acid etch remnants left within dental tubules could result in tooth sensitivity. After rinse, and prior to applying the bond, the etched area should be left gently dry, but not dessicate.

2) **Application of the bonding agent:** This can take two main forms: one-step, which combines the primer and bonding agent in a single bottle, and two-step, which keeps them separate. Additionally, self-etching systems have shown promise recently, and are less technique-

sensitive. The bonding agent should be applied in a very thin layer and the excess gently removed with a brush or air. After it is applied, it should be light-cured according to the manufacturer's recommendations, normally for around 10 seconds of continuous light.

3) **Restoration:** A solid or nanohybrid composite is placed on the tip of the crown and shaped around it. With solid material, this can be done with a plastic filling instrument or a brush coated with unfilled resin. Flowable composite on the other hand achieves a regular round shape on application. Once the composite is placed and shaped, it is light cured. The surface can then be smoothed and shaped with white stones, fine diamonds,

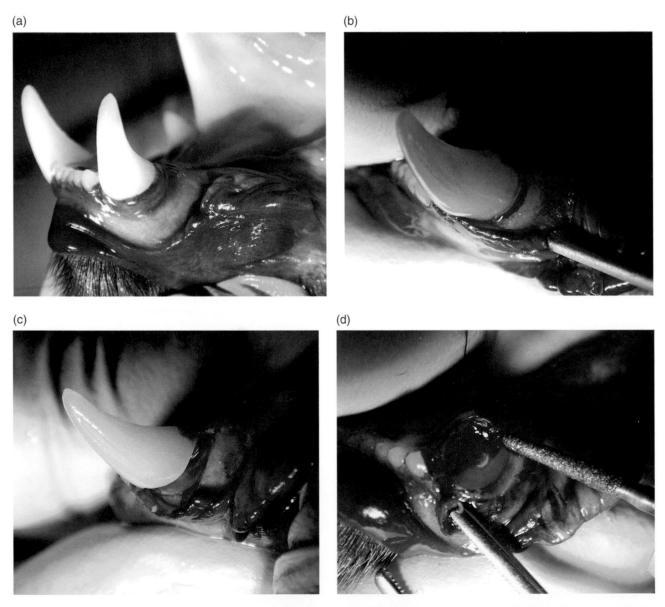

(a)

(b)

(c)

(d)

Figure 24.28 (a) Crown amputation of the mandibular canine tooth. (b) Designing the envelope flap. (c) Cutting the crown with a fissure bur. (d) Smoothing the cut edges. (e) Closure of access. (f) Postoperative radiograph. (g) Distant radiographic follow-up. Note the 404 was extracted.

(e)

(f)

(g)

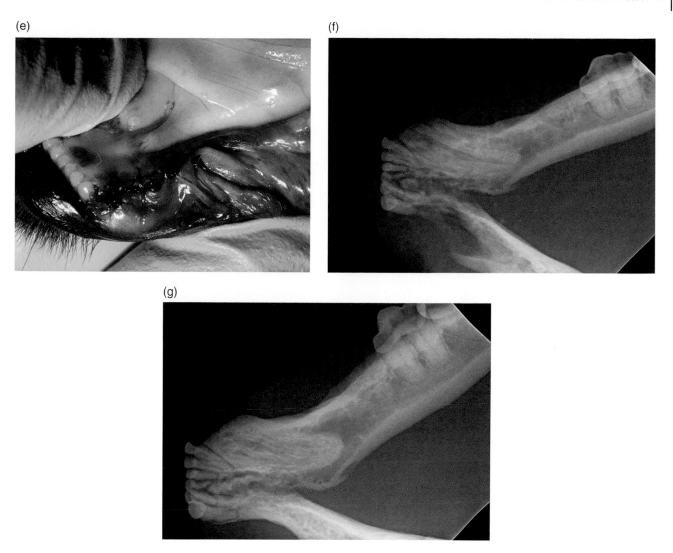

Figure 24.28 (Continued)

or sanding discs. Once finished, a layer of unfilled resin should be applied to smooth the final restoration (Niemiec 2014) (Figure 24.31).

Gingivectomy and **gingivoplasty** are usually performed together and are used to reshape the gingiva and reestablish the normal depth of the gingival sulcus (Figure 24.32). Numerous techniques are available, including cold steel, diamond bur, electrosurgery, and laser (Force and Niemiec 2009). The first step is to outline the incision line in order to achieve the new free gingival margin approximately 1–2 mm coronaly to the cemento-enamel junction. As plaque may interfere with wound healing, strict but disciplined home care must be recommended, through brushing should begin no sooner than 14 days after surgery. Application of oral cleansing gel (Maxiguard, Addison labs) three or four

times a day seems to be the best solution in the recovery period (Gorrel and Hale 2012).

A **buried knot suture** is particularly indicated when there is a need to reduce a surface area of potential plaque accumulation or contacting tissues (e.g., tongue). It also helps reduce the incidence of foreign bodies (e.g., hair) becoming attached to the suture. The most common applications are quadrant extraction in caudal stomatitis, palatal surgery, and persistent deciduous dentition extraction. This technique requires similar principles to general suturing in the oral cavity (Pippi 2017). The difference is that the first pierce of the needle is from the inside and the knot is tightened within the wound. In this author's experience, this technique does not change the healing time, and patients end up with much less entrapped foreign material at the wound margins (Figure 24.33).

Pharyngotomy is potentially indicated when performing oral fracture repair requiring occlusion control or when

(a)

(b)

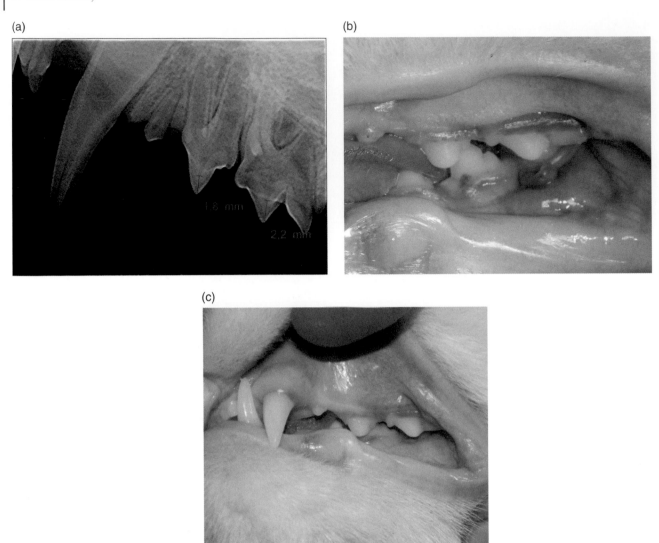

(c)

Figure 24.29 Odontoplasty of 207, 208. (a) Radiographic assessment of the maximum extension of the crown reduction. (b) Result of odontoplasty. (c) At four weeks' follow-up.

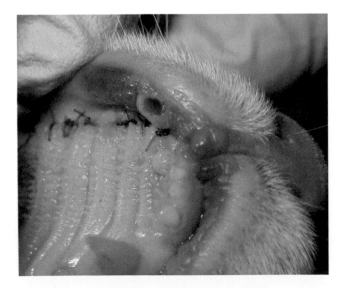

Figure 24.30 Traumatization of the upper lip by the mandibular canine tooth after right maxillary canine tooth extraction.

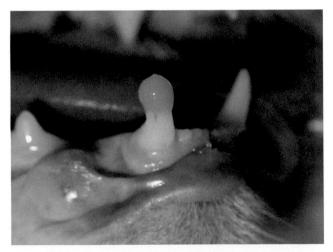

Figure 24.31 Composite buildup on a mandibular canine crown is placed to avoid traumatisation of the upper lip after ipsilateral maxillary canine tooth extraction.

(a)

(b)

(c)

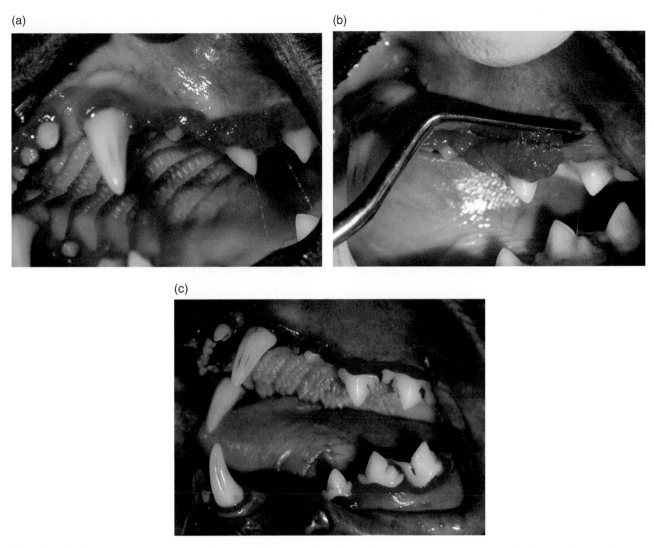

Figure 24.32 Hyperplastic gingiva associated with juvenile gingivitis requires (a) gingivectomy or gingivoplasty, which can be performed with a (b) Kirkland knife. This procedure results in (c) normal gingival sulcus depth.

(a)

(b)

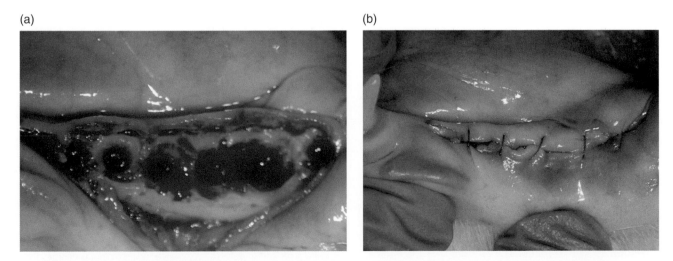

Figure 24.33 Closure of a (a) surgical extraction flap should preferably be done using a (b) buried knot suture technique.

access to oral structures must be very comfortable. It involves making a surgical incision into the pharynx in order to allow placement of an endotracheal tube or feeding tube (Figure 24.34). This tube is then removed immediately after surgery. Possible indications include maxillofacial trauma repair, temporomandibular joint luxations, palatal surgery for palatal tumors, and cleft palate. **Pharyngostomy** is a similar procedure performed when longer-term tube placement is required (e.g. feeding tube placement). Both are contraindicated if any proliferative lesions or other pathologies are present in the surgical area of the skin. Complications of pharyngotomy and pharyngostomy are related to injury of anatomic structures at the area of surgery: tonsils, hyoid bones, jugular vena, salivary glands, lingual arteria, or hypoglossus nerve (Gawor and Gawor 2014). An alternative to the above is oesophagostomy procedure (Fink et al, 2014).

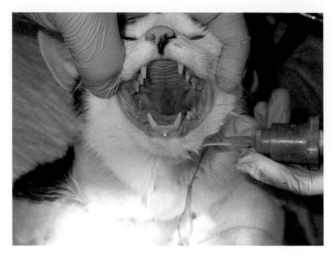

Figure 24.34 Pharyngotomy intubation.

References

Aguiar, J., Chebroux, A., Martinez-Taboada, F., and Leece, E.A. (2015). Analgesic effects of maxillary and inferior alveolar nerve blocks in cats undergoing dental extractions. *J. Feline Med. Surg.* 17 (2): 110–116.

Arzi, B., Clark, K.C., Sundaram, A. et al. (2017). Therapeutic efficacy of fresh, allogeneic mesenchymal stem cells for severe refractory feline chronic gingivostomatitis. *Stem Cells Transl. Med.* 6: 1710–1722.

Bar-Am, Y., Pollard, R., Kass, P., and Verstraete, F. (2008). The diagnostic yield of conventional radiographs & computed tomography in dogs & cats maxillofacial trauma. *Vet. Surg.* 37: 294–299.

Bar-Am, Y., Pollard, R.E., Kass, P.H., and Verstraete, F.J.M. (2008). The diagnostic yield of conventional radiographs and computed tomography in dogs and cats with maxillofacial trauma. *Vet. Surg.* 37: 294–299.

Beebe, D.E. and Gengler, W.R. (2007). Osseous surgery to augment treatment of chronic periodontitis of canine teeth in a cat. *J. Vet. Dent.* 24 (1).

Bell, C.M. and Soukup, J.W. (2015). Histologic clinical and radiologic findings of alveolar bone expansion and osteomyelitis of the jaws in cats. *Vet. Pathol.* 52: 910–918.

Bonner, S.E., Reiter, A.M., and Lewis, J.R. (2012). Orofacial manifestations of high-rise syndrome in cats: a retrospective study of 84 cases. *J. Vet. Dent.* 29 (1): 10–18.

Clarke, D.E. and Caiafa, A. (2014). Oral examination in the cat. A systematic approach. *J. Feline Med. Surg.* 16: 873–886.

DuPont GA. Crown amputation with intentional root retention for dental resorptive lesions in cats. *J Vet Dent.* 2002 Jun;19(2):107–10. PMID: 12108128.

Emily, P. (1992). Feline malocclusions. *Vet. Clin. North Am. Small Anim. Pract.* 22 (6): 1454.

FAB. (2008). WellCat for Life. Available from https://www.yumpu.com/en/document/read/7727281/wellcat-for-life-isfm (accessed July 5, 2020).

Fink, L., Jennings, M., and Reiter, A.M. (2014). Placement of esophagostomy feeding tubes in cats and dogs. *J. Vet. Dent.* 31: 133–138.

Force J, Niemiec B. Gingivectomy and Gingivoplasty for Gingival Enlargement. *Journal of Veterinary Dentistry.* 2009;26(2):132–137. doi:10.1177/089875640902600213

Gawor J (2017). Tooth resorption in cats affected by osteomyelitis of the jaws. Proceedings of the 26th EVDF, Malaga, May 18–20, 2017, 86.

Gawor, J. and Gawor, M. (2014). Faryngotomia i faryngostomia w zabiegach stomatologicznych i chirurgii szczękowej. *Mag Wet* 23 (200): 654–660.

Gaynor, J.S., Dunlop, C.I., Wagner, A.E. et al. (1999). Complications and mortality associated with anesthesia in dogs and cats. *JAAHA* 35: 13–17.

Gorrel, C. (2015). Tooth resorption in cats pathophysiology and treatment options. *J. Feline Med. Surg.* 17: 37–43.

Gorrel, C.E. and Hale, F.A. (2012). Gingivectomy and gingivoplasty. In: *Oral and Maxillofacial Surgery in Dogs and Cats* (eds. V. FJM and M.J. Lommer), 167–174. Philadelphia, PA: W.B. Saunders.

Gracis, M., Molinari, E., and Ferro, S. (2015). Caudal mucogingival lesions secondary to traumatic dental occlusion in 27 cats: macroscopic and microscopic description, treatment and follow-up. *J. Feline Med. Surg.* 17: 318–328.

Hennet PR, Camy GA, McGahie DM, Albouy MV. Comparative efficacy of a recombinant feline interferon omega in refractory cases of calicivirus-positive cats with caudal stomatitis: a randomised, multi-centre, controlled, double-blind study in 39 cats. J Feline Med Surg. 2011 Aug;13(8):577–87. doi:

Jennings, M.W., Lewis, J.R., Soltero-Rivera, M.M. et al. (2015). Effect of tooth extraction on stomatitis in cats: 95 cases (2000–2013). *J. Am. Vet. Med. Assoc.* 246 (6): 654–660.

Lewis, J., Tsugawa, A., and Reiter, A. (2007). Use of CO2 laser as an adjunctive treatment for caudal stomatitis in a cat. *J. Vet. Dent.* 24 (4): 240–249.

Lewis, J., Eked, A., Shofer, F. et al. (2008). Significant association between tooth extrusion and tooth resorption in domestic cats. *J. Vet. Dent.* 25 (2): 86–95.

Lommer, M. (2013). Efficacy of cyclosporine for chronic refractory stomatitis in cats: a randomised placebo controlled duble blinded clinical study. *J. Vet. Dent.* 30 (1): 8–17.

Lommer, M.J. (2013). Oral inflammation in small animals. *Vet. Clin. Small Anim.* 43: 555–571.

Millela, L. (2015). Occlusion and malocclusion in the cat what's normal, what's not and when's the best time to intervene? *J. Feline Med. Surg.* 17: 5–20.

Niemiec, B. (2014). *Veterinary Restorative Dentistry for the General Practitioner*. San Diego, CA: Practical Veterinary Publishing.

Niemiec, B.A. (2016). *Feline Dentistry Fro the General Practitioner*. San Diego, CA: Practical Veterinary Publishing.

Perry, R. (2015). Globe penetration in a cat following maxillary nerve block for dental surgery. *J. Feline Med. Surg.* 17: 66–72.

Perry, R. and Tutt, C. (2015). Periodontal disease in cats back to basics – with an eye on the future. *J. Feline Med. Surg.* 17: 45–65.

Pippi, R. (2017). Post-surgical clinical monitoring of soft tissue wound healing in periodontal and implant surgery. *Int. J. Med. Sci.* 14 (8): 721–728.

Reiter, A. (2014). Open wide. Blindness in cats after use of mouth gag. *Vet. J.* 201: 5–6.

Roza, M.R., Silva, L.A.F., Barriviera, M. et al. (2011). Cone beam computed tomography and intraoral radiography for diagnosis of dental abnormalities in dogs and cats. *J. Vet. Sci.* 12 (4): 387–392.

Rusbridge, C., Heath, S., Gunn-Moore, D.A. et al. (2010). Feline orofacial pain syndrome (FOPS): a retrospective study of 113 cases. *J. Feline Med. Surg.* 12 (6): 498–508.

Stebbins, K.E., Morse, C.C., and Goldschmidt, M.H. (1989). Feline oral neoplasia: a ten-year survey. *Vet. Pathol.* 26 (2): 121–128.

Verstraete, F.J., Kass, P.H., and Terpak, C.H. (1998). Diagnostic value of full-mouth radiography in cats. *Am. J. Vet. Res.* 59 (6): 692–695.

Vnuk, D., Pirkic, B., Maticic, D. et al. (2004). Feline high-rise syndrome: 119 cases (1998–2001). *J. Feline Med. Surg.* 6 (5): 305–312.

Wiggs, R.B. and Lobprise, H.B. (1997). Domestic feline oral and dental disease. In: *Veterinary Dentistry: Principles and Practice* (eds. R.B. Wiggs and H.B. Lobprise), 483–485. Philadelphia, PA: Lippincott-Raven.

Winer, J.N., Arzi, B., and Verstraete, F.J.M. (2016). Therapeutic management of feline chronic gingivostomatitis: a systematic review of the literature. *Front. Vet. Sci.* 3: 54.

Part IV

When to Call the Specialist

25

A Brief Introduction to Specific Oral and Dental Problems that Require Specialist Care

Jerzy Gawor

Veterinary Clinic Arka, Kraków, Poland

25.1 Introduction

The majority of daily veterinary dentistry (approximately 75%, in this author's experience) is made up of diagnostics, prophylaxis, and extractions. All other aspects of the discipline require advanced training, instrumentation, and technology. As they are less often performed, they frequently cause confusion and complications. Even experienced surgeons perform some procedures only rarely (in which case, it is worth practicing the relevant techniques on a cadaver before progressing to the live patient). If, based on the preoperative radiograph, it can be deduced that a case will be challenging, or if the practitioner is unskilled in the procedure or does not have access to the appropriate equipment, referral should be considered. This is much preferable to placing the patient's health and welfare in jeopardy.

A specialist is a veterinarian who, because of their experience, is prepared to negotiate numerous complications. Complications often arise when proper medical standards are not followed, but they can also occur due to the coincidence of unfavorable factors. Even a simple and common complication such as a root fracture during extraction can become a serious challenge when the root tip is pushed to the mandibular canal or nasal cavity. All potential complications should be considered prior to surgery, and a decision made about referring the case to a specialist before an irreversible problem occurs.

Some veterinarians are concerned that if they cannot offer advanced therapy, clients will lose confidence in their skills. Therefore, they see referring patients to a specialist as compromising their professional image. Finances may add an additional layer of complication: they see it as better to perform a simple procedure (e.g., extraction) instead of advanced therapy (e.g., root canal, periodontal surgery) in

order keep the income in-clinic rather than referring the patient out.

In general, both situations are incorrect, though there are always exceptions. The assumption that owners will expect all possible conditions to be managed by a general practitioner is erroneous in most cases. In this author's experience, clients are usually quite grateful to the referring veterinarian when their pet receives optimal treatment on time and in good condition. (From the specialist's perspective, it is important to express gratitude and credit to the cooperating veterinarian. This subject will be more widely discussed in the next chapter.) One exception is when the condition is very painful or life threatening, in which case the primary goal of treatment should be to relieve pain. In addition, the owner may have financial, schedule, or travel restrictions, though this should not be assumed.

25.2 Skills and Services

Specialists can offer a larger range of treatments than general practitioners, and it is their duty and privilege to present all available options for the management of a patient's condition. According to C. E. Harvey, "extraction is, in a way, an admission of failure for a dentist" (Harvey and Emily 1993). If a tooth can be saved and preserved, the option should always be made available. Offering extraction as the only solution for a dental problem is inappropriate.

There is nothing wrong with trying something for the first time, but if the trial is based only on theoretical knowledge, it can be frustrating for the operating veterinarian and create complications for the patient. In this author's experience, the best results are obtained by following these steps: reading, attending a lecture or online presentation,

The Veterinary Dental Patient: A Multidisciplinary Approach, First Edition. Edited by Jerzy Gawor and Brook Niemiec.
© 2021 John Wiley & Sons Ltd. Published 2021 by John Wiley & Sons Ltd.
Companion website: www.wiley.com/go/gawor/veterinary-dental-patient

assisting a specialist, performing cadaver practice, being supervised by a specialist, and then finally doing the procedure as the prime operator.

Every general practitioner is expected to provide the following dental services:

- Regular oral examinations as part of the clinical examination (e.g., at the time of vaccination or well-pet examination).
- Determination and application of the oral health index (OHI).
- First aid in oral or maxillofacial emergencies.
- Interpretation of preoperative blood profiles prior to all planned and emergency dental procedures that require sedation or anesthesia.
- Regular dental prophylaxis, including a thorough examination in conscious and sedated patient, dental charting, supragingival and subgingival scaling, polishing, gingival sulcal lavage, and charting of oral assessment results.
- Dental radiology and radiography at a quality level allowing for diagnosis and further consultation.
- Simple dental extractions.
- Prophylactic promotion and establishment of a home-care program, including tooth brushing, dietary support, dental chews and toys, and regular rechecks.

General practitioners should also have the knowledge and skills to:

- Identify basic orodental pathologies.
- Evaluate an occlusion.
- Identify oral structures on clinical and radiographic assessment.
- Perform tumor nodulus metastasis (TNM) evaluation of oral masses.
- Provide diagnostic protocol in maxillofacial injuries.

Some recommendations for the general practitioner who wants to improve their dental skills:

- When presented with an unknown oral pathology, never take the "wait and see" approach.
- Develop your skills, stay current with publications and books, and take part in dental promotions, discussions, and wet-labs.
- Training on cadavers will show you how far you can go. Ask a specialist to evaluate your work. Follow the gold standard for procedures even when working with cadavers.
- Tooth is not bone and gum is not skin. Oral surgery has numerous differences compared to orthopedic and soft-tissue surgery.
- Follow suggestions in the WSAVA Global Dental Guidelines.
- Do not use human dentists without experience in the veterinary field as a referral source – though they may provide a good knowledge of dental materials and instruments.

Any procedure can become advanced and complicated due to its complexity, technique sensitivity, or problems occurring intraoperatively. Management of such situations is easier for a specialist, who by definition is prepared and competent to deal with a wide range of clinical variations and unexpected scenarios. Any specialist will be capable of:

- Repairing oral and maxillofacial fractures.
- Endodontic procedures (root canal treatment).
- Oral and maxillofacial surgery, including palatal, temporomandibular joint (TMJ), and oncologic surgery.
- Orthodontics: preventive, interceptive, and corrective.
- Restorations of hard dental tissue damage.
- Periodontal surgery.
- Difficult extractions and management of their complications, including surgical extractions, oronasal fistulas (ONFs), and full-mouth extractions in cats and dogs.

25.3 Cases

The following cases are all examples that would benefit from referral. Note, however, that many more situations exist where a specialist might offer additional options and decrease the failure rate.

25.3.1 Case 1

Dog. Border collie. 1.5 years. Intact male. Complicated crown-root fracture of 208 with significant damage of distal root. Radiologic evaluation showed good condition of the mesial part of the tooth. The possible options for treatment included resection of the distal part followed by endodontic therapy of the mesial part or surgical extraction. Both procedures can be classified as advanced dentistry (Figure 25.1).

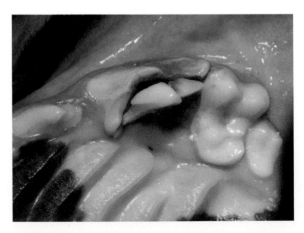

Figure 25.1 Complicated crown-root fracture of 208.

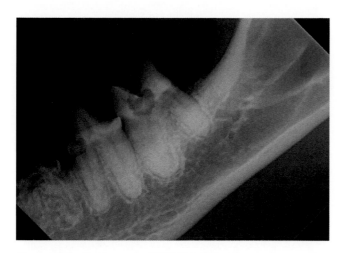

Figure 25.2 Radiograph of 307, 308, 309 with type 1 resorption present in 308, 309 and type 2 affecting 307.

25.3.2 Case 2

Cat. Norwegian forest. 13 years. Castrated male. Tooth resorptive lesions in the left mandibular third and fourth premolars and first molar (307, 308, 309). Type 1 resorption present in 308, 309, type 2 affecting 307. Surgical extraction of 308 and 309 and crown amputation of 307 is the only option to relieve pain and infection in this patient. The dental radiograph confirms presence of ankylosis and necessity of complete removal of the roots of 308, 309. The radiographic findings confirm that this will be a very difficult extraction. Postoperative dental radiographs are strongly encouraged to confirm complete removal of the teeth (Figure 25.2).

25.3.3 Case 3

Dog. Weimeraner. Two years. Castrated male. Squamous cell carcinoma. T3b, N1a, M0; III stage of growth. Wide resection of the tumor (2–3 cm margin) via a rostral mandibulectomy is the best treatment option. Following oncologic surgery standards, with respect to oral structures, proper closure and functionality of the remaining jaw are necessary for an acceptable final result (Figure 25.3).

25.3.4 Case 4

Cat. Persian. Eight months. Intact female. Traumatic class IV malocclusion with both side-to-side and rostrocaudal direction. Possible treatment options include orthodontic corrective treatment, crown height reduction followed by vital pulp therapy, and extraction of affected tooth with odontoplasty of lower canine to protect upper-lip entrapment. All should be performed by a specialist (Figure 25.4).

25.3.5 Case 5

Dog. Maltese. Eight years. Intact male. Nonstable mandibular fracture with root tip present in the fracture line. Treatment of the affected molar is required before stabilization of the fracture. Endodontic therapy with or without distal root resection must be done prior to fracture reduction and fixation (Figure 25.5).

25.3.6 Case 6

Dog. Yorkshire terrier. Six years. Intact male. Periodontal disease with pathologic pockets, gingival recession, and alveolar bone destruction of the maxillary incisors with 50% attachment loss. This problem can be solved either by extraction of the affected teeth or, if the patient qualifies, the owner is capable of daily home care, and the veterinarian is skilled, arrest and management of the disease by advanced procedures such as subgingival debridement, open curettage, root planning, teeth splinting, or periodontal flap surgery (Figure 25.6).

25.3.7 Case 7

Dog. German shepherd. Eight months. Intact female. Complicated crown fracture of canine tooth, which occurred two months prior to presentation. Radiographic assessment reveals periapical rarefaction and an open apex. The only treatment option for tooth salvage includes an apexification procedure, which requires access to endodontic instrumentation, sophisticated dental radiography, and certain materials (e.g., mineral trioxide aggreggate [MTA]) Alternatively, the tooth could be extracted (Figure 25.7).

25.3.8 Case 8

Cat. Domestic shorthaired. Eleven months. Spayed female. Palatal defect subsequent to high-rise syndrome. There were three previous unsuccessful surgeries. The next attempt is planned using an auricular cartilage graft (Figure 25.8).

25.3.9 Case 9

Dog. Golden retriever. Five years. Castrated male. Canine tooth (204) luxation subsequent to a dog fight. Reduction of the malpositioned tooth, intraoral stabilization, and subsequent endodontic treatment is required to save the tooth (Figure 25.9).

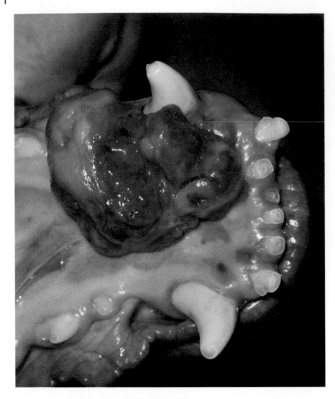

Figure 25.3   Squamous cell carcinoma of left rostral mandible. Clinical assessment: T3b, N1a, M0.

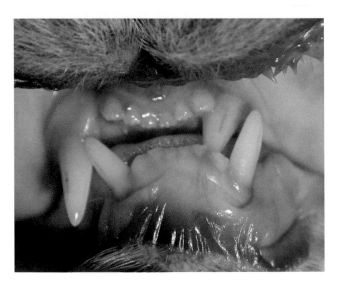

Figure 25.4   Class IV malocclusion in both side-to-side and rostrocaudal direction.

25.3.10   Case 10

Dog. Greyster. Five years. Male. Living in a kennel. Cage biter. Possible endodontic treatment of the fractured maxillary canine tooth (104) and prosthetic reinforcement of the mandibular canine tooth crown (404) with possible full jacket crown. A conservative composite restoration is not strong enough to avoid future damage (Figure 25.10).

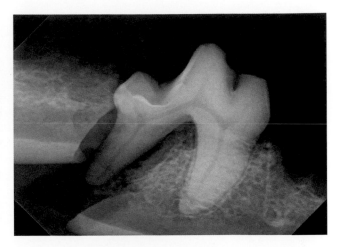

Figure 25.5   Nonstable mandibular fracture with root tip present in the fracture line.

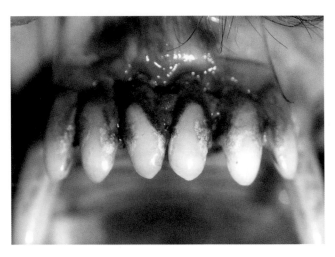

Figure 25.6   Periodontal disease with pathologic pockets, gingival recession, and alveolar bone destruction of the maxillary incisors with 50% attachment loss.

25.3.11   Case 11

Cat. Siamese. Four years. Spayed female. Left mandibular fracture involving the canine tooth (304) and a complicated crown/root fracture of the third premolar (307). This situation requires mandibular fracture stabilization, followed by endodontic treatment of 304 and extraction of damaged 307 when the stabilization is removed (Figure 25.11).

25.3.12   Case 12

Cat. Domestic shorthaired. Eight years. Intact female. High-rise syndrome after falling from the sixth floor. The pet suffers from the inability to close the mouth due to TMJ luxation, as well as numerous teeth fractures. Treatment requires surgical reduction of TMJ

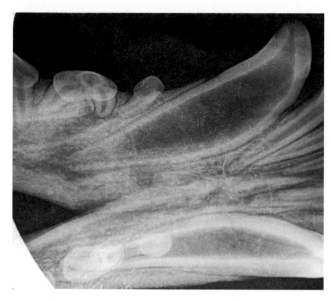

Figure 25.7 Complicated crown fracture of canine tooth 404 in 8 months old dog. Periapical rarefaction and an open apex indicate complicated pulp gangrene of immature tooth.

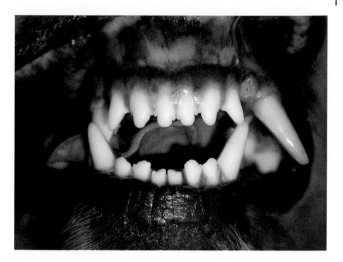

Figure 25.9 Left maxillary canine tooth (204) luxated after a dog fight.

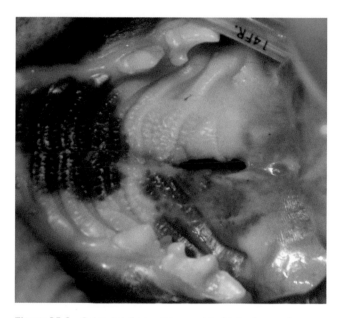

Figure 25.8 Palatal defect subsequent to high-rise syndrome, unsuccessfully treated three times.

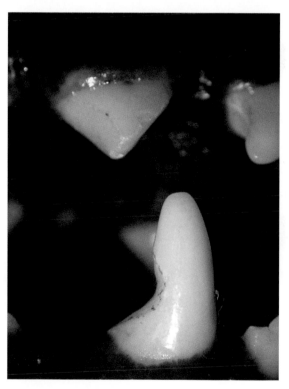

Figure 25.10 Right maxillary canine tooth (104) fracture and right mandibular canine tooth (404) with abrasion. Both require treatment.

luxation, maxillomandibular fixation, and temporary pulp dressing followed by extractions or endodontic treatment at the time of stabilization removal (Figure 25.12).

25.3.13 Case 13

Dog. Boxer. Four months. Cleft palate. It is very important to realize that the first surgical attempt has the highest chance for success, so long as it is properly performed. Because other abnormalities can be associated with cleft

palate, 3D diagnostic imaging is recommended to provide the whole diagnostic picture (Figure 25.13).

25.3.14 Case 14

Cat. Persian. Two years. Castrated male. Inability to open mouth three months after maxillofacial injury. Diagnostic imaging revealed TMJ pseudoankylosis caused by fusion of the right zygomatic arch with ipsilateral coronoid process.

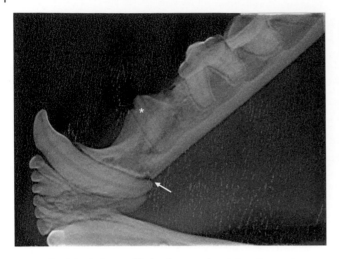

Figure 25.11   Left mandibular fracture involving the canine tooth (304) (arrow) as well as 307 which has a complicated crown/root fracture (asterisk).

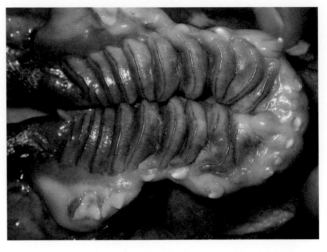

Figure 25.13   Cleft palate in a four-month-old boxer puppy.

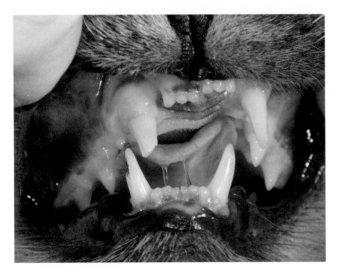

Figure 25.12   TMJ luxation causing inability to close the mouth, additionally right maxillary canine tooth (104) fracture is visible.

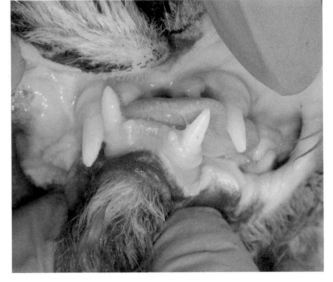

Figure 25.14   Cat with inability to open mouth three months after maxillofacial injury.

Treatment consists of careful surgical excision of the involved fused maxillofacial structures (Figure 25.14).

25.3.15   Case 15

Dog. Schnauzer. Eight months. Intact female. Bilateral impaction of the mandibular canine teeth. An alternative to extraction would be orthodontic extrusion of the impacted teeth (Figure 25.15). However, even surgical extraction of these teeth should be performed by a specialist.

25.3.16   Case 16

Cat. Domestic shorthaired. Two year. Spayed female. Lower-lip avulsion. Surgical debridement and reconstruction

of the lip attachment is the correct treatment for recovery of function and quality of life. Due to the traumatic origin of the damage, a thorough 3D imaging of the head is indicated (Figure 25.16).

25.3.17   Case 17

Cat. Domestic shorthaired. Eleven years. Castrated male. Buccal alveolar bone expansion and infra bony pocket of mandibular left canine (304). Reduction of the pocket with osteoplasty is an option for saving the tooth. Extraction of mandibular canines should not be the treatment of choice if realistic salvation options exist (Figure 25.17).

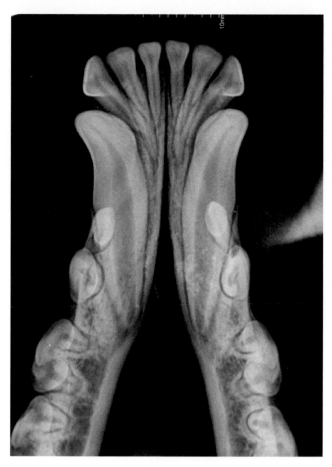

Figure 25.15   Bilateral impaction of the mandibular canine teeth.

25.3.18   Case 18

Dog. Mixed breed. Eight years. Spayed female. Significant periodontal pocket on the palatal aspect of the left maxillary canine (204). There is no oro-nasal communication. To save the tooth, advanced periodontal treatment (periodontal flap surgery, open root planning, and guided tissue regeneration) is necessary (Figure 25.18).

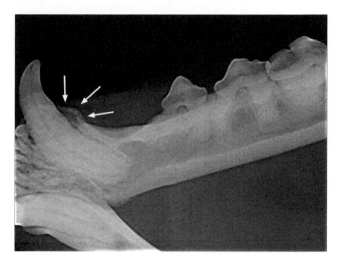

Figure 25.17   Buccal alveolar bone expansion and infra bony pocket of the mandibular left canine (304) (arrows).

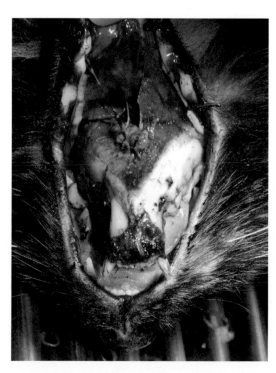

Figure 25.16   Cat with lower-lip avulsion

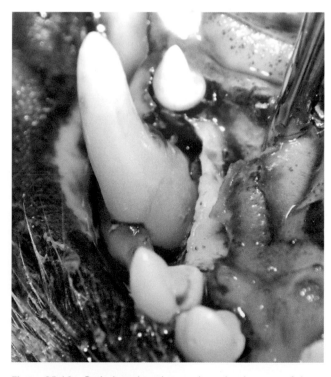

Figure 25.18   Periodontal pocket on the palatal aspect of the left maxillary canine (204).

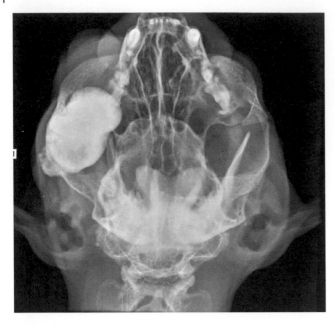

Figure 25.19 Mass localized under the zygomatic arch, affecting the eye (exophthalmos) and causing pain and disfunction of occlusion.

25.3.19 Case 19

Cat. Thirteen years. Castrated male. Maxillofacial mass (fibroma ossificans) localized under the zygomatic arch, affecting the eye (exophthalmos) and causing pain and dysfunction of occlusion. Excision of the tumor with eye

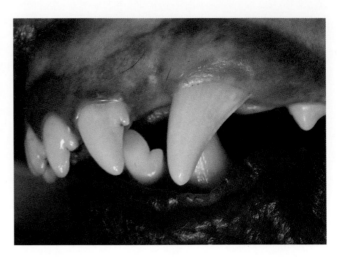

Figure 25.20 Class II malocclusion causing palatal defect.

enucleation is the best treatment option, providing the cat with comfort and functionality (Figure 25.19).

25.3.20 Case 20

Dog. German shepherd. Seven months. Intact male. Class II malocclusion (an abnormal rostrocaudal relationship between the dental arches, in which the mandibular arch occludes caudal to its normal position relative to the maxillary arch) causing palatal defect. Reduction of the mandibular canine crown height combined with vital pulp therapy would resolve the palatal trauma (Figure 25.20).

Further Reading

Bellows, J. (2004). Small Animal Dental Equipment, Materials and Techniques. *Blackwell.*

Harvey, C.E. and Emily, P.P. (1993). *Small Animal Dentistry.* St. Louis, MO: Mosby.

Holmstrom, SE; Frost, P; Eisner, ER. (2004). Veterinary Dental Techniques for the Small Animal Practitioner,3rd ed. Philadelphia: WB Saunders.

Mulligan, TW; Aller, MS; Williams, CA. (1998). Atlas of Canine and Feline Dental Radiography, Trenton. Veterinary Learning Systems.

Niemiec, BA. (2013) Veterinary Periodontology. Ames, Wiley Blackwell.

Niemiec, BA. (2013) Veterinary Orthodontics. Practical Veterinary Publishing. USA, San Diego.

Reiter, A; Gracis, M. (2018). BSAVA Manual of Canine and Feline Dentistry and Oral Surgery 4th edition BSAVA Publication.

Tutt, C. (2006). Small Animal Dentistry a manual of techniques. Blackwell Publishing.

Verstraete, FJM. (2012). Lommer MJ Oral and ~Maxillofacial Surgery in Dogs and Cats. 1st edn Saunders, Elsevier, Edinburgh.

Wiggs, RB; Lobprise, HB. (2019). Veterinary Dentistry: Principles and Practice, Wiley.

26

How to Cooperate with a Specialist

Brook Niemiec

Veterinary Dental Specialties and Oral Surgery, San Diego, CA, USA

26.1 Introduction

This chapter will be much less about the veterinary dental patient, though the benefit to the patient is central to the discussion. The specialization process is very long and difficult, and requires a significant investment in funds, time, and energy following veterinary school. Therefore, not everybody will decide to pursue this option. To be a specialist is to be competent in the entire discipline of dentistry (i.e., oral surgery, periodontology, restorative dentistry, endodontics, prosthodontics, and orthodontics), including theory, practice, materials, and techniques. In addition, due to the complex cases that are common to our profession, veterinary dental specialists are required to have an increased level of skill with general anesthesia. Nevertheless, a well-educated general practitioner can provide quality dental care for the majority of patients.

Because dental and oral problems are incredibly common in dogs and cats, it is important to provide quality service in resolving the most common oral diseases. Thanks to numerous workshops, training sessions, seminars, and so on, the number of veterinarians skilled in dental procedures is growing. Thus, there is a room for both the first-contact veterinarian, who may also effectively manage the most common dental diseases, and the specialist, who is dedicated to solving the more complicated cases. It is very important for both to realize how these two tiers of competence complement each other.

While board-certified veterinary dentists are still somewhat rare (approximately 190 worldwide at the time of this writing), most major metropolitan areas in North America and Europe have at least one. When seeking advice or referral for veterinary dentistry or oral surgery, it is always recommended to seek out an American Veterinary Dental College (AVDC) or European Veterinary Dental College (EVDC) diplomate. Even if none are available in your geographic

area, don't forget that some clients will be willing to travel long distances for proper care. This author routinely has clients drive five or six hours, and has treated patients in his California practice from Alaska, Japan, Mexico, and Korea. If a diplomate is still not an option, look for a Fellow of the Academy of Veterinary Dentistry. In addition, some countries (e.g., Australia, New Zealand, Germany) offer advanced certificates in veterinary dentistry. If none of these is an option either, locate a "dental enthusiast" as a final option.

26.2 What You Should Do

There are several keys to proper cooperation with a specialist. Paying decent attention to these areas will smooth the referral, improve communication, save time for everyone involved, and possibly save the client money and the patient additional therapy.

First and foremost, the specialist will often rely on the general practitioner for pre-anesthesia examination and testing. While always important, this is absolutely critical in cases where the client is traveling a long distance or surgery is planned on the first specialist visit. If a possible anesthesia concern is not discovered until the time of surgery, it will put the client, patient, and specialist in a bind. The client will likely have taken time off work and possibly driven some distance for the consultation, while the specialist likely scheduled out several hours for the surgery, and if it is not performed, it will affect their income. This leads to three possibilities, all of which are less than ideal:

- **Perform the work-up for the concern that day:** This negatively affects the specialist's and client's scheduling. In addition, testing is likely more expensive when performed same-day at a referral center. Finally, this is income that we as specialists would prefer the general practitioner to have.

- **Refer back to the general practitioner for the work-up:** Again, this negatively affects the client and specialist, as well as delaying care, causing suffering to the patient.
- **Perform the procedure regardless:** This increases the anesthetic risk.

Thus, a complete physical examination should be performed by the referring veterinarian, concentrating on the cardiopulmonary systems. Take particular care when examining the heart for arrhythmias and murmurs.

If a patient who would benefit from dental or oral surgical therapy has a systemic issue, this is another indication for a dental specialist. Veterinary dentists can perform dental procedures faster than general practitioners in the vast majority of cases. In addition, those in referral hospitals often have access to other specialists (e.g., cardiologists, anesthesiologists) and to advanced anesthesia techniques and monitoring, which can make anesthesia safer.

Ideally, all preoperative testing should be performed by the referring veterinarian and forwarded to the specialist prior to the consultation. If you have any question to regarding to what tests the specialist would like to run, feel free to call their office. In general, a complete blood count (CBC) and chemistry, and ideally a urinalysis and T4, is recommended/required prior to general anesthesia. Further testing (thoracic radiographs, cardiac or internal medicine work-up) is based on these tests and the physical exam.

Another thing that greatly improves the referral process is an accurate diagnosis. It is not unusual in veterinary dental referral practice for the client to want an estimate *prior* to seeing the specialist. While we try avoid this in practice if at all possible, it is sometimes a necessity. Therefore, having a good working diagnosis will assist in creating an approximate cost for the client. This is especially true if the condition has been discovered under general anesthesia at the general practice. All teeth that require treatment should be listed, and if at all possible dental radiographs and pictures should be included with the referral paperwork.

Finally, we request that general practitioners not attempt a procedure for which they are not trained (see Chapter 25). We understand that complications can arise with any surgical procedure, and in general a good specialist can help smooth over any client concerns. Prior to any procedure, you should think about the clinical problem that is to be managed as a complex challenge, not as being easy and predictable. Any operation can become a difficult one when unexpected complications arise. Tooth extraction is not generally considered advanced dentistry, but on occasion

complications can occur (e.g., a root fragment pushed to the mandibular canal) that are difficult to manage and require specialized skills and equipment.

It is always harder to fix a failed procedure than to perform it correctly in the first place. For example, retained roots are much more difficult to find and extract than an intact tooth. Another common issue is chronic oronasal fistula or palate defect repair. Each successive surgery makes closure more challenging due to tissue damage and scarring. Therefore, if your first attempt fails, all subsequent ones likely will as well. This author has been the fifth veterinarian performing the ninth surgery on a patient with a chronic oronasal fistula (ONF). The client was very frustrated, to say the least.

The other issue is that by the time the patient is referred, the client may have run out of funds to deal with the problem. When I was in general practice, I would refer many patients to specialists early in the course of treatment because even though they might have been more expensive initially, they could diagnose and treat conditions more efficiently and less expensively than I could due to their greater experience.

26.3 What to Expect from the Specialist

First, you should expect timely and complete communication with respect to diagnosis and treatment, particularly regarding any follow-up that you might need to perform. Ideally, you should receive the records by email on the day of surgery. If you have issues with a specialist's communication, please contact them. Referring doctors often have different ideas about how they wish to be communicated with: some want a phone call, some *do not* unless it is critical, and some don't care one way or the other. If you are dissatisfied by our communication, we wish to know about it!

Some veterinary dental specialist centers provide a referral form that can be uploaded from their website (Figure 26.1), or even have online referring. Use of such a form makes life easier and reduces the chances of miscommunication.

Next, you should expect to have your questions answered in a timely fashion. We understand that there is a plethora of new knowledge in all specialties, and it is impossible for a general practitioner to keep abreast of all areas. In general, specialists are happy to assist you to stay current. However, as human beings, we do tend to be more responsive to good referring veterinarians. If a veterinarian calls who routinely refers, we will do everything in our power to contact them ASAP, but if someone rarely (or never) refer cases, they may not be our priority – especially if they call frequently.

Patient Referral Information

Owner's Name:_____ Date of Referral:_____

Owner's Phone:(Hm#)_____ (Cell#)_____ Referring Doctor:_____

Referring Hospital:_____ (Hospital Phone#)_____

Pet's Name:_____ Age:_____ Sex:_____ Weight:_____ Breed:_____

Referred for: 1._____

2._____

3._____

Brief history of current problems:_____

_____

_____

_____

Diagnostic Test Results *(PLEASE ATTACH A COPY OF MOST RECENT BLOOD TESTS, LAB RESULTS, AND RADIOGRAPHIC FINDINGS)*:

_____

_____

_____

_____

Treatments & Medications Administered (list **ALL** drugs prescribed, including dosage and duration):_____

_____

_____

_____

PLEASE INSTRUCT PET OWNERS TO CONTINUE GIVING ALL MEDICATIONS AS PREVIOUSLY PRESCRIBED

Comments:_____

_____

_____

Endodontics, Periodontics, Orthodontics, Oral Surgery, Crowns, Restoratives & Oral Radiography

* Locations of our four practices are on the back of this sheet *

Figure 26.1 Referral form, Arizona Veterinary Dental Specialists.

Finally, you should expect continuing education (CE) or continuing professional development (CPD) from your specialist. If your local referral hospital does not routinely put on lectures or send out newsletters, ask for them. This interaction can greatly improve the veterinarian–specialist relationship. It is in the best interest of the patient if the first-contact veterinarian can properly manage problems requiring immediate treatment. Therefore, specialists spend time teaching veterinary colleagues and nurses how to diagnose and treat emergency cases. Online learning is a common means of cooperation, though this can have certain limitations, which must be understood (Figure 26.2).

26.4 Conclusion

We think of general practitioners as our partners in oral health. With our advanced training, we can provide the latest therapies – as well as traditional ones – in the most efficient and atraumatic ways. For those interested in specialty work, the referral should be made. We ask you to perform the necessary preoperative work-up, and we promise to provide timely and accurate communication.

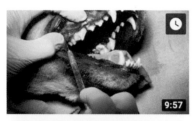

Veterinary Dentistry - Nerve Blocks for Oral Surgery for Dogs and Cats
VeterinaryDentistry • 154 tys. wyświetleń • 7 lat temu

Local nerve blocks in veterinary **dentistry** for oral surgery in **dogs** and cats. For veterinary **dental** courses, labs and classes please ...

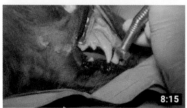

Veterinary Dental Maxillary Canine Tooth Extraction in a Dog
VeterinaryDentistry • 173 tys. wyświetleń • 7 lat temu

For veterinary **dental** courses and webinars please visit: http://veterinarydentistry.net/

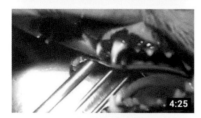

Canine Tooth Extraction
Suburban Animal Clinic • 138 tys. wyświetleń • 8 lat temu

Dr. Missy Shardy walks you through an **extraction** of a diseased **canine tooth** in a **dog**.

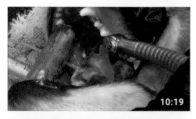

Surgical Tooth Extraction at Poulsbo Animal Clinic
Poulsbo Animal Clinic • 31 tys. wyświetleń • 4 lata temu

Watch Dr. Craig Adams of Poulsbo Animal Clinic step-by-step as he extracts an upper 4th premolar from a **dog** named Riley.

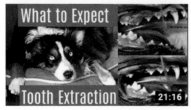

What to Expect - Dog Tooth Extraction
Animal Scholar • 7,4 tys. wyświetleń • 12 miesięcy temu

What happens when your **dog** needs to have a **tooth** extracted? Here's an explanation on what to expect before and after surgery, ...

Figure 26.2   Example of e-learning available on YouTube.

Useful Algorithms for the Management of Oral Problems
Jerzy Gawor

Oral Health Index

Ranking of evaluated parameters identified during oral cavity assessment and interview

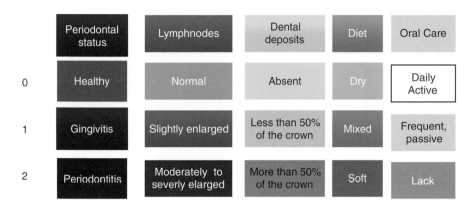

	Periodontal status	Lymphnodes	Dental deposits	Diet	Oral Care
0	Healthy	Normal	Absent	Dry	Daily Active
1	Gingivitis	Slightly enlarged	Less than 50% of the crown	Mixed	Frequent, passive
2	Periodontitis	Moderately to severly elarged	More than 50% of the crown	Soft	Lack

Summary: possible score: 0–10 subdivided into three categories of the patients:

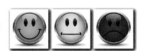

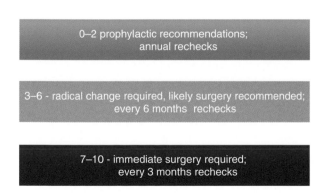

0–2 prophylactic recommendations; annual rechecks

3–6 - radical change required, likely surgery recommended; every 6 months rechecks

7–10 - immediate surgery required; every 3 months rechecks

Periodontal diseases 1

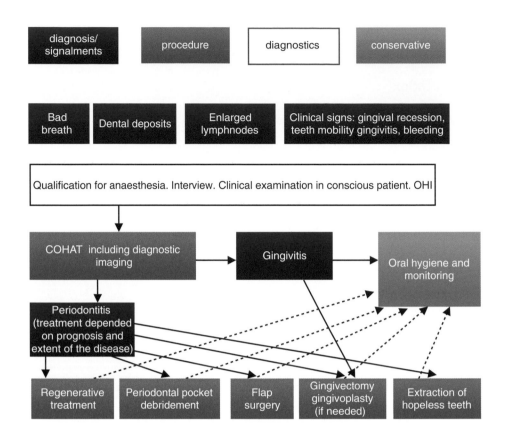

Periodontal diseases 2

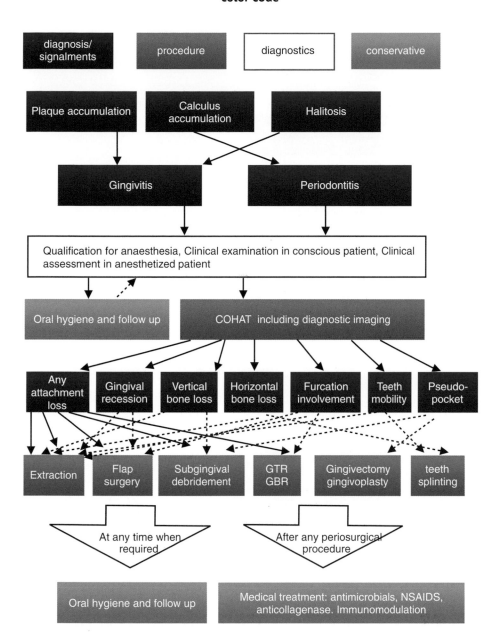

High Rise Syndrome or Head injury

color code

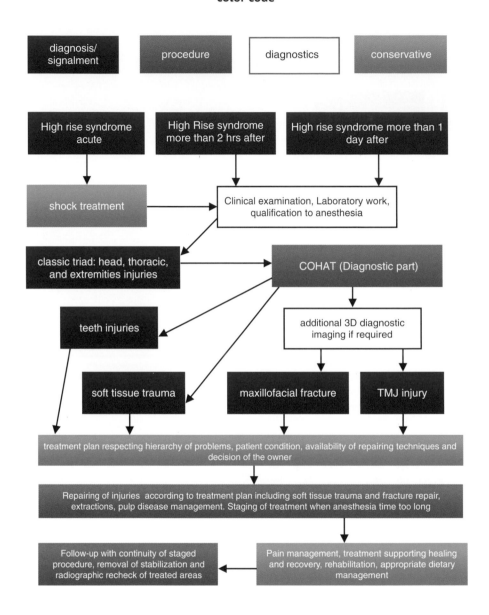

Teeth injuries

color code

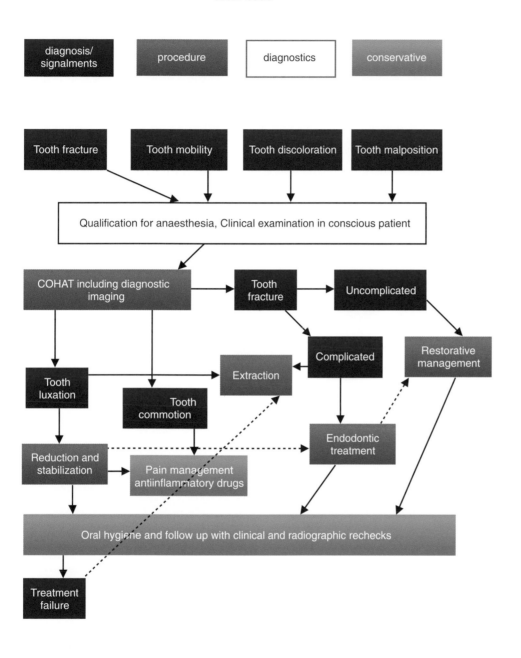

Pulp disease

color code

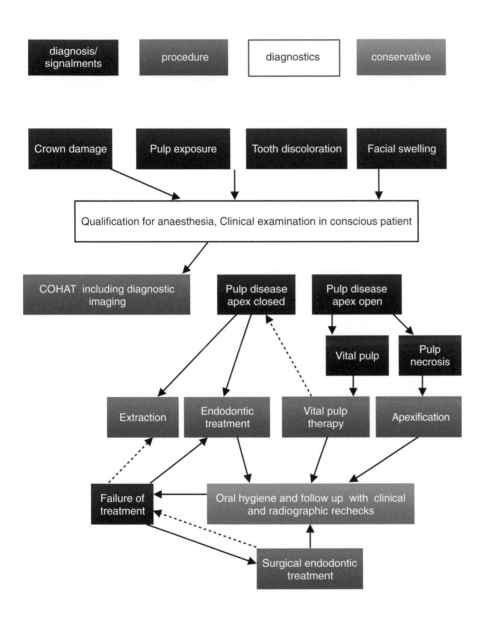

| diagnosis/signalments | procedure | diagnostics | conservative |

Crown damage — Pulp exposure — Tooth discoloration — Facial swelling

Qualification for anaesthesia, Clinical examination in conscious patient

COHAT including diagnostic imaging — Pulp disease apex closed — Pulp disease apex open

Vital pulp — Pulp necrosis

Extraction — Endodontic treatment — Vital pulp therapy — Apexification

Failure of treatment — Oral hygiene and follow up with clinical and radiographic rechecks

Surgical endodontic treatment

Oral mass

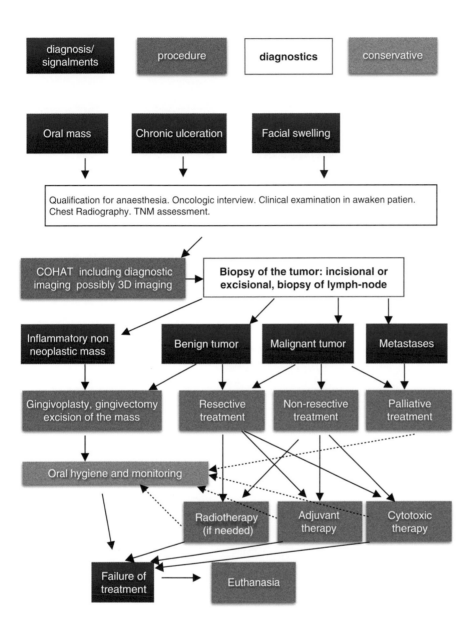

Orthodontics

color code

| diagnosis/ signalment | procedure | diagnostics | conservative |

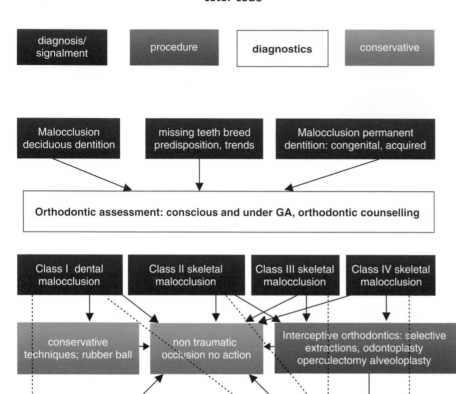

Inflammatory feline oral diseases

color code

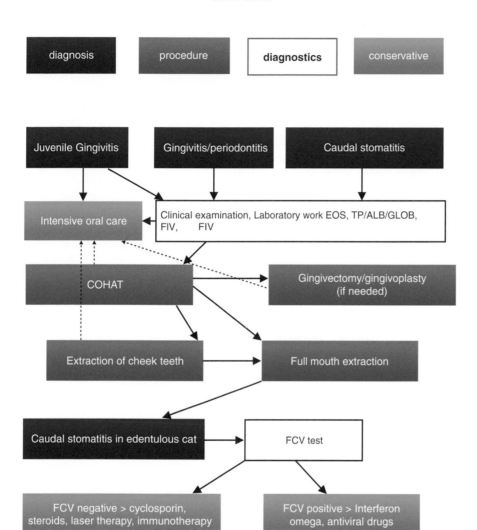

Teeth resorption

color code

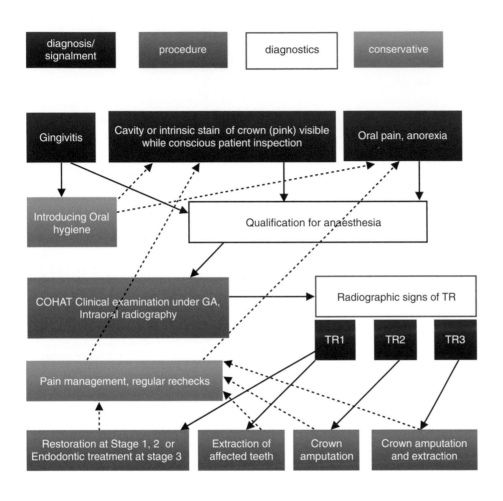

| diagnosis/ signalment | procedure | diagnostics | conservative |

Appendix A

Drugs and Doses

Margo Karriker

University of California Veterinary Medical Center, San Diego, CA, USA

Anti-inflammatory Drugs

Drug name	Mechanism of action	Dose (F = feline, C = canine)	US trade names	References
Carprofen	NSAID; non-selective COX inhibitor	C: 4.4 mg/kg PO or SQ every 24 hours; or 2.2 mg/kg PO or SQ every 12 hours. SQ doses should be administered 2 hours prior to procedure. F: 4 mg/kg SQ or IV, given preoperatively at the time of induction of anesthesia	Rimadyl; generic	Plumb's Veterinary Drugs. Brief Media. 2019 Rimadyl injection package insert. Zoetis. May 2019. Rimadyl caplets package insert. Zoetis. May 2019.
Deracoxib	NSAID; COX-2 selective	C: For pain and inflammation: 1–2 mg/kg PO every 24 hours for 3 days F: None	Deramaxx	Deramaxx package insert. Elanco US.
Firocoxib	NSAID; COX-2 selective	C: 5 mg/kg PO every 24 hours for 3 days for postsurgical pain and inflammation F: None	Previcox	Previcox package insert. Boehringher Ingelheim. December 2018.
Grapiprant (Galliprant)		C: 2 mg/kg PO once daily.		Galliprant package insert. Elanco US.
Meloxicam	NSAID; COX-2 selective	C: 0.2 mg/kg IV, SQ, or PO once; after 24 hours, followed with 0.1 mg/kg PO every 24 hours F: 0.3 mg/kg SQ once	Metacam, generic	Metacam injection package insert. Boehringer Ingelheim Vetmedica, Inc. September 2019. Metacam oral suspension package insert. Boehringer Ingelheim Vetmedica, Inc. August 2019.
Robenacoxib	NSAID; COX-2 selective	C: 2 mg/kg SQ or PO every 24 hours. SQ doses should be administered 45 minutes prior to the procedure. F: 2 mg/kg SQ every 24 hours for 3 days; 1 mg/kg PO every 24 hours for a maximum of 3 days. First dose should be administered 30 minutes prior to procedure.	Onsior	Onsior injection package insert. Elanco US. Onsior tablets package insert. Elanco US.
Corticosteroids	Consult pharmacology reference of choice.			

The Veterinary Dental Patient: A Multidisciplinary Approach, First Edition. Edited by Jerzy Gawor and Brook Niemiec.
© 2021 John Wiley & Sons Ltd. Published 2021 by John Wiley & Sons Ltd.
Companion website: www.wiley.com/go/gawor/veterinary-dental-patient

Analgesics

Drug name	Mechanism of action	Dose (F = feline, C = canine)	US trade names	References
Nocita (bupivacaine liposomal)	No acceptable doses at this time.			
Bupivicaine/ lidocaine	local analgesic	C: 1-2mg/kg F: 1mg/kg		Plumb DC. Bupivacaine. https://www.plumbsveterinarydrugs.com/#!/monograph/Ljf37PSR3g/. Updated July 2017. Accessed October 2020
Buprenorphine (including Simbadol)	Opioid, mu partial agonist	C: (using Simbadol): 0.02mg/kg IM C: 0.01–0.03 mg/kg SQ, IV up to every six hours 0.12mg/kg OTM up to every six hours F: Using SIMBADOL 1.8 mg/mL injection: 0.24 mg/kg SQ every 24 hours for up to three days; administer the first dose approximately one hour prior to surgery Using Buprenex or generic 0.3 mg/mL injection: 0.01–0.03 mg/kg SQ, IV or OTM up to every six hours	Simbadol, Buprenex, generic	Simbadol injection package insert. Zoetis. July 2017. Ko, J. C., Freeman, L. J., Barletta, M., et al. (2011). Efficacy of oral transmucosal and intravenous administration of buprenorphine before surgery for postoperative analgesia in dogs undergoing ovariohysterectomy. *J. Am. Vet. Med. Assoc.*, 238(3): 318–328. Plumb DC. Buprenorphine. Plumb's Veterinary Drugs. https://www.plumbsveterinarydrugs.com/#!/monograph/8r3dFe6zhm/. Updated June 2019. Accessed October 2020.
Butorphanol	Opioid, agonist/ antagonist	C: 0.1–0.5 mg/kg SQ, IV, or IM up to every 2 hours or as CRI of 0.1–0.4 mg/kg/hour F: 0.4 mg/kg SQ up to every 6 hours for 4 days; First dose should be at least 20 minutes prior to procedure	Torbutrol, Torbugesic, Dolorex, generic	Torbugesic-SA injection package insert. Zoetis. July 2019. Plumb DC. Butorphanol Tartrate. Plumb's Veterinary Drugs. https://www.plumbsveterinarydrugs.com/#!/monograph/qZ8Rb9KuWc/. Updated December 2019. Accessed October 2020.
Codeine	Opioid, mu agonist	C: Combined with acetaminophen, 1-3mg/kg PO q 8 hours		Plumb DC. Codeine. Plumb's Veterinary Drugs. https://www.plumbsveterinarydrugs.com/#!/monograph/QKJzRidEUS/. Updated March 2020. Accessed October 2020.
Fentanyl (including Recuvyra)	Opioid, mu receptor agonist	Using transdermal patch: 1–5 mcg/kg/hour; duration of analgesia is up to 96 hours Using injection: 2–10 µg/kg IV or as a CRI F: Using transdermal patch: 12 µg per cat/hour; duration of analgesia up to 96 hours Using injection: 2–10 µg/kg IV or as a CRI	Duragesic, Sublimaze, generic	Bellei, E., Roncada, P., Pisoni, L., et al. (2011). The use of fentanyl-patch in dogs undergoing spinal surgery: plasma concentration and analgesic efficacy. *J. Vet. Pharmacol. Ther.*, 34(5): 437–441. Plumb DC. Fentanyl Transdermal Patch. Plumb's Veterinary Drugs. https://www.plumbsveterinarydrugs.com/#!/monograph/HhKoswRxVt/. Updated August 2017. Accessed October 2020. Plumb DC. Fentanyl Citrate Injection. Plumb's Veterinary Drugs. https://www.plumbsveterinarydrugs.com/#!/monograph/Gs92zeeJLI/. Updated April 2020. Accessed October 2020.

Drug name	Mechanism of action	Dose (F = feline, C = canine)	US trade names	References
Gabapentin	Structurally related to GABA; however, analgesic and anticonvulsant mechanism of action is unknown	C: 10–20 mg/kg PO q 8 hours; 30 mg/kg PO q 6 hours may be required F: 10–20 mg/kg PO q 8 hours	Neurontin, generic	KuKanich, B. (2013). Outpatient oral analgesics in dogs and cats beyond nonsteroidal antiinflammatory drugs: an evidence-based approach. *Vet. Clin. North Am. Small Anim. Pract.*, 43(5): 1109–1125. Plumb DC. Gabapentin. Plumb's Veterinary Drugs. https://www.plumbsveterinarydrugs.com/#!/monograph/CSJtfV8dnf/. Updated September 2019. Accessed October 2020.
Hydromorphone	Opioid, mu receptor agoninst, delta receptor agonist	C: 0.05–0.1 mg/kg SQ, IM, or IV up to every 2 hours or as a CRI F: 0.05–0.1 mg/kg SQ, IM, or IV up to every 2 hours or as a CRI		Bateman, S. W., Haldane, S., and Stephens, J. A. (2008). Comparison of the analgesic efficacy of hydromorphone and oxymorphone in dogs and cats: a randomized blinded study. *Vet. Anaesth. Analges.*, 35(4): 341–347.
Methadone HCl	Opioid, mu receptor agonist; NMDA inhibitor	C: 0.1–0.5 mg/kg SQ, IM, or IV up to every 4 hours or as a CRI F: 0.05–0.5 mg/kg SQ, IM, or IV up to every 4 hours or as a CRI	Generic	Plumb DC. Methadone HCl. Plumb's Veterinary Drugs. https://www.plumbsveterinarydrugs.com/#!/monograph/Ez66Xm6taB/. Updated March 2020. Accessed October 2020.
Morphine sulfate	Opioid, mu receptor agoninst, delta receptor agonist	C: 0.5–2 mg/kg SQ, IM, or IV up to every 2 hours; or as a CRI of 0.1–0.2 mg/kg every hour F: 0.05–4 mg/kg SQ IM, or IV up to every 3 hours	Generic	Plumb DC. Morphine sulfate. Plumb's Veterinary Drugs. https://www.plumbsveterinarydrugs.com/#!/monograph/5BqpZtqbxG/. Updated August 2017. Accessed October 2020.
Tramadol	Opioid, mu receptor agonist	C: 4–10 mg/kg PO every 6–12 hours F: 1–2 mg/kg PO q 12–24 hours	Generic	KuKanich, B. (2013). Outpatient oral analgesics in dogs and cats beyond nonsteroidal antiinflammatory drugs: an evidence-based approach. *Vet. Clin. North Am. Small Anim. Pract.*, 43(5): 1109–1125.

Anesthetics/Sedatives

Drug name	Mechanism of action	Dose (F = feline, C = canine)	US trade names	References
Acepromazine maleate	Phenothiazine neuroleptic agent	C: 0.55–0.6 mg/kg SQ, IM, or IV; 0.55–2.2 mg/kg PO F: 1.1–2.2 mg/kg SQ, IM, or IV	PromAce injectable, generic	PromAce injectable package insert. Boehringer Ingelheim Vetmedica Inc. August 2019. PromAce tablets package insert. Boehringer Ingelheim Vetmedica Inc. June 2012.
Alfaxalone	Neuroactive steroid	C: For induction: 1.5–4.5 mg/kg IV without a preanesthetic; 0.2–3.5 mg/kg IV with a preanesthetic For maintenance anesthesia: 1.2–2.2 mg/kg IV over 60 seconds, every 6–8 minutes. F: For induction: 2.2–9.7 mg/kg IV without a preanesthetic; 1.0–10.8 mg/kg IV with a preanesthetic For maintenance anesthesia: 1.1–1.5 mg/kg IV over 60 seconds, every 7–8 minutes	Alfaxan injectable	Alfaxan Multi-dose injectable package insert. Jurox Pty. Ltd.
Dexmedetomidine	Synthetic alpha$_2$ adrenoreceptor agonist	C: For sedation and analgesia: 500 mcg/m^2 IM; 375 mcg/m^2 IV For preanesthesia: 125–375 mcg/m^2 IM F: 40 mcg/kg IM	Dexdomitor injection, generic	Dexdomitor injection package insert. Zoetis. August 2013.
Diazepam	Benzodiazepine	C: 0.1–0.5mg/kg IV F: 0.1–0.3mg/kg IV	Valium	Plumb DC. Diazepam. Plumb's Veterinary Drugs. https://www.plumbsveterinarydrugs.com/#!/monograph/x9Kt8MPnT1/. Updated June 2019. Accessed October 2020.
Etomidate	non-barbiturate anesthetic	C and F: 0.5–2 mg/kg IV	Amidate	Plumb DC. Etomidate. Plumb's Veterinary Drugs. https://www.plumbsveterinarydrugs.com/#!/monograph/MTfSgjwZnr/. Updated July 2017. Accessed October 2020.
Ketamine	NMDA-Receptor Antagonist	C: 5–7mg/kg IM (in combination) F: 22–33 mg/kg IM (single agent); 5–7mg/kg IM (in combination)	Ketaset	Ketaset package insert. Zoetis. June 2019 Plumb DC. Ketamine. Plumb's Veterinary Drugs. https://www.plumbsveterinarydrugs.com/#!/monograph/imxUTZ1jdB/. Updated August 2018. Accessed October 2020.
Midazolam	Benzodiazepine	C and F: 0.1–0.3mg/kg SQ, IM or IV	Versed	Plumb DC. Midazolam. Plumb's Veterinary Drugs. https://www.plumbsveterinarydrugs.com/#!/monograph/4yqiVGLueS/. Updated February 2020. Accessed October 2020.

Drug name	Mechanism of action	Dose (F = feline, C = canine)	US trade names	References
Propfol	Sedative hypnotic	C and F: For induction: 3.2–7.6 mg/kg IV to effect For maintenance: 1.7–3.2 mg/kg IV		Propoflo-28 package insert. Zoetis Inc. October 2019.
Tiletamine/Zolazepam	Anesthetic/tranquilizer combination	C: 9.9–13.2 mg/kg IM F: 9.7–11.9 mg/kg IM	Telazol	Plumb DC. Tiletamine/zolazepam. Plumb's Veterinary Drugs. https://www.plumbsveterinarydrugs.com/#!/monograph/0QaV5IcknK/. Updated October 2017. Accessed October 2020. Telazol package insert. Zoetis. June 2019
Telazol				
Trazodone	5-HT2A and 5-HT2C (serotonin) antagonist/reuptake inhibitor	C: 3–5mg/kg PO q 12 hours F: 50mg/cat PO q 12-24 hours	generic	Plumb DC. Trazodone. Plumb's Veterinary Drugs. https://www.plumbsveterinarydrugs.com/#!/monograph/ba9xQv20CJ/. Updated June 2019. Accessed October 2020.

Appendix B

Instruments Handling and Sharpening

Jerzy Gawor

Veterinary Clinic Arka, Kraków, Poland

B.1 Introduction

In Chapter 1, we advised you to invest in high-quality equipment and instrumentation, using distributors that provide very good service. Quality instruments are more resistant to rust and damage, and provide better procedure outcomes if used properly. In addition, immediate service or replacement when instruments break is crucial for continuity of dental care (Figure B.1).

Even the best instruments from the best brands require maintenance and sharpening. This will increase their lifespan and improve the quality of service. They should be maintained as close as possible to their original state in terms of shape and design. Working with sharp instruments is more efficient, faster, and more tissue-friendly, and minimizes chronic wrist and hand injuries and fatigue.

Before sharpening, instruments should be cleaned and sterilized to avoid contamination of the sharpening kit by dirt or contagious debris. However, sterilization blunts the working edges, necessitating further sharpening. The use of proper disinfectant or cleaning media, brushes, and wipes (ideally, the ones recommended by the manufacturer) is strongly recommended. The quality of water used during the depuration process is important, as poor water composition can affect both the process itself and the appearance of the instruments.

Numerous dental procedures involve the use of chemical compounds that can be damaging to instruments if not carefully removed from their surfaces after use. In particular, the chlorides are dangerous and may cause pitting, even of stainless steel. Any remnants of dental materials must be removed from instrumentation immediately following a procedure. Tap water contains chemicals that can cause staining or corrosion of instruments, so for particularly precious instruments, a final rinse with demineralized water is recommended.

Machine-based cleaning is convenient and improves cleaning standards, but it requires additional counter space. In addition, machine cleaning is of value only when there are enough instruments to warrant it. Fragile instrumentation must be placed in organizers to ensure its stabile position and lack of movement during the cleaning process.

Ultrasonic cleaning is recommended for all instruments that have microscopic areas where debris can accumulate (e.g., saw blades, burs, serrated cutting edges, etc.) (Figure B.2).

Visual inspection of cleaned instruments is important and any inadequate cleaning must be repeated. This is a good opportunity to identify damaged or broken instruments (Figure B.3).

Cassettes, boxes, and organizers help in organizing the kits needed for specific surgical procedures. Additionally, they keep instruments in position, reducing the risk of mechanical damage of fragile parts by friction or frequent contact.

Mineral deposits can be removed by acid-based detergents, following manufacturer's recommendations. Silicate build-up can be removed by hydrofluoric acid-containing agents. If there is any doubt, it is best to contact the manufacturer prior to attempting to remove or treat any corrosion, stains, and so on.

B.2 Sterilization

Steam sterilization of specula and mirrors should not be done too often, as they can become dull. Instruments that are thermostable can be autoclaved according to manufacturer's instructions, though handpieces and "elbows" (hinges) can only undergo this treatment at up to 134 °C and for minimal durations.

Dry heat can be used for all dental instruments except turbines, grips, and contra-angles

The Veterinary Dental Patient: A Multidisciplinary Approach, First Edition. Edited by Jerzy Gawor and Brook Niemiec.
© 2021 John Wiley & Sons Ltd. Published 2021 by John Wiley & Sons Ltd.
Companion website: www.wiley.com/go/gawor/veterinary-dental-patient

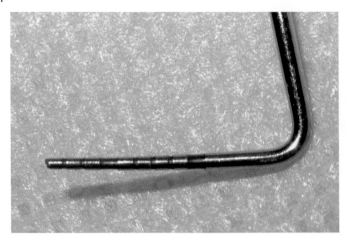

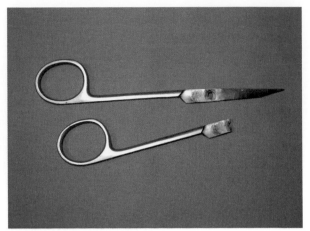

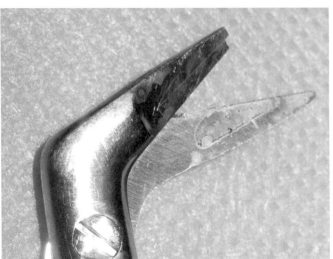

Figure B.1 Broken instrument examples.

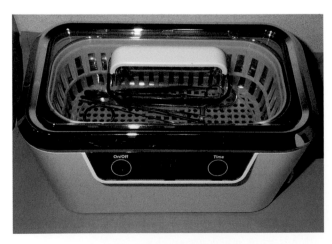

Figure B.2 Ultrasonic cleaning is very useful for small instruments with areas prone to entrapping debris.

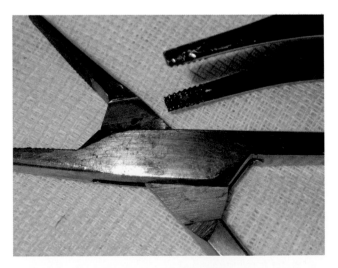

Figure B.3 Careful inspection after cleaning is necessary for quality control and to reveal breakage.

Gas sterilization methods are rarely used in veterinary dentistry, but they may be utilized for certain things, such as implants containing polymers and metal.

B.3 Sharpening

Sharp-edged instruments must be sharpened on a regular basis (Hale 2004). This includes scalers, scissors, curettes, luxators, and elevators. The most common advice is to sharpen them after each use; in the case of curettes, it may be best to sharpen them every 10–15 working strokes (Niemiec 2012). The best way of determining the sharpness of a curette or scaler is to use an acrylic test stick. Here, the instrument is held in a modified pen grasp, with the face plane perpendicular to the long axis of the stick. If the cutting edge bites into the acrylic, the instrument is sharp. If it does not bite in but slides along the acrylic, the instrument is dull (Figure B.4).

Sharpening is easier when using a specific dental instrument sharpening kit, which will include a selection of stones and oil (Figure B.5). Instruments can be sharpened using several different types of stones in several different shapes:

- **Arkansas Stones:** Natural stone used for routine sharpening and finishing, available in flat and conical shapes.
- **India Stones:** Synthetic stone used for recontouring of a dull instrument, available in cylindrical (used for toes and faces) and wedge (used for edges, toes, and faces) shapes.
- **Ceramic Stones:** Synthetic stone used for routine sharpening and finishing of an instrument.

Cleaned and sterilized scalers and curettes should be sharpened before each use with a flat stone. The goal of sharpening is to retain the 70–80° angle between the face and the lateral surface of the working tip, or a 110° angle between the face and the stone (Figure B.6).

It is critical to know what type of curette is being sharpened in order to properly maintain the cutting edge. For Gracey curettes (area-specific), only the lower edge of the face should be sharpened, while for universal curettes and scalers, sharpening can be carried out on all sharp edges.

Luxators and elevators also need to be sharpened regularly, using a cylindrical Arkansas stone and oil. The tip of the elevator should be sharpened on the convex side (Figure B.7), while the luxator should be sharpened on the concave one (Figure B.8). If the working part is significantly damaged, it should be professionally repaired or returned to the manufacturer.

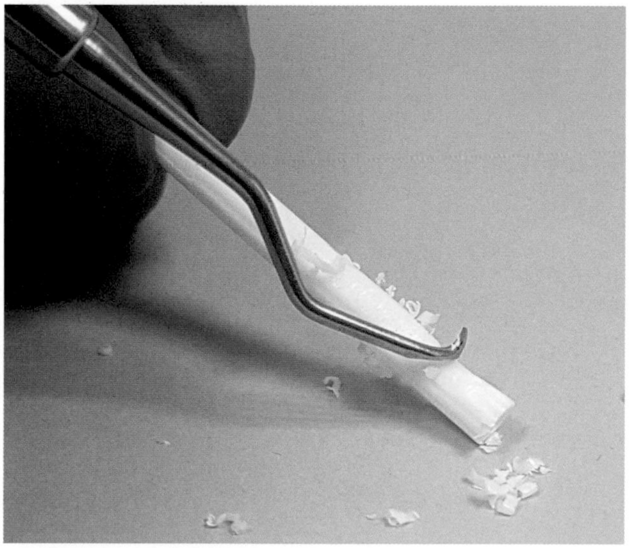

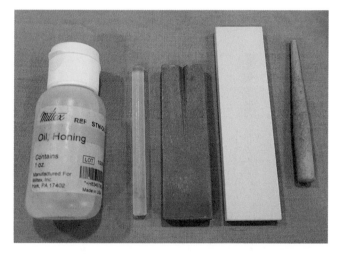

Figure B.5 Sharpening equipment includes: oil, acrylic stick and selection of stones.

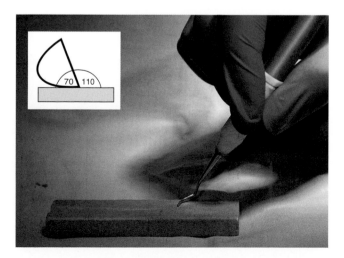

Figure B.6 A 110° angle should be maintained between face of a currette and the sharpening stone.

Figure B.4 Acrylic stick test of sharpness.

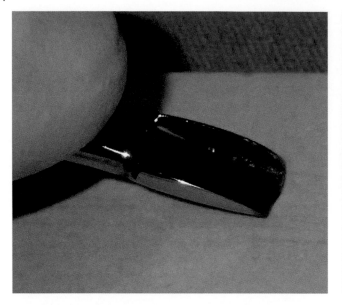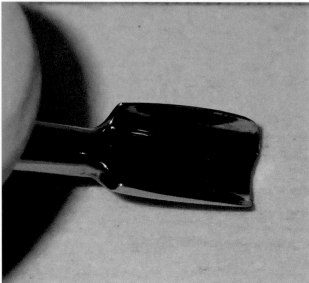

Figure B.7   The tip of an elevator should be sharpened on the convex side.

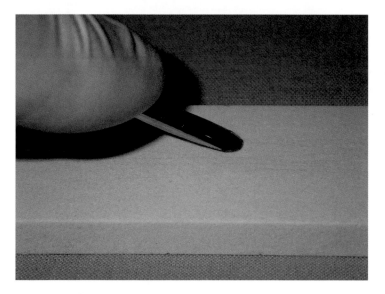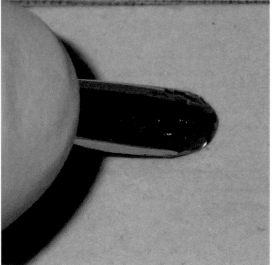

Figure B.8   A luxator should be sharpened on the concave side.

Commercial sharpening machines are available, but using them requires skill and experience (Figure B.9). Without these, the risk of irreversible damage is significant.

Videos are available on YouTube showing correct instrument sharpening techniques.

B.4   Maintenance of Power Equipment

Radiography Equipment

The surface of the arms and the generator head must be wiped with disinfectant after each use. The phosphoric plates require caution, but if dirt is identified they should be cleaned with disposable wipes (e.g., for glasses) and then dried. Both the sensor and the phosphoric plates should be protected during cleaning by single-use sleeves or pouches. The sensor should be cleaned with unkinked wire. Protective containers can be used for safe storage during cleaning.

Ultrasonic Scalers

All scaler tips should be sterilized after each use. Their length and shape should be checked on a frequent basis,

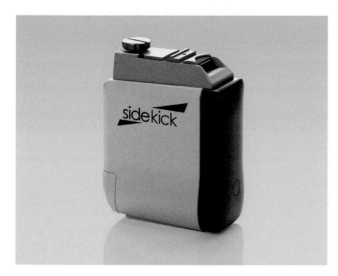

Figure B.9   Mechanized Hu-Friedy sharpener for sharpening scalers and currettes.

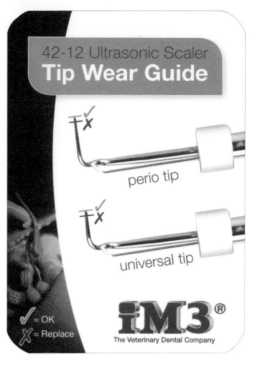

Figure B.10   Testing card for checking the quality of ultrasonic scaler tips.

looking in particular for any damage incurred. Manufacturers offer printed cards you can check the tip against to know when it is time to replace it (Figure B.10).

Handpieces

The manufacturer's instructions will provide specific care tips. All handpieces should be cleaned and disinfected after each use. Additionally, both slow- and high-speed handpieces should be lubricated daily, with the oil placed in the appropriate air inlet hose: normally, the smaller one of the 2 larger holes. In case of having numerous handpiece, a reasonable solution is to use the professional Handpiece Cleaning and Lubrication Unit.

Compressor

In oil compressors it is necessary to check the oil level, it is non needed in oil free ones. At the end of each day, the pressure should be lessened, while the fluid should be drained from the air reservoir regularly (e.g., once a week), following manufacturer's instructions. If the compressor is kept outside of the clinic, low temperatures may cause freezing of the liquid, preventing delivery of air pressure.

References

Hale, F.A. (2004). Instruments sharpening. Available from http://www.toothvet.ca/VSTEP/i%20-%20sharpening.pdf (accessed July 5, 2020).

Niemiec, B.A. (2012). *Veterinary Periodontology*. Hoboken, NJ: Wiley.

Appendix C

Abbreviations and Dental Charts

Jerzy Gawor

Veterinary Clinic Arka, Kraków, Poland

**AVDC Abbreviations for use in Case Logs
Equine and Small Animal**

This list of abbreviations has been recommended by the Nomenclature Committee and approved by the AVDC Board. The list is in alphabetical order.

Anatomical items are shown in **bold**.

Conditions and diagnostic procedures appropriate for use in the Diagnosis column of a case log entry are shown in left side.

Treatment procedures and related items suitable for inclusion in the Procedure column in the case log entry are shown in the middle.

Note: Use of other abbreviations in AVDC case logs is not permitted – write out the whole word if it must be included in an entry.

For further information on the use of particular definitions, visit the Nomenclature page on the AVDC website.

		Definition
A		**Alveolus**
AB		Abrasion
ABE		Alveolar bone expansion
ALV		Alveolectomy/alveoloplasty
ANO		Anodontia
AOS		Alveolar osteitis
AP		**Apex**
	AP/X	Apicoectomy
APN		Apexification
AT		Attrition
ATE		Abnormal tooth extrusion

		Definition
B		Biopsy
	B/B	Bite biopsy
	B/CN	Core needle biopsy
	B/E	Excisional biopsy
	B/I	Incisional biopsy
	B/NA	Needle aspiration
	B/NB	Needle biopsy
	B/P	Punch biopsy
	B/S	Surface biopsy
BR		Bite registration
BRI		Bridge
BTH		Ball therapy
BUC		Buccotomy
BUP		Bullous pemphigoid
C		**Canine**
CA		Caries
	CA/INF	Infundibular caries (equines)
	CA/INF/D	Distal infundibular caries
	CA/INF/M	Mesial infundibular caries
	CA/PER	Peripheral caries (in equines)
CB		Crossbite
	CB/C	Caudal crossbite
	CB/R	Rostral crossbite
CC		Calcinosis circumscripta
CEJ		**Cementoenamel junction**
CFL		Cleft lip
	CFL/R	Cleft lip repair
CFP		Cleft palate

The Veterinary Dental Patient: A Multidisciplinary Approach, First Edition. Edited by Jerzy Gawor and Brook Niemiec.
© 2021 John Wiley & Sons Ltd. Published 2021 by John Wiley & Sons Ltd.
Companion website: www.wiley.com/go/gawor/veterinary-dental-patient

		Definition			Definition
	CFP/R	Cleft palate repair		CR/T	Temporary crown
CFS		Cleft soft palate		CR/XP	Crown reduction
	CFS/R	Cleft soft palate repair	CS		Culture/sensitivity
CFSH		Soft palate hypoplasia	CT		Computed tomography
	CFSH/R	Soft palate hypoplasia repair		CT/CB	Cone-beam CT
CFSU		Unilateral cleft soft palate	CTH		Chemotherapy
	CFSU/R	Unilateral cleft soft palate repair	CU		Contact mucositis or contact mucosal ulceration
CFT		Traumatic cleft palate	**D**		**Diastema**
	CFT/R	Traumatic cleft palate repair		D/O	Open diastema
CHO		Calvarial hyperostosis		D/ODY	Diastema odontoplasty (or widening)
CL		Chewing lesion		D/V	Valve diastema
	CL/B	Chewing lesion (buccal mucosa/cheek)	DC		Diagnostic cast
	CL/L	Chewing lesion (labial mucosa/lip)		DC/D	Die
	CL/P	Chewing lesion (palatal mucosa/palate)		DC/SM	Stone model
	CL/T	Chewing lesion (lingual/ sublingual mucosa/tongue)	DI		Discharge
				DI/ND	Right nasal discharge
CMO		Craniomandibular osteopathy		DI/NS	Left nasal discharge
				DI/NU	Bilateral nasal discharge
COM		Commissurotomy		DI/OD	Right ocular discharge
CON		**Condylar process of the mandible**		DI/OS	Left ocular discharge
				DI/OU	Bilateral ocular discharge
	CON/X	Condylectomy	DMO		Decreased mouth opening
COO		Condensing osteitis	DP		Defect preparation (prior to filling a dental defect)
COR		**Coronoid process of the mandible**	**DT**		**Deciduous tooth**
	COR/X	Coronoidectomy		DT/P	Persistent deciduous tooth
CPL		Cheiloplasty/ commissuroplasty	DTC		Dentigerous cyst
				DTC/R	Dentigerous cyst removal
CR		**Crown**	**E**		**Enamel**
	CR/A	Crown amputation		E/D	Enamel defect
	CR/AC	**Anatomical crown**		E/H	Enamel hypoplasia
	CR/C	Ceramic crown (full)		E/HM	Enamel hypomineralization
	CR/C/P	Ceramic crown (partial)		E/P	Enamel pearl
	CR/CC	**Clinical crown**	EM		Erythema multiforme
	CR/L	Crown lengthening	ENO		Enophthalmos
	CR/M	Metal crown (full)	EOG		Eosinophilic granuloma
	CR/M/P	Metal crown (partial)		EOG/L	Eosinophilic granuloma (lip)
	CR/P	Crown preparation		EOG/P	Eosinophilic granuloma (palate)
	CR/R	Resin crown (full)			
	CR/R/P	Resin crown (partial)		EOG/T	Eosinophilic granuloma (tongue)
	CR/RC	**Reserve crown**	ER		Erosion
	CR/PFM	Porcelain fused to metal crown (full)	ESP		Elongated soft palate
				ESP/R	Elongated soft palate reduction
	CR/PFM/P	Porcelain fused to metal crown (partial)	EXO		Exophthalmos

		Definition
F		Flap
	F/AD	Advancement flap
	F/AP	Apically positioned flap
	F/CO	Coronally positioned flap
	F/EN	Envelope flap
	F/HI	Hinged (overlapping) flap
	F/IS	Island flap
	F/LA	Laterally positioned flap
	F/RO	Rotation flap
	F/TR	Transposition flap
FB		Foreign body
	FB/R	Foreign body removal
FOD		Fibrous osteodystrophy
FOL		Folliculitis
FRE		Frenuloplasty (frenulotomy, frenulectomy)
FT		Fiberotomy
FX		Fracture (tooth or jaw; see T/FX for tooth fracture abbreviations)
	FX/R	Repair of jaw fracture
	FX/R/EXF	External skeletal fixation
	FX/R/IAS	Interarch splinting (between upper and lower dental arches)
	FX/R/IDS	Interdental splinting (between teeth within a dental arch)
	FX/R/IQS	Interquadrant splinting (between left and right upper or lower jaw quadrants)
	FX/R/MMF	Maxillomandibular fixation (other than muzzling and interarch splinting)
	FX/R/MZ	Muzzling
	FX/R/PL	Bone plating
	FX/R/WIR/C	Wire cerclage
	FX/R/WIR/O S	Intraosseous wiring
GC		Gingival curettage
GE		Gingival enlargement (in the absence of a histological diagnosis)
GF		Graft
	GF/B	Bone graft
	GF/C	Cartilage graft
	GF/CT	Connective tissue graft
	GF/F	Fat graft
	GF/G	Gingival graft
	GF/M	Mucosal graft
	GF/N	Nerve graft

		Definition
	GF/S	Skin graft
	GF/V	Venous graft
GH		Gingival hyperplasia
GR		Gingival recession
GTR		Guided tissue regeneration
GV		Gingivectomy/gingivoplasty
HC		Hypercementosis
HS		Hemisection
HYP		Hypodontia
I1,2,3		**Incisor**
IM		Detailed imprint of hard and/or soft tissues (e.g., individual teeth or palate defect)
	IM/F	Full-mouth impression (i.e., imprints of teeth of upper and lower dental arches)
IMP		Implant
INF		**Infundibulum**
IOF		Intraoral fistula
	IOF/R	Intraoral fistula repair
IP		Inclined plane
	IP/AC	Acrylic inclined plane
	IP/C	Composite inclined plane
	IP/M	Metal (i.e., lab-produced) inclined plane
ITH		Immunotherapy
LAC		Laceration
	LAC/B	Laceration (cheek skin/buccal mucosa)
	LAC/G	Laceration (gingiva/alveolar mucosa)
	LAC/L	Laceration (lip skin/labial mucosa)
	LAC/O	Laceration (palatine tonsil/oropharyngeal mucosa)
	LAC/P	Laceration (palatal mucosa)
	LAC/R	Laceration repair
	LAC/T	Laceration (lingual/sublingual mucosa)
LE		Lupus erythematosus
LIN		**Tongue**
	LIN/X	Tongue resection
LIP		**Lip/cheek**
	LIP/X	Lip/cheek resection
LN		**Lymph node** (regional; i.e., facial, mandibular, parotid, lateral, and medial retropharyngeal)
	LN/E	Lymph node enlargement

		Definition
	LN/X	Lymph node resection
M1,2,3		**Molar**
MAL		Malocclusion
	MAL1	Class 1 malocclusion (neutroclusion; dental malocclusion with normal upper/lower jaw length relationship)
	MAL1/BV	Buccoversion
	MAL1/DV	Distoversion
	MAL1/LABV	Labioversion
	MAL1/LV	Linguoversion
	MAL1/MV	Mesioversion
	MAL1/PV	Palatoversion
	MAL2	Class 2 malocclusion (mandibular distoclusion; symmetrical skeletal malocclusion with the lower jaw relatively shorter than the upper jaw)
	MAL3	Class 3 malocclusion (mandibular mesioclusion; symmetrical skeletal malocclusion with the upper jaw relatively shorter than the lower jaw)
	MAL4	Class 4 malocclusion (asymmetrical skeletal malocclusion in a caudoventral, side-to-side, or dorsoventral direction)
	MAL4/DV	Asymmetrical skeletal malocclusion in a dorsoventral direction
	MAL4/RC	Asymmetrical skeletal malocclusion in a rostrocaudal direction
	MAL4/STS	Asymmetrical skeletal malocclusion in a side-to-side direction
MAR		Marsupialization
MET		Metastasis
	MET/D	Distant metastasis
	MET/R	Regional metastasis
MMM		Masticatory muscle myositis
MN		**Mandible/mandibular**
	MN/FX	Mandibular fracture
MRI		Magnetic resonance imaging
MX		**Maxilla/maxillary**
	MX/FX	Maxillary fracture
N		**Nose/nasal/nasopharyngeal**
	N/EN	Rhinoscopy
	N/LAV	Nasal lavage
	N/NS	Naris stenosis
	N/NS/R	Naroplasty
	N/NPS	Nasopharyngeal stenosis

		Definition
	N/NPS/R	Nasopharyngeal stenosis repair
	N/POL	Nasopharyngeal polyp
	N/SCC	Nasal SCC (check abbreviations under OM for other tumors)
OA		Orthodontic appliance
	OA/A	Orthodontic appliance adjustment
	OA/AR	Arch bar
	OA/BKT	Bracket, button or hook
	OA/CMB	Custom-made OA/BKT
	OA/EC	Elastic chain, tube or thread
	OA/I	Orthodontic appliance installment
	OA/R	Orthodontic appliance removal
	OA/WIR	Orthodontic wire
OAF		Oroantral fistula
	OAF/R	Oroantral fistula repair
OC		Orthodontic counseling
ODY		Odontoplasty
OFF		Orofacial fistula
	OFF/R	Orofacial fistula repair
OLI		Oligodontia
OM		Oral/maxillofacial mass
	OM/AA	Acanthomatous ameloblastoma
	OM/AD	Adenoma
	OM/ADC	Adenocarcinoma
	OM/APN	Anaplastic neoplasm
	OM/APO	Amyloid-producing odontogenic tumor
	OM/CE	Cementoma
	OM/FIO	Feline inductive odontogenic tumor
	OM/FS	Fibrosarcoma
	OM/GCG	Giant cell granuloma
	OM/GCT	Granular cell tumor
	OM/HS	Hemangiosarcoma
	OM/LI	Lipoma
	OM/LS	Lymphosarcoma
	OM/MCT	Mast cell tumor
	OM/MM	Malignant melanoma
	OM/OO	Osteoma
	OM/OS	Osteosarcoma
	OM/MTB	Multilobular tumor of bone
	OM/PAP	Papilloma
	OM/PCT	Plasma cell tumor

		Definition
	OM/PNT	Peripheral nerve sheath tumor
	OM/POF	Peripheral odontogenic fibroma
	OM/RBM	Rhabdomyosarcoma
	OM/SCC	Squamous cell carcinoma
	OM/UDN	Undifferentiated neoplasm
OMJL		Open-mouth jaw locking
	OMJL/R	Open-mouth jaw locking reduction
ONF		Oronasal fistula
	ONF/R	Oronasal fistula repair
OP		Operculectomy
OR		Orthodontic recheck
OS		Orthognathic surgery
OSN		Osteonecrosis
OSS		Osteosclerosis
OST		Osteomyelitis
PA		**Periapical**
	PA/A	Periapical abscess
	PA/C	Periapical cyst
	PA/G	Periapical granuloma
	PA/P	Periapical pathology (if a distinction between granuloma, abscess or cyst cannot be made)
PCB		Post-and-core build-up
PCD		Direct pulp capping
PCI		Indirect pulp capping
PD		Periodontal disease
	PD0	Clinically normal
	PD1	Gingivitis only (without attachment loss)
	PD2	Early periodontitis (<25% attachment loss)
	PD3	Moderate periodontitis (25–50% attachment loss)
	PD4	Advanced periodontitis (>50% attachment loss)
PDE		Acquired palate defect
	PDE/R	Acquired palate defect repair
PEC		Pericoronitis
PEO		Periostitis ossificans
PH		**Pulp horn (in equines, numbered by the du Toit system)**
	PH/D	Pulp horn defect
PHA		**Pharynx**
	PHA/IN	Pharyngitis
PM1-4		**Premolar**
POB		Palatal obturator

		Definition
PRO		Professional dental cleaning (scaling, polishing, irrigation)
PTY		Ptyalism
PU		**Pulp**
	PU/M	Mineralization of pulp
	PU/S	Pulp stone
PV		Pemphigus vulgaris
PYO		Pyogenic granuloma
R		Restoration (filling of a dental defect)
	R/A	Filling made of amalgam
	R/C	Filling made of composite
	R/CP	Filling made of compomer
	R/I	Filling made of glass ionomer
RAD		Radiography
	RAD/SG	Sialography
RBA		Retrobulbar abscess
RCR		Retained crown-root or clinical crown-reserve crown or clinical crown-reserve crown and root
RCT		Standard root canal therapy
	RCT/S	Surgical root canal therapy
RO		**Root**
RO/AC		**Anatomical root**
RO/CR		**Clinical root**
	RO/X	Root resection/amputation
RP		Root planing
	RP/C	Closed root planing
	RP/O	Open root planing
RPA		Retropharyngeal abscess
RR		Internal resorption
RTH		Radiotherapy
RTR		Retained root or reserve crown
S		Surgery
	S/M	Partial mandibulectomy
	S/MB	Bilateral partial mandibulectomy (removal of parts of the left and right mandibles)
	S/MD	Dorsal marginal mandibulectomy (marginal mandibulectomy, mandibular rim excision)
	S/MS	Segmental mandibulectomy (removal of a full dorsoventral sement of a mandible)
	S/MT	Total mandibulectomy (removal of one entire mandible)
	S/P	Partial palatectomy

		Definition
	S/X	Partial maxillectomy
	S/XB	Bilateral partial maxillectomy (removal of parts of the left and right maxillae or other facial bones)
SCI		Scintigraphy
SG		**Salivary gland**
	SG/ADC	Salivary gland adenocarcinoma (check abbreviations under OM for other tumors)
	SG/ADS	Sialadenosis
	SG/IN	Sialadenitis
	SG/MAR	Marsupialization
	SG/MUC/S	Sublingual sialocele
	SG/MUC/P	Pharyngeal sialocele
	SG/MUC/C	Cervical sialocele
	SG/NEC	Necrotizing sialometaplasia
	SG/RC	Mucous retention cyst
	SG/SI	Sialolith
	SG/X	Salivary gland resection
SHE		Shear mouth (increased occlusal angulation of equine cheek teeth)
SIN		**Sinus**
	SIN/CF	**Conchofrontal sinus**
	SIN/CF/F	Conchofrontal sinus flap
	SIN/CMX	**Caudal maxillary sinus**
	SIN/EN	Sinoscopy
	SIN/F	Sinus flap
	SIN/IN	Sinusitis (e.g., SIN/IN/RMX = rostral maxillary sinusitis)
	SIN/LAV	Sinus lavage
	SIN/MX/F	Maxillary sinus flap
	SIN/RMX	**Rostral maxillary sinus**
	SIN/SP	**Sphenopalatine sinus**
	SIN/TRP	Sinus trephination
	SIN/VC	**Ventral conchal sinus**
SR		Surgical repositioning
ST		Stomatitis
	ST/CS	Caudal stomatitis
SYM		**Mandibular symphysis**
	SYM/R	Mandibular symphysis repair
	SYM/S	Mandibular symphysis separation
T		**Tooth**
	T/A	Avulsed tooth
	T/CCR	Concrescence
	T/DEN	Dens invaginatus
	T/DIL	Dilaceration
	T/E	Embedded tooth

		Definition
T/EL		Tooth elongation (abnormal intraoral and/or periapical extension of the coronal and/or apical portions of the tooth; e.g., T/EL/CC = elongation of the clinical crown)
	T/FDR	Fused roots
	T/FUS	Fusion
	T/FX	Fractured tooth (see next seven listings for fracture types)
	T/FX/EI	Enamel infraction
	T/FX/EF	Enamel fracture
	T/FX/UCF	Uncomplicated crown fracture
	T/FX/CCF	Complicated crown fracture
	T/FX/UCRF	Uncomplicated crown-root facture
	T/FX/CCRF	Complicated crown-root fracture
	T/FX/RF	Root fracture
	T/GEM	Gemination
	T/I	Impacted tooth
	T/LUX	Luxated tooth
	T/MAC	Macrodontia
	T/MIC	Microdontia
	T/NE	Near pulp exposure
	T/NV	Nonvital tooth
	T/PE	Pulp exposure
	T/RI	Tooth reimplantation (for an avulsed tooth)
	T/RP	Tooth repositioning (for a luxated tooth)
	T/SN	Supernumerary tooth
	T/SR	Supernumerary root
	T/TRA	Transposition
	T/U	Unerupted tooth
	T/V	Vital tooth
	T/XP	Partial tooth resection
TMA		Trauma
	TMA/B	Ballistic trauma
	TMA/E	Electric trauma
	TMA/BRN	Burn trauma
	TMA/R	Trauma repair
TMJ		**Temporomandibular joint**
	TMJ/A	Temporomandibular joint ankylosis (true or false)
	TMJ/A/R	Temporomandibular joint ankylosis repair
	TMJ/D	TMJ dysplasia

		Definition			Definition
	TMJ/FX	Temporomandibular joint fracture	XSS		Open extraction of a tooth
	TMJ/FX/R	Temporomandibular joint fracture repair		XSS/APX/R PL	Extraction of a tooth after apicoectomy and repulsion
	TMJ/LUX	TMJ luxation		XSS/BUC	Transbuccal extraction of a tooth after buccotomy
	TMJ/LUX/R	Temporomandibular joint luxation reduction		XSS/BUC/A LV	Transbuccal extraction of a tooth after buccotomy and alveolectomy
TON		**Palatine tonsil**		XSS/COM	Transbuccal extraction of a tooth after commissurotomy
	TON/IN	Tonsillitis		XSS/COM/A LV	Transbuccal extraction of a tooth after commissurotomy and alveolectomy
	TON/X	Tonsillectomy			
TP		Treatment plan		XSS/MIB	Extraction of a tooth via minimally invasive buccotomy (small incision made for introduction of straight instrumentation to elevate, section, or drill into a cheek tooth for the purpose of facilitating its transoral extraction)
TR		Tooth resorption			
TRP		Trephination			
TS		Trisection			
TT		Temporal teratoma			
US		Ultrasonography			
VPT		Vital pulp therapy			
X		Closed extraction of a tooth (without sectioning)		XSS/RPL	Extraction of a tooth after repulsion
XS		Closed extraction of a tooth (with sectioning)	**ZYG**		**Zygoma (zygomatic arch)**
	XS/ODY	Removal of interproximal crown tissue to facilitate transoral extraction of a tooth		ZYG/X	Zygomectomy

Dental Charts

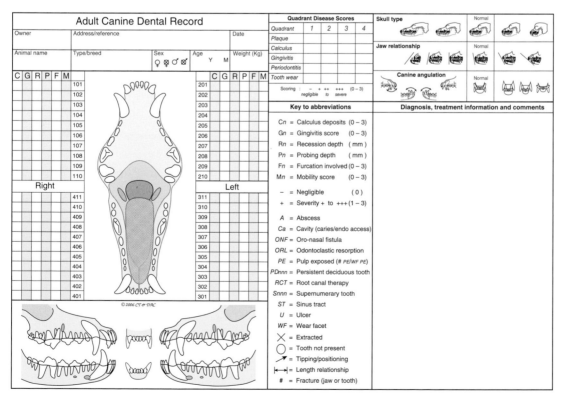

Source: Courtesy of David Crossley.

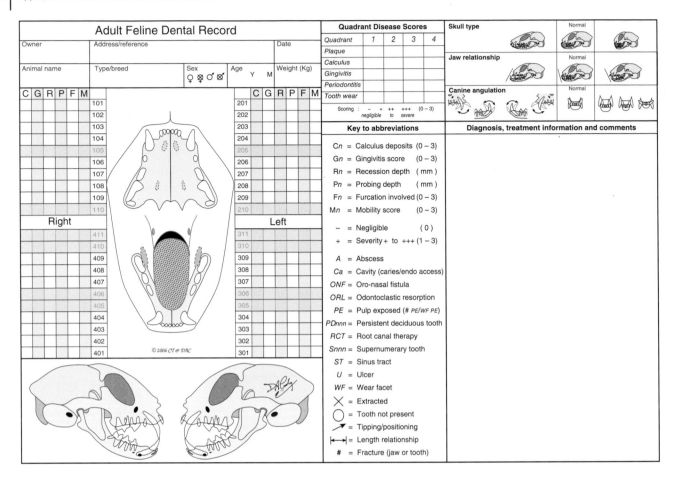

Adult Feline Dental Record

Owner	Address/reference		Date
Animal name	Type/breed	Sex ♀ ⊗ ♂ ⊗	Age Y M	Weight (Kg)

C	G	R	P	F	M			C	G	R	P	F	M
						101	201						
						102	202						
						103	203						
						104	204						
						105	205						
						106	206						
						107	207						
						108	208						
						109	209						
						110	210						

Right   **Left**

						411	311						
						410	310						
						409	309						
						408	308						
						407	307						
						406	306						
						405	305						
						404	304						
						403	303						
						402	302						
						401	301						

© 2006 CT & DAC

Quadrant Disease Scores

Quadrant	1	2	3	4
Plaque				
Calculus				
Gingivitis				
Periodontitis				
Tooth wear				

Scoring : – + ++ +++ (0 – 3)
negligible   to   severe

Key to abbreviations

Cn = Calculus deposits (0 – 3)
Gn = Gingivitis score (0 – 3)
Rn = Recession depth (mm)
Pn = Probing depth (mm)
Fn = Furcation involved (0 – 3)
Mn = Mobility score (0 – 3)

– = Negligible (0)
+ = Severity + to +++ (1 – 3)

A = Abscess
Ca = Cavity (caries/endo access)
ONF = Oro-nasal fistula
ORL = Odontoclastic resorption
PE = Pulp exposed (# PE/WF PE)
PDnnn = Persistent deciduous tooth
RCT = Root canal therapy
Snnn = Supernumerary tooth
ST = Sinus tract
U = Ulcer
WF = Wear facet
✕ = Extracted
◯ = Tooth not present
↗ = Tipping/positioning
↔ = Length relationship
= Fracture (jaw or tooth)

Skull type
Normal

Jaw relationship
Normal

Canine angulation
Normal

Diagnosis, treatment information and comments

Source: Courtesy of David Crossley.

Brook Niemiec, Dip. AVDC, Dip. EVDC, Fellow AVD
Allen Skinner, Dip AVDC
Natalie Henderson, DVM
Cody Fielder, DVM

www.DogBeachVet.com

Patient Name:
_____
Patient #:
_____
Date:
_____

Skull Type:	Mandibular Symphysis:	Occlusion:	Oral Exam Findings:		
O Brachycephalic	O Intact	O Ideal/Normal	AB- Abrasion	LAC- Laceration	T/FX/EF- Enamel Fracture
O Mesocephalic	O Separation	O MAL/1-Neutroclussion	AT- Attrition	O- Missing Tooth	T/FX/ EI- Enamel Infraction
O Dolichocephalic	O Laxity	O Distoversion	CA- Caries	OM- Oral Mass	T/FX/UCF- Uncomplicated Crwn Fracture
Temporomandibular	- Mild/Mod/Severe	O Labioversion	CWD- Crowding	PE- Pulp Exposure	T/FX/CCF- Complicated Crwn Fracture
Palpation:	**Upper Airway:**	O Linguoversion	E/D- Enamel Defect	RD- Retained Deciduous Tooth	T/FX/UCRF- Uncomplicated Crwn-Rt Fracture
O Normal	O Elongated Soft Palate	O Mesioversion	E/H- Enamel Hypocalcification/Hypoplasia	RO- Rotated Tooth	T/FX/CCRF- Complicated Crwn-Rt Fracture
O Pain	O Palate Defect	O Rostral Crossbite	FB- Foreign Body	SE- Supraerupted	T/FX/RF- Rt Fracture
O Crepitus	O Stenotic Nares	O Caudal Crossbite	GH- Gingival Hyperplasia/Hypertrophy	SN- Supernumerary	T/ LUX- Luxated Tooth
O Clicking	O Tonsilitis	O MAL/2-Mand Distocclusion	GR- Gingival Recession	ST/CU- Contact Ulcer Stomatitis	T/NV-Non- Vital Tooth
O Inhibited	O Oroantral Fistula (OAF)	O MAL/3-Mand Mesiocclusion	IE- Infraerupted	T/A- Avulsed Tooth	TR- Tooth Resorption
O Luxated	O Oronasal Fistula (ONF)	O Edentulous			

Tooth #	110	109	108	107	106	105	104	103	102	101	201	202	203	204	205	206	207	208	209	210
Furcation (F)																				
Periodontal Dz (PD)																				
Mobility (M)																				

Buccal →
Palatal →

Lingual →
Buccal →

Tooth #	411	410	409	408	407	406	405	404	403	402	401	301	302	303	304	305	306	307	308	309	310	311
Furcation (F)																						
Periodontal Dz (PD)																						
Mobility (M)																						

Radiograph:	Exodontia:	Other Surgical:	Subgingival:
DTC- Dentigerous Cyst (suspect)	CRA- Crown Amputation	BG- Bone Graft	RP/C- Root Planing Closed
FX- Fracture	CRR- Crown Reduction	OAF/R- Oroantral Fistula Repair	RP/O- Root Planing Open
pRC- Prev Root Canal Therapy	X- Simple Closed Extract	ONF/R- Oronasal Fistula Repair	**Subgingival Antibiotics:**
RTR- Retained Tooth Root	XS-Non-Sx Extract with Sectioning		CLIN- Clindoral
SYM- Symphyseal Separation	XSS-Surgical Extraction	**Suture:**	DOX- Doxirobe
-Type 1 / 2 / 3	O Buccal Cortical Bone Removal	O Chromic Gut___	**Cleaning:**
T/E- Embedded Tooth	O Alveoloplasty	O Monocryl___	PRO-Perio Prophylaxis
T/I- Impacted Tooth			O Hand Scaling
TR- Tooth Resorption	**Periodontal Surgery:**		O Ultrasonic Scaling
pVP- Prev Vital Pulp Therapy	GV- Gingivoplasty/Gingivectomy	**Diagnostics:**	O Subgingival Curettage
	OP- Operculectomy	B/E- Biopsy Excisional	O Chlorhex/Pumice Polish
		B/I- Biopsy Incisional	O Fluoride
	Restoration:	CS- Culture/Sensitivity	O OraVet
	BD- Bonded Sealant		

Comments:_____
_____
_____
_____

VETERINARY DENTAL SPECIALTIES & ORAL SURGERY
www.DogBeachVet.com

Brook Niemiec, DVM, Dip. AVDC, Dip. EVDC, Fellow AVD
Robert Furman, BVMS, MRCVS, Dip. AVDC
Allen Skinner, DVM, Dip AVDC

Patient Name:
_____

Patient #:
_____

Date:

Skull Type:	Mandibular Symphysis:	Occlusion:	Oral Exam Findings:		
O Brachycephalic	O Intact	O Ideal/Normal	AB- Abrasion	LAC- Laceration	T/FX/EF- Enamel Fracture
O Mesocephalic	O Separation	O MAL/1-Neutrocclussion	AT- Attrition	O- Missing Tooth	T/FX/ EI- Enamel Infraction
O Dolichocephalic	O Laxity	O Distoversion	CS-Caudal Stomatitis	OM- Oral Mass	T/FX/UCF- Uncomplicated Crwn Fracture
Temporomandibular	-Mild/Mod/Severe	O Labioversion	CWD- Crowding	PE- Pulp Exposure	T/FX/CCF- Complicated Crwn Fracture
Palpation:	**Upper Airway:**	O Linguoversion	E/D- Enamel Defect	RD- Retained Deciduous Tooth	T/FX/UCRF- Uncomplicated Crwn-Rt Fracture
O Normal	O Elongated Soft Palate	O Mesioversion	E/H- Enamel Hypocalcification/Hypoplasia	RO- Rotated Tooth	T/FX/CCRF- Complicated Crwn-Rt Fracture
O Pain	O Palate Defect	O Rostral Crossbite	FB- Foreign Body	SE- Supraerupted	T/FX/RF- Rt Fracture
O Crepitus	O Stenotic Nares	O Caudal Crossbite	GH- Gingival Hyperplasia/Hypertrophy	SN- Supernumerary	T/ LUX- Luxated Tooth
O Clicking	O Tonsilitis	O MAL/2-Mand Distocclusion	GR- Gingival Recession	ST/CU- Contact Ulcer Stomatitis	T/NV- Non-Vital Tooth
O Inhibited	O Oroantral Fistula (OAF)	O MAL/3-Mand Mesiocclusion	IE- Infraerupted	T/A- Avulsed Tooth	TR- Tooth Resorption
O Luxated	O Oronasal Fistula (ONF)	O Edentulous			

Tooth #	109	108	107	106	104	103	102	101	201	202	203	204	206	207	208	209
Furcation (F)																
Periodontal Dz (PD)																
Mobility (M)																

Buccal →
Palatal →

Lingual →
Buccal →

Comments:_____
_____
_____
_____

Radiograph:	Exodontia:	Other Surgical:	Subgingival:
DTC- Dentigerous Cyst (suspect)	CRA- Crown Amputation	BG- Bone Graft	RPC- Root Planing Closed
FX- Fracture	CRR- Crown Reduction	OAF/R- Oroantral Fistula Repair	RPO- Root Planing Open
pRC- Prev Root Canal Therapy	X- Simple Closed Extract	ONF/R- Oronasal Fistula Repair	**Subgingival Antibiotics:**
RTR- Retained Tooth Root	XS- Non-Sx Extract with Sectioning		CLIN- Clindoral
SYM- Symphyseal Separation	XSS- Surgical Extraction	**Suture:**	DOX- Doxirobe
-Type 1 / 2 / 3	O Buccal Cortical Bone Removal	O Chromic Gut___	**Prophylaxis:**
T/E- Embedded Tooth	O Alveoloplasty	O Monocryl___	PRO- Perio Prophylaxis
T/I- Impacted Tooth			O Hand Scaling
TR- Tooth Resorption	**Periodontal Surgery:**	**Diagnostics:**	O Ultrasonic Scaling
pVP- Prev Vital Pulp Therapy	GV- Gingivoplasty/Gingivectomy	B/E- Biopsy Excisional	O Subgingival Curettage
	OP- Operculectomy	B/I- Biopsy Incisional	O Chlorhex/Pumice Polish
		CS- Culture/Sensitivity	O Fluoride
	Restoration:		O OraVet
	BD- Bonded Sealant		

Tooth #	409	408	407	404	403	402	401	301	302	303	304	307	308	309
Furcation (F)														
Periodontal Dz (PD)														
Mobility (M)														

Appendix D

List of Hereditary Problems and Breed Predispositions in Dogs and Cats

Jerzy Gawor

Veterinary Clinic Arka, Kraków, Poland

No.	Breed	Required diagnostic method and record	Problem	Ranking of clinical importance
Dogs				
1.	Akita inu	C, Ph	Uveodermatologic (UV) syndrome	3
		X	Temporomandibular joint (TMJ) dysplasia (Figure D.1a,b); open mouth locking	2
2.	American cocker spaniel	X	TMJ dysplasia; open mouth locking	2
3.	Basset hound	X	TMJ dysplasia; open mouth locking	2
4.	St. Bernard's	C, Ph	Cheilitis due to macrocheilia	1
		C, Ph	Cleft tongue, bifid tongue	3
5.	Boxer	C, X	Supernumerary teeth (Figure D.2.a,b),	1
		C, Ph	Cleft palate (Figure D.3)	3
		C, Ph	Gingival hyperplasia	1
		C, X	Impacted teeth	2
		X	Dentigerous cyst	2
		C, Ph	Elongated soft palate, stenotic nostrils, brachycephalic obstructive airway syndrome (BOAS) (Figure D.4.a,b,c)	2
6.	Brittany spaniel	C, Ph	Cleft palate	3
7.	Boston terrier	C, Ph	Elongated soft palate, stenotic nostrils BOAS	2
8.	English bulldog	C, Ph	Elongated soft palate, stenotic nostrils BOAS	2
		C, Ph	Supernumerary teeth,	1
		C, Ph	Wry mouth	2
9.	French bulldog	C, Ph	Elongated soft palate, stenotic nostrils BOAS	2
		C, X	Teeth crowded (Figure D.5)	1
10.	Bullterrier	C, Ph	Lingually displaced canines, narrow-base canines (Figure D.6)	1
11.	Bullmastif	C, X	Idiopathic calvariar hyperostosis (Figure D.7)	2
12.	Cairn terrier	X, H	Craniomandibular osteopathy (CMO) (Figure D.8)	3

(Continued)

The Veterinary Dental Patient: A Multidisciplinary Approach, First Edition. Edited by Jerzy Gawor and Brook Niemiec.
© 2021 John Wiley & Sons Ltd. Published 2021 by John Wiley & Sons Ltd.
Companion website: www.wiley.com/go/gawor/veterinary-dental-patient

No.	Breed	Required diagnostic method and record	Problem	Ranking of clinical importance
13.	Cavalier King Charles spaniel	C, Ph, H	Plaque-associated stomatitis	2
		C, Ph	Lip-fold dermatitis (Figure D.9)	1
		X	TMJ dysplasia, open-mouth locking	3
		C, Ph H	Eosinophilic granuloma complex with oral expression (Figure D.10)	2
14.	Italian greyhound	C, R	Mesioversion of the maxillary canine teeth, lance teeth (Figure D.11)	2
		C, Ph, X	Odontodysplasia (Figure D.12a,b)	2
		C, G	Familial enamel hypoplasia	2
15.	English cocker spaniel	C, Ph	Lip-fold dermatitis	1
		X	Abnormalities in skull development	2
16.	Collie	L	Gray collie syndrome	3
		C, X	Lance teeth	2
		C, H	Gingival hyperplasia	1
17.	Dalmatyńczyk	C, X	Caries	1
		C, H	Gingival hyperplasia	1
18.	Doberman	G	Von Willebrand's disease	3
		C, H	Gingival hyperplasia	1
19.	Great Dane	C, H	Gingival hyperplasia	1
20.	Dog de Bordeaux	C, H	Gingival hyperplasia	1
21.	Chinese crested dog	C, X	Oligodontia (Figure D.13a,b,c)	2
22.	Longhaired dachshund	C, X	Lance teeth	2
		C, Ph	Retrogenia (Figure D.14)	2
		C, Ph	Lingually displaced canines, narrow-base canines	2
23.	Shorthaired dachshund	C, X	Lance teeth	2
		C, Ph, X	Lingually displaced canines, narrow-base canines	2
		C, Ph, X	Periodontopathy of the palatal aspect in maxillary cuspids	1
24.	Kerry blue terrier	C, X	Oligodontia	1
25.	Labrador retriever	X	TMJ dysplasia; open-mouth locking	3
26.	Lhasa apso	C, X	Teeth crowded	1
		C, X	Retained teeth	2
		X	Dentigerous cyst	2
27.	Maltese	C, Ph, H	Chronic ulcerative periodontitis/stomatitis (CUPS) (Figure D.15)	2
28.	Pug	C, Ph	Elongated soft palate	2
29.	Anatolian shepherd	C, Ph	Ankyloglossia (Figure D.16)	1
30.	German shepherd	C, Ph	Retrogenia	2
		C, Ph	Lingually displaced canines, narrow-base canines	2
		L	Masticatory muscle myositis (MMM)	3
31.	Tervuren	C, Ph	Vitiligo (Figure D.17)	1
32.	Pointer	C, Ph	Retrogenia	2

No.	Breed	Required diagnostic method and record	Problem	Ranking of clinical importance
33.	Poodle standard	C, Ph, X	Periodontopathy of the palatal aspect in maxillary cuspids	1
		C, X, Ph	Hypoplasia enameli	2
34.	Rottweiler	C, Ph	Vitiligo	1
		L	MMM (Figure D.18)	2
35.	Samoyed	C, L	UV syndrome	3
		G	Amelogenesis imperfecta (Figure D.19)	2
36.	Irish setter	C, X	Supernumerary teeth,	1
		C, Ph	Lip-fold dermatitis	1
		C, X	TMJ dysplasia; open-mouth locking	3
37.	Shar-pei	C, Ph	Tight-lip syndrome	2
		C, Ph	Retrogenia	2
		C, Ph	Lingually displaced canines, narrow-base canines	2
38.	Sheltie	C, X	Lance teeth	2
39.	Shi-tzu	X	Dentigerous cyst	2
		C, X	Teeth crowded	1
		C, X	Periodontal disease	1
40.	Springer spaniel	C, Ph	Lip-fold dermatitis	1
		C, X	TMJ dysplasia; open-mouth locking	3
41.	Siberian husky	C, Ph, H	Plaque associated stomatitis	1
		C, L	Uveodermatologic syndrome; UV syndrome	3
		C, H	EGC with oral expression	2
42.	Large Schnauzer	C, Ph	Microcheilia	2
43.	Miniature Schnauzer	C, Ph	Microcheilia	2
		G	Myotonia congenita	3
44.	Tibetan terrier	C, X	Delayed teeth eruption	2
45.	Scottish terrier	X, H	CMO	3
		C, Ph, H	Plaque-associated stomatitis	1
46.	Weimeraner	X	TMJ dysplasia; open-mouth locking	3
47.	West Highland white terrier	X, H, L(G)	CMO	3
48.	Wheaton terrier	C, Ph	Delayed teeth eruption	2
49.	Yorkshire terrier	C, X	Deciduous teeth persistence	2
		C, Ph	Teeth crowded	1
		C, Ph, H	Plaque associated stomatitis	1
50	Nova Scotia duck tolling Retriever	C, G	Cleft lip/palate	2
Cats				
1.	Persian	C, X	Brachycephalism (mouth breathing)	2
		C, X	Malocclusion class III mandibular mesiocclusion	1
		C, X	Teeth crowded	1

(Continued)

No.	Breed	Required diagnostic method and record	Problem	Ranking of clinical importance
2	Exotic	C, X	Brachycephalism (mouth breathing) (Figure D.20)	2
		C, X	Malocclusion class III mandibular mesiocclusion	1
		C, X	Teeth crowded (Figure D.21)	1
3.	Maine Coon	C, X, L(H)	Juvenile gingivitis	1
		C,X,L(H)	Malocclusion resulting from impingement of the maxillary fourth premolar (108/208) on the oral mucosa around the mandibular first molar (309/409) (Figure D.22)	1
		C,X,L(H)	Malocclusion class III mandibular mesiocclusion	1
4.	British shorthaired	C, X, L(H)	Juvenile gingivitis	1
		C, X, L(H)	Malocclusion causing impingement of the maxillary fourth premolar (108/208) on the oral mucosa around the mandibular first molar (309/409) (Figure D.23)	1
5.	Norwegian forest cat	C, L(H)	Eosinophilic granuloma complex with oral expression (Figure D.24)	I
6.	Siamese	C, L(G)	Feline muccopolysaccharidosis	3
			Cleft palate	2
			Juvenile gingivitis	
7.	Burmese	C, X	Feline orofacial pain syndrome	2
		C,X,L(G)	Craniofacial deformity; Burmese head defect	3

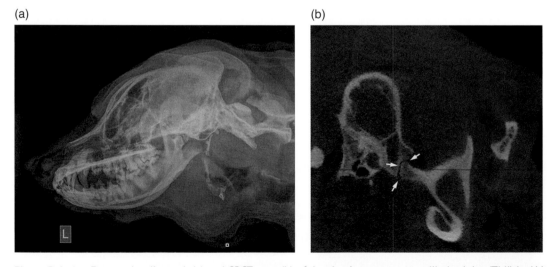

(a)   (b)

Figure D.1a,b Extraoral radiograph (a) and CBCT scan (b) of dysplastic temporo-mandibular joint (TMJ) in Akita inu dog.

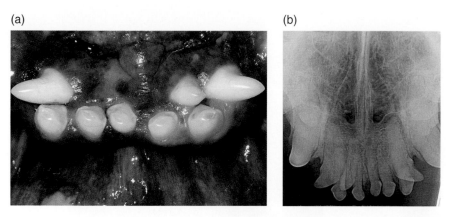

Figure D.2a,b   Supernumerary maxillary incisors teeth in Boxer. Clinical (a) and radiographic (b) assessment.

Figure D.3   Cleft palate in boxer puppy.

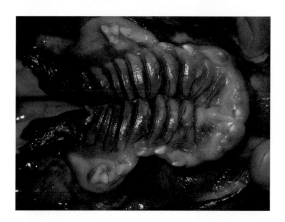

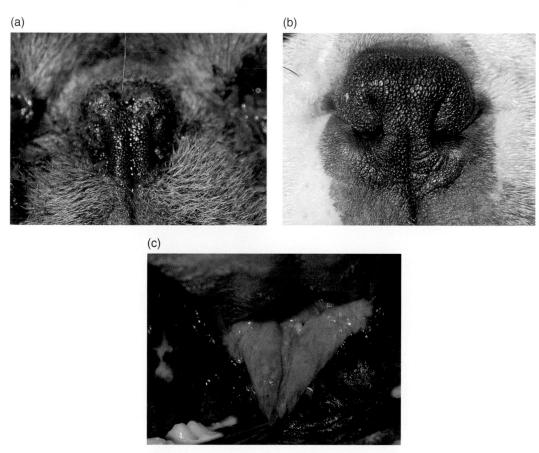

Figure D.4a,b,c   Brachycephalic Obstructive Airway Syndrome (BOAS) can be diagnosed in any brachycephalic breeds and may include stenotic nostrils: examples in a Persian cat (a) and a Shi-Tzu dog (b) as well as elongated soft palate (c).

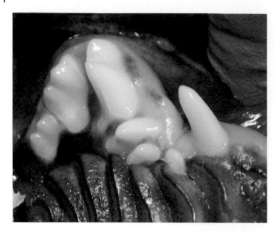

Figure D.5 Teeth crowding in maxillary dentition typical for brachycephalic breeds due to shortened upper jaw.

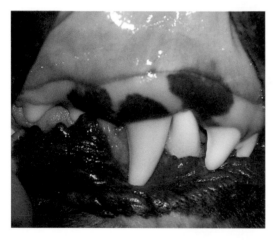

Figure D.6 Lingually displaced right mandibular canine tooth (404) in Bullterrier.

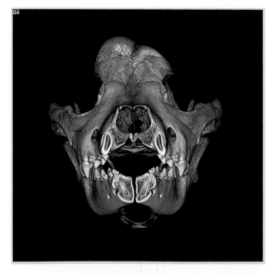

Figure D.7 Infantile Cranial Hyperostosis (ICH) in a bullmastiff

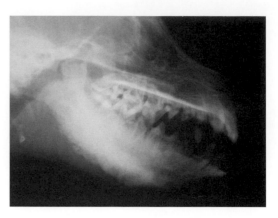

Figure D.8 Craniomandibular Osteopathy (CMO) in a Cairn Terrier causing significant change of mandibular bone tissue.

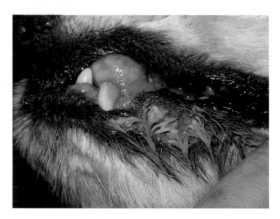

Figure D.9 Lip-fold dermatitis in a Cavalier King Charles Spaniel

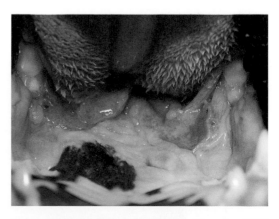

Figure D.10 Eosinophilic Granuloma Complex (EGC) causing proliferative palatal lesion in Cavalier King Charles Spaniel (b)

Figure D.11 Mesioversion of left maxillary canine tooth (204) in an Italian Greyhound.

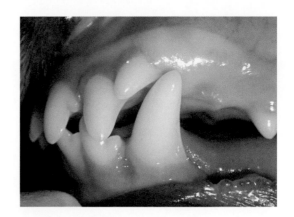

(a)

(b)

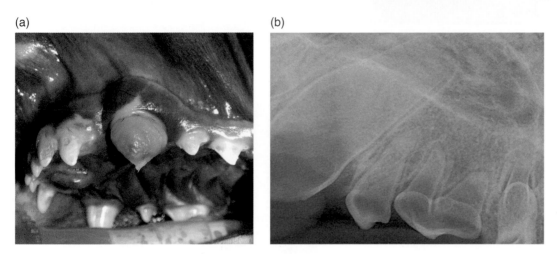

Figure D.12a,b Odontodysplasia present in entire dentition. Clinical picture (a) and radiographic appearance (b)

(a)

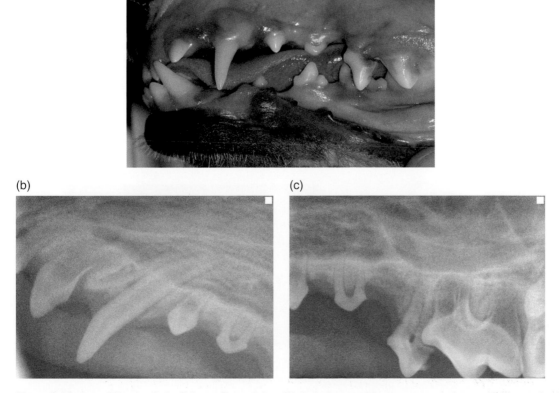

(b)

(c)

Figure D.13a,b,c Oligodontia in Chinese Crested dog. Clinical picture with numerous persistent deciduous dentition (a) and radiographs (b,c)

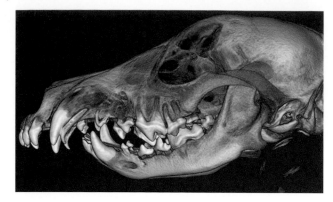

Figure D.14   Significant retrogenia in longhaired dachshund

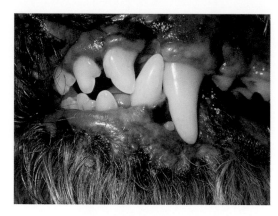

Figure D.17   Vitiligo affecting formerly pigmented mucosa in Tervueren

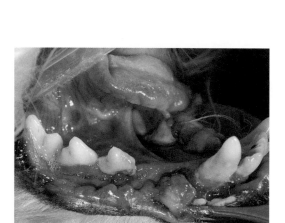

Figure D.15   Chronic Ulcerative Paradental Stomatitis in a Maltese

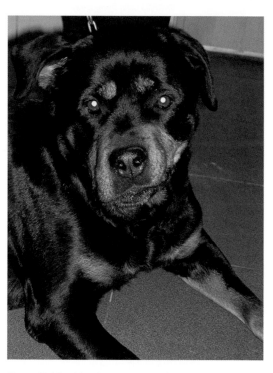

Figure D.18   Masticatory Muscle Myositis affecting a Rottweiler

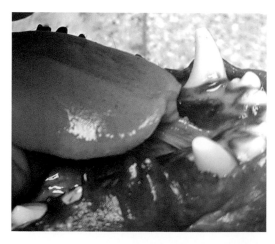

Figure D.16   Ankyloglossia in an Anatolian shepherd [Courtesy of dr Efe Onur]

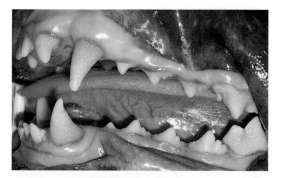

Figure D.19   Amelogenesis imperfecta affecting the entire dentition in Samoyed.

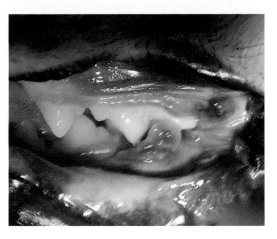

Figure D.20   Feline brachycephalism. CBCT reconstruction of exotic cat scull. Note the significantly reduced size of nasal cavity

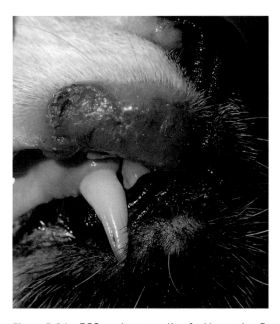

Figure D.23   Malocclusion resulting from impingement of the fourth maxillary premolar in mucosa at the area of opposed molar tooth in a British shorthaired cat creating a pyogenic granuloma.

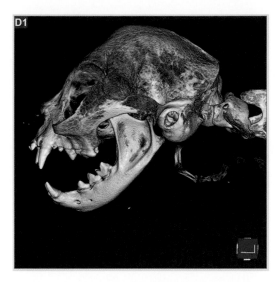

Figure D.21   Mandibular incisor teeth crowding in a Persian cat

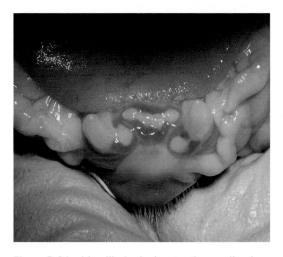

Figure D.24   EGC on the upper lip of a Norwegian Forest Cat.

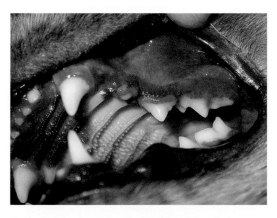

Figure D.22   Juvenile gingivitis in Maine Coon

Appendix E

Tolerance of Malocclusion and Dental Abnormalities in Dogs

Jerzy Gawor

Veterinary Clinic Arka, Kraków, Poland

Scissor bite and full dentition (42 teeth) are required in approximately 75% of the registered dog breeds in the Federation Cynologique Internationale (FCI). Deviations from this are considered a fault, and in most cases result in disqualification from the breeding stock.

However, some patterns of FCI allow or even require the acceptance of a different shape of occlusion and tolerate some missing teeth. The following derogations were derived directly from the breed standards available at www.fci.be.

FCI number	Breed	Tolerance in occlusion	Other dental tolerances
186	Affenpinscher	Slight retrogenia required	
7	Airedale Terrier	Scissor bite or level bite	
255	Akita	Level bite or delicate progenia is a small problem	
46	Appenzell Cattle Dog	Level bite is accepted	
63	Austrian Black and Tan Hound	Scissor bite or level bite	
64	Austrian Pinscher	Level bite is accepted	
163	Basset Hound	Scissor bite or level bite	
271	Bearded Collie	Level bite is accepted	
44	Beauceron		Missing first premolar is accepted
81	Belgian Griffon	Delicate progenia is required	
15	Belgian Shepherd Dog	Level bite is even preferred by livestock herders	Absence of two premolars 1 (2 P1) is tolerated; molars 3 (M3) are not taken into consideration
45	Bernese Mountain Dog		Missing third molars is accepted
215	Bichon Frise	Incisors must be in contact	
10	Border terrier	Level bite is accepted	
140	Boston Terrier	Progenia is required; teeth should not be visible	
191	Bouvier des Flandres	Level bite is accepted	
144	Boxer	Progenia is required; teeth should not be visible	

(Continued)

The Veterinary Dental Patient: A Multidisciplinary Approach, First Edition. Edited by Jerzy Gawor and Brook Niemiec.
© 2021 John Wiley & Sons Ltd. Published 2021 by John Wiley & Sons Ltd.
Companion website: www.wiley.com/go/gawor/veterinary-dental-patient

FCI number	Breed	Tolerance in occlusion	Other dental tolerances
80	Brussels Griffon	Delicate progenia is required	
149	Bulldog	Progenia is required; teeth should not be visible	
157	Bullmastiff	Level bite is required	
273	Canaan Dog	Scissor bite or level bite	
87	Catalan Sheepdog		Blunt canines are accepted
335	Central Asia Shepherd Dog		Fault is small dentition, stained teeth, missing premolar
246	Cesky Terrier	Scissor bite or level bite	
218	Chihuahua	Scissor bite or level bite	Missing premolars accepted
137	Chien des Pyrenees	Level bite is accepted	
288	Chinese Crested Dog	Scissor bite or level bite	Missing premolars accepted
198	Coarse Haired Italian Hound	Level bite is accepted	
283	Coton de Tulear	Incisors must be in even line	
277	Croatian Sheepdog	Level bite is accepted	Missing first premolar is accepted
116	Dogue de Bordeaux	Progenia is required 0.5–2 cm; teeth should not be visible	
308	Dutch Smoushond	Level bite is accepted	
225	Fila Brasileiro		Missing first premolar is accepted
299	German Hound	Scissor bite or level bite	
103	German Hunting Terrier		Missing third molars are accepted
235	German Shepherd		Missing first mandibular premolar is accepted
58	Great Swiss Mountain Dog		Missing first or second premolar is accepted, third molars are not taking into account
132	Hamilton Stovare	Level bite is accepted	
213	Hannoverian Scenthound	Scissor bite or level bite	
214	Hellenic Hound	Scissor bite or level bite	
57	Hungarian Shorthaired Pointing-Dog	Retrogenia with overjet 2 mm is accepted	
239	Hungarian Wire-haired Pointing Dog	Progenia over 2 mm is not accepted	
302	Irish Glen of Imaal Terrier	Level bite is accepted	
40	Irish Soft Coated Wheaten Terrier	Scissor bite or level bite	
160	Irish Woolfhound	Level bite is accepted	
206	Japanese Chin	Level bite is required; delicate retrogenia or progenia is accepted; scissor bite is accepted	
262	Japanese Spitz	Level bite or delicate progenia is a serious problem	
278	Karst Shepherd Dog	Level bite is accepted	
128	King Charles Spaniel	Delicate retrogenia is required	
192	Kromforhrlander	Level bite is accepted	
118	Large Munsterlander	Level bite is accepted	Missing first premolar is accepted
227	Lhasa Apso	Reverse scissor	
141	Long-haired Pyrenean sheepdog	Level bite is accepted	

FCI number	Breed	Tolerance in occlusion	Other dental tolerances
321	Majorca Shepherd Dog	Retrogenia with overjet 3 mm is accepted	Shortened cuspids crown is not tolerated
264	Mastiff	Slight retrogenia is accepted	
234	Mexican Hairless Dog		Missing all premolars is accepted; missing incisors are accepted
238	Mudi	Retrogenia with overjet 2 mm is accepted	
197	Neapolitan Mastiff	Level bite or scissor bite; progenia is accepted	
314	Nederlandse Kooikerhondje	Level bite is accepted	
50	Newfoundland	Level bite is accepted	
265	Norwegian Lundehund	Level bite is accepted	
312	Nova Scotia Duck Tolling Retriever	Progenia is accepted	
294	Otterhound	Significant retrogenia or progenia is a problem	
310	Peruvian Hairless Dog		Missing one premolar or molar is accepted
24	Poitevin	Delicate progenia should be accepted	
333	Polish Greyhound	Level bite is accepted	Missing first premolars
172	Poodle	Significant retrogenia is not accepted	All incisors, canines, and molars must be present • Absence of 2PM1 is not taken into account • Absence of one or two PM2, if symmetrical, is accepted • Absence of M3 is not taken into account
147	Rottweiler	Level bite is accepted	
193	Russian Hunting Sighthound, Borzoi	Scissor bite or level bite	
212	Samoyed	Level bite is accepted	
41	Sarplaninac	Level bite	
150	Serbian Hound	Level bite is accepted	
279	Serbian Mountain Hound	Progenia is a serious problem but do not disqualify	
229	Serbian Tricolor Hound	Level bite is accepted	
82	Small Braband Griffon	Delicate progenia is required	
60	Small Swiss Hound	Level bite is accepted	
326	South Russian Ovtcharka		Teeth: White, big, fitting closely. The incisors are set regularly and close in scissor bite Faults: Teeth too small and spaced, yellow, or prematurely worn. Broken teeth but not impeding a correct closure of the jaws. Lack of premolars Severe faults: Everything which does not correspond to a perfect closure of the teeth but not impeding a correct closing of the teeth in scissor bite. Decayed teeth. Incisors set irregularly
91	Spanish Mastiff	Level bite is accepted	Missing one premolar is accepted
59	Swiss Hound	Scissor bite or level bite	

(Continued)

FCI number	Breed	Tolerance in occlusion	Other dental tolerances
252	Tatra Shepherd Dog	Level bite is accepted	
231	Tibetan Spaniel	Delicate retrogenia is required	
209	Tibetan Terrier	Delicate progenia should be accepted	
85	West Highland White Terrier	Level bite is accepted	

Appendix F

Assisted Feeding in Dental Patients

Michał Jank[1] and Jerzy Gawor[2]

[1] *Division of Pharmacology and Toxicology, Department of Preclinical Sciences, Institute of Veterinary Medicine, Warsaw University of Life Sciences (WULS-SGGW), Warsaw, Poland*
[2] *Veterinary Clinic Arka, Kraków, Poland*

Nutrition is an important element of perioperative care which is often neglected. In some clinics, it is a task of veterinary nurse to obtain an accurate diet history, understand the metabolic effects of anesthesia, and appropriately implement assisted feeding or diet recommendations. Also, the identification and preemptive treatment of pets at risk for malnutrition prior to or following a surgical procedure can significantly improve recovery and reduce morbidity.

Due to the nature and localization of oral pathologies, dental patients frequently require different forms of assisted feeding. This assisted feeding in some cases requires only the change of the texture of food – instead of hard/dry food (kibble), semi-moist (canned) or liquid food is required, whereas other patients require tube feeding or even parenteral nutrition. The veterinarian must always select the most natural method of food intake by animal. One of the key factors which must be taken into consideration in patients with reduced ability to ingest is the physiological role of food in the alimentary tract as well as the mechanical and paracrine stimulation of gastrointestinal tissues by the food ingredients. A reduction in ingesta significantly reduces the digestive and absorptive activity of many different cells and reduces the ability of the patient to recover quickly once the ability to eat normally returns (Kawasaki et al. 2009).

F.1 Change in Food Texture

Numerous common oral and maxillofacial procedures may impair the mastication ability of the patient. These procedures include, but are not limited to: maxillofacial injuries, teeth fractures or extractions, and soft tissue/periodontal surgeries. In these cases, the functional discomfort may limit the patient's ability for proper mastication. Therefore, offering semiliquid or liquid food facilitates swallowing and enables enteral nutrition (Figure F.1). Typically, the body condition of the patient is normal, without excessive muscle or cachexia, this there are no specific nutritional requirements for offered food.

The diet should just fulfill the nutritional requirements of the patient according to its physiological state and age. The texture is one of the key aspects of nutrition. Therefore, dry pet food (kibble) should be replaced with soft food. This can take the form of canned food, or the kibble can be soaked in warm water to soften it. Further, proper mixing or grinding may be required to facilitate swallowing. Canned nutrition is available in a semiliquid, fine-ground form which is complete and balanced and do not require excessive chewing during ingestion.

F.2 Tube Feeding

Some animals are not able to voluntarily intake food following oral surgery, thus tube feeding is necessary. Assisted feeding (parenteral or enteral) is recommended if an animal has not consumed adequate calories for three to five days (including presurgical period) due to poor appetite or medical conditions preventing intake. Patients requiring tube feeding may suffer from malnutrition but maintain a fully functional alimentary tract (normal integrity, motility, and enzymatic activity), so the main task of the practitioner is to deliver the food to stomach. Those techniques ensure the most natural means of patient feeding and delivery of nutrients to the GIT as well as the whole body (Parker and Freeman 2014). In the majority of cases, tube

The Veterinary Dental Patient: A Multidisciplinary Approach, First Edition. Edited by Jerzy Gawor and Brook Niemiec.
© 2021 John Wiley & Sons Ltd. Published 2021 by John Wiley & Sons Ltd.
Companion website: www.wiley.com/go/gawor/veterinary-dental-patient

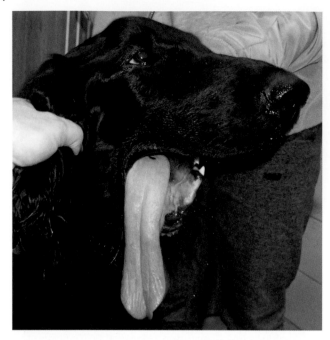

Figure F.1 Four year-old flat coated retriever nine months after mandibulectomy.

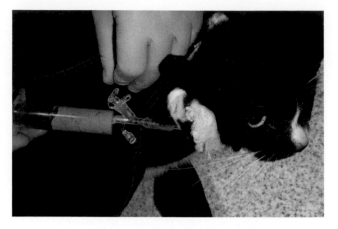

Figure F.3 Esophageal feeding tube placed immediately after mandibulectomy in a cat. Administering Hill's A/D diet.

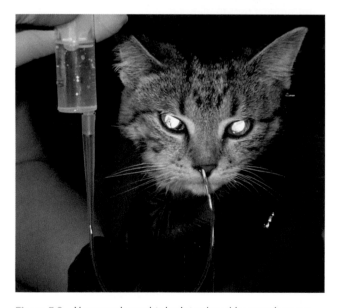

Figure F.2 Nasoesophageal tube introduced in conscious cat.

feeding is less stressful for the patient than syringe feeding. In addition, syringe feeding is not possible in some cases. When tube feeding is instituted, two aspects must be considered: proper tube placement and appropriate nutritional administration.

Nasal feeding tubes are usually only recommended for short-term nutritional support (5–10 days) which is sufficient for initial healing of large surgical wounds and/or for restoration of appetite following the procedure (Saker and

Remillard 2010) (Figure F.2). It is important that the tube does not interfere with nor prevent normal oral food intake. Placement of nasoesophageal feeding tubes has several advantages:

1) simple to place
2) minimal to no sedation is necessary
3) requires no special equipment.

Verification of tube placement within the esophagus requires radiography or an end-tidal carbon dioxide monitor. Tubes placed within the gastrointestinal tract should yield no carbon dioxide when checked (Johnson et al. 2002). Disadvantages of nasoesophageal tubes include patient discomfort and the exclusive use of liquid diets as the tubes used for this technique typically measure 3.5–5 Fr.

Esophageal feeding tubes are recommended for critically ill animals and have almost completely replaced pharyngostomy tubes. They are also easy to place, require only brief anesthesia, and can accommodate more calorically dense diets (i.e. >1 kcal/ml), making them ideal for patients that have feeding-volume limitations. Tubes ranging from 12 to 19 Fr are commonly used and patient discomfort is not usually an issue. The larger diameter tube allows for administration of semiliquid food. However, it is recommended to thoroughly soften the food with water and mix it thoroughly in order to avoid tube blockage. The most common complications associated with esophageal tubes are obstruction and cellulitis at the stoma site. The proper technique of tube placement is described elsewhere (Fink et al. 2014).

Once the tube is placed, the proper diet must be selected. Many companies offer special diets in powdered form which need to be reconstituted before administration. The easier way is to apply available liquid diets (Figure F.3).

F.3 Evaluation of Nutritional Needs of Animal

Once the method of feeding and type of the food is selected, the daily nutritional requirement of animal must be calculated. This is based on the body weight of animal as well as its body condition. The basis for calculation of daily nutritional requirement is the resting energy requirement (RER) of the animal. For this purpose, one can use exponential equation, $RER = 70 \times body\ weight^{0.75}$ or, if the body weight is between 2 and 45 kg using following formula: $RER = (30 \times body\ weight) + 70$. The result obtained is in kilocalories (Chan and Freeman 2006). After calculation of RER, the amount of each nutrient should be adjusted based on the caloric value of each ingredient.

In recent years, additional nutritional considerations for immune modulation (glutamine, arginine, omega-3 fatty acids, and nucleotides) in humans and animals during recovery from GI surgery has anecdotally demonstrated positive effects on reducing postoperative complications and shortening hospital stay; however, strong evidence is lacking. Glutamine is a conditionally essential amino acid and rapidly proliferating cells like enterocytes and lymphocytes preferentially use glutamine as an energy substrate and may enhance nutritional status and recovery. Arginine is also a conditionally essential amino acid that can accelerate wound healing by enhancing collagen production and influencing host immunity. Caution should be used with supplementing arginine because it may worsen inflammatory responses in critical patients. Omega-3 fatty acids include eicosapentaenoic acid (EPA) and docosahexaenoic acid (DHA) which are found in fish oil and are generally dosed through fish oil supplements. The general role of omega-3 fatty acids is inhibiting inflammation through several molecular pathways (Sobotka 2013).

F.4 Nutritional Challenges in Veterinary Dental Patients

Before performing any surgical procedure, it is important to collect data such as body condition score, muscle condition score, body weight, diet, treats, medications/supplements, and any recent changes in appetite or GI function. These will help formulate appropriate feeding recommendations both pre- and post-surgery.

The majority of dental patients require procedures which are performed under general anesthesia. Thus, nutritional questions will arise as in any anesthetized patient which must be answered before the procedure. Anesthetic and sedative medications reduce or eliminate airway protective reflexes that normally prevent regurgitation of gastric contents into the lungs. Consequently, complications of anesthesia may include intraoperative aspiration or gastroesophageal reflux (GER), which could potentially cause esophagitis or, when severe enough, esophageal strictures (Savvas et al. 2016). Scheduled surgical procedures should be performed on patients with an empty alimentary tract, ergo the veterinarian must decide when to stop feeding as well as when to reinitiate. In the recent years, the length of the fasting period before anesthesia significantly decreased. The absence of the food in the alimentary tract has destructive influence on GIT morphology and function (Sanderson et al. 2017). Without food, the length of the intestinal villi decreases significantly, and the production of digestive enzymes is also reduced. GIT juices (especially pancreatic juice) comprise substances with trophic influence on enterocytes and the composition of GIT microbiome is changed by the prolonged inactivity of alimentary tract. This results in changes which affect the recovery of the patient after procedure. The longer the inactivity of alimentary tract, the more significant the negative changes are and the longer period of recovery to a normal physiological state. That is why current approach to such patients is to withdraw the food as late as possible before the surgical procedure and start re-alimentation as fast as possible after. One study compared dogs given half of their daily estimated energy requirement (EER) in canned food 10 hours prior to an elective surgery to those given their EER 3 hours before the surgery (Savvas et al. 2016). The 10-hour fasting group had significantly increased incidence of GER when compared to the 3-hour fasting group. The current recommendation of AAHA for fasting of dogs prior to anesthesia suggests 4–6 hours in case of healthy animals, 1–2 hour for animals younger than 8 weeks or <2 kg of body weight, and 6–12 hours in case of patients with history or risk of regurgitation (Grubb et al. 2020).

The problem of fasting length is much more complicated in case of patients with coexisting diseases or senior animals. In case of patients with coexisting diseases influencing animal metabolism, the fasting should be long enough to avoid unnecessary vomiting before anesthesia. If patient is suffering from diabetes mellitus, the length of fasting depends on the number of meals (hours of feeding) and timing of the procedure. Blood glucose levels should be monitored before, during, and after procedure. Anesthesia impairs the body's response to insulin, which may contribute to hyperglycemia during and following surgery (Kim et al. 2016) in both healthy and diseased patients. In addition to anesthesia's effect on insulin, the normal mechanisms for maintaining glucose homeostasis become ineffective during the perioperative period due to the action of catabolic hormones increasing glucose and minimizing the effects of insulin. Blood glucose concentrations increase from hepatic glycogenolysis and gluconeogenesis as a response to metabolic stress caused by surgery. Generally, patients with diabetes receive on the day of the procedure half of the normal insulin dose and the last meal could be offered two hours before procedure at latest. Such two to four hours fasting period is recommended by AAHA (Grubb et al. 2020) and the last meal should be offered as ½ of regular meal in the form of wet food with pate consistency. In case of hypoglycemia, a small amount of water with glucose could be considered or dextrose in lactated Ringer solution could be given intravenously. After completion of the procedure, the glucose level should be measured and in case of hypoglycemia, proper action must be taken (i.e. administer a small amount of glucose). However, the procedure depends on individual patients.

From the nutritional point of view, a history of pancreatic diseases (especially acute pancreatitis) in a patient undergoing general anesthesia is of particular concern. Since the systemic hypotension is considered to be one of the potential causes of pancreatitis, the strict monitoring of the patient during anesthesia, especially cardiovascular function, is critical (Gaschen 2010). It is theorized that impairment of the blood microcirculation in pancreas during surgery could be one of the causes of acute post-op pancreatitis and the occurrence of this disease postsurgically precludes the early reintroduction of feeding the patient. That is why in patients at risk of pancreatic disease, the nutritional preparation for surgery should be based on feeding digestible carbohydrates (starch) in order to avoid overstimulation of pancreas. On the other hand, the chronic pancreatic insufficiency results in significant changes in intestinal microbiome (pancreatic juice contains an antibacterial factor which regulates the proliferation of different bacterial strains in the intestine) (Hamada et al. 2018), so in such patients, it would be beneficial to implement beneficial probiotic bacteria to the diet used for refeeding after procedure in order to restore proper composition of microbiome.

In senior animals, the presurgical nutritional approach depends on the clinical condition of the patient; however, no dramatic changes of the food are recommended. Once animal is healthy, the standard recommendations for the fasting prior to anesthesia should be followed.

The postoperative nutritional approach has changed significantly in the last few years. The current approach to such patients is focused on as quick as possible return to normal feeding (Corbee and Van Kerkhoven 2014). The reasons for this are as follows:

- The postsurgical period is characterized by nutritional and metabolic changes which lead to a catabolic state.
- Appetite reduction.
- Negative energy balance.

One of the side effects of general anesthesia is postsurgical ileus resulting from impaired GIT motility (Carroll and Karim 2009). Even in healthy dogs, contraction of the stomach, duodenum, and jejunum/ileum are reduced after 12–24 hours of fasting. Also, early nutrition after surgery may limit the risk of decreased GI motility and direct stimulation of mucosa causes endocrine stimulation supporting GI recovery (Sanderson et al. 2017). Early caloric requirement also decreases mortality rate and shortens the length of hospital stay in dogs and cats. That is why the length of fasting period before the surgery has been gradually reduced in recent years.

In patients which still have the ability to voluntary ingest, a small meal should be offered directly after complete recovery from anesthesia (Figure F.4a and b). In case of patients after receiving a professional dental cleaning without tooth extraction or other extensive dental procedures, quick return to normal feeding is recommended. This quickly restores the normal function of the GIT and promotes microbiome stability. The role of the latter is much more important than it was previously believed since it influences the gut-associated lymphoid tissue as well as local and systemic immunity of the body.

After extensive procedures (extraction of multiple teeth, fracture stabilization after maxillofacial injuries, and oncologic surgery), it is recommended to offer liquid or semiliquid foods. You can offer the food if animal is eating on his own or use force-feeding (synergy, nasal tube, etc.) if it is necessary. It strongly depends on the patients. Sometimes additional subcutaneous or intravenous fluid therapy is necessary.

How to treat "healthy" patients

- It is recommended to take a nutritional history for all patients and ask whether it is going to tolerate the change of nutrition for pre- and postsurgical period. Such change includes introduction of new food from one week before procedure to two to four weeks after procedure. This makes it possible to introduce a diet with increased calorie level, wet foods for convalescing patients (Recovery [Recovery]; Convalescence [Royal Canin], CN [Purina], a/ [Hills]) or intestinal diets (moderately high energy level, high digestibility diets which help to avoid postsurgical diarrheas: Gastrointestinal [Royal Canin], EN [Purina], i/d [Hill's], etc.)
- If possible, the wet food with uniform texture should be offered – pate, fine-ground cans, or crushed chunks in gravy. Carefully mixed and ground homemade food is also an option.
- If the patient does not tolerate wet food, dry pet food soaked with water could be offered. Dry pet food may

(a)

(b)

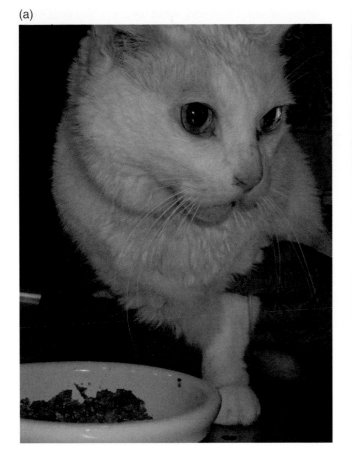
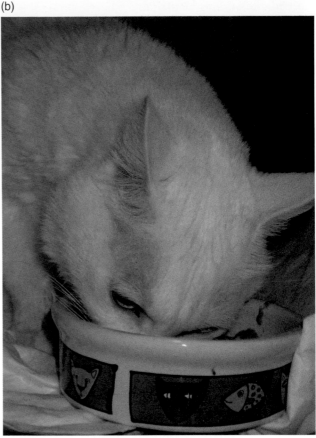

Figure F.4   Food presented one hour after recovery from anesthesia (a) and voluntary eating (b).

also be soaked with some liquid diets, i.e. Recovery (Royal Canine), Oralade, etc.

- Following oral surgery, it is recommended to feed soft and not-irritating foods (foods should not inducing dust, the powders, powdered toppers, and additives should be avoided) for several days. In dogs, sage or chamomile infusions maybe considered since they are supporting the process of mucosal healing.

Treating "sick" patients

- Recommendations for "sick" patients regarding food type are similar as for "healthy" patients, with the exception of diet type change. It is recommended to keep the patients on the same diet which after the procedure could be fortified with some fluids (i.e. Duphalyte in cats with chronic kidney failure). The only accepted change is to replace dry diet with wet diet or with dry soaked diet.
- In cats with chronic kidney failure, who following the procedure become completely anorectic, it is recommended to start intravenous or enteral tube feeding. In case of complete lack of appetite, it is possible to give small amounts of instant recovery diet, because complete absence of the food intake for several days could lead to hepatic encephalopathy.

How to manage patients without teeth

If a dental procedure results in extraction of all teeth, the postsurgical nutrition may become complicated, especially in patients which before procedure were fed only with dry pet food. The risk of undernutrition is especially high in patients which previously were not eating wet food, are resistant to eat any type of wet food, and their body condition before the procedure was not ideal (below 3/5). In such a situation, it is recommended to offer soaked intestinal or recovery dry diets. These diets are highly digestible because they contain extremely small amounts of fiber, but in order to be properly digested should be thoroughly ground before administration. This should improve the process of digestion and absorption of nutrients. Sometimes in small breed dogs, also soaked dry intestinal diet for cat could be solution.

How to improve food palatability:

- Mix dry food with wet food.
- Addition of meat (cooked is preferred in order to avoid bacterial contamination) or meat broth to offered food.
- Addition of warm water to wet food.
- Addition of highly palatable foods, such as liver, cooked meat, sugar (dogs), honey (dogs), yogurt (if there is no nutritional contraindications).

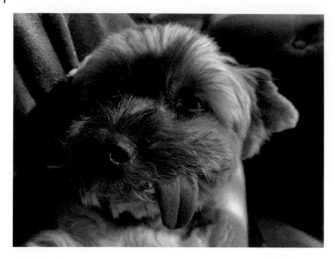

Figure F.5 Teethless dogs often have a protruded tongue but they quickly adapt to proper food intake.

- Warming of wet food (especially for cats).
- In some cases, pharmacological stimulation of appetite (Cyproheptadine: syrup 0,4 mg/ml; tablets – 1–4 mg PO (dog); 2 mg/cat/12 h; mirtazapine in tablets 15 mg, 30 mg, 45 mg: ¼ tabl. 15 mg –dog <7 kg b.w.; ½ tabl. 15 mg – dog 8–15 kg b.w.; 1 tabl. 15 mg – dog 16–30 kg b.w.; 2 tabl. 15 mg – dog>30 kg b.w.; megestrol acetate (40 mg/ml) – 5 mg/kg b.w. PO 1×d) or force feeding is necessary. In the latter, the patient receives the food from syringe or through tube.

Commercial pet food for dental patients

- Liquid diets fulfilling requirements of recovery or high energy diets, i.e. Instant – Convalescence.
- Wet foods for recovering healthy animals: Convalescene (dogs), Recovery (dogs/cats), CN (dogs/cats), a/d or i/d (dogs/cats); gastrointestinal; EN Purina.
- Wet foods for recovering sick animals
  - Chronic kidney failure (CRF): Renal (RC), cans: NF (Purina), Renal (RC), k/d (Hill's)
  - Pancreatic disorders: liquid: Low fat (RC); cans: low fat (dog) RC, i/d low fat Hill's; Kot: Gastrointestinal moderate RC, i/d Hill` s, Sensitivity RC
  - Diabetes: the best option is to give currently offered diet; cans: diabetic (safe since contain no sugar, gastrointestinal should not be used).

References

Carroll, J. and Karim, A. (2009). Pathogenesis and management of postoperative ileus. *Clin. Colon Rectal Surg.* 22 (1): 47–50.

Chan, D.L. and Freeman, L.M. (2006). Nutrition in clinical illness. *Vet. Clin. Small Anim.* 36 (2006): 1225–1241.

Corbee, R.J. and Van Kerkhoven, W.J.S. (2014). Nutritional support of dogs and cats after surgery or illness. *Open J. Vet. Med.* 4: 44–57.

Fink, L., Jennings, M., and Reiter, A.M. (2014). Esophagostomy feeding tube placement in the dog and cat. *J. Vet. Dent.* 31 (2): 133–138. https://doi.org/10.1177/089875641403100215.

Gaschen, F. (2010). Pancreatitis. In: Canine and Feline Gastroenterology (eds. P. Lecoindre, F. Gaschen, E. Monnet, et al.), 377–384. Wolter Kluwer France.

Grubb, T., Sager, J., Gaynor, J.S. et al. (2020). 2020 AAHA anesthesia and monitoring guidelines for dogs and cats. *J. Am. Anim. Hosp. Assoc.* 56: 1–24. https://doi.org/10.5326/JAAHA-MS-7055.

Hamada, S., Masamune, A., Nabeshima, T., and Shimosegawa, T. (2018). Differences in gut microbiota profiles between autoimmune pancreatitis and chronic pancreatitis. *Tohoku J. Exp. Med.* 244: 113–117.

Johnson, P., Mann, F., Dodam, J. et al. (2002). Capnographic documentation of nasoesophageal and nasogastric feeding tube placement in dogs. *J. Vet. Emerg. Crit. Care* 12 (4): 227–233.

Kawasaki, N., Suzuki, Y., Nakayoshi, T. et al. (2009). Early postoperative enternal nutrition is useful for recovering gastrointestinal motility and maintaining the nutritional status. *Surg. Today* 39 (3): 225–230. https://doi.org/10.1007/s00595-008-3861-0. Epub 2009 Mar 12. PMID: 19280282.

Kim, S.P., Broussard, J.L., and Kolka, C.M. (2016). Isoflurane and sevoflurane induce severe hepatic insulin resistance in 7a canine model. *PLoS One* 11 (11): e0163275.

Parker, V.L. and Freeman, L.M. (2014). Jak wprowadzić odżywianie dojelitowe do swojej praktyki. *Weterynaria po Dyplomie* 15 (2): 8–16.

Saker, K.E. and Remillard, R.L. (2010). Critical care nutrition and enteral assisted feeding. In: Small Animal Clinical Nutrition, 5e (ed. M.S. Hand), 440–476. Topeka: Mark Morris Institute.

Sanderson, J.J., Boysen, S.R., McMurray, J.M. et al. (2017). The effect of fasting on gastrointestinal motility in healthy dogs as assessed by sonography. *J. Vet. Emerg. Crit. Care* 27 (6): 645–650.

Savvas, I., Raptopoulos, D., and Rallis, T. (2016). A "light meal" three hours preoperatively decreases the incidence of gastro-esophageal reflux in dogs. *JAHAA* 52 (6): 357–363.

Sobotka, L. (2013). Podstawy żywienia klinicznego. IV wydanie. Scientifica. Kraków.

Index

a

Acid etching   355–356
Actinobacteria   77
Actinomyces   225
Active home care   62
Acute jaw-motion disorders
  jaw-locking syndrome   327, 330
  TMJ fractures   329
  TMJ luxation   327–329
Adenocarcinboma   201, 202
Against medical advice (AMA)
      release form   263, 264, 319
Alfaxalone   141, 173–175, 177,
      178, 185, 190–193, 390
Allodynia   141–143
Alveolar bone loss   123, 126, 305,
      324, 351, 353
  chronic   239
Alveolar osteomyelitis   128, 129
Amantadine   148, 160
Amelogenesis imperfecta   224,
      416
American Animal Hospital
      Association (AAHA)   29,
      173
American Heart Association
      (AHA) guidelines   88–89
American Society for the
      Prevention of Cruelty to
      Animals (ASPCA)   110
American Veterinary Dental
      College (AVDC)   373
Anaerobic bacteria   212

Anaerobic infection   91, 123, 291
Analgesics   388–389
  administration of   141, 154
  assessment of pain   145
  cardiac and respiratory
      function   184
  classic   141
  fast-acting antibiotics and   320
  nociceptive process   141
  opioid   155, 184
  preventive   146
  provision of   140
  receive   146
  sedative   171–173
  traditional   352
Anatomic anomalies   250–251
Anesthesia   233–234, 242,
      390–391
  balanced anesthesia   146, 189,
      192, 193, 195, 196
  induction   174–175
  laboratory testing   170
  management   171–174, 176
  patient history/physical
      exam   169–170
  record   169
Anesthesia-free dentistry (AFD)
  animal welfare   114, 115–116
  teeth cleaning without
      anesthesia   115–116
Anesthesia induction
  alfaxalone   174
  endotracheal tube   175

  etomidate   175
  facemask   175
  hypoventilation   181
  mucous membrane   175
  neuroactive steroid   174
  recovery   182–183
Anesthetic management
  drugs selection   171
  inhalant anesthetic
      maintenance   176
  intravenous catheter
      placement   173
  pre-induction support   173–174
  premedication   170–171
  protocols creation   173
Angiotensin-converting enzyme
      (ACE)   184, 189
Animal welfare
  AWNA options   110
  challenges   109
  ethics   109
  Five Animal Welfare Needs
      109–111, 116
  Five Freedoms   110–111
  optimal oral health   116
  prevalence of dental
      disease   111
  proper therapy   116
  QOL measurement tools   111
  regular dental
      examination   116
  root of   109
  term   109

The Veterinary Dental Patient: A Multidisciplinary Approach, First Edition. Edited by Jerzy Gawor and Brook Niemiec.
© 2021 John Wiley & Sons Ltd. Published 2021 by John Wiley & Sons Ltd.
Companion website: www.wiley.com/go/gawor/veterinary-dental-patient

Animal welfare needs assessment (AWNA) 110
Ankyloglossia 221, 222
  Anatolian shepherd 416
Antibacterial ingredients, nutritional products 79
Anticholergics 171
Anti-epileptic drugs 195
Anti-inflammatory drugs 387
  analgesic and potential drugs 155
  corticosteroids 154–155
  EP4 receptor antagonists 152
  NSAID 151–152, 153, 154
Anti-inflammatory therapy 221
Antimicrobials
  bacteremia and infective endocarditis 94–97
  control
    infection (*see* Infection control)
    periodontal disease 96–97
    plaque 97–98
  general approach 87
  human dentistry (*see* Human)
  optimal duration and 87
  oral and dental infections 90–93
  oral infections associated with dental procedures 93–94
  oral microbiota, dogs and cats 87–88
  prevention and treatment of oral disease 87
  products, oral home care 63
Arkansas stones 395
Arrhythmic drugs 191–193
Aspergillus infection 224–225
Assessment and recognition, pain
  feline pain assessment 143
  oral cancer 144
  pain management 144
Association of American Feline Practitioners (AAFP) 152
Auscultation 233
Autosomal recessive amelogenesis imperfecta (ARAI) 221
Azotemia 185, 229

b
Bacteremia 212–213, 214
  causes 89
  culture 212
  duration of 88
  estimated rate, dogs and cats 212
  infective endocarditis and 94, 95
  prevention of 94–96
  procedure group in human dentistry 213
  reduce post-extraction 102
  teeth descaling 213
  transient 88, 211
Bacteremia and infective endocarditis
  ampicillin 95
  cats 94
  choosing drugs 95
  criteria 95
  cultured bacteria, periodontal abscess 95, 96
  dental prophylaxis 94
  diagnosis 94
  dogs 94
  gram-negative bacteria 95
  gram-positive cocci 95
  limitations 94
  oral and ocular surgery 208
  overuse of antimicrobials 94
  perioperative antimicrobial therapy 94
  periprocedure prophylaxis 95
  prophylaxis, orthopedic implants 96
  recommendations, AVDC 94–95
Balanced anesthesia 146, 189, 192, 193, 195, 196
Barrier sealant 66, 267, 285
Blood pressure measurement 189
Body temperature 7, 103, 181, 189, 192, 193, 233
Bonding agent 333, 334, 356
Bone sequestrum 320

Brachycephalic breeds 127, 196, 197, 324, 330, 340–341, 413, 414
Brachycephalic obstructive airway syndrome (BOAS) 196–197, 409, 413
Brachycephalic patients
  induction of anesthesia 196–197
  maintenance phase 197
  preoperative considerations 196
  recovery and postoperative management 197
  sedation 196
Bradycardia (beta blockers) 146, 147, 171, 172, 175, 189, 194, 195
Buccal alveolar bone expansion and infra bony pocket 370, 371
Buprenorphine 146, 149, 150, 156, 157, 161, 171, 172, 173, 178, 388
Buried knot suture 302, 357, 359
Butorphanol 146, 150, 151, 160, 171–173, 191–193, 195, 196, 388

c
Calcitonin gene-related peptide (CGRP) 140
Calculus formation
  bovine raw cortical 81
  development 80
  dogs and cats 80
  inorganic salts 80
  "natural" food eating 81
  scores 83
  sodium hexametaphosphate 81
  strategies 80–81
  type of chelating agent 81
Cancerogenic factor 128
Canine 245
Canine distemper 223
Canine leischmaniosis 225
Canine oral cavity microbiome 76

Canine tooth (204) luxation   367

Capillary refill time (CRT)   175

Capnography   179–181, 189

Cardiac disease
  anesthetic drugs   189–190
  balanced anesthesia   189
  continuous monitoring   189
  diagnostic procedures   189
  dogs
    DCM in   190–191
    MVI in   191–192
  emergency drugs   189
  goals   189
  HCM in cats   192–193
  hypotension   189
  induction of anesthesia   189
  intravenous access and
    endotracheal
    intubation   189
  oxygen supplementation   189
  pre-anesthetic evaluation   189
  stress   189
  ventilation and
    oxygenation   189

Cardiac system   319

Cardiac ultrasound   189

Cardiomyopathies   133

Carnassial   124

Carnivores   219

Catechin   79

Catecholamines   156, 172, 175, 194

Cat-friendly clinics   343

Caudal stomatitis   226
  clinical signs   344–345
  diagnosis   345
  etiology   344
  management   345
  medical therapy
    antibiotics/antiseptics   346
    anti-inflammatories   346–347
    cyclosporine   347
    doxycycline   347
    feline interferon omega   347
    lactoferrin   347
  surgical therapy   345–346

Caudoventral (204) luxation   328

Central nervous system (CNS)   319
  COX-1 enzymes   155
  gingivostomatitis in cats   141
  maropitant   161, 171
  nociceptive signalling   141
  obesity hypoventilation
    syndrome   183
  stabilization   319
  stressors   113

Ceramic stones   395

Certifications and
  specializations   5

Chinese Crested dog   415

Chlamydia   224

Chlamydia spp.   224

Chlorhexidine lavage   271

Chlorhexidine (CHX)
  solution   24, 25

Chronic grooming   226

Chronic kidney disease
  (CKD)   151, 214

Chronic oronasal fistula
  (ONF)   374

Chronic periodontal disease   128, 131, 141, 214

Chronic ulcerative paradental
  stomatitis (CUPS)   226
  maltese   416

Class II malocclusion   328, 372

Class IV malocclusion   367, 368

Cleft palates   251, 370

Client communication   242

Clinical assessment   137

Clostridium tetani   224

Clotting disorders   226

Cold steel   294

Cold sterilization   102

Commercial sharpening machines   396, 397

Communications
  content skills   32
  dental services   35
  empathy   33–34
  nonverbal and verbal   32, 33
  open-ended questions   32
  perceptual skills   32
  process skills   32

reflective listening   32–33

Complete blood count
  (CBC)   170, 319, 374

Complete oral health assessment
  and treatment
  (COHAT)   3, 50, 263, 269,
  378–383, 385, 386

Compliance
  actual   34
  adherence   28
  arterial   178
  client–pet and client–
    veterinarian bonds   29
  consultation process   31, 61
  geriatric patients   183
  home care   55, 224
  human–dog bond   29, 30
  miscommunication   32
  motivate client   267
  oral care   113, 131
  owner   29, 87, 104
  paternalistic   28–29
  percentage of pets,
    treatment   28
  rate   67
  with recommended
    therapy   270
  relationship-centered care   29
  thoracic   184
  tooth brushing   62
  treatment   149
  vessels   178

Complicated crown fracture of
  canine tooth   367, 369

Comprehensive oral health
  assessment and treatment
  (COHAT)   3, 50

Congenital feline
  hypothyroidism   228

Consulting room
  dental models and
    instruments   5, 6
  educational posters   7–9
  educational video   7, 10
  finger protection, oral cavity
    assessment   7, 10
  good-quality flat-screen
    computer monitors   7

Consulting room (*cont'd*)
  installation, list of useful
      equipment 7
  ISFM recommendations and
      standards 5
  presentation of radiographs 5
  safety consideration 7
  space 5
  standards of cat-friendly
      clinic 5, 6
  white board drawings 7
Continuing education (CE) 376
Continuing professional
      development (CPD) 376
  courses 5
  program 27
Continuous monitoring 189, 195
Corneal ulceration 202, 203, 207,
      208
Craniomandibular osteopathy
      (CMO) 134, 136, 219–222,
      414
Credentialed veterinary
      technicians/nurses
  anesthetized patient 53
  annual dental cleanings 49, 50
  color-coding system, follow-up
      visits 55
  concious animal
      assessment 51
  dental chart 51, 52
  diagnosis 49
  empowering 48
  history gathering 49–50
  home care instructions 55–56
  informational brochures,
      waiting room 56
  members 48
  modified pen grasp, scaling
      handpiece 54
  open-ended questions 50
  oral examination
  owner problems 50
  professional dental cleaning
      53–55
  responsibilities 49
  smile book creation 56
  treatment plan 51, 53

Crown amputation 340, 351,
      352, 355, 356, 367
Cryptococcus infection 225
Cytokines 142, 214

d
Day of surgery
  AMA 263
  anesthesia 263
  anesthesia record 266
  COHAT 263
  estimate and consent form 265
  pharmacologic plan 266
  procedures 264
  release form, AMA 264
  sedation 263
Dental burs 316
Dental charts 234, 235, 405–408
  abbreviations and 399–404
Dental extractions 305
Dental hypersensitivity 142
Dental operatory
  anesthesia equipment 10
  dental x-ray 7
  hazardous materials
      storage 10, 12
  hygienic requirements 10
  nitrogen and oxygen distribution
      7, 11
  patient protection, during
      sedation 7, 11
  procedures 7
  safety 10
  wall-mounted anesthesia
      machine 10, 12
  water usage 7, 11
  X-ray generator 10, 12
Dental/orofacial pain
  causes 142–143
  feline orofacial pain
      syndrome 143
  periodontal disease 143
  persistent postsurgical
      pain 142
  temporomandibular joint
      disorders 143
  treatment 145–146
Dental patient management

additional consultations 261
anesthesia, incidental
      finding 261, 263
consultation with pet owner
    GP perspectives 262
    specialist perspectives 261
follow-up 267
identifying problems 261
owner's initiative 261
routine oral examination 261
Dental patients and its general
      conditions
  brachycephalic 196–197
  cardiac disease 189–190
  DM 193–194
  history of seizures 195–196
  pregnant 194–195
Dental prophylaxis
  barrier sealant 285
  chlorhexidine lavage 271
  fluoride therapy (optional) 281
  periodontal evaluation 282
  postsurgical discharge 285
  presurgical exam and
      consultation 269–271
  probing 282, 282
  radiographs 283–285
  subgingival plaque and calculus
      scaling 274–279
  sulcal lavage 281
  supragingival
      cleaning 271–274
  treatment planning 285
  Triadan system 283
Dental radiography 202, 234,
      319, 366
  pathologic periodontal
      pockets 283
  preliminary radiographic
      assessment 284
Dental radiology 366
Dental services 35
Dentigerous cysts 135, 248
Dentoalveolar ankylosis 239,
      306, 308, 351, 355
Diabetes mellitus (DM) 184–185
  anesthetic management 185,
      194

blood glucose management 184–185

periodontal disease 214, 227–228

perioperative management 194

preoperative considerations 184, 193–194

recovery and postoperative management 194

Diagnostic kit

charting 17, 22

high-quality photography 17

magnification 17, 22

mirrors 17, 21

mouth props selection 17, 21

series of combined probes and explorers 17, 20

UNC probe and explorer 17, 19

Diagnostic testing 133

Diazepam 171, 191

Dilated cardiomyopathy (DCM)

predisposed breeds 191

systolic dysfunction 190–191

Drugs and doses

analgesics 388–389

anesthetics/sedatives 390–391

anti-inflammatory 387

Drugs selection, premedication

anticholergics 171

mild to moderate tranquilizers 171

moderate to heavy sedatives 172–173

sedative analgesics 171

suppression of vomiting 171

Dry heat sterilization 393

e

Echocardiogram (ECG) 170

Economic consequences 114

Education

associations 4

continuing education 4–5

e-learning concept 39, 41

evidence-based medicine concept 41

ex cathedra 41

face-to-face learning 39, 40

implementation 42

interactive session 39, 40

opportunities 4

postgraduate education and specialization 42

self-education 4

specialists 42

teaching (*see* Teaching veterinary dentistry)

theoretical and practical methods 41

Webinar in dentistry 39

WSAVA Dental guidelines team 43

E-learning 376

Electrocardiogram 179

Electrocardiography 189

Electrosurgery 294–297, 302, 357

Emergency drugs 189

Emergency referrals 319

Empathy

communications

centralized position of the patient 33, 34

identification, emotions 33

nonverbal behaviors, consultation 34

statement 33

trust 33

verbal behaviors, consultation 34

definition 30

Empiric therapy 202

Enamel hypocalcification/hypoplasia (EH) 223, 248, 250

Endodontic disease 123, 202, 250, 305

Endo-perio lesions 122

Endotoxins 213, 214, 277

Endotracheal tube 169

Entotoxins 213–214

Envelope flap 311

Eosinophilic granuloma complex (EGC) 226, 353–355

Eosinophils 226

Epidermolysis bullosa aquisita 226

Equipment considerations

consulting room 5–7

waiting room 5, 6

Eruptive gingivitis 251

Erythema multiforme (EM) 226, 400

Esophageal feeding 424

Etomidate 191, 193

Eucalyptus oil 79

European Veterinary Dental College (EVDC) 373

Excessive hemorrhage 241

Exophthalmos 201, 202, 203

Exposure keratitis 202, 203

Extraction kit 23, 24

Extra-oral implant infections

human dentistry 89–90

f

Feeding

change in food texture 423

dental patients 84

description 75

dry food 79, 83

forms of assisted feeding 423

nutrition 423

nutritional needs of animal (*see* Nutrition)

plaque index 80

soft food 79

tube feeding 423–424

Feline Advisory Bureau (FAB) 133

Feline brachycephalism 417

Feline calicivirus (FCV) 222, 223, 347

Feline chronic gingivitis stomatitis 226

Feline dentistry 339

3D imaging 340

acid etching 355–356

bonding agent 356

brachycephalic breeds 340–341

buried knot suture 357

cat-friendly clinics 343

caudal stomatitis (*see* Caudal stomatitis)

crown amputation 355

Feline dentistry (*cont'd*)
  dental care   344
  EGC   353–355
  FOPS   352
  gingivectomy   357
  gingivoplasty   357
  high-rise syndrome   343
  juvenile periodontal disease
        352–353
  odontoplasty   355
  oral tumors   343
  perianesthetic hazards   340
  pharyngostomy   360
  postoperative challenges   340
  preoperative actions   339–340
  pulp therapy/standard
        endodontic therapy   355
  radiography   340
  surgery   340
  tooth resorption (*see* Tooth
        resorption)
Feline herpesvirus-1   222
Feline immunodeficiency virus
        (FIV)   222, 223
Feline juvenile gingivitis   226
Feline leukemia virus
        (FeLV)   222
Feline lower urinary tract disease
        (FLUTD)   133
Feline oral cavity microbiome   77
Feline oral pain syndrome
        (FOPS)   122, 143, 339, 352,
        359
Fenestration   313, 314
Fentanyl   147, 156, 171, 172, 173,
        177, 192, 388
Fine-needle aspiration (FNA)
        techniques   302
First consultation, pet owner
  GP perspectives   263
  specialist perspectives   263
Flap closure   313
Fluorescein staining   201
Fluoride therapy   281
Food texture   423
Fractured maxillary canine tooth
        (104)   368
Fresh frozen plasma (FFP)   185

Full flap   313
Functional residual capacity
        (FRC)   183
Fusobacterium   224

g
Gabapentin   145, 148, 160–161,
        195, 389
Gas sterilization   395
Gastrointestinal (GI) tract   121
General practitioners   39, 42, 109,
        233, 261, 263, 351, 365, 366,
        374, 376
General veterinary practice
  adjustable table   11, 13
  clinic's investment plan   3–4
  COHAT   3
  communication with pet owner
        12–13
  considerations   3
  dental operatory   7, 10
  diagnostics   3
  education   4–5
  equipment
    considerations (*see* Equipment
        considerations)
    power dental   17, 19
    proper equipment (*see* Proper
        equipment)
    selection of   3–4
  ergonomic solutions   10
  extractions   3
  high-quality screen and medical
        database   13
  high-speed internet and
        computer database
        networks   11
  instruments and surgical
        kits   12
  organization, and
        functionality   10–14
  pathology   11, 13
  professional dental cleaning
        3, 4
  promotion   5
  prophylactic procedures   3
  radiography   4
  safe anesthesia   14

  size, height, air conditioning,
        light and intensity of water
        access   11
  VIN   3
Generalized amelogenesis
        imperfect, Akita Inu   224
Genetic and developmental
        disorders
  ankyloglossia   221, 222
  anti-inflammatory therapy   221
  ARAI   221
  cleft lip/palates   219, 220
  CMO   219–222
  hydrocephalus   219, 221
  malocclusion   219, 221
  microglossia/aglossia   219, 221
  MMM   219, 220
  muscle biopsy   220
  oral and maxillofacial
        assessment   219, 220
  QOL   219
  siamese twins   219
  TMJ dysplasia   219, 220,
        221–223
  Von Willebrand's disease   220
Genetic testing   137
Gentle patient elevation   237
Geriatric denistry
  alveolar bone atrophy   255
  ankylosis and teeth
        resorption   254
  malocclusions   253
  orodental structures, aging   253
  periodontal disease   252, 253
  quality of life (QOL)   252
  right maxillary canine tooth
        254
  squamous-cell carcinoma
        (SCC)   254
  transparent and brittle
        enamel   255
Geriatric patients   183
Gingival attachment   306
Gingival hyperplasia   134
Gingivectomy   212, 215, 252, 294,
        353, 357, 359
Gingivitis   212
Gingivoplasty   294, 353, 357

Glomerular filtration rate (GFR) 151, 173
Glucocorticosteroids 154, 155
Gram-negative bacteria 76, 88, 95, 212, 213, 214
Gram-positive bacteria 212

h

Handpieces maintenance 397
Head injury 320, 321, 323, 330, 380
Hemorrhage 95, 142, 159, 206, 240, 241, 242, 298, 305, 319, 317
Hemostasic techniques
    blood vessels 297
    palatal artery 298
    repairing fractures 297
    segmental mandibulectomy 298
Hepatic dysfunction 185
Hereditary diseases
    diagnostic methods 134
    FAB (cats) 133
    scale for the negative influence 134
    UV syndrome 134
Hereditary problems and breed predispositions
    amelogenesis imperfecta 416
    ankyloglossia, Anatolian shepherd 416
    BOAS 413
    chronic ulcerative paradental stomatitis, Maltese 416
    CMO in Cairn Terrier 414
    EGC 414
    extraoral radiograph and CBCT scan, Akita inu dog 412
    feline brachycephalism 417
    ICH in bullmastiff 414
    Italian Greyhound 415
    juvenile gingivitis in Maine Coon 417
    lingually displaced right mandibular canine tooth 414
    lip-fold dermatitis 414

list of 409–412
malocclusion 417
masticatory muscle myositis, Rottweiler 416
Norwegian Forest Cat 417
odontodysplasia 415
oligodontia, Chinese Crested dog 415
retrogenia in longhaired dachshund 416
supernumerary maxillary incisors teeth, Boxer 413
teeth crowding 414
    mandibular incisor 417
High-efficiency particulate air filter (HEPA) 271
High-rise syndrome 206, 321, 343, 368, 380
Hip dysplasia 133
Histopathological examination 133, 137
Home care. *see* Regular oral home care
Horner's syndrome 206, 207
Human
    antimicrobial
        administration 88
        extra-oral implant infections 89–90
        infective endocarditis 88–89
        oral infections 90
    ARAI 221
    dentistry 213
    medicine 215
    pathogens 99
    probiotic bacterial strains 77
Hydrocephalus 219, 221
Hydrodynamic theory 142
Hydromorphone 146, 147, 150, 161, 171, 172, 177, 389
Hyperalgesia 141
Hyperglycemia 193
Hyperostosis 228
Hyperparathyroidism 227, 228
Hyperphosphatemia 227
Hypertrophic cardiomyopathy (HCM) 129
    induction of anesthesia 193

maintenance phase 193
periodontal disease
preoperative considerations 192
recovery and postoperative management 193
sedation 192–193
Hypocalcemia 227
Hypothermia 53, 172, 176, 181–182, 233, 285

i

Iatrogenic complications 305
Iatrogenic jaw fracture 126
Iatrogenic orbital/brain damage 240–242
iM3 Vet-Tome 308–309
Immune-related disorders 226, 227
Immunological injury 214
Improper therapy and iatrogenic damage 236–242
    damage of structures and tissue adjacent 240
    iatrogenic failures 236
    iatrogenic orbital/brain damage 240–242
    improper/incomplete scaling 236–237
    mandibular canal/nasal cavity 240, 241
    oronasal fistulas 239
    pathologic mandibular fractures 239–240
    retained tooth roots 237–239
India stones 395
Infantile Cranial Hyperostosis (ICH) 414
Infection control
    autoclaved instruments 103
    basic measures, needlestick injuries 101
    cross-contamination, pathogens 99
    environmental cleaning and disinfection 101
    equipment, cleaning and disinfection practices 102

Infection control (*cont'd*)
  extensive infection-control
      guidelines   99
  facility design   100
  goals of cleaning, disinfection
      and sterilization   102–103
  hand hygiene   100
  intraoperative patient
      management   103
  PPE   99–100
  precautions   99
  pre-procedure biocide mouth
      rinse   101–102
  sharps handling   100–101
  surgical antisepsis   103
  surveillance   104
  transmission   99
  zoonotic infections   104
Infectious disease
  actinomyces   225
  amelogenesis imperfecta   224
  appetite/indigestion   224
  aspergillus infection   224–225
  canine distemper   223
  canine leischmaniosis   225
  chlamydia   224
  cryptococcus infection   225
  EH   223
  FCV   222, 223
  feline herpesvirus-1   222
  FeLV   222
  FIV   222, 223
  mycotic infections   224–225
  oral lesions   225, 226
  oral manifestations   223
  oral papillomatosis   222, 224
  regurgitation/vomiting   224
  tetanus   225
Infectious hepatitis   223
Infective endocarditis   88–89
Inflammatory bowel disease
      (IBD)   133
Inflammatory feline oral
      diseases   385
Inflammatory lesion   234, 235
Instrumentation
  chlorhexidine (CHX)
      solution   24, 25

diagnostic kit (*see* Diagnostic
      kit)
instrument care and sharpening
      (*see* Instruments handling)
oral surgery and dentistry   17
periodontal kit   24
personal protective
      equipment   24
pharyngeal packs   24, 25
plaque-disclosing solutions
      24, 25
polishing paste   24
proper grasp   17
surgical kit (*see* Surgical kit)
suture needles   24
types or brands   17
Instruments handling   24
  avoid contamination   393
  broken instrument
      examples   393, 394
  cassettes, boxes, and
      organizers   393
  damaging   393
  machine-based cleaning   393
  maintenance   393
  maintenance of power
      equipment
      (*see* Power equipment)
  mineral deposits   393
  and sharpening (*see* Sharpening)
  sterilization   393–395
  ultrasonic cleaning   393, 394
  visual inspection   393
Interceptive orthodontics   211,
      246
Intermittent positive-pressure
      ventilation (IPPV)   183
International Association for the
      Study of Pain (IASP)   139
International Renal Interest
      Society (IRIS)   152
International Society of Feline
      Medicine (ISFM)   5, 152
Intramuscular injection, cats
      193
Intraoral dental sinus
      drainage   125
Italian Greyhound   415

j

Jaw-locking syndrome   327, 330
Juvenile facial dermatitis   226,
      227
Juvenile gingivitis   352
  Maine Coon   417
Juvenile hyperplastic gingivitis
      353
Juvenile periodontal
      disease   352–353
Juvenile periodontitis   251, 252,
      353

k

Kennel assistants   47
Keratoconjunctivitis sicca
      (KCS)   202
Ketamine   145, 160, 174, 175,
      177, 178, 184, 191

l

Lactobacilli   77
Lasers   294
  electrosurgery   296
  excisional biopsy   295
Left mandibular fracture   368,
      370
Left maxillary canine tooth (204)
      369
Leptospira canicola   224
Lidocaine   155, 156, 160, 174,
      175, 177, 340, 388
Lifelong prophylactic
      program   267
Lingual mucosa   222, 223
Lipopolysaccharides
      (LPSs)   213–214
Liver   214
Local anesthetic
  adjuncts   156–157
  infraorbital block   157–158
  maxillary berve block   158–159
  middle mental canal injection
      157
  pain management   155
  palatine block   159
  pharmacology   155–156
  regional techniques   157
Locomotory system   319

Lower-lip avulsion 370
Luxation 307–309

m

MAC sparing technique 177
Maladaptive process 141, 141
Malignancies 236
Malocclusions 219, 221, 247
   adverse dental interlock 246, 249
   class II 249
   fracture 247, 249
   interceptive orthodontics 246
   tolerance and dental abnormalities, dogs 419–422
Malpractice
   anesthesia 233–234
   client communication 242
   error 233
   improper therapy and iatrogenic damage 236–242
   oral examination and diagnostics 234–237
   true 233
   in veterinary dentistry 233
Mandibular canal/nasal cavity 240, 241
Mandibular canine teeth 370, 371
Mandibular canine tooth crown 368
Mandibular fractures 239–240
Mandibular incisor teeth crowding 417
Mandibular tumor 234, 236
Marketing
   and communications skills (*see* Communications)
   compliance 28–30
   CPD program 27
   dental assessment and treatment 28
   dental services 35
   empathy 30
   logic 30, 32
   motivation 30
   problems, selling veterinary dental services 27, 28

real problem 28
recommendations, treatments 27
sellers 30
trust 30, 31
Maropitant 161, 171, 173, 177, 178, 184, 194, 196
Mask induction 175, 191, 193
Mastication 83, 124, 213, 251, 254, 423
Masticatory muscle myositis (MMM) 219, 220, 416
Maxillary molar teeth 240
Maxillary tooth roots 239
Maxillofacial injury 205–207, 370
Maxillofacial mass 372
Mean arterial pressure (MAP) 178
Mechanized Hu-Friedy sharpener 396, 397
Medetomidine 191
Melanoma malignum 234, 236
Meperidine 148, 150, 156, 173
Mesenchymal cells 161
Metabolic diseases 226–229
   clotting disorders 226
   congenital feline hypothyroidism 228
   diabetes mellitus 227–228
   hyperostosis 228
   hyperparathyroidism 227, 228
   oral mucosa 229
   osteopenia juvenalis 227
   punch test 227
   soft oral tissues 227
   uremic ulcerations and uremic mucositis 229
Methadone 146–148, 150, 156, 171–173, 177, 191–193
Microflora 211
Microglossia/aglossia 219, 221
Midazolam CRI 177
Minimum alveolar concentration (MAC) 146, 160, 195
Minimum anesthetic concentration (MAC) 172
Mitral regurgitation (MR) 191

Mitral valve insufficiency (MVI), dogs
   induction of anesthesia 191–192
   maintenance phase 192
   preoperative considerations 191
   recovery and postoperative management 192
   sedation 191
Morphine 146–150, 161, 171–173, 177, 178, 191
Mucogingival junction (MGJ) 313
Mucosal bleeding time (MBT) 227
Mucosal proliferation 229, 230
Mucous membrane pemphigoid 226
Multimodal analgesia 141
Multimodal monitoring 233
Multirooted teeth extraction 311
Muscle biopsy 220
Mycotic infections 224–225
Myocardial ischemia 192
Myxosarcoma 201, 202

n

Naloxone 151
Nasal/alveolar bleeding 242
Nasal cavity 241
Nasal feeding 424
Nasolacrimal disease 127, 202
Nasolacrimal duct 204, 205
Natural toothbrush 80
Neoplasia 127
Neural theory 142
Neuropraxia 229
Nonanesthetic dentistry (NAD) 114
Noninvasive blood pressure (NIBP) 178
Non-sales selling 30
Nonstable mandibular fracture 367, 368
Nonsteroidal anti-inflammatory drugs (NSAIDs) 140, 184

Nonsurgical (closed) extractions
alveolus   309–310
closure of the extraction site
310
consent   305
dental radiographs   305–306,
310
elevation   307–309
extraction   309
gingival attachment   306–307
luxation   307–309
pain management   306
Noxious stimuli   140, 141
Nursing   5
Nutrition
body weight of animal   425
challenges   426–428
definition   75
elements   75
elimination of dental
plaque   79–80
feeding, perioperative care   423
oral microflora modification
antibacterial ingredients,
products   79
saliva composition   78–79
targeting specific
bacteria   77–78
passive hygiene, chewing   83
products (*see* Nutritional
products)
Nutritional products
antibacterial ingredients   79
elimination of dental plaque
antiplaque agent   80
commercial dry dental
diets   80
dental bars, chews and
treats   80
dry food   79–80
soft food   79
VOHC acceptance   83
VOHC website   83

O

Obesity   183
Obesity hypoventilation
syndrome   183

Ocular inflammation   127
Odontoblastic transduction
theory   142
Odontogenic abscess   201, 202
Odontoplasty   355
Oligodontia, Chinese Crested
dog   415
Operculectomy   248
Ophthalmic abnormalities   201
Ophthalmic care   206–208
Ophthalmic considerations
maxillofacial trauma   205–207
ophthalmic care   206–208
ophthalmic manifestations
201–206
oral and ocular surgery
208–209
Ophthalmic manifestations
aerobic and anaerobic cultures
205
antimicrobrials and
anti-inflammatories   202
blood vessels and nerves   201
clinical presentations   201, 202
conjunctivitis and exophthalmos
204–205
corneal ulceration   202, 203
empiric therapy   202
epiphora and
conjunctivitis   201, 202
exophthalmos   201, 202, 203
exposure keratitis   202, 203
nasolacrimal disease   202
nasolacrimal duct   204, 205
oral neoplastic process   205
orbital abscess   204
orbital cellulitis   201, 202, 203
orbital floor   201, 202
periocular inflammation
201–202
periodontal disease   201, 202
prompt and recognition   201
retrobulbar abscesses   204
temporary tarsorrhaphies   202
tooth root abscesses   202, 204
uveitis   201
zygomatic salivary
mucoceles   205

zygomatic sialadenitis   204, 205
Opioids   192
acute pain management   146
fentanyl   147
hydromorphone   147
meperidine   148
methadone   147
morphine   147
tramadol   148
Oral and dental infections
abscess or foreign body   90
adjunctive treatment measure
90
clindamycin   93
common dental antimicrobials   91
culture   90–91
dental abscesses   92
dosing regimens   90
implant procedure   93
intramuscular
administration   93–94
intravenous administration   93
monotherapy   90
odontogenic abscess, cat   92, 93
osteomyelitis   91–92
Pasteurella   93
sample collection, anaerobic
transport media   91
selection of appropriate
drugs   90
therapy   94
Oral and maxillofacial surgery
3D reconstruction   293
access flaps   298
biopsy   302, 303
dedicated oral surgery   303
envelope flap   299
four-handed dentistry   292
gentle tissue handling   296–297
hemostasic techniques   297
infection control   291
line angles   298
numerous strains   291
pain management   291
periosteum   299
structure and anatomy   292–293
surgical techniques   294

techniques, instruments and
materials 293
treatment planning 292
tumors treatment 292
wound closure (*see* Wounds)
Oral and ocular surgery 208–209
Oral cancer 128
Oral cavity 201, 215, 219, 241
calculus formation, inhibition of
(*see* Calculus formation)
finger protection 7, 10
nutritional strategies (*see* Nutrition)
Oral cavity disorder
calculus 75
clinical features 75
microbiome 75–77
overview 75
Oral cavity microbiome
bacteria 75–76
canine bacterial 76
feline 77
insoluble salts deposition 76
nutritional interventions 75, 76
oral microflora 75, 76
Oral defense system 121
Oral disease
impacts 139–140
systemic complications
gingival epithelium 129
hypertrophic cardiomyopathy
129
pathogenesis 129
prosthetic surgery 131
Oral emergencies
3D imaging 323
acute jaw-motion disorders (*see*
Acute jaw-motion disorders)
analgesics 320
clinical assessment 323
complications/consequences of
head injury 330
dentinal bonding
indications 331
preservation 335
purpose 334
steps 334
diagnostic imaging
2D radiography 321

3D imaging 321
full mouth radiography 321
fast-acting antibiotics 320
fractures 324
high-rise syndrome 321
pathologic/insufficiency fracture
324–325
physical examination 323
soft tissue damage 326–327
symphyseal separation
335–336
tape muzzle application
cats 331
dogs 331
tape muzzle fixation 325–326
trauma management 321
treatment plan 323
Oral examination and diagnostics
234–237
Oral health 267
antibiotics 211
atheroma and thrombus
formation 214
bacteremia 212–213, 214
dental interventions 215
diabetes mellitus 214
and endotoxins 214
entotoxins 213–214
guidelines, veterinarian
anesthesia 215
classification systems 215
healing times, different
tissues 215
recommendations 215–216
tissue healing and
bacteremia 215
human medicine 215
immunological injury 214
impacts
chronic inflammation 121
systemic diseases 121
interceptive orthodontics 211
liver 214
and orthopedic implants 214
periodontal disease 214
risk factors 211
spaying/neutering 211, 212
steel implants 214

Oral health index (OHI) 261,
366, 377
Oral infections, prevention of 88,
90, 93–94
Oral lesions 219, 225, 226
Oral manifestations 223, 225
Oral mass 383
Oral microflora modification
77–78
Oral mucosa 229
Oral neoplasms 343
Oral papillomatosis 222, 224, 251
Oral pathology 121
Oral problems management
high rise syndrome or head
injury 380
inflammatory feline oral
diseases 385
oral health index 377
oral mass 383
orthodontics 384
periodontal diseases 378, 379
pulp disease 382
teeth injuries 381
teeth resorption 386
Oral soft tissues
cleft palates 251
eruptive gingivitis 251
juvenile periodontitis 251, 252
oral papillomatosis 251
Oral surgical general kit 20, 22
Orbital abscess 204
Orbital cellulitis 201, 202, 203
Orofacial pain
agonist/antagonist, partial
149–150
amantadine 160
anti-Inflammatory drugs 151
gabapentin 160–161
ì-Opioid Agonist/ê-Agonists,
partial 150–151
ketamine 160
local anesthetics 155
maropitant 161
opioid antagonists 151
opioids 146–149
systemic lidocaine 160
treatment 145–146

Oronasal fistulas (ONFs) 239, 305
  chronic infection 122
  clinical signs 122
  mucogingival flap 122
  oronasal communication 122
  periodontal disease 122
Orthodontics 384
Orthopedic implants
  oral health and 214
  prophylaxis 96
Osteomyelitis 305
  biofilm involvement 92
  empiric treatment 129
  German Shepherd 91, 92
  histopathologic
    assessment 128
  long-term injectable therapy 92
  oral and dental infections
    91–92
Osteopenia juvenalis 227
Osteosarcoma 201, 202
Oxygen saturation 192
Oxygen supplementation 189

p

Packed cell volume (PCV) 172
Pain management
  anesthetic techniques 140
  assessment/
    recognition 143–145
  dental 111, 112
  intraoperative analgesia 140
  local anesthetic 155
  NSAID 140
  opioids 146–149
  treatment 145–146
Panophthalmitis 207, 208
Pasteurella 93
Pathologic jaw fracture 124–127
  bone loss 127
  chronic periodontal loss 124
  iatrogenic jaw fracture 126
  mandibular fracture 126
  neoplasia 127
  prognosis 126
Pathologic mandibular
    fracture 126

Patient physiology
  diastolic pressure 178
  electrocardiogram 179
  noninvasive arterial blood
    pressure 178–179
  pulse oximeter 181–182
  systolic blood pressure 178
  ventilation 179–181
Patient welfare. *see also* Animal
    welfare
  AFD 114, 115–116
  behavior changes 112
  chronic stressors 112
  client education matters
    112–113
  etiologies 112
  Five Animal Welfare
    Needs 109, 110
    framework 111
  Five Freedoms 109–111
  handling techniques 113
  improved welfare
    outcomes 114
  infection and pain 109
  non-human mammals 111
  pain 111, 112
  procedural design 113–114
  quality and potentially
    QOL 109
  stimulation 112
  un- and undertreated dental
    disease 109
  untreated dental disease 112
  veterinary visit 113
Pediatric dentistry
  canine 245
  deciduous dental formulae 245
  feline 245
  oral soft tissues (*see* Oral soft
    tissues)
  persistent deciduous dentition
    245–249
  teeth eruption 245
Pemphigoid oral lesion 226
Pemphigus foliaceus lesion 226
Pemphigus vulgaris 226
Perception 140
Periapical abscess 124, 202, 320

Periapical lesions 122–124
  carnassial abscess 124
  distal root of mandibular 124
  endodontic infection 123
  facial infraorbital/
    carnassial 124
  intraoral dental sinus
    drainage 125
  nasal cavity filled with
    debris 123
  types 122
Periapical rarefaction 367, 369
Periodontal disease 121, 201,
    202, 214, 378, 379
  antimicrobial 96
  clindamycin local-delivery
    systems 96–97
  doxycycline use 96, 97
  human 96
  pathologic pockets 367, 368
  prevention or treatment 96
  pulse therapy 97
  veterinary patients 96
Periodontal probe 234
Periodontal therapy 269
Perio-endo lesions 122–124
Periostitis ossificans 250
Persistent deciduous dentition
  delayed eruption or
    impaction 245, 249
  dental formulae for cats and
    dogs 245, 246
  incorrect eruption path or
    ectopic position 245
  juvenile gingivitis 246–248
  malocclusions (*see*
    Malocclusions)
  operculectomy 248
  periodontal ramifications 246
  permanent teeth eruption 246
  unerupted teeth 248
Persistent postsurgical pain 142
Personal protective equipment
    (PPE) 99–100
Pet owners 57
Pharyngeal packs 24, 25
Pharyngostomy 360
Photographic documentation 137

Physiology of pain   140–141
Piezoelectric bone surgery   296
Plaque
  accumulation   75
  antimicrobials   97
  biofilm-embedded bacteria   97
  commercial products   98
  dental plaque   97
  description   97
  direct topical application   98
  eradication   97
  and gingivitis control   75
  oral administration of biocides
      97–98
  risk   84
Plaque-associated stomatitis   226
Plasmacytic inflammatory
      disease   133
PLUS midazolam   191
Polish Small Animal Veterinary
      Association (PSAVA)   135
Positive endexpiratory pressure
      (PEEP)   183
Postoperative dental
      radiographs   310
Power equipment
  configuration   17
  dental unit main board   17, 19
  mechanical scalers and
      polishers   17, 19
  maintenance of
      handpieces   397
      radiography equipment   396
      ultrasonic scalers   396–397
  manufacturers and
      specialists   17
Pre-anesthetic protocols   173
Predisposed breeds   191, 192, 220
Pregnant patients
  anesthetic management   195
  perioperative management   195
  preoperative considerations
      194–195
  recovery and postoperative
      management   195
Premedication   196, 211
  drugs selection
    anticholergics   171

mild to moderate tranquilizers
      171
  moderate to heavy sedatives
      172–173
  sedative analgesics   171–172
  suppression of vomiting   171
goals   171
maropitant   161
obese patients   184
opioids   146
pre-anesthetic drugs and doses
      170
pre-induction support   173
protocol   174
Preoperative dental radiographs
      237, 305–306
Presurgical exam and consultation
  HEPA   271
  preliminary assessment   269
  staff and patient protection   270
  visual educational
      materials   270
Preventive analgesia   146
Probiotic bacteria
  in humans   77
  periodontitis   78
Proper equipment
  advantages, 3D versus 2D imaging
      16, 18
  business plan   15, 16
  options   14
  radiography   16
  selection   14, 16
Prophylactic Program, oral health
  periodontal disease   59
  periodontal therapy   70
  regular dental examinations   59–60
  regular oral home care   61–70
Propofol   191, 193, 196
Prostaglandin (PG)   151
Pulp disease   382
Pulse oximeter   181, 189
Punch test   227

q
Quality of life (QOL)   122, 133,
      139, 219
  measures   111

optimum health and   109
primary care   14

r
Radiography   4, 7, 16, 27, 34, 41,
      53, 134, 189, 202, 246, 263,
      319, 321, 323, 336, 339, 340,
      341, 343, 349, 366, 367, 396,
      424
Receptionists
  acceptance of dentistry   45
  appointments and
      procedures   45
  client in clinic   45, 46
  guidance   46
  NAD procedure   45
  online scheduling   46
  oral examination and dental
      cleaning   45
  responsibility   46
  telephone conversation   45
  veterinary team.   46
  waiting room, clean and
      pleasing   46
Regular dental examinations
  dental deposits   59
  Dental Index app   60
  oral assessment   60
  oral health index   59–60
  oral health parameters   59, 60
  size, mandibular lymph
      nodes   59
Regular dental prophylaxis   366
Regular oral home care
  active home care   62
  antimicrobial products   63
  antiseptic rinses   65–66
  application of waxy barrier
      sealant   66
  brushing technique   63–65
  client discussion/
      instruction   61–62
  component of   61
  dental plaque identification   61
  dental treats and chews   67–69
  double-headed toothbrushes
      62
  fatty acids   70

Regular oral home care (*cont'd*)
  goal of home plaque control   62
  Hill's Dental Care T/D diet   67, 68
  human toothbrushes   62
  infant brush   62
  kibbles   67
  mechanized toothbrush, dogs   62, 63
  other supplements   70
  passive home care   66–67
  periodontal disease   61
  plaque off series   70
  probiotics   69–70
  tartar-control diets   67
  teaching tooth brushing   63, 64
  therapy   61
  tooth brushing   62
  toothpastes   63, 64
  types   62
  water additives   69, 70
Renal disease   185
Rescue kit   23, 24
Residual calculus   236
Resorption and periapical lesion   234, 235
Respiratory distress   196
Retained tooth roots   237–239
Retrobulbar abscesses   204
Rostrodorsal luxation   328
Rottweiler   416
Royal Society for the Prevention of Cruelty to Animals' (RSPCA)   110
Rubber jaw   227, 228

S
Saliva composition   78–79
Samoyed   416
Schirmer tear testing   201
Secondary MVI   191
Sedative analgesics   171–172
Seizures in dogs and cats
  induction of anesthesia   196
  maintenance phase   196
  preoperative considerations   195
  recovery and postoperative management   196
  sedation   195
Sequestrum   18, 128, 320
Sharpening   24
  acrylic stick test of   395
  Arkansas, India and ceramic stones   395
  elevator   395, 396
  equipments   395
  luxator   395, 396
  mechanized Hu-Friedy sharpener   396, 397
  sharp-edged instruments   395
Siamese twins   219
Single-root extractions   305
Skills and services   365–366
Slippage   241, 242
Small sharp elevators   237
Somatic signaling mechanisms   141
Specialists
  cases   366–372
  cooperation   373–374
  expect timely and complete communication   374–376
  skills and services   365–366
  veterinary dental   42
Special patient presentations
  cardiac disease   184
  diabetes mellitus   184–185
  geriatric patients   183
  hepatic dysfunction   185
  obesity   183–184
  renal disease   185
Specific oral bacterial strains   77
Squamous-cell carcinoma (SCC)   128
  left rostral mandible   367, 368
Stabilization   319
Standardization   291
Steam sterilization   393
Steel implants   214
Sterilization
  dry heat   393
  gas   395
  steam   393
Streptococcal species   77
Stress   7, 27, 32, 110, 112–114, 122, 129, 143, 146, 172, 175, 184, 189, 191–197, 214, 233, 263, 266, 285, 321, 340, 424, 426
Student Chapters of the European Veterinary Dental Society (SCEVDS)   42
Subgingival plaque and calculus scaling
  curettes   276
  dental cleaning   274
  gingival margin   276
  manual scaler   275
  manual subgingival scaling   278
  mechanical subgingival scalers   279
  modified pen grasp   276
  polishing   279, 280
  procedure   277
  residual plaque and calculus   279
  ultrasonic scalers   277
Sulcal lavage   281
Supragingival cleaning
  calculus accumulations   271
  cooling spray   272
  correct grasp, mechanical scaler handpiece   273
  hand scaling   274
  magnetostrictive units   271
  mechanical scalers   271
  piezoelectric units   271
  rotosonic scaling   273
  sonic scalers   271
Supragingival hand scaling274
Surgical (open) extractions
  envelope flap   311–313
  fenestrating the periosteum   313
  full flap   313
  hand instruments   314–315
  powered equipment   315–316
Surgical kit
  extraction forceps   23, 24
  medium/large   20
  oral surgical general kit   20, 22
  rescue kit   23, 24
  selection of burs for extraction   23, 24

tissue scissors   20
Surgical techniques
     cold steel   294
     laser   294, 295
     operating microscopy   294
     piezoelectric bone surgery   296
     scar tissue   295
Suture needles   24, 300
Systemic diseases
     immune-related disorders
          226, 227
     infectious diseases   222–226
     metabolic diseases   226–229
     toxic conditions   229
     traumatic conditions   229–230
Systemic lupus erythematosus   226
Systolic dysfunction   190

t

Teaching veterinary dentistry
     curriculum for DVM
          students   41
     day-one skills, dental
          procedures   38
     didactic learning   39
     education   37, 39–41
     elective/optional course   38
     Europe's University
          Curricula   37–38
     fields of   37
     framework, clinical
          assessment   37, 38
     OIE recommendations   38
     practical learning and
          training   37
     primary care   38
     theoretical part   41
     three practical cadaver-based
          sessions   41–42
     worldwide faculties   38
Teeth eruption
     functional post eruptive
          stage   245
     preeruptive stage   245
     prefunctional eruptive
          stage   245
Teeth injuries   381
Teeth resorption   386

Temporomandibular joint (TMJ)
     dysplasia   137, 219–223
Tetanus   225
Thermoregulation   172, 173, 219
Thiopental   192–193, 195, 196
Thorax system   319
Thrombocytopenia   226
Thyroid disorders   228
Tibial-plateau-leveling osteotomy
     (TPLO)   96
Tissue handling   296–297
     stay sutures   297
TMJ ankylosis   320
Tonometry   201
Tooth brushing   62, 213
Tooth resorption
     behavior changes   112
     clinical features   348
     diagnosis   351
     in dog   254
     evaluation of   17
     management   351–352
     in older cats   253
     osteomyelitis   129
     pulp exposure and   234
     severe   112
     type 2   350
     type I   349
Tooth resorptive lesions   367
Tooth root abscesses   202, 204
'To Sell Is Human'   30
Total intravenous anesthesia
     (TIVA)   175
Total plasma protein (TPP)   185
Toxic influence   229
Tramadol   148
Transduction   140
Transient receptor potential
     ankyrin 1 (TRPA1)   142
Transient receptor potential
     vanniloid 1 (TRPV1)   142
Transillumination   234, 237
Transmission   99, 100, 140, 141,
     145, 155, 213, 344
Traumatic class IV
     malocclusion   367
Traumatic conditions   229–230
Traumatic malocclusion   226

Trigeminal neuralgia   141
Trust
     array of thank-you pictures   30,
          31
     competence and belief   30
     Diplomas in the waiting room
          30, 31
Tube feeding
     esophageal   424
     GIT   423
     mandibulectomy   424
     parenteral or enteral   423
     presurgical period   423
Tumor nodulus metastasis
     (TNM)   366

u

Ultrasonic cleaning   393, 394
Ultrasonic scalers   396–397
Unerupted teeth   248
     dentigerous cysts   248, 250
     enamel hypoplasia/
          hypocalcification   248, 250
Uremic ulcerations and uremic
     mucositis   229
Uveitis   201, 214
Uveodermatologic (UV) syndrome
     134, 409, 411

v

Veillonella   77
Ventilation
     capnography   179, 180
     mainstream method   180
     patient's breathing   179
     pulsoximetry sensors   180
     sidestream measurement   181
Veterinarians
     overview   56
     procedures   56–57
     team members   56
Veterinary care assistants
     areas   47
     four-handed dentistry   48
     intraoperative   47, 48
     packing a dental kit   48
     postoperative   47, 48
     preoperative   47, 48

Veterinary dentistry
  antimicrobials
    bacteremia and infective
      endocarditis 94–97
    oral and dental infections 90–93
    oral infections associated with
      dental procedures 93–94
  communication (*see*
    Communications)
  marketing (*see* Marketing)
  teaching (*see* Teaching
    veterinary dentistry)
Veterinary Internet Network
  (VIN) 3
Veterinary Medical Board (VMB)
  234

Visual inspection 234–237, 393
VOHC seal of acceptance 82, 83
Von Willebrand's disease 134,
  220, 226, 227, 410

w

Waiting room 5, 6
Warfarin poisoning 229
World Organization for Animal
  Health 110
World Small Animal Veterinary
  Association (WSAVA)
  139
Wounds
  double-layer suturing 301
  maxillofacial surgery 300

oral cavity 302
palatal surgery 299
partial-thickness flap 300
standard interrupted
  sutures 302
surgical procedure 299
suturing material 300

x

Xylazine 191

z

Zinc salts 79
Zoonotic infections 104
Zygomatic salivary
  mucoceles 205